MOTOR LEARNING AND DEVELOPMENT

Second Edition

MOTOR LEARNING AND DEVELOPMENT

Second Edition

Pamela S. Haibach-Beach, PhD
College at Brockport

Gregory D. Reid, PhD
McGill University

Douglas H. Collier, PhD
College at Brockport

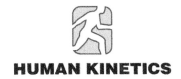

HUMAN KINETICS

Library of Congress Cataloging-in-Publication Data

Names: Haibach-Beach, Pamela S., 1977- author. | Reid, Greg, 1948- author. |
Collier, Douglas Holden, 1953- author.
Title: Motor learning and development / Pamela S. Haibach-Beach, Greg W.
Reid, Douglas H. Collier.
Description: Second edition. | Champaign, IL : Human Kinetics, [2018] |
Includes bibliographical references and index.
Identifiers: LCCN 2016057736 (print) | LCCN 2016057736 (ebook) | ISBN
9781492536598 (print)
Subjects: | MESH: Motor Activity | Motor Skills | Human Development | Age
Factors
Classification: LCC BF295 (ebook) | LCC BF295 (print) | NLM WE 103 | DDC
152.3/34--dc23
LC record available at https://lccn.loc.gov/2016057736

ISBN: 978-1-4925-3659-8 (print)

Acquisitions Editor: Bridget Melton; **Developmental Editors:** Ragen Sanner and Carly S. O'Connor; **Managing Editors:** Carly S. O'Connor, Anna Lan Seaman, and Kirsten E. Keller; **Copyeditor:** Patsy Fortney; **Indexer:** Dan Connolly; **Permissions Manager:** Dalene Reeder; **Graphic Designer:** Dawn Sills; **Cover Designer:** Keith Blomberg; **Photograph (cover):** © Human Kinetics; **Photographs (interior):** left photo on p. 34 © Doug Collier; right photo on p. 34 Bananastock; all other photos © Human Kinetics; **Photo Production Manager:** Jason Allen; **Senior Art Manager:** Kelly Hendren; **Illustrations:** © Human Kinetics, unless otherwise noted; **Printer:** Total Printing Systems

Printed in the United States of America   10   9   8   7   6   5   4

The paper in this book is certified under a sustainable forestry program.

Human Kinetics
1607 N. Market Street
Champaign, IL 61820
USA

United States and International
Website: **US.HumanKinetics.com**
Email: info@hkusa.com
Phone: 1-800-747-4457

Canada
Website: **Canada.HumanKinetics.com**
Email: info@hkcanada.com

E6895

Tell us what you think!
Human Kinetics would love to hear what we
can do to improve the customer experience.
Use this QR code to take our brief survey.

To my mom, who has instilled in me a lifelong love of learning.

—Pam Haibach-Beach

To my grandchildren, Jacob Liam Reid, Chloe Evelyn Reid, and Ethan Gregory Reid, whose motor learning and development continue to amaze and amuse.

—Greg Reid

To my parents, Martin and Barbara Collier, who have always modeled and gently moved me toward a lifelong joy of movement.

—Doug Collier

CONTENTS

PREFACE

Whether it be outsmarting the opponent on the field of play or simply walking down the street, we are consistently faced with the challenge of solving movement problems. When we walk down the street, we often have to avoid obstacles or other pedestrians while keeping in mind the wet, slippery pavement. In a competitive sporting environment, we may have to consciously think about faking out an opponent. No matter the setting, our skill level, or our age, we cannot avoid the fact that movement is a vital part of our lives and affects us in terms of our overall physical well-being, our intellectual functioning, and the development of our social skills. These effects are ever present—and ever changing—and take place over the course of our lives.

Clearly, then, how we develop, in addition to our previous movement experiences, affects how we acquire new motor skills and how we refine old skills. The learning of new motor skills and the refinement and adjustment of existing motor skills are critical aspects of our lives—aspects that we don't always appreciate. When performing everyday movements, we often do not appreciate how difficult it is to coordinate our limbs so that we can execute activities. As an example, we use a knife and fork to eat without giving these actions a second thought. This was a very difficult task when we were small children, however. We had to learn how to control both limbs in a coordinated fashion to cut meat and feed ourselves. Over time, though, this initially challenging feat became second nature, and the frustration caused by the complexity of these actions was soon forgotten. That feeling of frustration in learning those

early everyday tasks returns, however, if as adults we must relearn these basic movements following a serious accident or medical event (such as a stroke). The intense physical and occupational therapy required to relearn even the simplest of tasks reminds us of the intricacy of motor skills. No matter the time of life—infancy through old age—the ongoing interactions between our ever-changing abilities, the environment, and the task we're solving at the moment determine how we proceed.

Motor Learning and Development, Second Edition, provides a framework for understanding both fields and for exploring how motor learning and motor development interact with and affect each other. Having a thorough understanding of the factors that "push" the development of motor skill across the life span will better prepare you to teach movement skills effectively to learners at any chronological age and at any skill level. *Motor Learning and Development, Second Edition,* examines the development of movement skill in humans from infancy to older adulthood (referred to as life span motor development) and examines how having different motor, cognitive, and social abilities affects how, when, and why we learn motor skills. As movement educators, we must understand the complexities of teaching movement skills to people of various backgrounds, interests, experiences, and abilities. As we have noted, learning a motor skill (or a combination of motor skills) can be quite challenging, and many elements must be taken into consideration. *Motor Learning and Development, Second Edition,* guides you in an accessible and interesting manner into the fields of motor development and motor learning.

The book includes a variety of methods to facilitate learning and keep you engaged with the material.

Motor Learning and Development, Second Edition, is an undergraduate text written for students and professionals pursuing careers in physical education, athletic training, early childhood education, gerontology, kinesiology, special education, adapted physical education, primary and secondary education, physical therapy, occupational therapy, and related fields. The text presents a strong theoretical foundation in an engaging and accessible way. You will learn how to develop, implement, and critically assess motor skill programs for learners at all developmental levels.

Although the fields of motor learning and motor development have been addressed in a variety of undergraduate texts, none have merged these two fields into one textbook. *Motor Learning and Development, Second Edition,* fills this void. The content is based on the latest research in the fields of motor development and motor learning. This text also provides a framework for developing movement programs that facilitate skill acquisition for all types of learners—from those with significant disabilities to elite athletes. This book also prepares you for meeting national standards and Praxis exams.

Life Span Perspective

This book adopts a life span perspective that goes beyond the developmental and neuromotor changes associated with childhood and younger adulthood. This perspective provides an in-depth look at all ages throughout the human life span, including the many large life changes associated with younger and older adults. These changes can include leaving home, entering the workforce, getting married, and having children. We also examine the social and psychological changes associated with life transitions. Societal mores and expectations can have a huge impact on the motor development of various cohorts. For instance, in today's highly technological age, adolescents are much more likely to spend a larger portion of their free time playing with cell phones, iPods, and video games than participating in physical activity. On the other hand, many adults have changed their focus to health and wellness, which has resulted in a surge of people who are eating healthier meals, giving up unhealthy habits such as cigarette smoking, and participating in more physical activity. These healthy decisions are certainly having a large impact on older adults' motor development and on slowing their rate of functional decline. However, what motivates an adolescent to participate in sport or physical activity may be of little interest to a middle-aged adult or, indeed, a child.

It is important to take a broad view and consider many variables when examining individual motor development and performance. This book details these variables to prepare movement educators to teach motor skills to a broad array of people representing many ages, developmental levels, and degrees of physical proficiency in a variety of settings, including educational, athletic, clinical, and fitness settings.

Changes to the Second Edition

Motor Learning and Development has undergone a thorough revision since the first edition, including a reorganization of the structure of the book, the addition of three new chapters and several new ancillaries, updated material based on the latest research, and revised examples throughout the book. A main focus of these changes has been to more thoroughly cover both motor learning and motor development as well as to unite these fields to best prepare practitioners to devise developmentally appropriate programs for people of any age or skill level. Much of the content in part I has been reorganized, and a new chapter, Understanding Movement Control, has been added. The theories outlined in chapter 1 of the first edition have been moved to a new chapter titled Theoretical Constructs in Motor Behavior, which focuses solely on the theories. Parts II and III have been reorganized to reflect similar topics rather than separate age groups as in the first edition. These changes have enabled us to better infuse the two fields of motor learning and motor development. In addition, two more chapters have been added: chapter 6, Infant Motor Development, and chapter 18, Devising a Plan.

New ancillaries in the second edition include laboratories and PowerPoint presentations for each chapter and video clips for chapters 6, 7, and 17. This edition has also been updated with the latest research and includes new opening vignettes for each chapter.

Organization

Part I, Theory and Foundational Concepts, provides a basic outline of the fundamental concepts in motor learning and motor development. Chapter 1 introduces the subfields of motor behavior, motor control, motor learning, and motor development, as well as important concepts and terminology. Chapter 2 emphasizes movement control, including reaction time, attention, arousal, sensory contributions, and memory. The major tenets and theoretical perspectives from the fields of motor behavior are explained in chapter 3. Chapter 4 discusses motor skill progression as well as three models of motor learning stages. Instructors who have a thorough understanding of the strengths and shortcomings of each model will have more and better-developed tools to engender positive behavioral, cognitive, and physical changes in performers. It is at this point (chapter 5) that we discuss important methodological considerations, including how to measure and assess

motor learning and organize the learning experience to facilitate positive transfer and long-term retention.

Part II, Life Span Physical Activity and Movement, provides a solid background on movement patterns across the life span, from infancy to older adulthood. Chapter 6 examines infant motor development, including prenatal growth and development, spontaneous and reflexive movements in early infancy, and the development of motor milestones. Chapter 7 picks up where chapter 6 ends by examining fundamental motor skills developed during childhood, including locomotor and manipulative skills. The development of fundamental movement skills is essential to healthy development in childhood. Children who are given a strong movement foundation will have the skill sets and the confidence to be physically active with their families, with peers, and on their own. Chapter 8 explores physical activity and movement in young, middle, and older adulthood. The discussion focuses first on physical activity in adulthood and peak athletic performance, and then explores the changing movement patterns observed in older adults.

Part III, Functional and Structural Constraints, examines the changing individual constraints throughout the life span. Chapter 9 discusses some of the structural factors that constrain the acquisition and development of movements throughout childhood and adolescence. Chapter 10 discusses the physiological changes that affect physical function and movement, including age-related changes in the skeletal, muscular, cardiovascular, nervous, endocrine, and sensory systems. Movement educators who work with older adults must understand the effects of aging on the physiological systems and the impact these changes have on movement. Chapters 9 and 10 address how structural constraints may interact with functional factors (the focus of chapters 11 through 13), tasks, and environments. Chapters 11 through 13 examine the potential affective, cognitive, behavioral, and psychomotor differences that affect the learning of movement skills over the life span. Chapter 13 discusses a variety of psychological, sociological, and cognitive variables in adulthood. It is important to distinguish psychological and sociocultural factors in adulthood from those that are present in childhood and adolescence, because they change considerably.

Part IV, Designing Developmentally Appropriate Programs, gets you ready to prepare, design, and implement developmentally appropriate movement programs. Chapter 14 examines the physical, affective, and instructional dimensions that affect motor learning, and prepares you to structure the environment appropriately with these factors in mind. Chapter 15 discusses prepractice considerations, including how to set goals and introduce motor skills through the use of demonstrations, verbalizations, attention directing, and physical guidance. The discussion continues in chapter 16, which addresses the design and structure of effective practice sessions. Topics include variable practice, practice specificity, part and whole practice, and practice distribution. Just like practice, feedback should be designed around the person and the task. Chapter 17 discusses the functions and types of feedback as well as effective feedback scheduling. The book closes with a new chapter, Devising a Plan, which brings all of the book's concepts together to help you design developmentally appropriate programs. The chapter includes examples of developmentally appropriate programs as well as case studies.

Pedagogical Features

Many features throughout the book will help you understand the concepts introduced in each chapter.

- *Opening vignette:* Each chapter opens with a vignette, a practical example that introduces one or more of the main concepts explored in the chapter.

- *Research Notes:* Each chapter includes sections that present important research experiments. Many of these research notes have been updated for the second edition.

- *Try This:* This feature supplements the text with a variety of short applications that you can perform at home or at your desk. Answering questions will help you think critically about the concepts.

- *What Do You Think?:* Each chapter includes opportunities to stop and think about the material. This feature provokes critical thinking and stimulates further thought about the material. You can answer these questions on your own or discuss them in class.

- *Summary:* A brief summary of the key elements and concepts is provided at the conclusion of each chapter.

- *Supplementary Activities:* Two additional activities are presented at the conclusion of every chapter. These are intended either as outside activities or as classroom laboratory activities.

- *Glossary:* Key terms and concepts are printed throughout the text in bold type for emphasis and are defined at the end of each chapter.

Note: In this text we use English measurements followed by metric conversions in parentheses. The exception is with yards, which convert to approximately the same number of meters.

Web Resource

The student web resource includes laboratories for each chapter, the What Do You Think? and Try This activities, and videos for chapters 6, 7, and 17 with accompanying study questions. The labs provide experiential learning for difficult concepts or topics and typically require some equipment and additional space such as a gymnasium or outside area. The videos accompany the laboratory activities for chapters 6, 7, and 17, and can be used as part of a lecture.

When an activity, form, or video mentioned or appearing in a chapter is available on the web resource, you will see an icon that looks like this:

The web resource can be accessed by visiting www.HumanKinetics.com/Motor LearningAndDevelopment. If you purchased a new print book, follow the directions included on the orange-framed page at the front of your book. That page includes access steps and the unique key code that you'll need the first time you visit the *Motor Learning and Development* website. If you purchased an e-book from HumanKinetics.com, follow the access instructions that were e-mailed to you following your purchase.

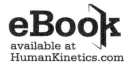

available at
HumanKinetics.com

LETTER TO INSTRUCTORS

Although there are many excellent books that examine motor development from a life span perspective and books that explore the field of motor learning, there is not, to our knowledge, a book that combines the two. You will find that *Motor Learning and Development, Second Edition*, achieves the goal of combining the two fields in an accessible and interesting way, and explains how motor development and motor learning inform each other and intersect.

Those with a thorough understanding of the multiple factors that set in motion the development of motor skills from infancy to older adulthood are in a good position to teach movement skills efficiently and to individualize their instruction. This individualization is a point of emphasis throughout the text, given the complexity of teaching learners of various backgrounds, interests, abilities, and ages. Furthermore, learners' abilities and interests are hardly static; rather, they are very dynamic. Thus, to work with learners at all life stages, we must be continually aware of the ongoing interactions between ever-changing abilities, an ever-changing environment, and the tasks at hand. The intersection of these three factors determines how to proceed.

And so, this textbook—based on the latest research in the fields of motor learning and motor development—provides both the theoretical foundation and applied information for developing movement programs for all types of learners—from those with identifiable disabilities to those at both ends of the ability spectrum.

Motor Learning and Development, Second Edition, is divided into four parts. Part I, Theory and Foundational Concepts, lays the groundwork by outlining the fundamental concepts of motor control, motor learning, and motor development. Part II, Life Span Physical Activity and Movement, provides a solid background in physical activity and movement patterns from infancy through older adulthood, examining not only *what* skills are developed but also *how* they are developed. Part III, Functional and Structural Constraints, delineates the constraints that may, in combination, hinder or promote optimal development. The fourth and final part, Designing Developmentally Appropriate Programs, gives detailed information that prepares students to organize, develop, implement, and evaluate movement programs for a variety of learners. Although the material that precedes part IV has a direct bearing on the development of appropriate programs, the students need not have read every chapter of the text to benefit from part IV.

Although this textbook is written from a life span perspective and details how skill is acquired over the course of one's life, a particular course may emphasize a certain time frame. If, as an example, motor learning and motor development in school-age children and adolescents is the focus of the course, you may decide to bypass chapters 8, 10, and 13. The same applies to a course focusing more on adult development and aging. In this case, the emphasis may be on chapters 8, 10, and 13 in addition to parts I and IV. As noted in the sample syllabus, the material in *Motor Learning and Development, Second Edition*, can be taught over the course of a 15-week semester.

Each chapter in *Motor Learning and Development, Second Edition*, has the following features that engage students in their reading and help them to understand the concepts.

Motor Learning and Development Syllabus

Week	Day	Topic	Assignments and readings
Part I Theory and Foundational Concepts			
1	1	Introduction to course	Syllabus
	2	Perspectives in motor behavior	Chapter 1; Try This and SA 1 or 2
	3	Perspectives in motor behavior	Chapter 1; lab
2	1	Understanding movement control	Chapter 2; Try This
	2	Understanding movement control	Chapter 2; SA 1 or 2
	3	Understanding movement control	Chapter 2; lab
3	1	Theoretical constructs in motor behavior	Chapter 3; Try This
	2	Theoretical constructs in motor behavior	Chapter 3; SA 1 or 2
	3	Theoretical constructs in motor behavior	Chapter 3; lab
4	1	Stages of skill acquisition	Chapter 4; Try This and SA 1 or 2
	2	Stages of skill acquisition	Chapter 4; lab
	3	Assessing motor learning	Chapter 5; Try This
5	1	Assessing motor learning	Chapter 5; SA 1 or 2
	2	Assessing motor learning	Chapter 5; lab
	3		Exam I
Part II Life Span Physical Activity and Movement			
6	1	Infant motor development	Chapter 6; Try This
	2	Infant motor development	Chapter 6; SA 1 or 2
	3	Infant motor development	Chapter 6; lab
7	1	Fundamental skills in childhood	Chapter 7; Try This
	2	Fundamental skills in childhood	Chapter 7; SA 1 or 2
	3	Fundamental skills in childhood	Chapter 7; lab
8	1	Movement in adulthood	Chapter 8; Try This and SA 1 or 2
	2	Movement in adulthood	Chapter 8; lab
	3	Movement in adulthood	Midterm
Part III Functional and Structural Constraints			
9	1	Physical development	Chapter 9; Try This
	2	Physical development	Chapter 9; SA 1 and 2
	3	Physical development	Chapter 9; lab
10	1	Physical aging	Chapter 10; Try This and SA 1 or 2
	2	Physical aging	Chapter 10; lab
	3	Cognitive development	Chapter 11; Try This and SA 1 or 2
11	1	Cognitive development	Chapter 11; lab
	2	Psychosocial and social–affective development	Chapter 12; Try This and SA 1 or 2
	3	Psychosocial and social–affective development	Chapter 12; lab
12	1	Psychosocial and cognitive factors in adulthood	Chapter 13; Try This and SA 1 or 2
	2	Psychosocial and cognitive factors in adulthood	Chapter 13; lab
	3		Exam
Part IV Designing Developmentally Appropriate Programs			
13	1	Physical, affective, and instructional factors	Chapter 14; Try This and SA 1 or 2
	2	Physical, affective, and instructional factors	Chapter 14; lab

Week	Day	Topic	Assignments and readings
	3	Prepractice considerations	Chapter 15; Try This and SA 1 or 2
14	1	Prepractice considerations	Chapter 15; lab
	2	Practice	Chapter 16; Try This and SA 1 or 2
	3	Practice	Chapter 16; lab
15	1	Feedback	Chapter 17; Try This and SA 1 or 2
	2	Feedback	Chapter 17; lab
	3	Devising a plan	Chapter 18; case studies
16			Final exam

SA = Supplemental Activities

- *Chapter objectives:* Each chapter begins with approximately six learning objectives related to the most important concepts. These objectives guide the students' reading and allow you to spend less class time lecturing and more time on interactive, student-focused learning activities and skill development. If you believe that the best approach to teaching the material is to use the lecture as your primary methodology, the chapter objectives provide a road map for both you and the students.

- *Research Notes:* Research experiments pertinent to the chapter material are presented throughout the text. Beyond their importance to the fields of motor learning and motor development, these research notes allow you to engage the students in debates and discussions about topics such as research design, the appropriateness of the question (i.e., why is this a good question to ask—or is it?), what the next question might be, and how to design the next question. Students can work on these questions and others during or outside of class, either individually or in small groups. Much of the research presented can lead to robust debate.

- *What Do You Think?:* This feature gives students the opportunity to think about the course content both critically and creatively. Examples include thinking back to how the students acquired a challenging skill, considering how to teach a diverse group of learners, and explaining how plasticity is demonstrated when a stroke patient regains the ability to hit a slice backhand. The key point is to stimulate critical thinking. Students can use this feature individually, in pairs, as a group, or in a class discussion either inside or outside of the classroom.

- *Try This:* This feature engages students in a practical application that clarifies a given concept. Students actively engage in a physical activity to attain a more thorough understanding of the concept at hand. This feature stimulates critical thinking and can be incorporated into the course either in or outside of the classroom.

- *Supplemental Activities:* At the end of each chapter, two activities are provided that can be completed as either classroom laboratory activities or at-home activities. These activities give students a chance to deepen their understanding of the topics presented in the chapter.

- *Key terms:* Key terms are the most important concepts in the chapter and appear in bold text. They are defined at the end of each chapter.

Five ancillaries facilitate the teaching of this material:

- *Instructor guide:* This ancillary includes sample answers to the What Do You Think? sections and, as appropriate, the Try This activities. It also includes troubleshooting tips for each chapter and its labs.

- *Test package:* This ancillary includes 170 multiple-choice, true-or-false, and short-answer questions and their answers. These test questions can be used for building quizzes or as a supplement to your own exam questions.

- *Laboratories:* Labs for chapters 1–17 are available to students through the web resource. The labs engage students in practical applications of important concepts from the chapters; they require more time and preparation than the Try This activities. Most labs require students to complete an activity, record their data, and for some, calculate and compare their data to class data. Instructor's tips for the labs are available in the instructor's guide.

- *Presentation package:* PowerPoint presentations are available for each chapter and include objectives, important figures and tables, key concepts, and summary points.

- *Video clips:* Video clips are available in the web resource for chapter 6, Infant Motor Development; chapter 7, Fundamental Skills in Childhood; and chapter 17, Feedback. The Study Questions links in the web resource contain questions focused on these videos, but you can use these videos to demonstrate these reflexes, motor milestones, and motor skills as you see fit.

The ancillaries are available at www. HumanKinetics.com/MotorLearningAnd Development.

We hope we have laid some groundwork for using *Motor Learning and Development, Second Edition,* in your course, allowing you to teach and, more important, engage students in these essential subjects. Be sure to familiarize yourself with the text so that you can manage your time to ensure that you cover the appropriate material for your course. Clearly, you will need to determine the amount of time required for covering each chapter and concept. Keeping track of material that required more time or less time to cover than you anticipated will help you make informed changes to future courses.

How much time you take to cover material from the text is, of course, an individual decision that has much to do with your pedagogical philosophy and course content goals.

We wish you the best as you use the first textbook to combine the fields of motor learning and motor development.

ACKNOWLEDGMENTS

Motor Learning and Development, Second Edition, is a comprehensive book, combining two fields of study into one textbook. We have presented the material that we felt was most relevant and current, while also unifying these two fields. There are many topics covered throughout this book, so for some areas we have called on the expertise of others. Therefore, we are grateful to colleagues who have provided input. In particular, we would like to extend our deep appreciation to Dr. Melanie Perreault for her contributions to chapter 2, Understanding Movement Control, and to Dr. Stephen Gonzalez for his invaluable advice on psychosocial assessments and related references. We are also deeply grateful to our colleagues and students who read drafts of the content and provided editorial suggestions throughout the process.

In addition, we would like to acknowledge those who made possible the photos used in chapter 7 and the cover: the children, who demonstrated the fundamental motor skills during the photo shoot; the parents, who facilitated their children's involvement; and Jim Dusen, whose photography was exceptional.

PART I

Theory and Foundational Concepts

In the first chapter of this section, we define the three fields of motor behavior: motor control, motor learning, and motor development. The key terms of each field are explained, and some core areas of research in each field are introduced. Motor skill classification, including sport skills, developmental classifications, single-dimensional classifications, and multidimensional classifications, is also detailed in this chapter. The classification of motor skills is important for any movement educator with an interest in rehabilitation, education, or athletics, because the appropriate practice and feedback schedules often depend on the type of motor skills.

Chapter 2 examines the many factors involved in understanding movement control, including reaction time, attention, arousal, sensory contributions, and memory. Because these factors have a profound impact on movement throughout the life span, they are discussed throughout the book. We then turn to the theoretical constructs of motor behavior, as well as the evolution of the field of motor development from its inception in the late 18th century to the present day, in chapter 3. The three main theoretical constructs that drive research in motor behavior (the information-processing theory, ecological approach, and dynamic systems approach) differ not only in the way they define development and learning, but also in how they examine behavior.

In chapter 4, we examine the developmental and motor learning stages. First, we use Clark's mountain of development to explain how skills evolve from prenatal development through skill proficiency. This is followed by a discussion of the stages of learning, including Fitts and Posner's, Bernstein's, and Gentile's learning stages, providing a framework for categorizing the skill level of learners from novices to experts. These models enable practitioners to assess the level of the learner and, more appropriately, to prepare practice sessions.

Part I concludes with methodological considerations (chapter 5), including how to measure and assess motor learning. Indicators of motor learning beyond basic performance measures are described (the best indicator of motor learning is performance following a retention interval). Also examined is transfer of learning, which is a critical component of learning a motor skill. Practitioners need to know how to promote positive transfer in any setting.

PERSPECTIVES IN MOTOR BEHAVIOR

Chapter Objectives

After reading this chapter, you should be able to do the following:

- Define the fields of motor learning, motor control, and motor development.
- Explain the importance of motor skill classification.
- Classify motor skills using single-dimensional and multidimensional classifications.
- Distinguish between motor skills and abilities.
- Understand Fleishman's taxonomy.
- Understand the evolution of motor development.
- Explain why the fields of motor behavior are important for teaching and assessing motor skills in sport, physical activity, and health professions.

Is Nathaniel's Improvement Motor Learning or Motor Development?

Nathaniel, an energetic toddler, loved to play with balls of many shapes and sizes. To encourage his motor skill development, his mom would ask Nathaniel to throw the balls to her, and then catch them when she would throw them back. In only a couple of months, his throwing had improved considerably. Nathanial was now able to throw three times farther and was throwing with much better form. In this example, a young child demonstrated significant improvement in his motor skills over a relatively short period of time. Would these changes be considered motor learning or motor development?

Practitioners need to understand not only motor learning and motor development, but also how each field influences the other. These two fields are strongly related but often separated in textbooks. This chapter provides a background for each of these fields, discussing the main motor learning and development concepts, tenets, and theoretical frameworks. Subsequent chapters use a life span perspective to explain how to prepare, implement, and assess motor skill programs for anyone regardless of age, developmental level, or motor skill. In the opening scenario, a mom taught her son how to throw and catch a ball, and the child exhibited significant improvement. Can this improvement be attributed solely to practice effects (motor learning), or, because toddlers develop and grow at such a rapid rate, was it due to growth and maturation (motor development)?

Defining Terms in Motor Behavior

A full understanding of the fields of motor behavior is necessary before designing, implementing, or assessing a motor skill program. **Motor behavior** is an umbrella term for the fields of motor control, motor learning, and motor development. **Motor control** researchers investigate the neural, physical, and behavioral aspects of human movement. An understanding of all three fields—motor learning, motor development, and motor control—optimizes skill acquisition. **Motor learning** is the study of the processes involved in the acquisition of a motor skill and the factors that enhance or inhibit the ability to perform a motor skill. Researchers in the field of **motor development** examine the products and underlying processes of motor behavior changes across the life span. (See table 1.1 for a summary of each field.)

A practitioner with a strong background in motor behavior has a solid foundation in how humans develop across the life span; can explain why particular behaviors have manifested; and can design programs that assess, diagnose, or teach motor skills for the purposes of instruction or rehabilitation. In this book, the term *practitioner* refers to any type of movement educator, including physical education teachers, clinicians, trainers, instructors, and coaches. Let's take a closer look at the fields of motor behavior.

Motor Control

Motor control is a subdiscipline of motor behavior that focuses on the neural, physical, and behavioral aspects of human movement. One area of study for motor control researchers is the role of the neurological system in the function of the body. Some researchers examine reaction time as an indicator of processing speed and nerve conduction velocities under varying conditions. Researchers in the field

Table 1.1 Summary of the Fields of Motor Behavior

Field	Key points
Motor control	Addresses the underlying processes of movement. Investigates the degrees of freedom problem (how the system is able to constrain the number of degrees of freedom to produce a coordinated movement pattern). Examines the serial order problem (sequencing and timing of movement behaviors). Investigates the perceptual–motor integration problem (how perception and action are incorporated).
Motor learning	Addresses the process of acquiring a capability for producing skilled actions. Is a direct result of practice and not due to maturation or physiological changes. Cannot be observed directly. Results in relatively permanent changes in the capability for skilled behavior.
Motor development	Addresses the performance product (outcome) and process (underlying mechanisms). Addresses successive development (following in uninterrupted order) and systematic development (step-by-step procedures). Is related to, but not dependent on, age.

of motor control also investigate how the system moves in a controlled and coordinated fashion. Even fundamental motor skills and movements are quite complex. The number of movement possibilities is nearly infinite because of the degrees of freedom available. The field of motor control deals with three core issues: the degrees of freedom problem, the serial order problem, and the perceptual–motor integration problem. This section provides a brief overview of these motor control problems.

Degrees of Freedom Problem

Degrees of freedom are the number of independent elements that must be constrained to produce coordinated motion (Bernstein, 1967). At the joint level, there are dozens of movement possibilities even for simple actions such as reaching for a glass. Minimally, the wrist, elbow, and shoulder are involved in the reach, each of which has multiple axes of rotation. If the person is standing during the reach, the hips, knees, and ankles are also involved in coordinating the movement. At the muscular level, the number of movement possibilities, or degrees of freedom, increases to the hundreds. If extended to the neuronal level, there could be millions, if not billions, of movement possibilities.

Coordination involves constraining the number of degrees of freedom to decrease the complexity of the movement task so as to produce a movement pattern and achieve

Coordination

Exercise 1.1

Generally, coordination is thought of as performing an activity more fluidly through practice, but our limbs are already coordinated to perform actions together, such as the right arm and the left arm or even the upper body with the lower body. To see for yourself, try each of these activities and notice how the limbs influence each other.

1. Writing activity:
    a. Regardless of your hand dominance, write your name backwards with your left hand. How difficult was this task? Did you have to concentrate on what you were doing? Did you think about which direction the letters should be going? Perhaps you even made an error and one of your letters was in the correct direction rather than backwards.
    b. Now take a second writing utensil in your right hand (you should have one in each hand). While writing backwards with your left hand, write forwards with your right hand. Were you able to accomplish this task? Was it harder or easier than only writing backwards with your left hand? Try it a second time and see if you can do it faster while thinking only about writing with your right hand. Were you able to increase the speed and complete both tasks while not even thinking about the harder task?
2. Hand and foot activity: Make circular motions clockwise in the air with one foot. After you've done that for a little while, add drawing 6s in the air with your finger while continuing to make circular clockwise motions with your foot. What happened when you added the second task?
3. In both activities, did you notice that your limbs are coordinated with each other? How did the hand and foot activity compare with the writing activity?

a task goal (Sparrow, 1992). Coordination involves bringing parts into proper relationship (Turvey, 1990). Increased coordination leads to a more positive task outcome. But in addition to coordinating the body parts, the person must also complete the task with **control**. The person must be able to manipulate the movements in such a way as to meet the demands of the task. For example, a dancer can coordinate her body parts to execute all of the correct steps. However, what distinguishes her as a dancer is her ability to accentuate certain movements while also moving with style and grace, making each movement appear seamless and effortless. A softball pitcher must constrain his degrees of freedom by deciding when to initiate the pitch and the speed of the pitch. The timing, the initiation and release, and the speed of the pitch are all variables of control.

Serial Order Problem

The **serial order problem** refers to the sequencing and order of movement behaviors. The timing and order of an activity are critical for nearly every movement we produce. Think about the importance of the sequence of sounds in speech or the movements in walking, running, or throwing. In speech, if the order is changed, the sounds and meanings of the words and sentences change. For example, a speech error would occur if you misspoke by saying *dirthbay* instead of *birthday*. Errors in speech that result from exchanging letters in adjacent words have been termed **spoonerisms** after an Oxford professor, William Spooner, who was known to often make such errors (Rosenbaum, 2010). He has been quoted as having made the slip "You hissed all my mystery lectures" instead of "You missed all my history lectures." In general, these sequencing errors occur in a specific way. Consonants switch with other consonants, vowels with other vowels, and even nouns with nouns and verbs with verbs.

Serial order errors are not limited to speech. People make performance-related action errors all the time. Have you ever put something away in an obviously wrong place (e.g., silverware in the trash instead of the dishwasher), missed your exit when driving, or sent a text to the wrong person? These errors occur when we are not paying attention to what we are doing. With these errors, you clearly knew what you intended to do. The problem arose because you were thinking about the action rather than the specifics of the task. For example, you could visually identify the dishwasher and the trash, but perhaps were more focused on the goal of clearing the plate and not on what you were throwing away. This type of error is referred to as an **action slip**.

Everyone makes these errors from time to time. So, why are they particularly interesting? These examples indicate that people prepare an action plan in advance, rather than planning and then executing one thought at a time (Lashley, 1951); this allows us to be much more efficient with our actions.

The serial order problem has also been found in the production of correct, or accurate, movements through coarticulation. **Coarticulation** refers to the simultaneous motions that occur in sequential tasks (Rosenbaum, 2010). This means that we are preparing for subsequent movements rather than completing one movement before preparing for the next. Coarticulation suggests that we preplan activities to move efficiently. Preparing simultaneous movements enables us to type fast, speak clearly, and transport objects efficiently. Learning how to write involves the ability to write one letter while also preplanning how to produce the following letters. The way the letter is formed actually changes based on the following letters. Research suggests that this coarticulation of writing reaches an adult level at around the age of nine (Kandel & Perret, 2015). Coarticulation also occurs in grasping. The position we use to grasp an object depends on where we are going to move the object. In a study by Cohen and Rosenbaum (2004), participants were asked to grasp a plunger

Action Planning

Exercise 1.2

Look in the mirror and say the word *twilight*. Did you notice that your lips rounded prior to producing the *t* sound? Look at your lips as you say the words *gold* and *cupid*. Did you notice the same thing? These examples indicate that there is an action plan for the entire word prior to the utterance of the first sound. If each sound were planned separately, your mouth would not have changed shape until after the *t, g,* or *c* sounds.

1. What are some other words in which you can notice a preparatory action plan?
2. Provide examples of performances other than typing and grasping in which movements are prepared in advance. What is this called?
3. What are some examples of action slips that you have experienced?

and place it to either a high or a low final position. The position of the grasp on the plunger changed based on the final position. Participants grasped the plunger high when they were going to place the plunger in a low position; conversely, they grasped it low when placing it in a high position. Refer to exercise 1.2 for a speech example of coarticulation.

Perceptual–Motor Integration Problem

As the name implies, the **perceptual–motor integration problem** addresses how perception and motor control are integrated. For example, how is movement affected by perception, and conversely, how is what we perceive affected by our actions? This is not a which came first, the chicken or the egg kind of problem. Rather, perception and movement actually work together, continuously influencing one another. You may move closer to an object to see it better, or closer to a sound to hear it better. In those cases, movement improves perception.

Movement can also inform perception. Our perception is affected by our actual or intended actions. Hirsiger, Pickett, and Konczak (2012) examined the influence of size and weight cues on perception and action. Every day, we make inferences on the sizes and weights of objects. This information affects how we grasp things; whether we need two fingers, a full hand, or two hands; and how much force we need to exert. Perceptions of object weight are biased by expectations of size, and perceptions of object size are biased by expectations of the weight. Lighter objects are often perceived as being smaller than they actually are, whereas heavier objects are often perceived as being larger. Therefore, the perception of the size or the weight influences the action response to grasp and lift the object. This topic is discussed further in chapter 3.

Neurophysiological research has provided further insights into the perceptual–motor integration problem. It was discovered that the same motor neurons fired when macaque monkeys watched an activity being performed as when they were producing the movement themselves. This observation occurred by chance when one of the researchers picked up some food and ate it. The researcher noticed that the same neurons were firing that would be firing if the monkey were picking up food and eating it himself. These neurons are referred to as mirror neurons because they fire when people witness an action that they could perform themselves. Research on mirror neurons was conducted with ballet and capoeira dancers (Calvo-Merino, Glaser, Grezes, Passingham, & Haggard, 2005). The brain activity of the dancers was higher when they watched others performing the dances that they were skilled in (e.g., ballet dancers had more brain activity when watching ballet, and capoeira dancers had more brain activity when watching capoeira). The results further indicate that learning new motor skills can change the amount of neuronal firing during observations of those motor skills.

Motor Learning

Motor learning is a subdiscipline of motor behavior that examines how people acquire motor skills. Motor learning is a relatively permanent change in the ability to execute a motor skill as a result of practice or experience. This is in contrast to **performance**, the act of executing a motor skill that results in a temporary, nonpermanent change. One way to conceptualize this difference is to consider the change of state in an egg (Schmidt & Lee, 2014). When an egg is boiled, there is a permanent change in the state of that egg. The egg has irreversibly transformed into a solid. To conceptualize performance, we could make an analogy to water. When temperatures drop below 32 degrees Fahrenheit (0 °C), water solidifies to ice. This is not a permanent change, because water will convert back to its original form if temperatures increase again to above 32 degrees Fahrenheit. The permanent change that results from boiling an egg is analogous to the permanent change in the ability to perform a motor skill, or motor learning. The change in water resulting from temperature increases or decreases, on the other hand, is analogous to performance changes because of its lack of permanency.

Now let's return to the definition of motor learning. Recall that motor learning is the process of acquiring the ability to produce skilled actions. The first characteristic of motor learning is that a process is required to induce a change in the ability to perform skillfully. A process, in regard to acquiring a skill, is a set of events or occurrences resulting in a change in the state or end product. Dropping temperatures would be the process that causes water to change form. Drills in sport are processes with the goal of improving the capability to perform skillfully. For instance, soccer juggling is a common method (process) to improve ball control in soccer players. A player who tears her anterior cruciate ligament must undergo months of physical therapy (process) to rehabilitate her knee and regain her strength and flexibility. The goal of conducting a process is to increase the strength of this state, be it altering the temperature to change the state of water, or promoting motor learning through practice drills or physical therapy sessions.

Capability implies that skilled behavior *may* occur if the conditions are favorable. There is certainly no question that Jack Nicklaus acquired the capability to play the game of golf. However, even Nicklaus had his off days, although his off-day skills in golf most likely still far exceeded many, if not all, of our golf skills. Certain variables can prevent optimal performance even when the capability is attained, such as external conditions (e.g., rain, snow, sleet, cold, wind), motivation, wellness, or fatigue.

The second characteristic of motor learning is that it must occur as a direct result of practice. Motor learning is not due to maturation or physiological training. A change that occurs as a result of maturation is a motor development change. For instance, learning to walk is motor development, not motor learning, because it is a motor skill that all humans acquire; in contrast, learning to shoot a basketball requires practice and is due to motor learning.

The third characteristic of motor learning is that it cannot be observed directly. It can only be assumed based on long-term performance changes. Motor learning, like love or success, is a construct. It cannot be seen, but is assumed to have occurred when relatively permanent changes in the capability of skilled behavior are observed through performance changes. Motor learning is assumed to produce positive, irreversible effects in the capability for skilled behavior, meaning that these changes are not temporary, as reflected in the saying *It's like learning to ride a bicycle.*

Children and adults who are occupational or physical therapy patients may notice that they perform better in the therapy setting than they do at home. To facilitate the transition from the clinic to home and continue the benefits of therapy outside of the facility, therapists often teach patients activities they can practice at home. For example, school occupational therapists help children with fine motor delays improve skills such as writing, typing, and cutting. To continue the improvements when school is not in session or when the therapist is not available, the therapist should encourage young clients to create art projects that require fine motor control, such as drawing, cutting, and painting, and to work on their writing or typing as a form of at-home occupational therapy. Classifications of motor skills are important for both physical educators and health professionals who design and implement motor skill programs, because certain practice designs are more appropriate for particular skill classifications.

Skill Classification

Skills are the learned ability to bring about predetermined results with maximal certainty, often with a minimum outlay of time or energy (Knapp, 1963). An athlete or performer is considered **skillful** if he has achieved a criterion of excellence and is capable of performing at a high level the majority of the time. Motor skills have also been defined as activities that require a chain of sensory (vision, hearing, touch, smell), central (brain and nervous sys-

tems), and motor mechanisms whereby the performer is able to maintain constant control of the sensory input and in accordance with the goal of the movement (Argyle & Kendon, 1967). Physical activities can be classified into categories. Each activity is unique with respect to the structure of the task, task goals, and obstacles. Although physical activities have many unique qualities, there are also commonalities across activities, such that proficiency in one skill can lead to increased proficiency in another (i.e., positive transfer of learning).

Classifying skills is useful for teaching and learning. Practitioners who can appropriately classify skills are better able to adapt the learning experience to a changing environment, enabling better program design and maximizing motor learning. As discussed in chapters 15 through 17, practice sessions should be designed for particular skill classifications. The following sections examine motor skill classifications in terms of sport skills, movement taxonomies, single-dimensional classification, and multidimensional classification.

Sport Skills

Sport skills have been separated into three categories: cognitive, perceptual, and motor (Honeybourne, 2006). **Cognitive skills** refers to the intellectual skills of the mover. These are the skills that enable a performer to make decisions and solve problems. The cognitive skill of decision-making speed is critical for a quarterback in American football, who must make quick, effective decisions. **Perceptual skills** are those that involve interpreting and integrating sensory information to determine the best movement outcome. Attention and previous movement experiences also affect perceptual skills. For example, a soccer player assesses the position of defenders and teammates to determine whether to pass the ball to an open player or continue dribbling toward the goal. The speed and direction of the athlete's movements depend on the perceptual information she receives regarding the current situation. **Motor skills** are the physical elements that enable the movement. To put it simply, the activity could not be completed without the learned ability to coordinate the limbs to produce the action.

At young ages, basic skills provide the foundation for activities that require much more complicated sport-specific motor skills. These basic skills are termed **fundamental motor skills** and include activities such as overhand throwing, jumping, catching, kicking, and striking. By building a basis with these fundamental motor skills, people are able to perform a wide array of similar activities. For instance, a child who has learned how to jump, hop, and skip will be better able to perform more sport-specific activities such as the long jump, the high jump, and even the basketball layup. The fundamental skill of striking is useful in many sports, including hockey, golf, racket sports, softball, and baseball. Chapter 7 addresses the developmental progressions of several fundamental motor skills.

Movement Taxonomies

A **movement taxonomy** provides a framework for grouping motor skills into themes for teaching fundamental motor skills. **Taxonomies** are classifications of objects or events according to a common theme. In the developmental taxonomy, motor skills can be broken down into three groups: nonlocomotor stability, locomotor skills, and manipulative skills.

Nonlocomotor Stability **Stability** is the ability to maintain body position against the forces of gravity, which may include other circumstances that increase the difficulty of the task (Gallahue, Ozmun, & Goodway, 2012). Gymnasts must be able to maintain body position while holding the body's entire weight upright between two rings or while completing a balance beam routine; figure skaters must be able to maintain a static position while gliding across the ice; and divers must be able to

hold a vertical position while entering the water. Maintaining stability is fundamental for not only most sport-related motor skills, but also many functional skills. It is also critical to maintain stability while reaching high for a can in a cupboard or unexpectedly stepping onto ice.

Locomotor Skills **Locomotor skills** are gross motor skills in which the goal of the movement is body transport. Locomotor skills cannot be developed separately from stability. The body must be stabilized before a proficient locomotor pattern can be performed. Body transport can occur when a person is moving from point A to point B, or during sporting activities such as a racquetball match, a gymnastics routine, or a soccer game.

Typically developing infants progress through a developmental sequence of body transport. When they are very young, they are not strong enough or coordinated enough to locomote using their feet, so they learn other methods for transporting their bodies from one point to another. Young infants begin body transport by learning how to roll over. This usually begins around 3 months of age, when most infants can roll from their backs or abdomens onto their sides. Infants then progress to using their arms and knees to transport their bodies by crawling (body drag) at 6 to 8 months and by creeping (quadruped movement, abdomen off the floor) around age 8 to 10 months. After infants have increased their abdominal and leg strength as well as their coordination, they can pull to a standing position (7 to 9 months), walk with assistance (9 to 10 months), and then finally perform bipedal walking alone (12 to 14 months).

Manipulative Skills **Manipulative skills** use smaller muscle groups and enable people to explore the world, bringing objects closer and feeling their size and texture to identify them. Some physical activities are specifically geared toward the manipulation of objects (e.g., archery and marksmanship). In these tasks, even slight adjustments to the movement can compromise the performance outcome considerably.

Although tasks can be classified as manipulative or locomotor, they rarely occur as one or the other in complete isolation during recreation or sporting activities. Most advanced motor skills require the ability to control all three of the skill elements, whereas fundamental motor skills focus more on individual elements. For example, a basketball player is manipulating the basketball while also transporting the body closer to the basket; a bowler manipulates the bowling ball, adjusting the amount of spin and force at the release point, while also transporting the body closer to the pins; and even in billiards, while players are eyeing up the point of contact for the stick, they must also transport the body to that position. When designing a practice sequence or teaching a new skill, especially to a young child or someone with few movement experiences, a practitioner would do well to simplify the task by focusing on only one aspect of the movement at a time and to take each of the three developmental taxonomies into consideration. The sequence should begin with a stable task. As the performer increases in proficiency, more difficulty can be added, such as increased locomotion and manipulation of an implement. The following list presents an example of teaching a child how to kick a ball using the developmental taxonomy.

Developmental Taxonomy Progression for Kicking a Ball

Step 1: Kick a stationary ball into a goal while standing still.

Step 2: Take a step and kick a stationary ball into a goal.

Step 3: Run and kick a stationary ball into a goal.

Step 4: Dribble the ball and kick into a goal.

Step 5: Dribble the ball and kick into a goal that is being guarded.

Single-Dimensional Classification

The first step in learning a new motor skill is to understand the basic elements and sequence of the movements. Movements can be broken down into particular situations, including game strategies, rules, and goals. It is also important to break the activity down further into simple units, or the basic skills. In this section, skills are classified according to movement precision, environmental predictability, time constraint taxonomy, and the nature of the skill.

Movement Precision Motor skills can be classified by the size of the muscle groups being used to produce the movement pattern and consequently the precision of the movement. Skills in which large muscle groups produce the movement, such as the quadriceps, hamstrings, and gluteus maximus, tend to be much larger, less precise movements. These motor skills are classified as **gross motor skills**. Skills in which precise movements are critical to perform with increased accuracy and control use smaller muscle groups and are categorized as **fine motor skills**. Dialing a phone number, playing the piano, and typing are skills that require precise movements of smaller muscle groups. This classification is important for developmental sequencing. Children are generally less able to control smaller muscle groups and are thus taught activities that involve larger muscle groups, such as running and jumping, before they are taught how to coordinate their limbs to perform fine motor skills such as in drawing, writing, and playing games (e.g., jacks or marbles). Practitioners preparing motor skill programs for very young children should keep this concept in mind.

Environmental Predictability Skills can also be classified according to the predictability of the environment. Skills used in a task that takes place in a stable environment in which objects or events are also stationary are considered **closed**

skills. With closed skills, the performer's goal is to perform the movement correctly and then replicate the action; an example is performing a foul shot in basketball. Foul shots are not constrained by time or space, and the environment is stable. The shooter does not have to pay attention to defenders trying to steal the ball or block the shot, and the distance to the hoop and the height of the hoop remain stable. On the other hand, **open skills** occur in an environment in which objects, people, and events are constantly changing. These skills require that the mover be much more attentive to the environment, constantly monitoring the situation for changing conditions. A hockey slap shot is considered an open skill, because the environment is highly unpredictable.

Skills classified according to the predictability of the environment occupy a continuum. No skills are entirely closed, because there are always some conditions that will change; however, for closed skills, the predictability is much greater than it is for open skills. Bowling would be placed more toward the closed end of the continuum because the skill is completed inside a building, and the pins remain stationary for each frame. Gutters are the only obstacle, and they too remain stable. The only condition that can vary is the number of pins that remain after each attempt and perhaps the amount of background noise, which is presumably much less than during a Division 1 collegiate American football game. Figure 1.1 provides several examples of motor skills on the open–closed continuum.

Golf is an example of a sport that is performed in a somewhat predictable environment compared to team sports. Golfers can benefit from practicing with added pressure or the element of surprise.

Golf is often practiced in a very controlled and predictable facility (i.e., driving range), and then played in a much less predictable environment (i.e., golf course). Golfers are often not prepared for playing under the increased pressure and environmental conditions they may face during a match. Tiger Woods has exceptional focus even under intense pressure but didn't become a highly skilled professional golfer by practicing only in controlled environments. Earl, Tiger's father, a Green Beret in the U.S. Army, learned to shoot a rifle during simulated war games rather than in controlled, predictable environments. When Tiger was a young child, Earl prepared him for unpredictable situations by distracting him during golf rounds. Tiger would also play under various weather conditions, day or night. At times, Earl would talk during Tiger's swing. These distractions taught him to tune out environmental influences, preparing him to play championship golf matches under unpredictable and often distracting circumstances.

Tiger Woods' story is only one example of how manipulating the environment can help learners perform better. Amateurs of any sport or recreational activity may believe that they simply choked under pressure, although there are ways to minimize this occurrence. Most often, amateurs do not have experience in stressful, competitive environments, whereas professionals are very familiar with varied conditions and pressure situations.

Preparing the learning environment requires an understanding of the fundamental differences between game and motor tasks. This is also important for rehabilitation, because the clinical environment is much more controlled than the real world. Therapists must prepare their clients to function in unpredictable

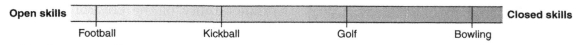

| Open skills | | | | Closed skills |
| Football | Kickball | Golf | Bowling | |

Figure 1.1 Examples of skills on the open–closed continuum. All motor skills fit somewhere between open and closed on the continuum. For instance, no skills are entirely closed skills. Every skill has at least some aspects that are somewhat variable or unpredictable.

environments with changing surfaces of support including rough terrain, potholes, unexpected slippery surfaces, and unpredictable events.

An additional element of environmental predictability is **intertrial variability**, which refers to any change that occurs between trials (i.e., practice attempts). A skill with high intertrial variability has aspects that change with every performance attempt. Intertrial variability can be present in both open and closed skills. The closed skill of batting in T-ball has no intertrial variability, whereas a pitch in baseball has high intertrial variability. Each pitch is unique, requiring the batter to adapt to the changing conditions. The key to success in T-ball batting is consistency. Functional tasks can also have varying levels of intertrial variability. Walking up the stairs at home or across a room should have relatively low intertrial variability, whereas walking on the busy sidewalks of Manhattan would have high intertrial variability. Every day a person's path would have to be different to avoid bumping into people or objects along the way.

Although open skills always include at least some intertrial variability, most closed skills have little to no intertrial variability. They are often performed in a stable environment in which most factors are predictable. In some closed skills, intertrial variability adds to the challenge of the task, as in golf. After each golf putt, the distance, angle, and position of the ball in relation to the hole is different. There are no defenders or other variable conditions except for the weather. The terrain may also change with differing obstructions (artificial) and impediments (natural) across the course. This variability adds to the complexity of the task, making it more challenging and interesting to the performer and the observer.

Time Constraint Taxonomy The difficulty of a task can be determined by its pacing. Tasks with time constraints are less complex than tasks without them. **Self-paced tasks** are initiated by the mover (e.g., golf, darts, archery). Basketball players shooting foul shots often engage in preliminary routines prior to shooting. They can adopt a routine because the shot is not constrained by time; instead, accuracy is the key. Other skills do not have the luxury of self-pacing. A pitcher determines when to initiate the pitch, so the pitch is self-paced. The batter's movements are **externally paced tasks** because she is responding to the pitched ball. She does not have the luxury of swinging whenever she desires. Instead, she must swing when the ball reaches the plate, which is determined by the release, speed, and

WHAT DO YOU THINK?

Exercise 1.3

1. Chris spends many hours a week practicing his golf swing at his local driving range, mastering techniques such as his grip, his posture, and the basics of the swing. Although he can perfect his swing on a practice tee, he experiences problems when transferring to a golf course. Why does he perform so well at the driving range, yet has problems when playing on a course?

2. What components in racket sports are (a) self-paced and (b) externally paced?

3. Name two games or sports that are entirely self-paced and two games or sports that are entirely externally paced.

4. Name two everyday or functional tasks that are self-paced and two functional tasks that are externally paced.

trajectory of the pitch. Performing a penalty kick in soccer is another example of a self-paced movement; however, the goalie's response is externally paced by the kicker. Most functional tasks and physical and occupational therapy treatments are internally paced, such as writing, brushing teeth, and performing muscle-strengthening exercises. Driving, on the other hand, is a combination of the two. You choose your speed, to some degree, and your route; but you must stop at red lights and wait for the green before continuing while varying your speed based upon the traffic.

Nature of the Skill A fourth method for defining skills is by the nature of the task. Fitts and Posner (1967) defined tasks by the beginning and end points of the movements. A **discrete motor skill** is one in which the beginning and end points are clearly defined. These movements are generally short in duration and have a distinct difference between their initiation and termination. A photograph taken during the beginning of the movement for a discrete skill would be qualitatively different from a photograph taken at the conclusion of the movement (see figure 1.2). The two photographs would illustrate undoubtedly different things. An observer would also easily be able to determine which photograph was taken at the beginning of the movement and which was taken at the end. Another key component of discrete skills is a period of time that must elapse before a subsequent movement must occur. For instance, a quarterback in American football must wait to receive a ball before passing. Some examples of discrete skills are throwing, kicking, punching, shooting, and catching.

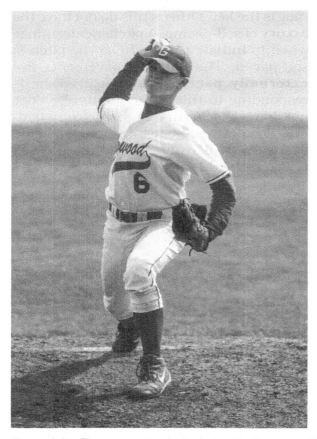 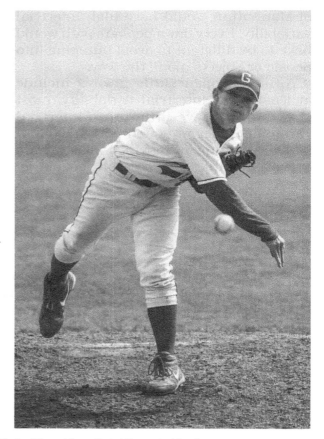

Figure 1.2 The movement at the beginning of a throw is qualitatively different from that at the end of the throw.

Exercise 1.4

Provide one example of each of the following classifications of skills, and define each of your examples as either self-paced or externally paced.

1. Discrete open skill
2. Discrete closed skill
3. Continuous open skill
4. Continuous closed skill
5. Serial open skill
6. Serial closed skill

Continuous motor skills do not have clearly defined beginning and ending points. These tasks are longer in duration, and the mover is in constant motion (Fitts & Posner, 1967). Continuous motor skills appear as repetitive movements. The movements are generally simple and are continuously repeated, as in running, swimming, cross-country skiing, and bicycling. Looking at a photo of a child riding a bicycle, it is difficult to determine whether she is at the beginning or end of the movement. **Serial motor skills** are motor skills that include a series of discrete skills that must occur in a specific sequence. If the order of the movements can be altered, the task would not be classified as a serial task. The triple jump, consisting of an approach, hop, skip, and jump, is an example of a closed serial skill. If the sequence were altered to a hop, approach, jump, and skip, this combination would no longer be considered the triple jump. A basketball layup is an example of an open serial skill when performed in a game because defenders can alter the timing and position of the movement. Serial skills can be thought of as a string of beads. Each component can be performed separately as a discrete skill, such as catching, dribbling, jumping, and shooting. Serial skills require that the performer not only be skillful at the discrete skills independently, but also be able to transition from one movement to the next in the proper sequence.

Multidimensional Classification

Practitioners lead learners through a progression of movements to perform an open skill proficiently. It is best to place learners in a closed environment in which much of the task can be simplified and controlled before progressing to a more challenging and adaptable open environment. Gentile (2000) designed a classification system for gradual progressions from closed to open environments. **Gentile's taxonomy**, which is useful for individualizing motor skill progressions, uses two main categories to assist in program development: the environmental context and the action requirements. Gentile's classification system was developed for physical therapists, but is widely used by physical educators, trainers, and coaches as well.

Environmental Context The environmental context consists of two factors: regulatory conditions and intertrial variability. **Regulatory conditions** are the environmental factors specific to a particular skill or sport. For example, some of the regulatory conditions in soccer are the size of the field, the height and width of the goal, and the size and weight of the ball. These conditions typically are the same for any soccer game regardless of where it is played. Regulatory conditions standardize how a person must adapt to a given situation to produce a successful outcome.

Gentile (2000) classified regulatory conditions as either moving or stationary. Stationary regulatory conditions, such as the pins in bowling, require considerably less skill than moving regulatory conditions, such as the clay targets in skeet shooting. Stationary regulatory conditions in the absence of intertrial variability represent a closed skill, whereas moving regulatory conditions that include intertrial variability represent an open skill (Adams, 1999). Stationary regulatory conditions with intertrial variability require moderately closed skills. Figure 1.3 gives an example of a motor skill in each of the four categories. The complexity of T-ball is lower than that of batting with a machine because the regulatory conditions are stable and there is no intertrial variability (i.e., the ball is in the same position for every attempt). A ball that is hanging on a rope will be in a different position every time, but the regulatory conditions are stationary. The most complex task is batting a pitched ball. The ball is moving, and the trials are variable.

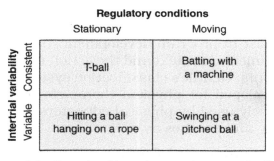

Figure 1.3 Examples of the environmental context of Gentile's (2000) multidimensional classification system.

Action Requirements Gentile (2000) used two classifications to define the action requirements of a skill: body orientation and manipulation (figure 1.4). **Body orientation** is classified as either body transport (during sporting activities, such as a basketball layup or a triple jump) or body stability (as in archery). Body orien-

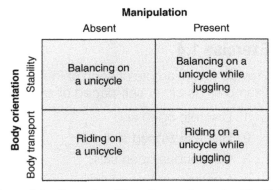

Figure 1.4 Examples of the action requirements of Gentile's (2000) multidimensional classification system.

tation is an important component in exercises used in therapy settings. Body transport activities include locomotor exercises (e.g., crawling, walking, jumping), whereas body stability activities include many balance exercises. Activities that require body transport are higher in complexity than activities that can be completed in a stable body position. When someone must manipulate an object (e.g., racket, bat, or ball) or an opponent (e.g., in wrestling, boxing, or karate), the task is considered higher in complexity. The person must not only adjust or maintain body posture and position (or both) but also manipulate and control an implement (e.g., tennis ball) or a person (e.g., in judo).

Gentile's taxonomy combines the four classifications for the environmental context with the four classifications of the action requirements to create a 16-category system for classifying motor skills. Examples of motor skills for each category are depicted in figure 1.5. Motor skills become increasingly complex from the upper-left quadrant of the taxonomy to the lower-right quadrant. The push-up, in the first quadrant (upper left), is the task lowest in complexity. There is little variability in performing a push-up from trial to trial. When performing successive push-ups, the performer simply needs to repeat the previous movement until either reaching muscle failure or achieving a goal. No body transport or object manipulation is required. Throwing an American football pass, in the last quadrant (lower

Action requirements

		No body transport or object manipulation	Object manipulation but no body transport	Body transport but no object manipulation	Both body transport and object manipulation
Closed skills	Stationary and consistent	Push-up	Decline sit-ups with a medicine ball	Triple jump	Javelin throw
Moderately closed skills	Stationary and variable	Balancing on one foot with different shoes on	Playing cricket with darts	Completing an obstacle course	Salsa dancing in an empty dance studio
Moderately open skills	Moving and consistent	Sitting on an exercise ball	Hitting a tennis ball served from a pitching machine	Running in the woods	Kicking a ball to an unguarded goal
Open skills	Moving and variable	Doing a push-up on an exercise ball	Skeet shooting	Dancing in a crowded club	Throwing a football pass

Environmental conditions (left axis)

Increasing complexity (right axis)

⟵——————— Increasing complexity ———————⟶

Figure 1.5 Examples of motor skills in each category of Gentile's (2000) multidimensional classification system. Note that this figure illustrates the classification of a variety of motor skills rather than progressions of one motor skill.

right), is considered highest in complexity. A quarterback must be able to anticipate the receiver's position and the time and location of the pass. A quarterback must also be able to adapt to various environmental conditions with each performance attempt while transporting his body and manipulating the ball.

Gentile's taxonomy is particularly useful in therapy settings. By manipulating the environment or changing the task requirements, the activity can be progressed. For example, if the goal is to help a five-year-old child with left hemiplegic cerebral palsy climb a ladder to a slide, the task or the environment (or both) can be manipulated to create progressions to help the child succeed. One activity could be a stability task with a manipulation requirement in a closed environment: the child could stand in front of bilateral stationary upright poles and work on maintaining a static grasp on the poles with both hands. The therapist could minimize distractions by conducting the sessions in a quiet and private area

of the clinic. In addition, a nonslip material could be wrapped around the pole to improve grip. Progressions could include controlling the grasp and releasing the poles with one hand and then the other. In addition, the speed could be changed and the distractions could be increased (Kenyon & Blackinton, 2011).

Activities could be planned for all 16 categories for a particular motor skill; however, it is not likely to be necessary. A performer who can complete the fundamental movement pattern consistently and under variable conditions is prepared to begin at the ninth category, which is for a motor skill that is moving, is consistent, and does not involve body transport or object manipulation. If the motor skill is a closed skill, then the practice should be designed for only the first eight categories. Gentile's taxonomy enables an instructor to implement a precise skill progression appropriate for learners of all developmental levels to enable them to progress to their desired levels of difficulty.

Skill Versus Ability

Abilities differ from skills in the sense that skills are learned, whereas abilities are a product of both learning and genetics (Fleishman, 1964). Skills describe a level of proficiency on a specific motor task, whereas abilities are part of a person's traits that affect the capability to become skillful when learning a new motor task. **Abilities** can be defined as genetically predetermined characteristics that affect movement performance, such as agility, coordination, strength, and flexibility. Abilities are enduring and, as such, are difficult to change in adults.

Early researchers in the area of motor abilities hypothesized the existence of only one **general motor ability** (Brace, 1927). This hypothesis was based on observations of accomplished athletes who were adept at many athletic events and also able to quickly learn new and unfamiliar motor skills. You likely know athletes in your age group who fit this description (e.g., the star high school quarterback who also led the basketball team to state championships and held the school batting average record). It may appear that many athletes are capable of performing very skillfully across many motor skills.

Research examining individuals' performances across activities supports the notion that every motor skill requires very specific abilities for skillful performance, and that each person has many independent abilities. This has been termed the **specificity hypothesis** (Henry, 1968). For example, abilities required for skilled race car driving include rate control, manual dexterity, stamina, control precision, and reaction time; a typist needs to have abilities in aiming and finger dexterity; a surgeon requires arm–hand steadiness and multilimb coordination; and a figure skater performing the triple axel requires abilities such as explosive strength, dynamic flexibility, gross body coordination, and multilimb coordination. These abilities were defined in Fleishman's (1962) taxonomy, which categorized abilities into either perceptual–motor abilities or physical proficiency abilities (see Fleishman's Taxonomy of Motor Abilities). Although it is doubtful that **Fleishman's taxonomy** is an exhaustive list of motor abilities, it does provide a framework for assessing individual differences.

Fleishman's Taxonomy of Motor Abilities

Perceptual–Motor Abilities

- Control precision: The ability to make highly controlled movements with larger muscle groups (e.g., hockey puck handling).
- Rate control: The ability to make continuous anticipatory adjustments in relation to a moving target (e.g., Formula 1 racing).
- Aiming: The ability to make accurate hand movements directed at small targets (e.g., texting).

- Response orientation: The ability to make quick decisions in the presence of multiple response options; also referred to as choice reaction time (e.g., quarterback in American football).
- Reaction time: The ability to react as quickly as possible to gain an advantage; also referred to as simple reaction time (e.g., sprinting).
- Manual dexterity: The ability to manipulate large objects with the hands (e.g., dribbling a basketball).
- Finger dexterity: The ability to manipulate small objects with the fingers (e.g., typing).
- Arm–hand steadiness: The ability to move the hand and fingers precisely without regard to strength or speed (e.g., performing surgery).
- Wrist and finger speed: The ability to move the fingers and wrist rapidly (e.g., speed stacking).

Physical Proficiency Abilities

- Strength
  - Explosive strength: The ability to exert maximal energy in one explosive act; commonly known as *power* (e.g., standing long jump).
  - Static strength: The ability to exert maximal force against an immovable or heavy object (e.g., dynamometer).
  - Trunk strength: The ability to exert repeated strength using the core muscles (e.g., pole vaulting).
- Flexibility and speed
  - Extent flexibility: The ability to move the body through a large range of motion (e.g., yoga).
  - Dynamic flexibility: The ability to make repeated flexing movements (e.g., squat thrusts).

RESEARCH NOTES

What Abilities Most Influence Soccer Performance?

A research study was conducted to examine the motor abilities that most strongly influence technique and performance in soccer (Talvoć, Hodžić, Bajramović, Jelešković & Alić, 2009). Soccer was chosen because it is generally considered an aerobic sport because of the size of the field and the duration of the game (90 minutes). Yet soccer also has anaerobic elements, such as sprints and jumps. In the study, 88 participants between the ages of 12 and 14 years completed 18 variables for motor abilities, such as foot tapping on the wall, body lift-ups from lying, and forward bends on the bench; two variables for functional abilities, a 12-minute run and six 50-meter runs; and 15 variables on soccer technique performance, such as inside-foot ball receiving, rolling dribbling, and heading.

The study question was, What abilities most influence soccer performance? The results revealed a strong influence of all of the abilities as a whole, indicating that soccer is a complex sport that may require the interaction of many underlying abilities for highly proficient performance. Moving beyond this general finding, the authors examined each ability at a one-variant level and found that the most important abilities were multilimb and gross body coordination, dynamic strength, and explosive strength. These results indicate that physical proficiency abilities may be more influential on soccer technique performance than perceptual–motor abilities, specifically those related to strength, endurance, and coordination.

- Speed of limb movement: The ability to make fast, gross, and discrete limb movements without regard to accuracy (e.g., throwing a javelin).
- Balance
  - Static balance: The ability to maintain body equilibrium in one position (e.g., standing still on one foot).
  - Dynamic balance: The ability to maintain balance while changing position (e.g., gymnastics).
  - Balancing objects: The ability to balance an external object (e.g., circus clown balancing a stick on his nose).
- Coordination
  - Multilimb coordination: The ability to coordinate movements of more than one limb simultaneously without moving the whole body (e.g., driving a manual car).
  - Gross body coordination: The ability to coordinate gross motor activity of the whole body (e.g., hurdling).
- Endurance
  - Stamina: The ability to prolong exertions of the entire body; cardiorespiratory endurance (e.g., running a marathon).

- Dynamic strength: The ability to exert repeated force; also referred to as muscular endurance (e.g., kayaking).

A person's abilities are shaped by biological and physiological factors (Fleishman, 1964). The composition of muscle tissue is certainly going to affect physical proficiency motor abilities such as strength, endurance, and flexibility. Physiological deficits in visual development would also limit perceptual–motor abilities, potentially affecting reaction time. Abilities are also affected by environmental factors. For example, children afforded formal education continue to develop their verbal and reasoning abilities throughout their academic years, just as children who participate in physical fitness–related or sport-related programs develop their motor abilities. The rate at which abilities develop varies across childhood and adolescence, both within individuals and across individuals. This is largely due to growth and maturation changes. The rate of development levels out between the ages of 18 and 22 years, and then remains relatively stable throughout adulthood (Fleishman, 1964).

WHAT DO YOU THINK?

Exercise 1.6

1. Choose one motor skill in which you consider yourself proficient. Name five of the motor abilities that would be most important to perform skillfully at that motor skill. Then, for each motor ability, rank yourself from 1 (very low ability) to 5 (very high ability).

2. Choose a motor skill at which you are not skillful. Name five of the motor abilities that would be most important to perform skillfully at that motor skill. For each motor ability, rank yourself from 1 (very low ability) to 5 (very high ability).

3. Did you notice a difference between your general ranking for the activity in which you are proficient and the one for the activity in which you are not proficient?

4. Do you think your underlying abilities influence the sports and activities you choose to engage in? What about the sports and activities you generally avoid? Explain your answer.

Occupational therapists often focus on improving motor abilities such as finger dexterity, arm–hand steadiness, and aiming; physical therapists often focus on control precision, multilimb coordination, dynamic flexibility, and dynamic balance. Some clients have lost some ability as a result of injury, whereas others may have a developmental disability.

Motor Development

Motor development is a subdiscipline of motor behavior that examines the age-related, successive changes that occur over the life span and the processes and factors that affect these changes. Changes that occur during a short period that are not associated with practice or experience, such as a child throwing farther or running faster between the ages of two and three, would likely be due to motor development.

Motor development is assessed according to the **product** (the outcome of performance) or the **process** (the underlying mechanisms of change). The amount of weight lifted or the distance a javelin is thrown are examples of movement products, whereas the action that was performed to produce the throw is a movement process. Motor development, however, is not simply change. Motor development must be organized and systematic, such as an infant progressing through the motor milestones of raising the head, to rolling over, to crawling, and then to walking. The changes also need to be successive—that is, they must occur in an uninterrupted order. Motor development, therefore, is systematic and marked by successive changes over time. Changes that occur as a result of practice or experience, however, are due to motor learning, not motor development. For example, if a physical education teacher instructs a student to snap his wrist in a squash swing as opposed to using a solid-arm swing in the tennis stroke, the resultant change would be considered motor learning. A therapist teaching alternative ways to lift objects overhead following a shoulder injury would also be dealing with motor learning rather than motor development.

Development can occur over various time periods, from very long time (phylogeny) to very brief in response to immediate task demands. **Phylogeny** refers to the evolutionary development of a species, which may take many hundreds, even thousands, of years. **Ontogeny** refers to development that occurs over the life span of one individual. The focus throughout this book is on ontogenetic development. A third level is local biology, including physiological changes such as respiration. Task demands are imposed on an immediate time scale, which can be as short as minutes or even seconds.

Although laypeople often use the terms *growth* and *development* interchangeably, they refer to different things. **Physical growth** refers to an increase in body size or in individual parts that occurs through maturation. However, the term *growth* is more inclusive of overall body changes, as defined by development. The process of development is not limited to the changes occurring during infancy and childhood. Development occurs throughout the life span as people continually undergo cognitive, physical, and psychosocial changes regardless of their age.

The term **maturation** refers to the fixed transitions or order of progressions that enable a person to progress to higher levels of function. Maturation includes internal processes that are unaffected by external factors such as the environment. Of course, aspects of the environment, such as learning experiences, parental influence, and physical surroundings, certainly can alter the timing of developmental transitions. A child who is given a ball during infancy is much more likely to be able to catch and throw at an earlier age than a child who is given only a doll. Not receiving a ball does not prevent the child from learning how to catch and throw, but will delay the development of these skills.

Aging refers to a process or group of processes occurring in living organisms that with the passage of time leads to a loss of adaptability, functional impairment, and eventually death (Spirduso, Francis, & MacRae, 2005). Aging is the progression of life from birth whereby a person matures, and this process continues through physical decline, ending with death. People are often classified by chronological age (see table 1.2) to avoid confusion in defining age groups. For instance, one professional may define a four-year-old as a child, whereas another professional may refer to a four-year-old as a preschooler. The importance of age classifications becomes even more prominent in the upper continuums of life, where age classification discrepancies can be as much as 20 years (i.e., when does old adulthood begin—at age 55, 65, or 75?).

The field of motor development combines biology, the study of the growth and maturation of living organisms, and psychology, the study of human behavior (Clark & Whitall, 1989). However, because the study of motor development must involve living humans, the research tends to focus more on the behavioral aspects and so is more aligned with psychology than with biology. The history of the field of motor development has commonly been divided into four periods: the precursor period, the maturational period, the normative period, and the process-oriented period (Clark & Whitall, 1989) (see table 1.3).

Precursor Period

The field of motor development has its roots in the precursor period, beginning in the late 18th century. During this time, the main method for studying motor development was through descriptive observations, with the focus on the product, or outcome of development. It was also during the precursor period that Charles Darwin developed one of the main arguments for understanding the processes of motor development, the nature versus nurture debate. The perspective that development occurs as a function of nature assumes that maturation occurs as a result of genetic or internal factors (Gesell, 1928, 1954). This view, known as the **maturational perspective**, became

Table 1.2 Age Classifications

Description	Age or transition marker
Newborn	Birth to 6 weeks
Infant	Age 6 weeks to age at walking
Toddler	Age at walking to 2 years
Preschooler	Age 3 to age at start of school
Young child	Age at start of school to 7 years
Child	Age 8 to 10
Preadolescent	Age 11 to onset of puberty
Adolescent	Onset of puberty to 20 years
Young adult	Age 21 to 40
Middle-aged adult	Age 41 to 60
Young-old adult	Age 61 to 74
Old adult	Age 75 to 99
Centenarian	Age 100+

Table 1.3 Periods in the Evolution of the Field of Motor Development

Period	Characteristics
Precursor (1787-1928)	Focus on product development Nature versus nurture argument
Maturational (1928-1946)	Focus on maturation
Normative (1946-1970)	Focus on movement skills in school-age children
Process-oriented (1970-present)	Hypothesis-driven research Emergence of the information-processing theory, ecological approach, and dynamic systems approach

quite popular in the 1930s during the maturational period. The **environmentalism perspective** assumes the converse: It is not heredity that molds the maturational process; rather, humans are nurtured by their environment. This argument ensued for many decades and continues to some degree even today. Charles Darwin did not believe that nature or nurture favors one developmental process over another. Instead, the environment (nurture) and genetic factors (nature) interact. Maturationists assume that a child born with the underlying abilities to excel at certain sports will eventually exhibit excellence in those sports. However, environmentalists propose that even basic skills must be developed. Either people who are not given the appropriate equipment or environment to learn such skills will be delayed in developing them, or the skills will never materialize.

Charles Darwin's work was seminal in the study of motor development. It provided insights into the effect of the environment on the animal. Darwin theorized about how animals adapt to changing environments and discussed developmental sequences found across species (Darwin, 1859, 1871, 1872). He also wrote about the importance of studying both the product of the behavior and the process.

Maturational Period

A boom in motor development studies occurred in the 1930s following the emergence of the field of developmental psychology. As the name of this period implies, the main focus was on maturation. Arnold Gesell led the maturationist movement, asserting that infant maturity is genetically predetermined, meaning that the infant moves from one developmental cycle to the next under the control of the central nervous system (composed of the brain and the spinal cord). Each cycle occurs in a very orderly and predetermined fashion; for example, infants roll over at around five months, sit up at six months, and stand at eight months. Maturationists assume that these transitions are set and controlled by nature. Children progress to the next step when they are ready. External influences are not included in these transitions; an internal clock, so to speak, simply determines precisely when the infant will progress. More recent research has shown that the environment can certainly influence the onset of these transitions. For instance, a child who never lies on his belly will crawl much later than a child who receives regular belly time. The child's environment has delayed this transition because the infant was not given the opportunity to strengthen the arm, leg, and core muscles necessary for crawling. Children who are blind have been found to be significantly delayed in reaching many milestones (Ribadi, Rider, & Toole, 1987), taking on average an additional five months to crawl and an additional eight months to walk in comparison with their sighted peers. It is doubtful that the delay is genetically predetermined. Rather, it is more likely that the delay results from the lack of visual stimuli that would motivate them to reach objects of interest.

Esther Thelen's research on the infant stepping reflex and walking was seminal in this area. According to the maturation perspective, infants do not walk following the disappearance of the stepping reflex until neuronal paths mature. The persistence of the stepping reflex had been viewed as an indication of a developmental delay. Thelen examined the effects of body build and arousal on infant stepping and found that the disappearance of the stepping reflex was due to increased body mass in proportion to strength (Thelen, Fisher, Ridley-Johnson, & Griffin, 1982). Infants decrease their number of steps simply because they do not have the muscle strength to lift their heavy legs.

Growth occurs in a **cephalocaudal** direction, meaning that the head develops first and distal structures grow more slowly. Essentially, growth occurs from the head to the foot. An infant can control movements of the head much earlier than movements of the trunk or limbs. For instance, the eyes and mouth develop more quickly than the hands and feet. Controlled eye movements can be seen postnatally at very early ages. On a personal note, one of the authors of this book was surprised to see that immediately following birth, her firstborn child was able to track his mother's eye movements. He would lie peacefully when eye contact was maintained, but would scream when eye contact was removed, even for just a moment. With respect to his vision, he was not only alert but also very aware of his surroundings. It was also quite clear that although he was able to control his eye movements, it would be quite some time before he could control his head, neck, trunk, and limb movements.

While growth is occurring in a cephalocaudal direction, it is concurrently developing in a **proximodistal** direction; as the body is growing from head to foot, the trunk is advancing at a faster rate than the limbs. This can be examined in the prehension, or grasping, stages in infants. Initially, infants attempt to grasp an object with the whole palm. As they mature, they begin to use three fingers and then finally add the thumb and forefinger.

A secondary focus during the maturational period was on motor learning (McGraw, 1935). McGraw explained that "maturation and learning are not different processes, merely different facets of the fundamental process of growth" (McGraw 1945/1969, pp. 130-131). Comparing the development of twins in a study in which one twin was taught motor skills and the other merely matured, McGraw found not only that the environment has a strong influence on motor development, but also that there appear to be critical periods in which improvement can be optimized through advanced opportunities and instruction (McGraw, 1935, 1940).

Normative Period

Following World War II, the study of motor development was largely influenced by several physical educators, with a focus on movement skills in school-age children. The focus was less on cognitive development and more on the physical aspects of development, which caused a shift from process- to product-oriented research. Physical educators and researchers were also interested in anthropometric measures (growth measures) through childhood and the role of maturation and strength changes in children (Clark & Whitall, 1989, p. 189). Part of this shift was due to physical educators' interests at the time. They wanted to improve motor skill instruction through understanding changes in motor performance (Halverson, 1970). Motor learning researchers focused on the processes underlying performance changes when new simple motor skills are learned and on the evaluation of such performances. Unfortunately, it was not until the 1980s that motor developmentalists and motor learning and control researchers began appreciating the value of each others' work (Clark & Whitall, 1989).

Process-Oriented Period

A reemergence of motor development research occurred in the early 1970s as psychologists developed a renewed interest in the field and much study focused on hypothesis-driven research. During this period, three theoretical constructs emerged, each of which is still prominent today: the information-processing theory, ecological approach, and dynamic systems approach. It is important to have a basic understanding of the theories that drive research in motor development and motor learning to understand and interpret experimental findings in these fields. These theories are discussed in chapter 3 and are the theoretical basis for this book.

Summary

This chapter provided a background for the fields of motor control, motor learning, and motor development. It is important to understand the similarities and differences between these fields of knowledge and to appreciate the importance of bringing them together when planning a motor skill program for learners of any age, developmental level, or background. It is also critical to understand the differences between growth and development and between learning and performance, because they are very often overlooked.

We all stop growing at some point, but we never stop developing. Many people falsely assume that development is confined to infancy and childhood; however, development occurs throughout the life span. Another common misconception is that performance changes equate to learning changes, but this is not always the case. Learning results in a permanent change in the ability to perform skilled movement, whereas performance changes are the observable products of movement. Shooting a one-time half-court shot for a million dollars and shooting a free throw shot the next day are examples of performance. In a moment of extreme luck, someone could make the million-dollar shot but not be able to make a foul shot the following day. This person's performance would not reflect learning because a permanent change in the capability to shoot a basketball has not occurred.

This chapter also discussed skill classifications and motor abilities. Practitioners who use a multidimensional system, such as Gentile's, can individualize practice sessions for learners at various skill levels. By progressing through these stages, people can gradually increase the difficulty of the task until they are ready for the full complexity of the motor skill. Practitioners need to understand that a client can acquire motor skills only once she has the underlying abilities; however, she can have the underlying abilities but not be skillful in a particular motor skill. Finally, this chapter also presented the historical progression of the field of motor development leading into the current theoretical perspectives that are explained in chapter 3.

ONLINE LEARNING

Visit the web resource at www.HumanKinetics.com/MotorLearningAndDevelopment for an accompanying lab activity and exercises from the chapter.

LEARNING AIDS

Supplemental Activities

1. Choose a motor skill that can be relearned or learned in physical therapy and one that can be learned in occupational therapy. Remember that physical therapy focuses on larger muscle group activities such as walking and balance, whereas occupational therapy works on smaller muscle group activities such as using the hands to eat or using scissors.
   a. Classify each motor skill and devise a list of several progressions to assist a client in improving each motor skill.
   b. Name five of Fleishman's underlying abilities that would be necessary to proficiently perform each of the motor skills.
2. Search the Internet for products related to motor development and make a list. Who are these products targeted toward? What age range are they designed for? Describe how the products are expected to help infants or children develop. Do you think these products will help infants or children develop the abilities or skills they are intended to develop? Why or why not?

Glossary

abilities—Genetically predetermined characteristics that affect movement performance such as agility, coordination, strength, and flexibility.

action slips—Performance-related errors that typically occur when the person is not consciously attending to the movement.

aging—A process or group of processes occurring in living organisms that, with the passage of time, lead to a loss of adaptability, functional impairment, and eventually death.

body orientation—A classification used in Gentile's taxonomy that includes both body transport (e.g., basketball layup, triple jump) and body stability (e.g., in archery, foul shot).

capability—In regard to motor skill acquisition, a quality that implies that skilled behavior *may* occur if the conditions are favorable.

cephalocaudal—Proceeding from the head to distal structures; development begins with the head, and distal structures grow more slowly.

closed skills—Skills used in a task that takes place in a stable environment in which objects or events are stationary.

coarticulation—Simultaneous motions that occur in sequential tasks.

cognitive skills—Intellectual skills that enable a performer to make decisions and solve problems.

continuous motor skills—Motor skills that do not have a clearly defined beginning or ending point because of their cyclical nature (e.g., running, swimming, juggling).

control—Manipulation of movements in such a way as to meet the demands of the task.

coordination—The act of constraining the number of degrees of freedom to decrease the complexity of the movement task to produce a movement pattern and achieve a task goal.

degrees of freedom—The number of independent elements that must be constrained to produce coordinated motion.

discrete motor skills—Motor skills that are short in duration and have clearly defined beginning and end points (e.g., throwing, catching, kicking).

environmentalism perspective—A perspective that assumes that heredity does not mold the maturational process; rather, maturation occurs as humans are nurtured by their environment.

externally paced tasks—Tasks performed in response to external stimuli (e.g., a batter responding to a pitch).

fine motor skills—Skills in which precise movements are critical for performing with increased accuracy and control, and which use smaller muscle groups.

Fleishman's taxonomy—A classification system for motor skills that identifies the underlying motor abilities necessary to perform successfully.

fundamental motor skills—Basic motor skills (e.g., throwing, jumping, striking) that are typically acquired by around the age of seven.

general motor ability—An early hypothesis that there is only one motor ability.

Gentile's taxonomy—Motor skill taxonomy that uses two main categories—the environmental context and the action requirements—to assist practitioners with program development.

gross motor skills—Skills in which large muscle groups (e.g., quadriceps, hamstrings, gluteus maximus) produce the movement, which tends to be large and not very precise.

intertrial variability—Any change that occurs between trials (i.e., practice attempts).

locomotor skills—Gross motor skills with the goal of body transport.

manipulative skills—Motor skills that involve the manipulation of an object.

maturation—The fixed transition or order of progression that enables a person to progress to higher levels of function.

maturational perspective—A perspective that development occurs as a function of nature (i.e., as a result of genetic or internal factors).

motor behavior—An umbrella term for the fields of motor control, motor learning, and motor development.

motor control—The study of the underlying neural, physical, and behavioral processes of movement.

motor development—The study of the products and underlying processes of motor behavior changes across the life span.

motor learning—The processes involved in the acquisition of a motor skill and the factors that enhance or inhibit the capability to perform a motor skill.

motor skills—Voluntary, goal-oriented physical elements that enable movement.

movement taxonomy—A framework for grouping motor skills into themes for teaching fundamental motor skills.

ontogeny—The level of development occurring over the life span of one individual.

open skills—Skills performed in an environment in which objects, people, and events are constantly changing.

perceptual–motor integration problem—Line of research in motor control that examines how perception and motor control are integrated.

perceptual skills—The ability to interpret and integrate sensory information to determine the best movement outcome.

performance—The act of executing a motor skill.

phylogeny—The evolutionary development of the history of a species, which can occur over many hundreds or thousands of years.

physical growth—An increase in body size or in individual parts that occurs through maturation.

process—A set of events or occurrences resulting in a change in the state or end product.

product—The outcome of performance.

proximodistal—In relation to development, the earlier advancement of the trunk than of the limbs.

regulatory conditions—The environmental factors specific to a particular skill or sport.

self-paced tasks—Tasks initiated by the mover (e.g., in golf, darts, archery); also referred to as internally paced tasks.

serial motor skills—Motor skills that include a series of discrete skills that must occur in a specific sequence.

serial order problem—The study of the importance of the sequencing, order, and timing of movement behaviors.

skill—The learned ability to bring about predetermined results with maximal certainty, often with minimal outlays of time or energy.

skillful—A criterion of excellence for performing a motor skill.

specificity hypothesis—The hypothesis by Henry that specific abilities are necessary to perform each motor skill proficiently.

spoonerisms—Speech errors that occur as a result of exchanging letters in adjacent words.

stability—The ability to maintain body position against forces of gravity, which may include other circumstances that increase the difficulty of the task.

taxonomies—Classifications of objects or events according to a common theme.

UNDERSTANDING MOVEMENT CONTROL

2

Chapter Objectives

After reading this chapter, you should be able to do the following:

- Understand factors associated with movement preparation.
- Compare theories of attention and illustrate how arousal levels affect performance.
- Explain sensory contributions to movement and balance.
- Differentiate between short-term, long-term, and working memory.

Performance Under Fire

Sheila is still in a state of shock and awe. Last night she witnessed a terrible car accident. The driver two cars in front of her drifted off the road, crashing into a tree. He was trapped in the car, and the engine was starting to smoke. After pulling over onto the shoulder of the road and turning on her hazard lights, she called 911. Within a few minutes, she heard sirens in the distance and saw the approach of flashing lights. A fire engine! From the sidelines, she watched amazed at the speed and precision with which the firefighters worked when they arrived on scene. Within no time at all, the driver was freed safely from the car and other firefighters worked to contain the fire beginning to burn from the engine. Even now, it all seems like a blur. She finds herself wondering how the firefighters were able to perform so well given the gravity of the situation. What if they had hesitated for even an instant? What if they had focused only on freeing the driver and ignored the smoke from the engine? What if . . . ?

We thank Melanie Perreault for her contributions to this chapter.

Many of you have probably been in a situation similar to Sheila's—witnessing an incredible feat of motor performance that leaves you dumbfounded: a NASCAR driver passing another car with only inches to spare, a soccer goalie making a save during a critical moment in the game, or an athletic training team responding in record time to a serious injury. However, the observable motor response is often only the tip of an iceberg. The processes under the surface that dictate the motor response are often more important than the execution.

Imagine being one of the firefighters in the preceding scenario. You arrive on the scene of a serious accident filled with twisted metal, smoke, an entrapped and possibly injured driver, and witnesses in various emotional states. Amid the chaos, you might find your heart rate begin to rise, your breathing rate increase, and your mind pulled in a hundred different directions. In this heightened physiological and psychological state, how can you pick out the most pertinent sensory information, determine the best course of action, and act accordingly, all in as little time as possible? What if you hesitate or fail to notice the smoke coming from the car's engine? These questions highlight some of the important considerations when preparing any motor response: reaction time, attention, arousal, and sensory contributions. These concepts are discussed in this chapter.

Reaction Time

When someone is preparing a motor response, speed is often a critical factor. In some sport contexts, such as swimming and track, the speed at which the person reacts to the starting signal (see figure 2.1) could be the difference between first place and second place. For the firefighters in the opening scenario, the speed at which they can assess the scene and decide on a course of action could be the difference between whether the driver of the car lives or dies. This element of movement preparation is termed **reaction time (RT)**. It is the measure of the time between the presentation of a stimulus and the initiation of a motor response. Although the processes involved during RT are not directly observable, RT provides an indication of the speed at which one makes a decision; however, it does not take into account whether the decision was correct or appropriate. A related term, **movement time**, is the observable movement; that is, the time from the initiation of the movement until it has been completed. When combined, these two measures make up the person's **response time** (see figure 2.1). Given the importance of RT in many situations, it is necessary to understand the factors that affect RT and how to use them effectively. These factors include the number of stimulus–response alternatives, the psychological refractory period, and stimulus–response compatibility.

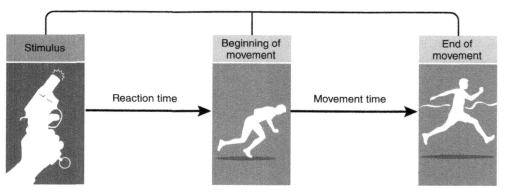

Figure 2.1 Reaction time begins immediately after the sound of the starter's gun and continues until the sprinter initiates a movement, at which time movement time begins. Response time includes reaction time and extends to the conclusion of the movement.

Stimulus–Response Alternatives

The simplest decisions in response to a stimulus require only one motor response. For example, when approaching a stop sign while driving, the only corresponding motor response is to bring the car to a stop. The reaction time to such an event is termed **simple reaction time** (or **simple RT**). In such cases, there is only one stimulus and one corresponding response option, and human RT is relatively short. However, what happens to RT when the driver approaches a stoplight? In this situation, the driver is now faced with a choice of three stimulus–response (S–R) options: green light, go; yellow light, slow down; red light, stop. This increase in the number of S–R alternatives, or **choice reaction time (CRT)**, has been shown to negatively affect RT. In a classic paper, W.E. Hick (1952), an experimental psychologist, found a logarithmic relationship between the number of S–R alternatives and choice RT. That is, as the number of S–R alternative increases, RT increases at a constant rate. This finding was later termed **Hick's law**.

Hick's law helps explain the importance of having a large repertoire of motor responses in any given situation. Let's consider the triple option in American football. This is an offensive scheme that allows for three players to run the ball, thus increasing the number of S–R alternatives. This play increases the amount of uncertainty for the defensive players, which will likely increase their RT to the play. However, strategies can be implemented to reduce the amount of uncertainty. Predicting a stimulus (**event anticipation**) or when it might occur (**temporal anticipation**), or both, can reduce the number of S–R alternatives. This is often achieved by picking up on precues in the environment (e.g., hip angle) that telegraph information pertinent to the situation. This, in turn, reduces the number of options that require a response. For example, the coaching staff might use scouting reports and game film in preparation for an upcoming game to identify tendencies of the opposing offense during certain game situations to narrow down the number of defensive responses. Likewise, an athletic trainer might use mental practice to run through common injury scenarios prior to a game to prime her responses to specific stimuli.

Although anticipating correctly can help reduce RT, it can have the opposite effect if done incorrectly. For example, Usain Bolt was disqualified from the 100-meter final

TRY THIS

Ruler Test

Exercise 2.1

1. To examine the difference between simple reaction time and choice reaction time, break up into pairs. Each pair of students has two rulers. (Yard or meter sticks could also be used.)

    a. Simple reaction time: One student (the experimenter) begins by holding a ruler vertically. The other student (the participant) places a thumb and forefinger at the bottom end of the ruler (at 0). The participant should leave approximately 1 inch (2.5 cm) of space between the thumb and the ruler and the finger and the ruler. The experimenter drops the ruler without warning, and the participant grasps it as quickly as possible (see figure 2.2). Record the number at the top of the position the participant grasps the ruler in the chart. Perform the experiment 10 times, then switch roles.

(continued)

b. Choice reaction time: The experimenter holds two rulers vertically, and the participant positions thumbs and forefingers at the end of each ruler (at 0). The experimenter randomly releases one of the rulers without warning. The participant grasps the ruler as quickly as possible. The participant may not grasp with both hands. If both hands grasp the rulers at the same time, the trial must be aborted. Record the value at the top of the position where the participant grasps the ruler into the chart, then switch roles.

2. Compare your results for simple reaction time versus choice reaction time.

3. Did you find it difficult to close only one hand during the choice reaction time test?

4. Explain why you are not permitted to grasp with both hands during the choice reaction time test.

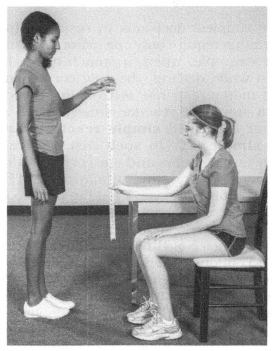

Figure 2.2 The ruler test can be used with a yardstick as shown. This picture illustrates a student grasping the yardstick after the experimenter has released it.

Trial	Simple reaction time	Choice reaction time
1		
2		
3		
4		
5		
6		
7		
8		
9		
10		
Mean		

of the 2011 IAAF World Championships because of a false start; he had incorrectly anticipated the timing of the starting gun.

Psychological Refractory Period

The way stimuli are presented can also affect RT. Often, stimuli requiring a response are presented at separate times. For example, during a point, a tennis player might first have to return a serve, next come toward the net for a short ball, and finally hit an overhead off a lob to end the point. However, when two stimuli are presented in quick succession, and they require different responses, processing a response to the first stimulus delays the response to the second stimulus. This delay, termed the **psychological refractory period (PRP)**, causes a marked increase in RT to the second stimulus. This delay is further compounded with age; that is, the PRP tends to affect older adults more than younger adults (Allen, Smith, Vires-Collins, & Sperry, 1998). The PRP is thought to result from a narrowing of attention to a single channel in which only one stimulus can be processed at a time (Smith, 1967). If the time given between stimuli is not sufficient, an attentional bottleneck occurs (see the section Attentional Capacity later in this chapter).

The PRP helps explain why faking works (see figure 2.3). Consider a tennis match in which Pete begins to move back after seeing his opponent, Andre, set up to hit a deep forehand shot. However, Andre changes his stroke just before contact with the ball, causing it to drop right over the net. As a result, Pete is not able to get to the ball in time. Because the PRP delayed Pete's RT to the drop shot, he was not able to respond quickly enough to make it to the ball. The fake must be believable, however, to work. If Andre had not presented a quality fake, Pete would likely not have been out of position because he would not have wasted time responding to it.

Stimulus–Response Compatibility

The amount of association between a stimulus and response can also affect RT. This association is termed **stimulus–response (S-R) compatibility**. The greater the amount of association, the shorter the RT even in a choice RT scenario. As mentioned previously, a driver approaching a stoplight has three S–R alternatives. However, for experienced drivers, the colors red, yellow, and green are highly associated with the corresponding responses of stop, slow down, and go. As a result, RT is relatively short even though there are multiple S–R options. In a similar vein, many manufacturers have designed vehicle backup camera displays that include red, yellow, and green zones to indicate how close the vehicle is to an object. The intention is to decrease the amount of time needed to

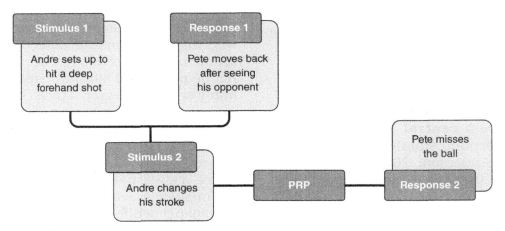

Figure 2.3 Time delay added by a psychological refractory period.

WHAT DO YOU THINK?

Exercise 2.2

1. Following are two images that illustrate various levels of stimulus–response compatibility. Describe the stimulus–response compatibility for each, including the stimulus and response and whether they are compatible.
   a. Stovetop
   b. Group exercise class

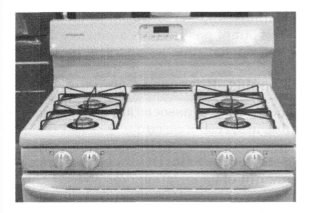 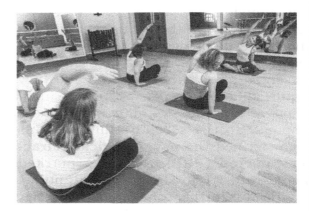

2. Provide another example that illustrates low stimulus–response compatibility and one that illustrates high stimulus–response compatibility.

react to objects that are close to the rear of the vehicle.

Attention

Attention is critical for effective decision making and motor performance. To fully understand how attention affects decision making and motor performance, we consider the three major characteristics of attention: capacity, selectivity, and focus.

Attentional Capacity

Most theories of attention propose that people have a **central limited capacity** when performing simultaneous activities (Magill & Anderson, 2013; Schmidt and Lee, 2011). In other words, the brain and central nervous system do not have a bottomless pit of space. If you have ever felt overloaded by visual and auditory

information, you realize that attention is limited. But the theories differ with regard to the extent and location of the limits. **Single-channel filter theories** propose that tasks are accomplished in serial order and that a bottleneck occurs at some point in information processing; at the bottleneck, the system can process only one task at a time (see figure 2.4). If the bottleneck occurs while a person is working on information detection (such as an air traffic controller), two tasks could not be performed simultaneously without many errors. However, a task that requires information detection might be more easily accomplished along with a task not depending on information detection, such as watching for a signal on a monitor while riding a stationary bike.

Consider a woman who is reading a newspaper while talking to a friend and watching television. According to the

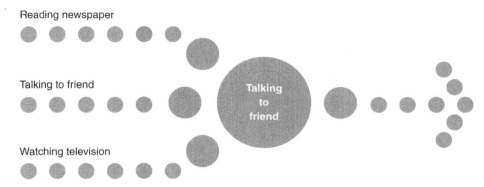

Reading newspaper

Talking to friend

Talking to friend

Watching television

Figure 2.4   Single-channel theory.

single-channel theory, she can attend to only one thing at a time. Perhaps she reads a couple of lines in the newspaper, but at this time isn't processing what is happening on the television or her friend's conversation. Her attention can then shift to her friend's conversation, but this comes at the cost of reading the newspaper.

Alternatively, Kahneman (1973) proposed a **central-resource capacity theory**. This is a more flexible system in which information-processing capacity can expand based on the individual, task, and situation. Kahneman asserted that attention requires cognitive effort. There is no particular bottleneck, but a more general pool of effort that can be strategically allocated to the activities. The person evaluates the amount of attention (e.g., cognitive effort) necessary to perform the tasks to determine whether she can do them simultaneously. The expansion and flexibility of the processing are not unlimited, and at some critical point, performance of one or more of the tasks will be adversely affected.

Finally, **multiple-resource theories** contend that we have several attention mechanisms, each with limited capacity (Magill & Anderson, 2013). Wickens (1980, 1992) posited that the mechanisms might be modalities (e.g., movement and speech), stages of information processing (e.g., perception or decision making), or codes of processing information (e.g., verbal codes or spatial codes). Tasks that require a common mechanism are difficult

to perform simultaneously, whereas those based on separate mechanisms can be performed simultaneously. This is similar to central-resource theory, but each mechanism has its own capacity limitations. When people exceed their capacity, **interference** occurs, meaning that they cannot do both activities without compromising one of them. You can try this while walking with a friend. If you ask your friend to answer math questions and progressively increase the difficulty of the questions, you will likely notice that your friend will either slow down, take longer to respond to the math questions, or make more math errors.

Attentional capacity is critical to understanding the importance of automaticity of performance. As some skills become automatized, people can attend to other aspects of the environment. For example, a basketball player must learn to dribble without looking at the ball before he can simultaneously dribble, run, view the positions of teammates and opponents, and contemplate the next move of passing, shooting, or continuing to dribble (refer to figure 2.5, *a* and *b*, for an illustration). Leavitt (1979) conducted a study with ice hockey players of different ages and experience levels as they skated for speed and performed one, two, or three simultaneous tasks, including visually identifying geometric shapes. The skating speed of young players decreased more than that of older and more experienced players when they were required to stick handle with a puck while simultaneously performing other tasks. Years of playing had provided the older players with a greater degree of automaticity of skating and even stick handling so that they were minimally affected by a visual identification task of naming geometric shapes projected onto a screen.

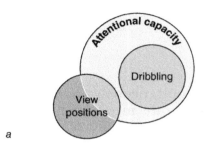

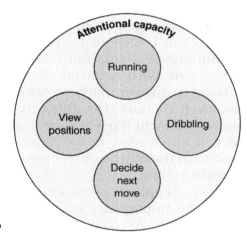

a

b

Figure 2.5 A young basketball dribbler *(a)* uses a lot of attentional capacity to just dribble the ball. Even just raising his head could cause him to lose control of the ball (interference). However, skilled basketball players *(b)* can dribble running down the court while looking at the other players and strategizing.

Selective Attention

In any performance context, an abundance of information is available to the performer. This information can be either relevant or irrelevant depending on the situation. Consider a typist in an open office. What information is available to her? The words she is typing, the computer monitor, a ringing telephone, and colleagues' conversations are just a few examples. To perform her task well, she needs to be able to attend to the relevant information (e.g., words) while filtering out the irrelevant (e.g., ringing telephone). This ability is known as **selective attention**.

A classic research study on selective attention comes from a series of experiments on speech recognition (Cherry, 1953). The author sought to answer the cocktail party problem; that is, "how do we recognize what one person is saying when others are speaking at the same time?" (pp. 975-976). To investigate this question, the author had participants listen to two messages simultaneously, one in each ear. Participants were instructed to attend to only one message for later recall and to reject the second message. The results indicated that participants had little to no trouble recalling the message while blocking out the other. Furthermore, very few participants could identify detailed characteristics about the rejected message, such as individual words, semantic meaning, and language. The findings from this research were later termed the cocktail party phenomenon.

WHAT DO YOU THINK?

Exercise 2.3

1. Do you believe that attention is flexible? Explain why or why not. Compare the attentional capacity theories: single-channel theories, central-resource capacity theory, and multiple-resource theories.

2. Consider the aforementioned theories of attention. How do they make you rethink how to teach your future students, patients, clients, or athletes?

Are You Listening to Me?

Exercise 2.4

How good of a listener are you? Are you so good that you can listen to two conversations at the same time? How about giving it a try. Break up into groups of three. One person is the listener, and the other two are the messengers. Each messenger plans a several-sentence message and delivers it into one of the listener's ears.

1. The first time around, the listener focuses on only one of the messages. Following the delivery of the message, the listener restates the message to the best of her or his ability. Then the listener recalls anything she or he can from the rejected message. How well was the listener able to recall each message?

2. The second time around, the messengers preplan new messages, and the listener tries to attend to both. How well was the listener able to recall each message this time around?

3. Were you surprised by any of the results?

Focus of Attention

Nideffer (1976) identified two dimensions along which attention can be focused: direction and width. *Direction* refers to the location of the focus, which can either be **internal** (within the person) or **external** (in the environment). *Width* refers to the amount or expanse of information attended to by the person, which can be either **narrow** (attending to specific cues) or **broad** (attending to the larger context). When combined, four attentional styles emerge: internal broad, internal narrow, external broad, and external narrow. Each type of attentional focus can be used in any performance context. For example, a basketball player performing a free throw could use any of the attentional styles shown in figure 2.6.

Some attentional foci are more helpful than others depending on their relevance to the task. For example, attending to the crowd is irrelevant when performing a free kick and can often be distracting. However, fixating on the formation of the wall has been shown to be effective for expert soccer players in free kick situations (Helsen & Pauwels, 1993).

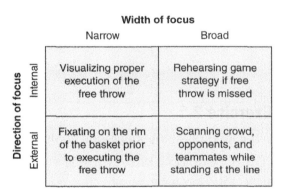

Figure 2.6   Attentional styles during a basketball free throw.

Although a player could attend to only one of the attentional foci, the attentional focus is more likely to shift throughout a performance. For example, a soccer player might first scan the field to get a complete picture of the situation, rehearse her role if the kick is recovered by the opposing team, visualize the execution of her kick, and finally fixate on the formation of the wall just before executing the kick. This shift in attentional focus is especially important when participating in many team sports. Because the environment is constantly in flux, a single attentional focus may prevent the performer from picking up on all of the relevant information available.

Attentional focus can also refer to how a person directs attention to the skill being performed. Under this view, an internal focus of attention occurs when the person attends to his body movements, whereas an external focus of attention occurs when he attends to the *effects* of his movements. For example, a basketball player performing a free throw might focus on making sure his wrist flexes when he releases the ball. This is an internal focus of attention because he is attending to the movement of his wrist. In contrast, he might focus on making sure the ball rotates backward when he releases it. This is an external focus of attention because he is attending to the *effect* of the wrist flexion (i.e., the spin of the ball) rather than the movement. Additional examples are listed in table 2.1.

A large body of evidence (see Wulf, 2013, for a review) has shown that an external focus of attention is more effective for motor learning and performance than an internal focus of attention. Wulf and colleagues (e.g., McNevin, Shea, & Wulf, 2003; Wulf, McNevin, & Shea, 2001) explained this effect using the **constrained action hypothesis**. They posited that an internal focus of attention constrains the motor system, which prevents the motor program from running off automatically; whereas an external focus of attention facilitates this automaticity. In recent years, Wulf and Lewthwaite (2010) extended this explanation with the **self-invoking trigger hypothesis**. They suggested that an internal focus of attention triggers people to engage in self-evaluation and self-regulatory processes in an attempt to gain control over their thoughts and feelings. If the addition of these processes extends the attentional capacity, automatic control of the motor program can become disrupted and lead to declines in motor performance.

WHAT DO YOU THINK?

Exercise 2.5

What kind of attentional focus shifts might occur for the following skills?

1. Driving on a busy highway
2. Pitching a baseball
3. Assessing an injured athlete
4. Mountain biking

Table 2.1 Research Examples Comparing Internal and External Attentional Focus

Task	Internal focus	External focus	Study
Ski simulator	Exert force on the outer foot.	Exert force on the outer wheels.	Wulf, Höß, & Prinz (1998)
Soccer instep kick	Remember to kick the ball with the instep.	Remember to kick the ball with the shoelaces.	Wulf, Wächter, & Wortmann (2003)
Biceps curl	Concentrate on the biceps muscles.	Concentrate on the curl bar.	Vance, Wulf, Töllner, McNevin, & Mercer (2004)
Golf pitch	Focus on the swinging motion of the arms.	Focus on the pendulum-like motion of the club.	Wulf & Su (2007)
Swimming: 16 m front crawl stroke	Arms: Pull the hands back. Legs: Push the insteps down.	Arms: Push the water back. Legs: Push the water down.	Freudheim, Wulf, Madureira, Pasetto, & Correa (2010)
Vertical jump	Concentrate on the tips of the fingers.	Concentrate on the rungs.	Wulf, Dufek, Lozano, & Pettigrew (2010)

Can Children Benefit From an External Focus?

Although the majority of research on attentional focus has looked at adult populations, recent findings also support the external focus advantage with children. For example, Perreault and French (2015) had 10- to 12-year-olds learn a modified basketball free throw over two days while receiving either internal (i.e., *Line up your hand and eye with the basket*) or external (i.e., *Focus on a spot just above the rim*) attentional focus feedback following every third practice attempt.

Following practice, participants returned approximately 24 hours later for a retention test. The results indicated that the external focus group had significantly better scores than the internal focus group had, illustrating the learning advantage associated with an external focus of attention. In addition, retrospective verbal reports from the participants following practice and retention provided support for the constrained action and self-invoking trigger hypotheses.

Arousal

Arousal is a term often used interchangeably with *anxiety*. Although related, these concepts have subtle, but distinct differences. **Arousal** is defined as "a general physiological and psychological activation, varying on a continuum from deep sleep to intense excitement"; whereas, **anxiety** is defined as "a negative emotional state in which feelings of nervousness, worry, and apprehension are associated with activation or arousal of the body" (Weinberg & Gould, 2015, p. 76). Thus, one who is anxious is also aroused; however, one who is aroused is not necessarily anxious.

The relationship between arousal and performance is often represented by the **inverted-U hypothesis** (Landers & Arent, 2010). As figure 2.7 illustrates, performance tends to increase as arousal increases, but only to a point. Once arousal surpasses the person's optimal arousal level, performance tends to drop off. The optimal arousal level largely depends on the person and the task being performed. Some people perform very well under high arousal conditions. Others, especially those with **trait anxiety** (a predisposition for anxiety in threatening situations), perform better under low arousal condi-

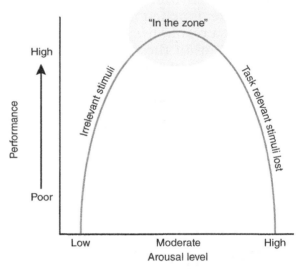

Figure 2.7 Effects of perceptual narrowing and the inverted-U hypothesis.

tions. One's arousal level at any point in time is referred to as **state anxiety**. Even people with relatively low trait anxiety may experience very high state anxiety in certain situations, such as taking exams or performing in front of an audience. The complexity of the task can also affect the optimal arousal level. Generally, tasks that are highly complex are performed more effectively under low arousal conditions (e.g., a chess game), whereas tasks that are low in complexity are performed more effectively under high arousal conditions (e.g., a bench press).

The role arousal plays in performance can be explained using the **cue-utilization hypothesis** (Easterbrook, 1959). Recall that in any performance context there are numerous stimuli in the environment, both relevant and irrelevant, that one can attend to. Under optimal arousal conditions, a person can selectively attend to the relevant stimuli while blocking out or ignoring the irrelevant. However, under low arousal conditions, attention broadens, resulting in focusing on both relevant and irrelevant stimuli. For example, a tennis player in a low arousal situation (e.g., competing against a low-skilled opponent) might start paying attention to irrelevant stimuli in the environment (e.g., fans in the stands or teammates playing on nearby courts). As a result, her attention may not be directed at all the relevant cues from her opponent, which ends up costing her a point. Conversely, under high arousal conditions, attention becomes overly narrowed, resulting in not focusing on all relevant stimuli. For example, the same tennis player in a high arousal situation (e.g., playing down a set) might miss important cues from her opponent (e.g., a poorly disguised drop shot) and not make it to the ball in time.

Sensory Contributions

Whether it's witnessing a traumatic accident (as in the example in the opening scenario of this chapter) or hearing oncoming traffic approaching, sensory information influences everything we do. We often move the way we do in response to the visual information we receive. We see a pass in the air and move to intercept it, we see a pothole and step around it, or we see something interesting and move closer for a better look. As such, it may not be surprising that vision is our predominant sensory system. In addition to the visual system, the somatosensory,

auditory, and vestibular systems provide critical information about our balance and position in space. This section provides a brief overview of these systems, focusing on their roles with balance and movement.

Exteroception

Exteroception provides information about the external environment related to the body. Vision is the predominant source of exteroceptive information, with an estimated 70 percent of sensory receptors residing in the eyes (Marieb, Wilhelm, & Mallatt, 2017).

Vision provides information about the environment with respect to the position of the head. To perceive an image visually, light enters the eye and passes to a light-sensitive membrane called the retina, forming an image. The image is then converted into nerve signals by light-sensitive cells called photoreceptors. The two types of photoreceptors are rods and cones. Rods and cones differ in their structures and functions:

Rods
- Are more numerous than cones.
- Provide peripheral vision.
- Detect movement.
- Perceive shades of gray (night vision).

Cones
- Are fewer and denser than rods.
- Enable acute vision (visual acuity).
- Operate best in bright lighting.
- Perceive color.

After the image is converted into nerve signals, the nerve signals are transmitted from the eye through the optic tract to the visual cortex of the brain. The nerve signals are actually sent to the opposite side of the brain, crossing the optic chiasm (figure 2.8). Thus, the nerve signals from the right side of the visual field go to the left side of the visual cortex, and vice versa. Finally, the brain interprets the nerve signals.

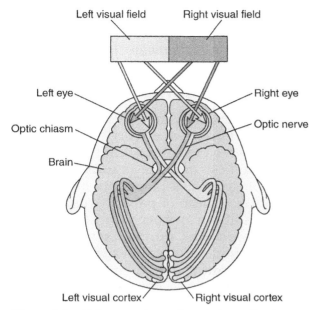

Left visual field   Right visual field

Left eye

Right eye

Optic chiasm

Optic nerve

Brain

Left visual cortex   Right visual cortex

Figure 2.8 Light enters the eye through the pupil and moves to the retina, where a visual image is formed. Photoreceptors convert the image into nerve signals, which are sent through the optic nerve and cross over the optic chiasm to the visual cortex to be interpreted.

Visual acuity refers to the sharpness of vision. Visual acuity allows us to see images such as faces and words on a page clearly. The two types of visual acuity are static and dynamic. **Static visual acuity** is the ability to clearly see a stationary image; it is most commonly assessed using the Snellen eye chart. **Dynamic visual acuity** is the ability to distinguish moving objects. Dynamic visual acuity is particularly important for athletes who must track an object or an opponent's position. Dynamic visual acuity develops at a later age than static visual acuity, reaching adult levels at around age 15 (Schrauf, Wist, & Ehrenstein, 1999). Girls tend to have worse static and dynamic visual acuity than boys have, which could affect sport performance, most notably in activities in which a moving object must be tracked. The delayed development of dynamic visual acuity may be a factor in the reduced participation of girls in some sports (Gallahue, Ozmun, & Goodway, 2012).

Another source of exteroception is hearing, or audition. Auditory information is often overlooked as an important factor in skillful movement; however, it is critical to both learning a movement pattern and performing skillfully. One of the most common methods of teaching a motor skill is verbal instruction. Think about it. Have you ever been taught a motor skill without the use of verbal cues, or at least some form of verbal instruction? Skilled performers also often use auditory signals during an activity to react quickly or as a frame of reference. For instance, a racquetball player may know the direction and speed of the ball simply from hearing the pitch of the bounce; a basketball makes different sounds depending on whether it hits the rim or the backboard or just the net (swoosh!); and a softball sounds different when it is caught in the palm of the glove rather than the pocket. Sounds can indicate the rhythm of movements as well. The rhythmic movement of a golf swing can be heard. Devices have even been made to help golfers learn the timing and rhythm of the golf swing by listening to a music file composed from the rhythm of skilled golfers.

Proprioception

Proprioception provides information about the state of the body itself, including the sense of movements and the relationship of body parts to one another. Proprioception is supported by Golgi tendon organs, muscle spindles, joint receptors, cutaneous receptors, and the vestibular apparatus. Because of proprioception, when we move, we know where our hands, limbs, and feet are with respect to one another without looking at them.

The **vestibular apparatus** found in the inner ear provides proprioceptive information by detecting head motion and the orientation of the head with respect to gravity, such as in a head tilt. The direction and rate of a spin is also provided by the semicircular canals. These three half-circle structures are oriented in three planes and filled with fluid to help us detect the direction and rotation of motion. The vestibular system not only provides information about the head, but is also a key contributor to static and dynamic balance.

Other proprioceptive structures are joint receptors, muscle spindles, Golgi tendon organs, and cutaneous receptors. **Joint receptors** are located in joint capsules and fire when the joint is in extreme positions, providing a protective function. **Muscle spindles** are embedded in muscle bellies and provide information about motion and joint positioning. Muscle spindles are most active when the muscle is stretched. Muscle information is also provided by **Golgi tendon organs**, which are located in the junction of the muscle and the tendon. The Golgi tendon organ responds to the intensity of the contraction and is most active when the muscle contracts. One proprioceptor that provides movement perception is located in the skin. The skin also contributes to proprioception via **cutaneous receptors** that signal a variety of perceptual states such as temperature, pain, and pressure. They are particularly important for our sense of touch. The highest concentration of cutaneous receptors in the body is in the fingertips, which is why we feel things much more acutely there than anywhere else on the body.

Poor proprioception has been linked to clumsiness in children (Li, Su, Fu, & Pickett, 2015) and adolescents (Visser & Geuze, 2000). Proprioception is critical to performing skillfully; it enables fluid movements by providing information about the relative positions of body parts to one another and in space, as well as the movements of the body (Haywood & Getchell, 2014). To fully develop proprioception, children must experience a wide variety of activities. In today's society, many children lack such experiences because of increased sedentary lifestyles and more urban environments. Children are spending less and less time playing outside and more time in passive activities such as watching television and playing video games. Limited active experiences can delay proprioceptive development and hinder the ability to learn more complex motor skills as children get older (Gallahue, Ozmun, & Goodway, 2012).

Memory

Memory, the ability to recall things, allows us to benefit from experience. When someone gives you a telephone number for later use, your first impulse may be to list it quickly in your cell phone directory or to write it on a piece of paper if your phone is not handy. If neither is available, you may rehearse the number several times with the hope of recalling it later; that is, you commit it to your memory. These three activities are conscious strategies you use because you realize the failings of the memory system. This section outlines some important ideas about how memory works and the role it plays in movement preparation.

Think about that phone number someone gave you. If you can dial it immediately, you do so quickly, knowing that it will remain with you for only a few more seconds before you forget it. Older models of memory distinguished between short-term and long-term memory (e.g., Atkinson & Shiffrin, 1968). In early computer terminology, these memory structures were described as the hardware of memory. Information moved from short-term to long-term memory via control processes such as rehearsal and practice. Control processes were considered the software of memory. **Short-term memory** was used when you dialed the number immediately. If you rehearse the number frequently and use it often, the number eventually finds its way into **long-term memory**, a permanent store. Long-term memory is reflected in the saying about riding a bicycle with reference to performing a task not attempted for many years. Adults actually do ride bicycles (and perform other skills) after many years of not riding. How are they able to do this? Quite simply, the movement skills of riding remain in the long-term memory store.

A more recent model of memory proposed by Baddeley (1986, 1995) has two structures: working memory and long-term memory. **Working memory** has some similarities to short-term memory, but the term *working* underscores the more active role of the control processes beyond those typically described under the term *short-term memory*. Working memory performs a number of functions, including temporarily storing recently presented material. It also retrieves information from long-term storage to solve problems, make decisions, and produce movement. Working memory is the structure in which memory control processes work to transfer information to long-term memory. We can think of working memory as a cognitive workspace (Magill & Anderson, 2013). Just before a hitter comes to the plate, the player at second base might review the batter's hitting tendencies stored in her long-term memory, couple that information with knowledge that a runner is on first base, and review her options if the ball is hit either slowly or sharply to her. Many of these cognitive activities are similar to the decision-making and attention processes previously described.

Working memory has been described in terms of both duration and capacity. Its duration is limited to 20 seconds. Adams and Dijkstra (1966) required blindfolded participants to move the handle of an apparatus on a trackway until it was physically blocked. After a retention interval, they tried to recall the movement by moving the handle back to the same point on the trackway. Results demonstrated that arm movements could be recalled very accurately if the retention interval was very short, but performance declined substantially in only 20 seconds.

It has long been argued that the capacity of working memory is seven items, plus or minus two (Miller, 1956). Thus, depending on the content and the person, capacity is between five and nine. Adults can usually remember a series of seven numbers without too much effort. Beyond that, the memory system is severely challenged. When researchers asked young gymnasts (Ille & Cadopi, 1999) and dancers (Starkes, Deakin, Lindley, & Crisp, 1987) to recall a movement sequence, the participants showed limits of six items and eight items, respectively. They were relatively experienced in the activity and could remember only a few movements in the correct order. Thus, practitioners should avoid lengthy sequential lists when teaching children.

Information that is practiced and used often finds its way into long-term memory (see figure 2.9). Long-term memory

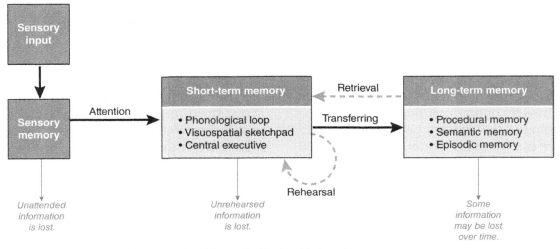

Figure 2.9 The process by which sensory input is eventually stored in long-term memory.
Adapted from Atkinson and Shiffrin 1968.

TRY THIS

Short-Term Memory Test

Exercise 2.6

Search for and take a short-term memory test on the Internet.

1. Compare your results with the answers at the conclusion of the test. How did you perform? Were you able to remember more than the average? Short-term memory is typically seven plus or minus two items. If you were able to remember more than the average, what are some strategies that you used? Explain.

2. Distinguish between short-term, long-term, and working memory.

3. What role does memory play in learning movements? How can you help students, athletes, patients, or clients remember movements?

contains past events and general knowledge. In terms of movement, knowledge includes the ability to perform physical skills such as swimming, bicycling, and skiing as well as declarative, procedural, and metacognitive knowledge (discussed in chapter 11). The capacity and duration of long-term memory are often considered unlimited, and long-term memory is relatively permanent.

Summary

Many factors are involved in understanding movement control, including reaction time, attention, arousal, sensory contributions, and memory. Speed is often a critical factor when preparing a motor response. This chapter discussed reaction time and the variables that affect it, including stimulus–response compatibility and the psychological refractory period. These factors are particularly evident in sport when a player is trying to gain an advantage over an opponent.

Attention and arousal are critical for effective decision making and motor performance. Although people have a limited attentional capacity, the capacity for performing a particular skill depends on the person's skill level. Highly skilled people require significantly less attentional capacity than novices; their skill frees up their attentional resources for dual tasks or strategies in sport contests. Attention is also selective, in that we choose what we attend to, as demonstrated in the cocktail party phenomenon.

Arousal is an important consideration for movement control because peak performance requires optimal levels of arousal. If arousal levels are too low, performers lack the focus necessary to perform well. In this case, they can be distracted by irrelevant stimuli such as sounds in the crowd. However, if arousal levels are too high, performers' attentional focus narrows and they can lose relevant information.

This chapter introduced sensory contributions to movement control including the visual, auditory, somatosensory, and vestibular systems. Each provides critical information for maintaining balance and movement control. The visual and auditory systems provide information about the environment, whereas the somatosensory and vestibular systems provide proprioceptive information. Through selective attention, sensory information is temporarily placed into short-term memory. This information is quickly lost unless it is rehearsed. If the information is rehearsed enough, it is placed into long-term memory. Information from long-term memory is retrieved by working memory to solve problems, make decisions, and produce movement. Each of these topics is further discussed in regard to motor development and aging in chapters 9 through 13.

ONLINE LEARNING

Visit the web resource at www.HumanKinetics.com/MotorLearningAndDevelopment for an accompanying lab activity and exercises from the chapter.

LEARNING AIDS

Supplemental Activities

1. Work with a partner and examine the effect of spinning on your vestibular system. Each of you should do one of the spinning activities.
    a. Person 1:
        1. Rapidly spin 20 times with eyes closed (or spin until you feel sufficiently dizzy); your partner can help, if needed.
        2. When you have finished spinning, open your eyes and turn toward your partner. Your partner throws a ball to you from approximately 20 feet (6 m) away. Catch the ball and throw it back to your partner. Continue this for about four catches and throws. Discuss your results. How accurate were your tosses? Did you catch the ball every time?
        3. An accurate toss is one in which the person can catch it without stepping or reaching. How accurate were the tosses and catches over time?
    b. Person 2:
        1. Rapidly spin 20 times with eyes closed (or spin until you feel sufficiently dizzy); your partner can help, if needed.
        2. When you have finished spinning, keep your eyes closed while your partner calls your name from approximately 10 feet (3 m) away. Try to walk as straight as possible toward your partner, who is calling your name. Describe the experience. Were you able to complete this task well—that is, did you walk in a straight line? Did you stumble?
        3. What is the main role of the vestibular system? Explain why you feel dizzy after spinning in relationship to the three sensory systems involved in balance: the visual, somatosensory, and vestibular systems.
2. Search YouTube for a video on selective attention tests (such as the original gorilla experiment). These videos illustrate that we can be blind to visual information when selectively attending to something else even if it is in the center of our visual field. Following these original experiments, this phenomenon has been demonstrated over and over again in many contexts. Work with a small group of students in your class to design your own selective attention video.

Glossary

anxiety—An emotional response to a perceived threat; can involve cognitive concerns or physiological reactions.

arousal—A general state of activation or excitability.

broad width of focus—Attending to the larger context, such as the scanning the field.

central limited capacity—A theory suggesting that human attention is limited because the central nervous system does not have endless space in which to process information.

central-resource capacity theory—Perspective on attention that is a more flexible system than the single-channel filter theories, in which information-processing capacity can expand based on the individual, task, and situation.

choice reaction time (CRT)—Time needed to react when there is more than one stimulus.

constrained action hypothesis—Perspective on attentional focus that posited that an internal focus of attention constrains the motor system, which prevents the motor program from running off automatically, whereas an external focus of attention facilitates this automaticity.

cue-utilization hypothesis—The hypothesis that the level of arousal influences attentional focus.

cutaneous receptors—Located in the skin; provide proprioceptive information in regard to temperature, pain, and pressure.

dynamic visual acuity—The ability to distinguish moving objects.

event anticipation—Anticipating what the stimulus will be (e.g., anticipating what pitch the pitcher will pitch).

external direction of focus—Attentional focus that is directed in the environment, such as focusing on the putt.

Golgi tendon organs—Located at the junction of the muscle and the tendon; respond to the intensity of the muscular contraction, providing proprioceptive information.

Hick's Law—A logarithmic relationship between the number of stimulus–response alternatives and reaction time, indicating that as the number of S-R alternatives increases, RT increases at a constant rate.

interference—A limitation on performance as a result of exceeding one's attentional capacity.

internal direction of focus—Attentional focus that is directed within the person, such as visualizing the movement.

inverted-U hypothesis—The idea that arousal and performance are related such that optimal performance is seen at a moderate level of arousal.

joint receptors—Located in the joint capsules; provide proprioceptive information in regard to joint position and fire when the joint is in extreme positions to serve as a protective function.

long-term memory—Information that is retained in memory relatively permanently.

memory—The ability to recall things; allows us to benefit from experience.

movement time—The observable movement; that is, the time from the initiation of the movement until it has been completed.

multiple-resource theories—Perspectives of attention that suggest that humans have several attention mechanisms (e.g., modalities, stages of information processing, codes of processing information), each with a limited capacity.

muscle spindles—Located within the muscle belly; provide proprioceptive information about motion and joint positioning and are most active when the muscle is stretched.

narrow width of focus—Attending to specific cues in the environment, such as focusing on a specific player.

proprioception—Provides sensory information about the state of the body itself, including the sense of movements and the relationship of body parts to one another.

psychological refractory period (PRP)—Time delay which occurs when two stimuli occur in quick succession and they require different responses; processing a response to the first stimulus delays the response to the second stimulus.

reaction time (RT)—The measure of the time between the presentation of a stimulus and the initiation of a motor response.

response time—The measure of the time between the presentation of a stimulus and the completion of the movement response (reaction time plus movement time).

selective attention—The ability to focus on selected sensory information while ignoring irrelevant information.

self-invoking trigger hypothesis—A perspective on attentional focus that suggested an internal focus of attention triggers people to engage in self-evaluation and self-regulatory processes in an attempt to gain control over thoughts and feelings.

short-term memory—Information that is only stored in memory for a relatively short period of time (typically 20-30 seconds).

simple reaction time (simple RT)—The time needed to react to a task with only one stimulus.

single-channel filter theories—Attention perspectives that propose a serial processing of tasks and the occurrence of a bottleneck at some point in information processing, a point at which the system can process only one task at a time.

state anxiety—Arousal level at a single point in time.

static visual acuity—The ability to clearly see a stationary image; commonly assessed using the Snellen eye chart.

stimulus–response (S-R) compatibility—The amount of association between a stimulus and response, which can also affect RT.

temporal anticipation—Anticipating when the stimulus will occur (e.g., when the pitcher will throw the pitch).

trait anxiety—Predisposition for anxiety in threatening situations.

vestibular apparatus—Located in the inner ear; provides proprioceptive information by detecting head motion and orientation of the head with respect to gravity (such as head tilt).

visual acuity—Sharpness of vision.

working memory—Performs an active role, including temporarily storing recently presented material, retrieving information from long-term memory storage to solve problems, making decisions, and producing movement.

THEORETICAL CONSTRUCTS IN MOTOR BEHAVIOR

3

Chapter Objectives

After reading this chapter, you should be able to do the following:

- Defend the theoretical constructs in motor behavior.
- Develop invariant features and parameters in generalized motor programs.
- Explain open-loop and closed-loop control.
- Differentiate information-processing theory and the ecological approach to perception.
- Construct the constraints model, such as how movement patterns are constrained by boundaries that limit movement possibilities.

Transitions

It is nothing short of remarkable witnessing a child's firsts—first smile, first time sitting up alone, first step, to mention only a few. They can certainly make us wonder what underlies these changes. Transitions are not limited to infancy and childhood, but continue across the life span. Maybe you recently learned how to juggle and struggled through many failed attempts before you could make several catches, then a few more; finally, you were able to juggle.

Transitions also occur following an injury such as a ligament tear. More and more baseball pitchers are undergoing surgery to repair the ulnar collateral ligament (UCL), which is commonly referred to as Tommy John surgery. Although this surgery is popular, the recovery is long and there are certainly no guarantees of returning to a preinjury level of play. Also, many variables can affect the recovery outcome. In the case of injury, rehabilitation drives movement pattern changes; whereas in the case of learning new movements, development, practice, or training induces change.

To explain what drives the many remarkable changes that occur throughout our life spans, three theoretical constructs were developed during the early part of the process-oriented period in the history of motor development theory, as discussed in chapter 1. These theoretical constructs—the information-processing theory, ecological approach, and dynamic systems approach—still drive research today. These theories differ in the way they define development and learning as well as in how they examine behavior. According to the **information-processing theory**, the brain receives, processes, and interprets information in order to send signals to produce skilled coordinated movements, similarly to how a computer functions. Proponents of the **ecological approach**, however, state that movement is much more complex than a simple input–output relay of information from the brain to the other systems. Instead, actions are determined by many internal factors (e.g., goals and capabilities) and external factors (e.g., what is available in the environment). The third theoretical perspective, the **dynamic systems approach**, has been viewed as an offshoot of ecological psychology. In this perspective, movement does not occur as a result of a set of instructions but rather as the result of the interplay of the task, the environment, and the individual. Movement is "softly" assembled, meaning that it emerges as a result of these three factors.

Information-Processing Theory

The basis of the information-processing theory is the idea that the brain acts like a computer, working as a receiver and processor of information (Fitts & Posner, 1967; Keele, 1973; Marteniuk, 1976; Schmidt, 1975a). A key area of this research addressed the processes involved in movement behavior. Although the process of development was a key area of interest in earlier research, there was a shift from investigating ontogenetic (life span) changes to processes of change within a life span such as memory, feedback, attention, and perception (Clark & Whitall, 1989).

A **generalized motor program (GMP)** is a representation of a pattern of movements that are modifiable to produce a movement outcome. A GMP can be thought of as a set of instructions stored in the brain. When we perform a particular skill, we retrieve this set of instructions, sending the message to the appropriate muscles. The time needed to organize a motor program depends on the complexity of the task; more complex tasks require more time to organize than less complex tasks do. Henry and Rogers (1960) illustrated this by measuring reaction time for three tasks varying in complexity. They found that reaction time (the time from the onset of a stimulus to the initiation of the response) increased with increasing complexity. When participants had to simply lift a finger from a switch, reaction time was only 165 milliseconds; but it went up to 199 milliseconds when the task increased in complexity to lifting the finger from the switch and then grasping a hanging tennis ball. It increased to 212 milliseconds for lifting the finger, striking the ball, pushing a button, and grasping another ball. These results indicate that movements are planned prior to initiating a response, because more time is required to prepare motor programs for more complex tasks.

To be classified into a particular GMP, an action must include **invariant features**—that is, features that cannot be modified between attempts. Invariant features are unique to their GMP much as the features of a person's signature are unique. If you were asked to write your name under varying conditions (e.g., with your dominant hand, with your nondominant hand, in large print or small print, or even with your feet), the general stroke and structure of your signature would be the same. Of course, the writing may be a bit sloppier with your feet, but it will still have the same general features as your signature with your dominant hand. The difference in the signatures is the effect of experience and reduced coordination and control in the nondominant limb, not the structure of the letters. A classic example that illustrates the effects of invariant features is shown in figure 3.1.

The three invariant features are the sequence of actions, relative timing, and relative force. If the sequence of a gymnastics routine were changed, it would no longer be the same routine. Additionally, if proportionally more time were spent on any one of these actions than on others (relative timing), the overall movement pattern would be compromised. A person can walk at many speeds; however, the relative timing will remain the same unless the person transitions to running. The same is true for relative force. To kick a ball harder, an athlete must proportionately increase the amount of force produced when planting the nondominant foot,

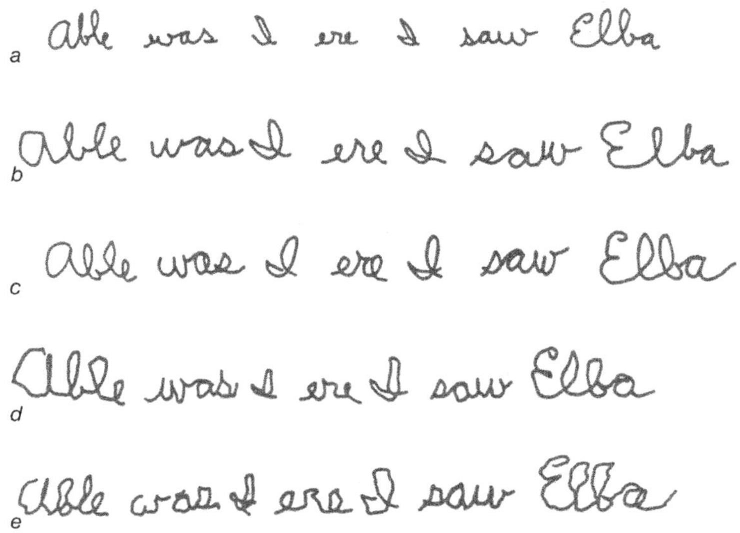

Figure 3.1 Invariant features affected this person's ability to write *(a)* with the right (dominant) hand, *(b)* with the wrist immobilized, *(c)* with the left hand, *(d)* with the pen gripped in the teeth, and *(e)* with the pen taped to the foot.

Reprinted, by permission, from M.H. Raibert, 1977, "Motor control and learning by the state space model," *Technical Report AI-TR-439* (Cambridge, MA: MIT Artificial Intelligence Laboratory), 50.

RESEARCH NOTES

Monkey Business

Polit and Bizzi (1978) investigated the notion of the GMP by deafferenting monkeys. Deafferentation is a technique whereby the sensory receptors are severed so that no proprioceptive feedback can be received. In other words, there is no longer any feeling in the deafferented limb. Polit and Bizzi trained several monkeys to perform pointing tasks. The monkeys were later deafferented, and their vision was blocked so that they could not see or feel where their deafferented limb was located. Following deafferentation, the monkeys were still able to accurately point to the target, without sensory feedback. These findings provide support for the notion of motor programs and the information-processing theory.

swinging the dominant foot back, swinging the dominant foot forward, and contacting the ball. Altering the relative timing or relative force will compromise the rhythm of the movement pattern.

The features that can be modified during the execution of a movement pattern are called **parameters**. Modifying parameters allows us to adapt our responses (e.g., walk at different speeds, shoot a basketball from different positions on the court, kick with more or less force). The three parameters are muscle selection, overall duration, and overall force. In the signature example in figure 3.1, similar features were found for writing with the dominant and with the nondominant hand. Writing with a different hand is a parameter change, not an invariant feature change, because of the use of different muscle groups. A quarterback in American football can throw a short pass to a running back or throw much farther for a Hail Mary pass to a wide receiver. The GMP used is the same whether you are unscrewing a very tight lid or a loose one, or whether you are kicking a penalty kick from the right or the left side of the goal.

As a reminder, GMPs are defined by their invariant features (nonflexible features) and parameters (flexible features). It is important to recognize the differences between invariant features and parameters; here is a quick recap of each:

Invariant Features

- Sequence of actions: An American football punt sequence is catch, approach, drop, kick.
- Relative timing: When you swing to hit a volleyball during a serve must be relative to the timing of your toss.
- Relative force: The force of your foot making contact with a ball during a kick should be relative to the force with which you approached the ball and the movement of your leg.

Parameters

- Muscle selection: The GMP is the same for throwing with your left hand as it is for throwing with your right hand.

- Overall duration: The GMP is the same for running slowly as it is for running faster.
- Overall force: The GMP is the same for batting with more overall force as it is for batting with less overall force.

Using parameters appropriate to the situation is particularly essential for open skills. Basketball players must vary each shot depending on their position relative to the basket, and shortstops in baseball must vary their throws to reach different bases. By practicing under varying conditions, learners develop rules or relationships that help them make appropriate movement responses. These are called **schemas**. Schemas develop over time through accumulated experiences within a generalized motor program. The more someone practices a GMP, the more developed the schema becomes, enabling the person to react more quickly and perform more accurately.

Modes of Control

Prior to executing a movement, the person must retrieve the appropriate GMP and choose the appropriate parameters for the situation. These decisions occur at a subconscious level and do not explain how the movement is controlled. There are many options for adapting any movement pattern, and as such, there is a wide variety of ways to control skill production. In a broad sense, two control systems underlie movements: closed-loop control and open-loop control.

Closed-Loop Control

Closed-loop control is used for relatively long-duration, continuous activities during which the person can make corrections based on feedback received while moving. In closed-loop control, the information used to make corrections travels through the stages of information processing. First, the information is processed and a motor program is initiated. Sensory information regarding the movement (i.e.,

When Is a Throw Not a Throw?

Exercise 3.1

Early motor program theories postulated that every task required a separate motor program. A new program was required to catch a tennis ball versus a softball, or to throw a ball 10 feet (3 m) rather than 15 feet (4.5 m). If a new program was required for every variation of a movement, an immense amount of space in memory would be needed for all the information. A theory of generalized motor programs was developed to address this issue. As long as a new coordination pattern was not required to perform a motor skill, it could be controlled by the same generalized motor program. To test this, try the following variations of throwing a small ball at a target. For *a* through *d*, the goal is to throw for accuracy; for *e*, the goal is to throw as hard as you can.

  a. Find a target that is only 5 feet (1.5 m) away and throw at it a few times.
  b. Take several big steps back so that you are 15 feet (4.5 m) from the target; then aim and throw at the target.
  c. From the same spot, aim and throw the ball more slowly.
  d. Using the same target and position, throw with your nondominant hand.
  e. Now take several big steps back until you are 30 feet (9 m) or more from the target, and throw as hard as you can at the target.

Answer the following questions based on your experience:

  1. Which of the throws were controlled by the same generalized motor program? If one or more was not, describe how you know that it was controlled by a different GMP.
  2. Which examples varied parameters? Describe how.

Answer these questions on a motor skill of your choice:

  3. Provide two examples of invariant features for a movement skill of your choice. Discuss why these features would place this movement into a different GMP.
  4. Now provide two examples of how you could vary this skill without compromising the movement pattern (parameters).
  5. If an adaptation in a motor skill has caused a change in the invariant features, should the learner practice under these conditions? Why or why not?

response-produced feedback) is compared to the desired movement, and corrections to the movement pattern can be made if necessary. For example, when you are walking to class, you have a plan for the route you are going to take, but you cannot plan exactly for the disturbances you may encounter, such as potholes, people walking toward you, and cars coming when you approach a crosswalk. When you encounter these things, you make adjustments, such as changing direction, slowing down, or even stopping. These changes occur throughout the execution of the movement of walking to class.

A thermostat is a good example of a closed-loop system. A thermostat regulates the room temperature based on the set temperature. It continuously monitors the temperature and makes a change only when the actual temperature doesn't match the set temperature. If the temperature is set to 68 degrees Fahrenheit (20 degrees Celsius), and the room temperature is detected to be 67 degrees, the heater will turn on. Once the heat reaches the desired temperature of 68 degrees, the heater turns off.

Open-Loop Control

Closed-loop control can only be used for slower actions that last long enough for feedback to be used during the movement. For movements that are more rapid and discrete, the control made is called **open-loop control**. To use open-loop control, the performer needs to preplan the movement by choosing a generalized motor program and then execute the action. A good example is composing a text message. You choose the person you are going to text, write your message, and send it. Once you click Send, you cannot go back and change the text. We've all sent that text to the wrong person, and there's simply no turning back. Perhaps there was an error in the text because you typed incorrectly or autocorrect changed what you wrote. If you want to make a change to your text, your only option is to send a follow-up text with the correct information. This action is not considered closed-loop because sending the subsequent text cannot eliminate and correct the original text. Open-loop control of movements is very common. Examples

include pressing an elevator button, heading a ball in soccer, flipping a light switch, and catching a line drive in baseball. Refer to figure 3.2, *a* and *b*, for a comparison of closed- and open-loop control.

In some cases, a modification of a rapid action can be made by making a quick adjustment following the initial movement. You may have started to shut a door and midway through realized that you didn't have your keys. If you made the adjustment quickly enough, you may have been able to prevent the door from shutting and locking you out. A good sporting example is the checked swing in baseball. The swing can be prevented if a second decision to not swing is made early enough. However, if the decision is made too late, the batter may not have enough time to check the swing. Nonetheless, the batter is aware that he should not have swung even as he is swinging, thus receiving response-produced feedback during the movement. This awareness, or feeling of incorrectness, is possible in many movements controlled by open-loop processes, such as knowing you made a poor basketball shot well before the ball reaches the basket.

Most activities incorporate both modes of control, such as the preceding texting example. Composing the text is controlled by closed-loop processes because you can make changes; however, pressing Send is

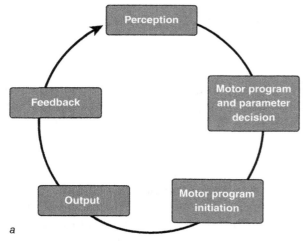

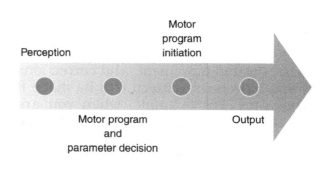

a

b

Figure 3.2 Systems of control can be *(a)* closed or *(b)* open.

Table 3.1   Comparison of Open- and Closed-Loop Systems of Control

Characteristics	Open-loop control	Closed-loop control
Speed of movement	Rapid	Slower
Accuracy of response	Less accurate	Very accurate
Feedback	Adjustments can't be made	Adjustments can be made

controlled by open-loop processes. When assessing how a movement is controlled, think about how long it takes to produce the movement. If there is time to make adjustments, then the movement is controlled by closed-loop processing. If the movement is very rapid and has a point of no return (i.e., there is no option to alter the movement while it is happening), then it is controlled by an open-loop process. For a comparison of open- and closed-loop control, see table 3.1.

Speed–Accuracy Trade-Off

Speed and accuracy are important in many motor skills, particularly those that have a temporal and spatial component such as in racket sports and fielding games. Although both accuracy and speed may be important in these motor skills, when a person focuses on one, the other is compromised—hence, the term **speed–accuracy trade-off**. For example, batters must be able to produce a quick and forceful swing that is also accurate. Given that pitchers can throw balls over 90 miles per hour (145 km/h) and batters are only 18 yards away, batters not only have minimal time to react but also must accurately position their bats to make contact with the ball.

Woodworth (1899) conducted some of the first research in motor behavior that focused on the relationship between speed and accuracy when drawing lines from one target to another. He found that accuracy diminished when speed or distance between targets increased. Fitts (1954) extended this research and discovered that speed decreased when either the distance between the targets was increased or the size of the targets was decreased when focusing on accuracy (see figure 3.3). Interestingly, this relationship exists only for spatial accuracy. In regard to temporal accuracy, such as the speed of a swing, accuracy improves with increased speed. Estimates of time are more accurate with less time than with more time. You could try this by estimating time with a stopwatch. Compare your estimates of shorter periods of time (e.g., one or five seconds) to longer periods of time (e.g., one minute). Were you more accurate estimating shorter periods of time or longer periods of time?

The effect of spatial and temporal accuracy instructions were examined in a speed–accuracy trade-off study in children (Rival, Olivier, & Ceyte, 2003). Children aged 6 to 10 years and adults completed three experimental conditions with different verbal instructions. The task was to

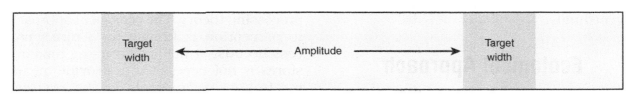

Figure 3.3   Fitt's tapping task in which participants tapped between the two target plates of varying widths separated by varying amplitudes using a stylus.

Haste Makes Waste

Exercise 3.2

1. On a piece of paper, draw five sets of two circles separated by approximately 5 inches (13 cm) for the first four sets and approximately 10 inches (25 cm) for the last set. The circles for the fourth set should be smaller in diameter. The circles are your targets. The task is to draw lines from one target to the other and continue moving back and forth under varying conditions, changing either the goal or the targets.

   a. Condition 1: Start with your pen in one circle in the first set of circles. Your goal is to move your pen back and forth from one circle to the other circle in the same set as *quickly* as possible. Do this at least 10 times.

   b. Condition 2: Starting with your pen in one circle in the second set of circles, move your pen back and forth from one circle to the other circle in the same set and back as *accurately* as possible 10 times. Your goal is to never go beyond the circles each time you go back and forth.

   c. Condition 3: Starting with your pen in one circle in the third set of circles, move your pen from one circle to the next circle and back as *quickly* and *accurately* as possible 10 times.

   d. Condition 4: Starting with your pen in one circle in the fourth set of cirlces, move your pen as *quickly and accurately* as possible back and forth from one to the other a total of 10 times.

   e. Condition 5: Starting with your pen in one circle in the fifth set of circles, move your pen back and forth as *quickly* and *accurately* as possible 10 times.

2. Discuss how your speed and accuracy changed in the varying conditions.

point to a lit target and (1) move as quickly as possible, (2) move as accurately as possible, or (3) move as accurately *and* quickly as possible. Reaction time was slower when participants were instructed to focus on accuracy or instructed to focus on both speed and accuracy. These results revealed that not only was the speed–accuracy trade-off present for all age groups, but all age groups were able to comply with the instructions and adapt their movements accordingly.

Ecological Approach

Perception, the act of attaching meaning to something, is essential and intricately linked to movement. Essentially, per-

ception enables us to interact with the environment in a meaningful way. For instance, we perceive the sizes of objects and determine how to adjust our grip to manipulate them. We perceive through our senses (vision, hearing, and kinesthesis), but perception is also affected by our personal experiences and understanding.

The relationship of perception and action is viewed very differently between the ecological approach and the information-processing theory. The ecological approach to perception is known as a *direct process* because it holds that using memory stores is not necessary to provide meaning to objects or events in the environment (Gibson, 1966). In contrast, the information-processing theory holds that action occurs as an *indirect process* of perception; that is, to act on the environment, a person must go through a series of steps. For instance, if a person comes across a steaming hot cup of coffee, he must first perceive the cup of coffee by locating memory stores of a cup of coffee. He then decides whether he wants to drink the coffee. If he is interested in drinking it, a message is sent from the brain to the limbs to reach for the cup of coffee. An example of this can be seen in figure 3.4.

Ecological psychologists explain that we do not go through a long series of processes to complete a task such as drinking a cup of coffee (see figure 3.4). Rather, we act on the environment in the manner afforded by the object. We cannot move without perceiving, just as we cannot perceive without acting. For example, a hiker walking through the woods who sees a fallen log does not see the log, perceive what it is, decide how to act on it, and then act on it. Instead, the log "affords" the hiker a place to sit. The perception and action are the same. **Affordances** are the action possibilities of the environment and task in relation to the perceiver's capabilities (Gibson, 1977, 1979). Perceiving and acting is guided by body-scaled ratios. For example, a person's leg length affects how that person climbs a set of stairs. Toddlers have much shorter legs and must compensate for a reduced ratio between leg length and the action space of the step height (Warren, 1984). Because children are tuned in to this body-scaled ratio, they do not have to learn new movement patterns as they growth and mature. Depending on individual differences and goals, action possibilities for a particular object can vary quite widely. A chair will most often afford a place to sit; however, a person who needs to reach for a high object may use a chair as a stool. A stool may afford small children a seat because of their shorter height and leg length; however, an adult might not be able to sit comfortably on a stool.

Ecological psychology rejects the idea that there is a need to search for memory stores for object representations. Instead, the acts of perceiving and moving occur simultaneously (Michaels & Carello, 1981). Objects are used to suit particular goals or needs (direct perception), not because there is a prior memory of using that object (indirect perception). This effect was illustrated in a locomotor task with toddlers and crawling infants ascending and descending a sloping walkway (Adolph, Eppler, & Gibson, 1993). Both groups overestimated their ability to ascend the slopes, but only the toddlers altered their movement patterns during the steeper descents. The toddlers often switched to a sliding movement, whereas the infants continued to crawl headfirst down the steep descents, often resulting in a fall. The infants hesitated only prior to the steeper descents, but did not attempt an alternate means of negotiating the slope.

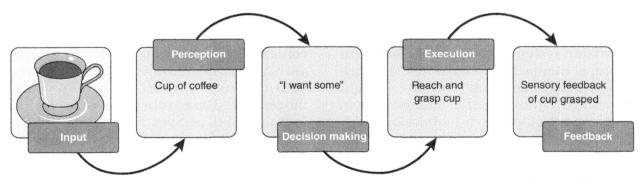

Figure 3.4 Example of an indirect process of action and perception as viewed by the information-processing theory. The person must perceive first, and then act on the environment.

Exercise 3.3

Affordances relate to action possibilities for a person and a particular environment. Movement patterns are specified by body-scaled ratios between the piece of equipment or elements in the environment and the size of the person. The following examples address how a person's size affects the person's movement pattern.

1. If an adult were teaching a six-year-old the basics of tennis, how do you expect their grips (both the adult's and the child's) to be affected if both use the same size racket? Discuss in terms of affordances.

2. How would you expect two-, four-, and eight-year-olds to catch a beach ball? A soccer ball? A Koosh ball?

3. Why is body scaling particularly important in physical therapy? Provide a couple of examples.

The toddlers, on the other hand, hesitated on the lower slopes and then switched to the more stable sliding method for the steeper slopes. These findings indicate that the perception of affordances (the degree to which a surface is walkable) is influenced by locomotor skills. Children learn how to perceive locomotion affordances through movement exploration.

Dynamic Systems Approach

During the early 1980s, Kugler, Kelso, and Turvey (1982) introduced the dynamic systems approach. They emphasized that movements are controlled by more than just the central nervous system; they are also controlled by interactions within various body systems as well as with the environment. For example, children's ability to jump high is affected by the muscular system (they need the strength to propel themselves into the air), the skeletal system (taller children have a height advantage in jumping), the adipose system (children with more body fat have more difficulty jumping high), and the neurological system (to coordinate the body to jump). In addition, the experience children have with jumping certainly influences their

capability to jump. Psychological factors such as motivation also affect how high children jump. They may jump significantly higher when a task is involved such as rebounding a basketball, or when given an incentive. Many factors are involved in how we move, which can cause us to move differently from one day to the next as a result of changes in the environment (physical or sociocultural), the task (goal, equipment, rules), or personal factors (motivation, attention, interest, fatigue).

The information-processing theory asserts that functioning occurs in a hierarchical manner; that is, all signals go to the brain and the brain issues commands to be sent to the muscles. However, the information-processing theory does not account for the continuous interaction of the person with the environment. Proponents of the dynamic systems approach contend that coordinated behavior occurs as a result of many variables that are continuously interacting to constrain movement. Researchers who favor the maturational perspective suggest that a predetermined plan specifies the sequence of movement behaviors. They suggest that movement is hardwired and preset, whereas the dynamic systems theorists suggest that movement emerges as a function of the person, the task, and the environment.

The dynamic systems approach characterizes movement as a self-organizing process. **Self-organization** is the system's ability to change states or acquire a new structure or pattern by itself. This perspective defines movement and coordination as a complex and evolving process. The system is constantly looking for stable states, or **attractors**. When the system is perturbed enough (e.g., if movement speed has increased or the person has been injured), the system will be disrupted and pushed into a new attractor, or stable, state (Thelen & Ulrich, 1991). An example of disruption as a result of injury is a racquetball player who suddenly cannot grip the racket tightly because of a strained ring finger. Interestingly, this looser grip results in a more mechanically efficient swing that can lead to the player swinging with more accuracy and velocity. Once the injured finger heals, the player, realizing the benefits, may stay with the new (and improved) grip. The finger injury perturbed her physical status (the system), pushing her to a new way of hitting the ball (a new attractor state).

Basic developmental phases such as sitting, crawling (belly on the ground), and creeping (belly off of the ground) can also be viewed as attractor states. During development, new attractors emerge as infants mature and increase strength and coordination, causing former attractor states to disappear. When infants are first learning to walk, they often switch back to their more comfortable state of creeping. However, after they have been walking for several months, they leave the attractor state of crawling and usually do not crawl except on rare occasions to negotiate the environment.

The stability of attractors has been compared to the depth of a basin or well; the deeper the well is, the more stable the behavior is (Ennis, 1992). Very stable patterns (deep wells) are quite difficult to change, such as a movement skill or pattern that is well learned; whereas shallow wells are volatile and very susceptible to switching into a new attractor state. A swimmer who has learned an unorthodox way of performing the butterfly stroke may have a difficult time using the correct technique introduced by a new instructor. The swimmer most likely will go through a period of slower sprint times and uncomfortable movement patterns before a phase shift pushes her movement pattern into a new attractor state. Physical therapists strongly encourage patients to walk without a limp so that they do not develop a stable pattern of limping once they have recovered from injury.

A **phase shift** is the change in a state that causes a shift or reorganization to a new attractor state, whereas **control parameters** are the variables that induce a shift to a new attractor state. Movement

WHAT DO YOU THINK?

Exercise 3.4

What would cause a change in self-organization in each of the following comparisons?

1. Compare hiking in the woods—encountering branches, fallen logs, and so on—to hiking in deep snow.
2. Compare dancing in a crowded club to dancing on an open floor.
3. Compare bench pressing at 60 percent of your max to bench pressing at 95 percent of your max.

speed, injury, weight, force, and sensory information can all act as control parameters. In the example of the racquetball player, the finger injury was the control parameter that caused a phase shift to a new grip. Increasing the speed on a treadmill can be a control parameter that causes a phase shift from walking to running. Control parameters can also limit or hinder performance. When this occurs, the control parameter is referred to as a **rate limiter**. Fear is a common rate limiter, because it often causes people to alter their movement patterns. A toddler who is afraid of being hurt by a thrown ball will likely close his eyes and protect his face rather than place his hands out in preparation to catch the ball. A bowling ball or a bat that is too heavy could also act as a rate limiter. Physical and occupational therapists work with patients to resolve some of the changes resulting from rate limiters. For example, a physical therapist may work with a stroke patient who must relearn how to walk or even pick up objects with the affected limb. Injuries and arthritis are other examples of rate limiters that physical or occupational therapists often encounter. Bench pressing with a comfortable weight is an example of a strong attractor. As the amount of weight is increased (control parameter), the person's form will become progressively less stable until at some point the person will change form to be able to continue to lift. The amount of increased weight that causes this change to poor form is an example of a rate limiter. The change from good form to bad form is an example of a phase shift. Following are brief descriptions and practical examples of these terms:

Attractor—A stable state, such as bench pressing with good form

Control parameter—The cause of a change, such as increasing the amount of weight used in a bench press

Rate limiter—The cause of a negative change, such as increasing the weight

used in a bench press beyond the capability of the lifter

Phase shift—A change that causes a shift to a new attractor, such as too much weight used in a bench press, which leads to a change in the lifter's form

Kugler. Kelso, and Turvey (1982) proposed that coordination is developed by changing constraints imposed by the interaction of the person with the environment, which they called the **constraints model**. Newell (1986) asserted that movement is constrained by boundaries that limit movement possibilities. These boundaries are termed **constraints**. People choose movement patterns based on the interaction of themselves, the task, and the environmental constraints (see figure 3.5).

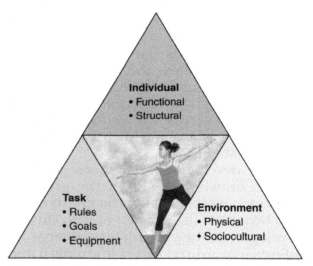

Figure 3.5 Model of the three constraints: individual, task, and environment.

Individual Constraints

Individual constraints are divided into two categories, structural and functional. **Structural constraints** include physical characteristics such as gender, height, weight, and body makeup. One would expect a 6-foot 5-inch (196 cm) man to perform very differently on a basketball court than a 4-foot 7-inch (140 cm) female. We would also expect the tall male and

Exercise 3.5

Because the goal of any motor skill program is to promote increased proficiency in motor skill performance, practitioners must understand what may limit the progression of a skill. For the following examples, list the potential rate limiters that are preventing or delaying progression in the motor skill.

1. An older adult can walk and climb stairs normally, but when descending must go down backward. What rate limiter is preventing him from moving forward when stepping downstairs?

2. An infant cannot hold her body upright to stand without supporting herself with a solid stationary object. What is preventing her from standing without support?

3. A four-year-old can hit a ball from a tee but cannot make contact with the ball when it is pitched to him. What rate limiters are preventing him from hitting the ball?

the petite female to move differently on the dance floor or even when walking down the street. **Functional constraints** include psychological and cognitive variables, such as motivation, arousal, and intellect. A dancer may perform a dance routine with more small errors when under much stress, ill, or fatigued, even though the structural constraints have not changed.

Task Constraints

Task constraints include the goals of the movement, rules, and equipment (Newell, 1986). All movement tasks are constrained by the goal of the movement. The goal of basketball is to outscore the opponent by shooting basketballs through a regulation-sized hoop while the other team is attempting to steal the ball. Because of this goal, athletes practice the motor skill of jump shooting. The rules of basketball also govern the body movements. Basketball players are allowed to take only one step after they have stopped dribbling. This rule adds to the complexity of the sport, preventing athletes from simply running up and down the court and requiring them to outsmart their opponents while dribbling. Finally, implements constrain movement possibilities. If the ball used in basketball were changed from a regulation size of 30

inches to 12 inches (76 to 30 cm), athletes would certainly have to alter their shots to accommodate this new task constraint.

Environmental Constraints

Environmental constraints are constraints that are external to the mover. These can be either physical or sociocultural. **Physical environmental constraints** include external conditions such as weather, temperature, lighting, floor surface, and step height. Tennis players play differently on grass courts than they do on clay or concrete courts. American football players change to shorter passes during rainy games because of the increased difficulty of grasping the wet ball. Physical environmental constraints do not affect only athletes; they affect us all every day. We walk differently on icy ground than on the beach. A high curb may be very difficult for someone in a wheelchair or on crutches to overcome. Even a young, able-bodied person may misjudge the curb and trip. **Sociocultural environmental constraints** are imposed by social and cultural norms and pressures. For instance, young women in some Eastern cultures may be less likely to participate regularly in sport than young women in the United States because

Constraints

Exercise 3.6

Individual Constraints

Place one hand over and behind your head and the other hand behind your back. Now attempt to grasp your fingers.

1. Were you able to accomplish this task? If not, what prevented you from grasping your fingers?
2. Would this be considered a structural or a functional constraint?

Task Constraints

Crumple up piece of paper into a ball and throw it into a basket (wastebasket if need be). Now throw a racquetball into the same basket from the same distance. Place the basket on top of a table or a shelf. Throw each ball into the basket again.

1. Did you use the same movement pattern for each ball? Describe your movement pattern(s).
2. Did you use the same movement pattern for each basket height? Describe your movement pattern(s).

Label the three types of task constraints. Provide an example of how you could vary one of these types of task constraints for a therapy related exercise or a physical education class activity.

Environmental Constraints

Shoot your paper ball and the racquetball into the basket again, this time with a fan blowing across the basket.

1. Did the added influence of wind influence the accuracy of your shot?
2. Did it affect both the paper ball and the racquetball?
3. Did you alter your movement pattern to overcome the increased airflow produced by the fan?

For further practice on the constraints, categorize each of the following as an individual, environmental, or task constraint.

a. Having the flu
b. Running into the wind
c. Brushing your teeth with an electric toothbrush rather than a regular toothbrush
d. Having stiff joints as a result of aging
e. Shooting hoops with the goals changed (e.g., playing P-I-G instead of a conventional game of basketball)
f. Hiking through rough terrain

Categorize each of the following as either a structural or functional constraint.

a. Lacking motivation
b. Having a broken leg
c. Being 5-foot 10-inches (178 cm) tall at the age of 12 years
d. Having poor flexibility
e. Being mentally fatigued

women with athletic builds are considered less attractive than thin women in those cultures. In the United States, women's participation in sport is rivaling that of men. This was not always the case, however. It was not until the passage of Title IX in 1972 that the gender gap in sport participation began to close. Prior to this educational amendment, women had far fewer opportunities for sport participation.

Summary

This chapter discussed the three main theoretical constructs that drive research in motor behavior: the information-processing theory, ecological approach, and dynamic systems approach. These perspectives differ not only in the way they define development and learning, but also in how they examine behavior. Some perspectives focus on particular age groups (e.g., maturational; see chapter 1), whereas others compare age differences (information processing) or examine how movement transitions emerge (dynamic systems and ecological approaches).

In the information-processing theory, movement patterns are defined as generalized motor programs (GMPs) that include variables that cannot be modified (invariant features) and variables that can be modified (parameters). It is important for learners to vary the parameters in practice to enhance their schema as well as increase their adaptability. However, they should not practice the movement pattern if there is a change in an invariant feature, because doing so will encourage incorrect form. Because of the many options for adapting any movement pattern, skill production is controlled in a wide variety of ways. In a broad sense, two control systems underlie movements: closed-loop control and open-loop control.

According to the ecological approach, perception and action are the same. We perceive objects as the actions they can afford us, and those perceptions and actions are guided by body-scaled ratios. Proponents of the dynamic systems approach contend that movement emerges as a function of the person, the task, and the environment. As individuals, we have our own unique structural and functional constraints, which are affected by changing task and environmental constraints. We encourage you to compare and contrast these theories and to examine development and learning from the theoretical perspective you find the most compelling.

ONLINE LEARNING

Visit the web resource at www.HumanKinetics.com/MotorLearningAndDevelopment for an accompanying lab activity and exercises from the chapter.

LEARNING AIDS

Supplemental Activities

1. In this chapter you learned about closed- and open-loop control. Many tasks have some components that are controlled by open-loop control and some by closed-loop control.
   a. Take 15 playing cards and, to the best of your ability, stack them to make a pyramid similar to the one in the illustration. Try this five times and record how many cards were stacked before they fell for each attempt. Break down card stacking into three components: (1) adjusting the cards in your hands, (2) leaning the cards, and (3) releasing the cards; label each as either open- or closed-loop control.

b. Take a coin and practice spinning it on a table and trapping it in a vertical position with your index finger. Perform this task 20 times and record the number of successful spins and successful vertical traps. Then break the task into three components: (1) spinning the coin, (2) preparing to trap the coin, and (3) trapping the coin; label each as either open- or closed-loop control.

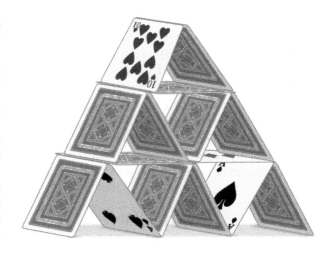

c. Choose a sport-related motor skill and explain which components are controlled by closed-loop control and which are controlled by open-loop control.

d. Choose an everyday activity and explain which components are controlled by closed-loop control and which are controlled by open-loop control.

2. Manipulating task and environmental constraints is an effective strategy for improving performance. Equipment can be changed so that it is appropriate for young learners or beginners. The rules can be adjusted so that learners can understand the basics without being overwhelmed. Activities can also be practiced in more predictable environments to enhance performance during skill acquisition.

a. Choose an activity and discuss several ways you could manipulate the environment and task (including the rules, goals, and equipment) to increase successful performances in beginning learners.

b. Discuss how you would progressively manipulate these constraints as the learners improve.

c. When could manipulating these constraints be ineffective and potentially even detrimental to skill learning?

Glossary

affordances—The action possibilities of the environment and task in relation to the perceiver's own capabilities.

attractor—A preferred state of stability toward which a system spontaneously shifts (dynamic systems approach).

closed-loop control—A type of control system that provides the opportunity to make continuous corrections based on feedback received during the movement.

constraints—Boundaries that limit a person's movement capabilities.

constraints model—A model of behavior asserting that coordination is developed by changing constraints imposed by the interaction of the individual with the environment.

control parameters—Variables that induce a shift from the current attractor state to a new attractor state.

dynamic systems approach—A perspective that addresses the interplay of the environment, task, and individual on skilled movement. Movement is the result of a self-organization of many systems, owing to interactions across these constraints.

ecological approach—A motor development or learning perspective that rejects the hierarchical view of the brain as the ultimate controller of movement. This perspective stresses the role of the environment as it interacts with the individual to produce fluid movement.

environmental constraints—Constraints that are external to the mover.

functional constraints—Individual constraints imposed by psychological variables such as motivation, arousal, and intellect.

generalized motor program (GMP)—A representation of a pattern of movements that is modifiable to produce a movement outcome; enables the production of skilled movement in the information-processing theory.

individual constraints—Boundaries imposed by the organism itself. *Also see* structural constraints and functional constraints.

information-processing theory—One of the theoretical constructs of motor behavior; it proposes that the brain receives, processes, and interprets information to send signals to produce skilled coordinated movements, similar to how a computer functions.

invariant features—Variables that cannot be modified between attempts (including the sequence of movements, relative force, and relative timing).

open-loop control—A type of control system for error correction that produces rapid, discrete movements; it requires preplanning of the movement.

parameters—Features that can be modified during the execution of a movement pattern (including muscle selection, overall force, and overall duration).

perception—The act of attaching meaning to something.

phase shift—The change in a state that causes a shift or reorganization to a new attractor state.

physical environmental constraints—External conditions that can aid or hinder movement patterns (e.g., weather, temperature, lighting, floor surface, step height).

rate limiter—A control parameter that limits or hinders performance.

schemas—Rules or relationships developed through accumulated experiences within a generalized motor program.

self-organization—A system's ability to change state or acquire a new structure or pattern of movement.

sociocultural environmental constraints—Constraints imposed by social and cultural norms and pressures.

speed–accuracy trade-off—Tendency for accuracy to be compromised when speed is increased (e.g. many errors) or speed to be sacrificed when focused on accuracy (e.g. movement is slowed down).

structural constraints—Individual constraints imposed by physical characteristics such as gender, height, weight, and body makeup.

task constraints—Constraints imposed by the task itself, including the goals of the movement, rules, and equipment.

4

STAGES OF SKILL ACQUISITION

Chapter Objectives

After reading this chapter, you should be able to do the following:

- Illustrate how motor skills progress through each period in the mountain of motor development.
- Compare and contrast three learning models—Fitts and Posner's, Gentile's, and Bernstein's. Generate a learner's behavioral characteristics for the stages of each learning model for specific motor skills.
- Prioritize the role of the practitioner according to each of the learning stages.

This is Harder Than I Thought!

Finn is a very athletic 14-year-old who decided to pick up a new sport, lacrosse. Although he is a skilled athlete who has played a lot of sports, he had a lot of difficulty with stick handling, particularly cradling the ball when he sprinted. Nearly every time he sprinted, he dropped the ball. Even with many acquired skills from playing years of basketball, baseball, and American football, cradling was a new skill for Finn. He had to learn to twist his hand back and forth in a rocking motion, but not too hard. Finn also had to learn that if he cradled closer to his face, the ball stayed in better and was harder to steal. After a few weeks of practicing drills, Finn noticed a big improvement in his stick handling, and with his improved skill level came improved confidence and enjoyment of this new sport.

The example in the opening scenario is certainly not unique to Finn. Whether you are highly skilled at many motor skills or not, everyone progresses through a series of stages when learning a new motor skill. The models discussed in this chapter address the stages of learning and provide a framework for categorizing the skill level of the learner from novice to expert. These models enable practitioners to assess the level of the learner and more appropriately prepare practice sessions. Those working with children must also understand motor skill development from infancy to adolescence. This chapter also examines how skills progress from prenatal development through skill proficiency using Clark's mountain of development.

Mountain of Motor Development

There is a misconception that maturation drives infant and child motor skill development (Clark, 2007). Although it may appear that a child has developed a new motor skill overnight, such as running, jumping, hopping, or catching, these skills do not magically appear. Motor skills must be taught and practiced (Drost, Brown, Wirth, & Greska, 2015). Children move the way they do because of individual and environmental constraints (Newell, 1984, 1986). Humans sit upright because of the biomechanical constraints of the human body and the gravitational forces imposed on the body. If gravitational forces were removed (as in outer space), it is unlikely that infants would acquire the ability to sit upright. Humans are born with preadapted motor behaviors that predispose particular reflexes and actions; nonetheless, these are either reinforced or modified by constraints in the environment. These preadapted motor behaviors prepare the infant for acquiring basic motor skills that generally develop during the first year of life. The acquisition of these motor skills does not occur through maturation alone; rather, these skills are honed by adapting

to changing constraints and through a learning process (Clark, 2007). As normally developing infants continue to grow, they are able to use these developmental skills to perform increasingly complex skills such as many sport-specific skills.

Clark and Metcalfe (2002) developed a life span view of motor skill development. In this framework, they defined separate periods in which typical patterns of motor skill development occur in a particular order (see figure 4.1). Clark and Metcalfe labeled this framework the mountain of motor development because each period builds on the previous period. This model describes motor skill development from birth to death, breaking down the development of skills into five periods.

The base of the mountain is the **prenatal period**, which consists of the last two trimesters of pregnancy. During this time, the fetus moves quite a bit. The next stage, the **reflexive period**, occurs following birth and lasts only two weeks. As suggested by the title of the stage, movements are reflexive as the newborn adjusts to many sensory changes such as bright lights and sounds. Following the first two weeks, the **preadapted period** begins. Infants start interacting with the environment by making goal-directed movements. During this period, phylogenetic motor behaviors prevail, such as sitting up, standing, crawling, and walking (refer to chapter 1 for the definition of phylogeny). When the infant can independently walk and self-feed—that is, perform the two fundamental skills necessary for basic survival—the infant has progressed to **fundamental motor patterns**. Fundamental motor patterns are basic movements such as throwing, catching, hopping, and jumping that form a base for more complex sport-specific movement patterns. These patterns are mature or well developed around the age of seven (Clark & Metcalfe, 2002; Gallahue, Ozumun, & Goodway, 2012).

From here, children typically pass a **proficiency barrier**, meaning they have exceeded a threshold of motor skill pro-

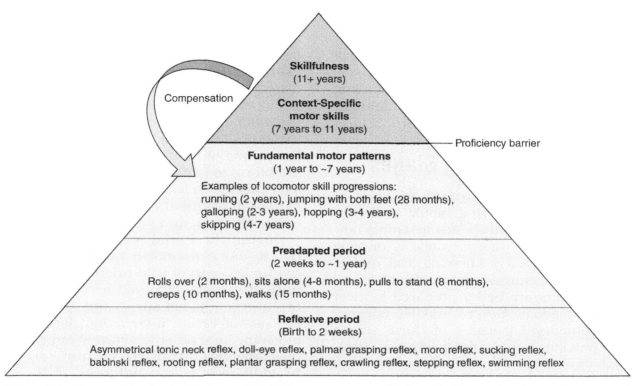

Figure 4.1 The mountain of motor development. *Note:* These ages are approximations. Each person is unique and progresses at his own rate.

Adapted, by permission, from J.E. Clark and J.M. Metcalfe, 2002, The mountain of motor development: A metaphor. In *Motor development: Research and reviews,* vol. 2, edited by J.E. Clark and J.H. Humphrey (Reston, VA: National Association for Sport and Physical Education), 163-190.

ficiency (Seefeldt, 1980). Once this proficiency barrier is surpassed, they begin to refine these fundamental motor patterns to movements specific for sports or other movement forms (e.g., a striking pattern may be modified for racket sports, baseball, or golf) and develop and maintain physical fitness (Stodden, True, Langendorfer, & Gao, 2013).

It should be noted that these motor skills do not develop naturally, but are the result of many constraints influencing the development of these skills (Newell, 1984, 1986). Movement experiences during early childhood are critical to the development of fundamental motor skills (Stodden & Goodway, 2007; Stodden et al., 2008). As such, not every child will pass the proficiency barrier at this age; those who don't may be delayed in their future development of related motor skills.

This period following fundamental motor patterns is termed the **context-specific**

motor skills period. The period at the peak of the mountain is the **skillfulness period**. This period does not distinguish between people of different skill levels (junior varsity, varsity, university, professional). To reach this period, a person needs to be skilled at the movement. In addition, skillfulness varies with each motor skill because no one is skillful in a wide variety of motor skills. A baseball player may be very fast and good at batting, catching, fielding, and throwing, but may not be a skillful swimmer or gymnast. As such, there is no single peak on the mountain; instead, there are many peaks of varying heights depending on the person's skillfulness in each activity (Goodway, Ozmun, & Gallahue, 2012). Those who aspire to reach the highest possible peak of the mountain must understand that this is a very long and demanding journey. People who incur an injury or must make some other adaptation as a result of the declines resulting from aging enter the **compensation period**. A full recovery from an injury may return someone to the former level of skillfulness. However, biological changes resulting from permanent injuries or aging effects may cause the person to remain at a lower position on the mountain.

Motor Learning Stages

Learners progress through a series of stages when improving motor skill proficiency, whether they are learning how to throw a ball, ride a unicycle, or type on a keyboard. By knowing and understanding the characteristics of each stage, practitioners are better prepared to meet learners' needs. Several models address the behavioral features of these stages and provide a unique perspective on them.

Fitts and Posner's Learning Stages

Fitts and Posner (1967) proposed a three-stage learning model (see the sidebar). Regardless of age or motor skill, all learners go through each of these stages when advancing from a novice to an expert level. This model classifies the stages around behavioral changes that can be observed in the performer. Practitioners have distinct roles at each level of learning.

Cognitive Stage

During the first stage, the **cognitive stage**, the learner's main goal is to understand the basic components of the motor skill movement pattern. This stage is termed the cognitive stage because learners require a considerable amount of mental activity to understand the movement pattern and appropriately coordinate their limbs. Novice learners often mentally verbalize their movements (e.g., a dancer may count the beats of the steps, or a triple jumper may say "Left, right, left, jump" to reinforce the movements until the pattern has been learned). During the cognitive stage, the learner often is easily confused and has many questions. If you were

water-skiing for the first time, you might have questions like these: *How do I position my feet? Do I bend my knees? How fast do I stand up when I'm being pulled out of the water?* Although experienced water-skiers do not even think about how to get out of the water, novice water-skiers must attend to the position of their body segments and the timing of their movements. Although attending to one's movements is a necessary process in learning any skill, it often causes movements to appear choppy, uncoordinated, and awkward.

During the initial stages of learning, people must attempt a number of techniques in a sort of trial-and-error process until they have achieved a certain level of success. It is not surprising, then, that the use of verbal instruction, feedback, modeling, and other teaching strategies is most effective during the cognitive stage. In addition to traditional forms of learning, recent research studies have found that reinforcement combined with passive movements can be as effective as active movements (Bernardi, Darainy, & Ostry, 2015). These findings are particularly significant for rehabilitation therapists, who often work with patients with limited mobility. It is during the cognitive stage that the largest gains in learning occur. Learners begin with very little knowledge of the motor skill and make rapid gains in performance as they learn the basics of the task.

Associative Stage

Once learners have a basic understanding of the task and have shown significant improvement in the movement pattern, they have progressed to the **associative stage** of learning. In this stage, the goal has shifted from learning how to solve the movement problem to refining the movement. Performance improvements are more gradual than those observed during the cognitive stage. Learners perform more consistently and can focus on error detection and correction. Because they do not have to focus as much on the production

Fitts and Posner's Learning Stages

Cognitive Stage (Beginner)

How do I produce this movement pattern?

Performer's Behavior

- Learning the fundamental movement patterns
- Engaging in high cognitive activity (attention to movement and self-talk)
- Exhibiting inconsistent performance
- Making many gross errors
- Experiencing the greatest performance improvements

Practitioner's Role

- Assisting the learner in understanding the movement pattern
- Using teaching strategies such as verbal instruction, demonstrations, and modeling, which are most effective during this stage

Associative Stage (Intermediate)

I've got it! Now, how do I get to the next level?

Performer's Behavior

- Exhibiting more consistent performance
- Making fewer errors
- Requiring fewer attentional demands
- Making more gradual performance improvements

Practitioner's Role

- Designing practice
- Facilitating error detection and correction

Autonomous Stage (Advanced)

I'm on top! How do I stay here?

Performer's Behavior

- Experiencing a high level of skill proficiency
- Performing largely automatically
- Making very few errors
- Performing very consistently
- Focusing on strategies

Practitioner's Role

- Designing practice
- Refining performance
- Motivating the performer

Exercise 4.1

Choose a motor skill in which you are moderately to highly skilled. Discuss the behavioral aspects of the performance for someone in each of Fitts and Posner's three learning stages, and develop strategies for instructing a learner in each stage (practitioner's role). An example is provided for the motor skill of juggling.

Juggling

Motor skill	Behavioral aspects		
	Cognitive	**Associative**	**Autonomous**
Juggling	• Makes very few catches. • Uses self-talk. • Has to focus attention. • Does not know how to compensate for poor tosses. • Experiences fast improvement after the movement pattern is learned. • Visually tracks ball movements.	• Is more confident. • Makes more consistent tosses. • Makes many more catches. • Shifts attention to the apex of the juggling trajectory. • Can detect errors but cannot always correct them while juggling.	• Is very confident. • Can perform multiple activities while juggling. • Can sustain the pattern for a long time.
	Practitioner's role		
	• Demonstrate how to juggle. • Provide verbal instructions. • Discuss the juggling pattern and the movement of the limbs. • Answer questions. • Provide a lot of feedback.	• Give feedback as requested. • Increase the challenges of the task (juggle under different conditions, focus on better control of the tosses, toss faster or slower). • Motivate the learner.	• Further increase the challenge. ○ Add distractions. ○ Add a secondary task. ○ Try a more difficult task (e.g., juggling with clubs or more balls). • Motivate the learner.

Chosen motor skill:

Behavioral aspects		
Cognitive	**Associative**	**Autonomous**
Practitioner's role		

of the movement, they can attend to other sources of information. The verbal component (self-talk) that was prominent in the cognitive stage is no longer present in the production of the movement pattern, because it is no longer necessary or beneficial.

The role of the instructor shifts when the learner is in the associative stage—from instructing to designing appropriate and effective practice sessions (see chapters 14-17). The learner understands the basic movement pattern, but still benefits from instructor feedback regarding errors and fine-tuning the movements.

Autonomous Stage

The final stage of learning in the Fitts and Posner model is the **autonomous stage**. To progress to the final stage, learners must practice for an extended period of time, often many years. Most people do not make it to the autonomous stage of learning. During this stage, the performer is so skilled that the movement appears automatic, or without thought, and almost effortless, and he may even be able to perform an additional task at the same time. An example is a circus performer riding a unicycle on a high wire while juggling. In this stage, the mover is able to focus on decision-making strategies, which are critical for high-level performance in open skills such as wrestling and rugby. This stage is reserved for very skilled performers and is considered the highest skill level. Performers in the autonomous stage consistently perform very well and are confident in their performance capabilities.

Although performers who reach this stage may be at the top of their game, this does not mean that instructors no longer play an important role. Although the amount of improvement may not be visible, performers can continue to fine-tune their performances in the autonomous stage. It is also important for instructors to assist in the maintenance of the performer's level of skill. The instructors should focus on designing practice schedules and maintaining the motivation levels of the performers. Not only is it difficult to reach the top; but also it is challenging to stay there!

Bernstein's Learning Stages

Another view of the learning stages is based on the degrees of freedom problem. Bernstein (1967) identified the challenge of organizing a complex structure of joints and muscles to produce smooth, goal-oriented movement as the degrees of freedom problem. Degrees of freedom are the number of functional units required to solve a movement problem (see chapter 1). Degrees of freedom can be thought of as the number of possible solutions to a performance task. Keep in mind that very few movements involve only one body segment, and many movements require whole body coordination. Using the notion of the degrees of freedom problem, Vereijken (1991) proposed a three-stage learning model using Bernstein's degrees of freedom.

TRY THIS

Observational Skills

Exercise 4.2

Go to an open gym, court, or field and observe a game. Try to find the most skilled and least skilled players. Describe specific behavioral characteristics of each of these players. Explain why you categorized them as most and least skilled.

- *Stage 1—Freezing the Limbs.* To perform a novel task, novices simplify the movement problem of having to control an overwhelming number of degrees of freedom by eliminating some of them. Novices do not understand the optimal method of managing these degrees of freedom in order to perform the new movement pattern, so they reduce these options to a more controllable number (Vereijken, van Emmerik, Whiting, & Newell, 1992). Vereijken described this process as "freezing the limbs." This is accomplished by keeping certain joint angles rigid throughout the movement or by temporarily coupling multiple joints so that they move as one segment. Although freezing the degrees of freedom simplifies the task, the movement appears very rigid, and the novice's ability to adapt to any unexpected changes is poor. For example, a young child uses only the arm to throw a ball. The legs and trunk are not used to assist in the throw, as they are in more advanced throwers. Inexperienced throwers also eliminate the backswing. The throw is completed almost exclusively at the elbow joint.

To assist beginners during the freezing the limbs stage, practitioners should simplify the task. Doing so encourages learners to focus on fewer degrees of freedom and increases their opportunities for success. For example, it would be more effective to instruct unskilled soccer players to keep the ball in the air by hitting it with only one leg than to encourage them to control the ball in the air with both legs, chest, shoulder, and head. Clinicians should begin rehabilitation with exercises that require only one plane of motion, fewer joints, or both. As learners or patients improve, difficulty can increase by encouraging movements that require more degrees of freedom.

- *Stage 2—Releasing the Limbs.* As learners become more comfortable with the basic movement pattern, they are able to gradually release the constraints imposed on the degrees of freedom. This makes the movement appear more fluid and allows them to gain more control over the production of the movement pattern. At this point, the degrees of freedom become incorporated into larger functional units of action, termed **coordinative structures**. Coordinative structures are formed by constraining or limiting potential options (e.g., muscles and joints) appropriately for a particular movement pattern. For instance, pole-vaulters form coordinative structures to be able to swing the trail leg forward and row the arms down while also keeping both arms and the left leg straight. Some coordinative structures appear at birth, providing the groundwork for phylogenetic motor behaviors (e.g., grasping, walking) that will develop later with growth and maturation.

Once learners have gained a basic level of proficiency, they use significantly more

RESEARCH NOTES

You're Staying Too Still!

A study completed several decades ago comparing novice and expert pistol shooters revealed that novices tightly locked the degrees of freedom in their arms, whereas experts did not show any locking of their upper limbs (Arutyunyan, Gurfinkel, & Mirskii, 1968, 1969). Instead, expert pistol shooters use compensatory actions in the arm, allowing them to perform with more arm control and less pistol motion. As suggested by Bernstein's learning model, the novice shooters simplified the task by freezing their limbs.

degrees of freedom than when they began practicing the motor skill. Practitioners should continue to encourage learners to increase their range of motion and, depending on the skill, the speed of the movement as their movements become smoother and more controlled.

• *Stage 3—Exploiting the Environment.* During the final stage of learning, the performer continues releasing degrees of freedom until all of the degrees of freedom necessary to accomplish the task have been released. At this point the performer is maximizing muscular efficiency through the use of the optimal number of degrees of freedom and is able to exploit environmental passive forces (i.e., gravity or inertia). Learners at this stage are considered experts. At this stage figure skaters can land impressive jumps, wide receivers in American football can make unbelievable catches while leaping into the air and avoiding defenders, and tennis players can maintain complete control of the flight patterns of the ball.

The main role of practitioners with learners in stage 3 is to design variable practice sessions that push them to continue extending their capabilities. Practitioners must keep the task interesting and fresh so that the learners stay motivated.

Evidence for Bernstein's Learning Stages

Researchers in one investigation examined the degrees of freedom by teaching participants how to operate a ski simulator apparatus. Initially, the participants moved very rigidly, fixing their lower limb joints (Vereijken et al., 1992). This enabled them to move with relatively high frequency (quick movements), but low amplitude (small side-to-side movements). The cross correlations were very high between joints during the early stages of learning. With practice, the cross correlations (couplings between joints) decreased, indicating that the degrees of freedom were being released. At this point, the participants were moving with more amplitude (covering more dis-

tance), but this came at the cost of frequency, meaning that they were unable to move back and forth at the same rate. As practice continued, the cross correlations continued to decrease and movement frequency continually increased, until the performers were able to move with the same or greater frequency as in the initial practice trials while maintaining large movement amplitudes. These results indicate that initially learners freeze their degrees of freedom to gain control over the movement. They do this because they are afraid of falling. As their confidence and familiarity with the task increase with practice, the number of degrees of freedom also increases.

Another research study compared dominant limb movements with nondominant limb movements during handwriting to investigate whether there was a difference in the number of degrees of freedom involved in the two limbs (Newell & van Emmerik, 1989). Limb dominance provides an opportunity to compare the effect of skill acquisition within the same participant. The investigators found that the nondominant limb used fewer degrees of freedom than the dominant limb did. These findings provide more evidence in support of Bernstein's (1967) learning stages by demonstrating that the degrees of freedom were released in the more practiced, dominant limb as opposed to the nondominant limb. These results were observed through high correlations between the joints in the nondominant limb. The authors also evaluated the independence between multiple joints. Cross correlations revealed the independence of two variables, with high cross correlations indicating that the variables are highly interdependent. In this case, if one body segment moved, such as the shoulder, then another body segment moved, such as the elbow. When the participants were writing with the nondominant limb, they were freezing their degrees of freedom. In contrast, when they were writing with the

Exercise 4.3

If you've ever watched people ice skate for the first time, you probably noticed how they stiffen their knees and move each leg as if it were a single segment. Their movements are very rigid and deliberate. Experienced ice skaters tend to move fluidly across the ice. Professional ice skaters are able to exploit the environment by propelling their bodies into the air, completing multiple turns and landing smoothly.

Swimmers have also been found to reduce their degrees of freedom when learning to swim (refer to the following table). Rather than freely moving their arms and legs, novice swimmers often move their arms in a short downward-pushing motion and their legs in a bicycle pattern, causing them to produce more of a doggy paddle than a fluid, advanced formal stroke. Stiffening limb movements causes the body to be in an upright vertical position, preventing much forward propulsion.

Think of two other activities in which Bernstein's learning stages are noticeably visible. Describe how the learner's movements appear in each of the three stages.

Motor skill	Stage 1: Freezing the limbs	Stage 2: Releasing the limbs	Stage 3: Exploiting the environment
Swimming	• Little to no arm or leg action occurs. • Arm action is a simple, short downward push. • Leg action is a circular bicycling action. • Overall, little to no forward propulsion occurs.	• More arm and leg action occurs. • Arms: Long push-pull • Legs: Bent-knee flutter kick • Overall: Rudimentary crawl	• Arms: Lift propulsion and bent elbow • Legs: Straight-leg flutter • Overall: Advanced crawl, rhythmic breathing

dominant limb, each body segment moved independently.

Evidence Against Bernstein's Learning Stages

In more recent years, the Bernstein learning stages have been challenged because they do not consider all influencing factors inherent in the performance of the motor skill (Newell & Vaillancourt, 2001). Completion of a motor skill occurs as the learner's characteristics (including structural constraints such as height and weight, and functional constraints such as motivation and movement experience), the task (goals, equipment, rules), and the environment (physical and sociocultural) interact. It was proposed that the order of the learning stages depends on the task goal and the constraints of the person.

To examine how changing the constraints of the task affects the behaviors evident in the learning stages, researchers had participants practice maintaining balance on a moving platform that oscillated in an anteroposterior direction (Ko, Challis, & Newell, 2003). In contrast to what happened in the study by Vereijken and colleagues, participants produced large ranges of motion at all joints, including the neck, hip, knee, and ankle. With practice, rather than increasing their joint motion, the participants decreased it. The learners were gradually freezing the degrees of freedom that were not essential for the task. They also decreased motion in some degrees of freedom, but not in others.

It appears that the participants were initially decreasing their degrees of freedom to find a new coordination mode, one that was more efficient and more stable (Newell, Kugler, van Emmerik, & McDonald, 1989). This new movement pattern would have a stronger attractor state (see chapter 3). Similar results were found in cellists: more skilled cellists used less elbow and wrist overall movement and less variability in comparison to novice cellists (Verrel, Pologe, Manselle, Lindenberger, & Woollacott, 2013). Higher skill in violin bowing was also associated with freezing degrees of freedom rather than releasing degrees of freedom, as Bernstein's learning model suggests (Konczak, Velden, & Jaeger, 2009). The main suggestion from these research studies is that there are many ways to solve a movement task. The most appropriate method for learning a new motor skill is determined by the interaction between the structural and functional constraints of the learner; the goals, equipment, and rules of the task; and the environmental constraints imposed on the learner.

Throwing Degrees of Freedom

Exercise 4.4

Throw a ball 5 to 10 times with as much force as you can using your dominant hand. Then switch hands and throw 5 to 10 times with your nondominant hand. Most likely, you were not able to throw the ball as far or as fast with your nondominant hand, but what about the movement characteristics of your throws? Describe what was different about the kinematics of your throws with your dominant hand versus your nondominant hand. You may find it easier to observe the differences in a friend. When did your friend use more degrees of freedom (e.g., contralateral step, increased range of motion of the arm)? Explain why there is a difference in the number of degrees of freedom used in each arm to accomplish the same task.

Gentile's Learning Stages

Gentile proposed a two-stage learning model (1972, 1987, 2000) to help practitioners by not only describing the nature of the movement, but also providing instructional strategies for each learning stage.

Getting the Idea of the Movement Stage

The first stage of learning is the **getting the idea of the movement stage**, which is similar to Fitts and Posner's cognitive stage of learning. During this stage the learner has two main goals: to understand the coordination required to perform the task and to determine the regulatory and nonregulatory conditions of the movement. Gentile used the term **regulatory conditions** to refer to conditions that provide relevant information for a motor skill. Regulatory conditions for the game of basketball include the ball, the positions of opponents and teammates, and the position of the player relative to the basket. To perform proficiently, a player must selectively attend to these important aspects. People depend on the external environment to produce successful movements (Chow, Davids, Button, & Koh, 2008). Regulatory conditions for a simple motor skill such as walking down the street include the surface of support (concrete, ice, gravel), other pedestrians, and objects along the path. The more complex motor skill of hitting a baseball with a bat requires the player to make contact with the ball; to do this, the player must understand both the positional (spatial) and the time (temporal) characteristics of the ball (Gentile, 2000). There is a much greater margin of error for a batter than for a walker. If the batter anticipates or misjudges the pitch, the bat will not make contact with the ball. The movement pattern executed by the batter depends on the spatial and temporal characteristics of the environment and the batter's spatial–temporal skills.

It is perhaps even more important for a learner to ignore nonrelevant cues, which Gentile refers to as **nonregulatory conditions**. Nonregulatory conditions distract learners from important relevant cues, preventing them from performing skillfully or even accomplishing the goal at all. Practitioners should emphasize the regulatory conditions during early skill acquisition to help learners avoid the acquisition of bad habits and to maximize learning during practice sessions. Learners who are easily distracted, especially children, should frequently be redirected toward the regulatory conditions. The learner must not only be able to selectively attend to the relevant cues (regulatory conditions) but also be able to ignore the irrelevant cues (nonregulatory conditions). A basketball player shooting a free throw must focus on the release of the ball and the rim of the basket while ignoring the sounds of the crowd screaming and stomping their feet on the bleachers. Most often, those distractions are not present during practice. The pedestrian needs to focus on oncoming traffic and traffic signals when crossing a busy street and avoid distractions from cell phone conversations, music, or other external noise. However, it is important for learners to practice under varying nonregulatory conditions to prepare for performances or real-world situations.

It is also critical to note that during the first stage of learning, the emphasis cannot be solely on the movement. Learners must be able to identify and select the regulatory conditions that influence their movement. This information is necessary for organizing a successful movement pattern.

The practitioner's role during Gentile's getting the idea of the movement stage is to clearly and concisely teach the learner how to perform the movement pattern. The practitioner should emphasize the basics of the task (e.g., goals and objectives) through demonstrations and verbal instructions. The learner's attention should be directed toward the relevant stimuli in the environment. For example, a batter should be told to focus on the pitcher's release point during the windup. Novice batters often alter their visual focus between the release point and the pitcher's head, whereas experts maintain a steady focus on the release point (Shank & Haywood, 1987). By focusing on the relevant stimulus (the release point), experts can accurately assess the pitch nearly 100 percent of the time, whereas novices who fluctuated between the head and the release point during the windup accurately identify only a little more than 50 percent of the pitches. Altering their visual focus causes novices to miss critical components of the pitch, which decreases their chances of making contact with the ball.

Fixation and Diversification Stage

Once learners understand the basic movement pattern, they advance to the second learning stage, the fixation and diversification stage. The key element during this stage is refining the movement pattern (similar to what occurs in Fitts and Posner's stage 2, the associative stage) and maintaining consistent performance (similar to what occurs in Fitts and Posner's stage 3, the autonomous stage). Gentile separates the stage into two subcomponents (fixation and diversification), depending on the predictability of the environment and the skill level of the performer (see figure 4.2).

• *Fixation.* When learning a closed skill, such as performing a power clean or playing billiards, the focus should be on consistency. The learner must refine the movement by determining how to most accurately perform the motor skill and then reliably replicate the action time and time again. Learners who are performing a routine, as in gymnastics, figure skating, and dance, practice and refine the movements until they can consistently perform the movement sequence well. In rehabilitation settings, therapists first assist patients in performing exercises under very controlled settings. Gentile refers to this subcomponent as the **fixation stage**, because learners are focusing on consistently reproducing a movement pattern. If, however, this was all they did, the performances would be very boring to watch.

• *Diversification.* Open skills, such as passing the puck to a teammate during a hockey game, progress to the subcomponent known as the **diversification stage** in which they are practiced in unpredictable environments. Successful performers of open skills must be very adaptable. Because they cannot predict how the opposing team will respond to their plays, they must alter their responses as play unfolds. When learning an open skill, learners must focus on diversifying their movement pattern by practicing the motor skill under many conditions. When learning a closed motor skill, the main objective is consistency, or in Gentile's terms, fixation. The objective in open motor skills is adaptability, or in Gentile's

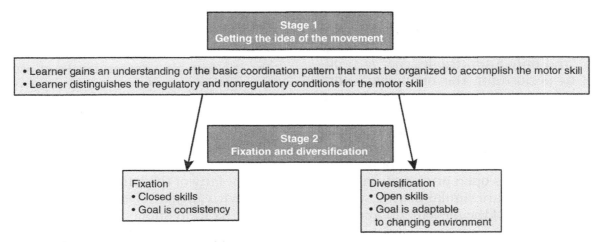

Figure 4.2 Gentile's two-stage learning model.

terms, diversification. Learners who can perform a motor skill very consistently only under predictable conditions will not be prepared when the environment unexpectedly changes. They must be able to make quick decisions and adapt their movement patterns to accommodate these changes. Patients undergoing physical or occupational therapy must not only learn how to perform the exercises in the controlled setting of the clinic, but more important, learn how to adapt the exercises so they can adapt to daily activities that will be performed at home or out in the community. Furthermore, the activities or motor skills they are learning or relearning must enable them to circumvent many obstacles and adjust to varying surfaces, slopes, and objects.

Once the learner has progressed to the second stage of learning, the fixation and diversification stage, instructional strategies should focus on refining the movement pattern until the learner can complete it consistently. Gentile refers to this as fixation. The movement pattern should be practiced repeatedly under similar regulatory conditions, whereas nonregulatory conditions should be varied. For example, during a closed skill such as bowling, the regulatory conditions (i.e., length of lane, size of gutters, number of pins, size of pins) should not be changed, but the nonregulatory conditions (i.e., crowd noise, fatigue level, motivation level, number of pins remaining) should be changed.

If the motor skill is an open skill, the practitioner will advance to the subcomponent known as the diversification stage after, and only after, the learner is proficient at performing the motor skill consistently using the subcomponent known as the fixation stage. Again, the fixation strategy includes teaching under similar regulatory conditions and variable nonregulatory conditions. Regardless of whether the motor skill is open or closed, instructional strategies are similar during stage 1, getting the idea of the movement, and then progress to stage 2, fixation and diversification. When practicing closed skills, the learner continues using the fixation strategy. For open skills, the practitioner should vary both the regulatory and nonregulatory conditions (diversification strategy) only after the learner can proficiently perform under stable regulatory conditions and variable nonregulatory conditions. For example, a punter in American football should be able to punt the ball consistently without defenders prior to trying punting with defenders. The following is an example of teaching a learner how to shoot a basketball using Gentile's learning stages.

Stage 1: Getting the Idea of the Movement

Teach the goal of a basketball shot.

Provide a demonstration (e.g., BEEF: balance, eyes on rim, elbow, follow-through).

Allow the learner to practice from the same position on the court repeatedly before moving to a different position.

Provide feedback regarding the shot—such as *Shoot with more arc, Increase the bend of your knees, Don't forget to follow through.*

Stage 2: Fixation Subcomponent

Vary practice conditions while remaining in a closed environment:

Practice shots without defenders at the foul line.

Practice when fatigued.

Practice under various motivation conditions.

Practice with crowd noise.

Practice under various levels of stress (e.g., provide incentives or punishments for missed shots, altering the importance of the shot).

Stage 2: Diversification Subcomponent

Vary practice conditions in an open environment (any of the following can be combined with any of the conditions in the stage 2 fixation subcomponent):

Add defenders.

Learn more plays.

Increase the pace of the game.

Link to Dynamic Systems Approach

The dynamic systems approach supports the changing dynamics and coordination patterns discussed in the three learning models. According to the dynamic systems approach (refer to chapter 3 for further information), learners begin producing a pattern of movement that is familiar to them, such as one from a similar motor skill (Zanone & Kelso, 1994). For instance, a skilled tennis player who has never played racquetball will likely swing at the racquetball with very little snap of the wrist. To control the ball in tennis, players are often initially taught to hit forehand and backhand with the whole arm from the shoulder. Because racquetball does not involve hitting the ball above a net into a court, the player can strategically hit the ball with great force against the wall. Racquetball players can generate more force and power by snapping the elbow and wrist when swinging at the ball. Swinging with the whole arm is a coordination pattern that is well developed in tennis players. This pattern would work on a racquetball court, but not well. This coordination pattern would be a strong attractor state with a deep well for a tennis player. As the player practices and progresses with the new game of racquetball, she is likely to vary her swing to accommodate the changing constraints of the enclosed court and the different elastic properties of the ball and the strings of the racket. With practice and instruction, the learner's swing would transition from the initial preferred coordination pattern of swinging with the whole arm to a new attractor state of swinging with more elbow and wrist action.

It is important to consider prior movement experiences before instructing a new motor skill. Prior movement experiences will strongly influence the coordination patterns that a learner adopts, for better

WHAT DO YOU THINK?

Exercise 4.5

Refer to the tennis and racquetball example discussed in the section Link to Dynamic Systems Approach.

1. What is the rate limiter (this term was introduced in chapter 3) for the tennis player who is learning how to play racquetball?

2. For tennis:

   a. At what stage (using Fitts and Posner's learning model) would you classify the athlete? Explain why.

   b. What instructional strategies would be most appropriate for the athlete? (*Hint:* The instructional strategies should depend on the stage of learning for each motor skill.)

3. For racquetball:

   a. At what stage (using Fitts and Posner's learning model) would you classify the athlete? Explain why.

   b. What instructional strategies would be most appropriate for the athlete? (*Hint:* The instructional strategies should depend on the stage of learning for each motor skill.)

or worse. A practitioner should be aware of the learner's prior movement experiences and adjust teaching strategies accordingly to maximize the rate of learning.

Practical Use of the Learning Models

These three learning models provide a multilevel perspective on motor learning. An emphasis on the impact the environment has on the learning process is stressed in both Bernstein's learning stages and Gentile's learning stages. In Bernstein's learning model, the individual's perception is affected by the changing dynamics of the environment. Gentile emphasized that instruction should be designed based on the predictability of environmental influences. Fitts and Posner's learning model defined cognitive and behavior processes across the skill level of the performer. A practitioner who understands how the environment affects the learning process will be able to manipulate the environment to optimize learning.

With initial instruction, the focus should be on the organization of the learner and then on the goal of the task. The practitioner should provide adequate instruction to get learners started performing the movement task, with the goal of allowing them to explore movement options while attempting to produce the basic coordination pattern. During this time, movement errors can be seen as positive because learners are discovering the patterns of movement that work and discarding those that do not. Novice performers generally show rapid improvements in performance. This rate of improvement gradually tapers off with continuing practice.

Learners who can perform the basic movement pattern should then focus on refining their movements to increase their probability of success. Once they can consistently produce a movement pattern, they can focus on adapting the movement pattern. This enables the learner to per-

form under various internal conditions (e.g., fatigue levels, motivation levels, the importance of the outcome) and external conditions (e.g., crowd noise; the position, angle, and distance of the movement; the positions of other players).

These three models provide a background to the cognitive and physical components of the learning stages as well as instructional strategies appropriate for each stage. A practitioner who fully understands the learning process will have the skills necessary to properly manipulate the learning environment and the learner (Rose & Christina, 2006).

Summary

Motor skill progression was defined developmentally by Clark and Metcalf (2002) as a mountain of motor development. Although people develop at different rates, the mountain of motor development illustrates how people progress from one stage to another and even incorporates descent down the mountain (although unintentional) following injury and declines due to aging (compensation).

Fitts and Posner (1967) developed a three-stage model for the acquisition of any motor skill. The first stage, the cognitive stage, is marked by many errors, inconsistencies, and self-talk. Once learners have learned the basic components of the task, they progress to the associative stage, in which the errors are few and less gross. The final stage, which many people never reach, is the autonomous stage. Vereijken (1991) proposed a three-stage model from Bernstein's notion of the degrees of freedom problem. In the first stage, novices tend to freeze their limbs to simplify the movement. As learners progress, they increase the number of degrees of freedom, creating more fluid movements. When they have achieved a high level of proficiency, they have reached the third stage, exploitation of the environment.

The third learning model, proposed by Gentile (1972, 1987, 2000), was intended to provide instructional strategies to practitioners. During the first stage, the getting the idea of the movement stage, learners focus on the movement basics. After they have acquired a basic concept of the movement pattern, they progress to the fixation and diversification stage. After achieving a high level of consistency by fixating on the same regulatory conditions, learners practice many movement modifications to prepare for unpredictable environments.

Each of these models contributes to our understanding of how people learn motor skills and helps the practitioner structure, design, and implement practice sessions with the goal of maximizing motor learning. By using a multilevel perspective, practitioners will have more tools to manipulate the environment to accommodate behavioral, cognitive, and physical changes in performers with increased skillfulness.

ONLINE LEARNING

Visit the web resource at www.HumanKinetics.com/MotorLearningAndDevelopment for an accompanying lab activity and exercises from the chapter.

LEARNING AIDS

Supplemental Activities

1. Bernstein's learning stages: YouTube has become a popular portal for searching for videos, from educational videos to cartoons to homemade videos. Many people, skillful or not, post videos of themselves performing. Search YouTube for three skill levels of soccer jugglers. Soccer juggling is an excellent example of Bernstein's learning stages because beginners generally limit their juggling to the use of only one leg, sometimes only the foot or the knee. As they increase their skill level, they begin to use more and more degrees of freedom by introducing more and more limb segments into their juggling.

   a. Were you able to find three soccer jugglers you would classify as being in stages 1, 2, and 3 of Bernstein's learning stages? Explain your rationale for these classifications. Describe the jugglers' behavioral characteristics.

   b. Search for other motor skills (e.g., ice skating, throwing a ball, skateboarding) that you could classify into Bernstein's three learning stages. Describe how the performances fit into these classifications.

2. Mountain of motor development: Choose two motor skills you would describe yourself as skillful in. Working backward down the mountain of motor development, explain what prior skills and experiences led you to achieve your level of proficiency. Start by defining how the motor skill is performed skillfully. For example, an experienced basketball player can perform a layup even when faced with a defender or increased game pressure, whereas a novice basketball player is unable to dribble to the basket and shoot. The novice must focus on the fundamental motor skill (e.g., dribbling or jumping). Work backward and describe the underlying motor skills and patterns required for your selected skills from the preadapted period to the skillfulness period.

   a. At what age did you become skillful?

   b. What context-specific skills that were critical to developing the level of skill you have now did you practice at an earlier age?

   c. Step back to fundamental motor skills. What fundamental motor skills were critical, and why?

> d. Ask your parents whether they did anything during the preadapted period that may have helped you advance your manipulative skills, postural skills, and locomotor skills.
>
> e. Use this information to fill out the following chart. Note: There's an example of a basketball layup included for each of the periods.

Motor skill	Skillfulness	Context-specific motor skills	Fundamental motor skills	Preadapted period
Basketball layup	Right, left, jump, shoot; pattern is performed well in spite of external influences (e.g., defenders)	Basketball shooting Stepping and shooting	Jumping Dribbling	Pull to stand Stand alone Walk with and then without assistance

From P.S. Haibach-Beach, G.D. Reid, and D.H. Collier, 2018, *Motor learning and development,* 2nd ed. (Champaign, IL: Human Kinetics).

Glossary

associative stage—The second stage in Fitts and Posner's learning model, in which the goal has shifted from solving the movement problem to refining the movement.

autonomous stage—The third and final stage in Fitts and Posner's learning model, in which the performer is at the highest level of motor skill proficiency.

cognitive stage—Fitts and Posner's first stage, in which the learner's main goal is to understand the basic components of the motor skill movement pattern.

compensation period—A period from Clark's mountain of motor development, which involves an adaptation to the environment as a result of an injury or declines resulting from aging.

context-specific motor skills period—A period of refinement of fundamental motor patterns as performers learn movements specific to sports or other movement forms; from Clark's mountain of motor development.

coordinative structures—Structures that occur when the degrees of freedom become incorporated into larger functional units of action to preserve a certain posture or movement.

diversification stage—Subcomponent of Gentile's second stage of learning in which open skills are practiced in unpredictable environments.

fixation stage—Subcomponent of Gentile's second stage of learning in which skills are practiced in a closed environment with a focus on consistency of the movement pattern.

fundamental motor patterns—Basic movements such as throwing, catching, hopping, and jumping that form a base for more complex sport-specific movement patterns.

getting the idea of the movement stage—Gentile's first stage of learning, similar to Fitts and Posner's cognitive stage of learning. During this stage the learner has two main goals: to understand the movement coordination required to perform the movement task, and to determine the regulatory and nonregulatory conditions of the movement.

nonregulatory conditions—Factors, unrelated to the movement task, that can distract the learner from important relevant cues, preventing skillful performances.

preadapted period—The mountain of motor development period in which infants start interacting with the environment by engaging in phylogenetic motor behaviors such as sitting up, standing, crawling, and walking.

prenatal period—The mountain of motor development period consisting of the last two trimesters of pregnancy in which the fetus moves quite a bit.

proficiency barrier—A hypothetical barrier used to describe a threshold of motor skill proficiency.

reflexive period—The mountain of motor development period following birth and lasting two weeks as the newborn adjusts to sensory input such as bright lights and sounds.

regulatory conditions—Environmental conditions that provide relevant information for motor skill performance.

skillfulness period—The period at the peak of the mountain of motor development in which a learner has acquired a high level of skill proficiency. This period does not distinguish between levels of performance, such as university and professional athletes.

5

ASSESSING MOTOR LEARNING

Chapter Objectives

After reading this chapter, you should be able to do the following:

- Describe multiple indicators of motor learning.
- Generate and interpret performance curves and explain the limitations.
- Assess transfer of learning and support positive transfer.
- Calculate retention and transfer measures.

Are All Athletic Wraps Created Equal?

Emily is majoring in athletic training and has learned how to wrap an ankle. She knows how to prepare the appropriate materials including tape adherent, heel and lace pads, prewrap, and athletic tape. She also has learned how to properly position the patient so that the foot is pointed upright at a 90-degree angle. Emily has practiced and is confident performing the steps involved in wrapping an ankle including spraying the adhesive, positioning the heel and lace pads, applying prewrap from the midfoot to the bottom of the gastrocnemius, applying anchor strips, attaching stirrups, placing three horseshoes to support the ankle, and finally taping the ankle in figure eights. Emily has practiced wrapping ankles countless times and is confident in her ability, but she has not learned how to tape a shoulder or other joints. Emily expects that her experience with wrapping ankles will help her learn how to tape other joints. This potential advantage would be considered positive transfer. Would you expect there to be a benefit from her knowledge of wrapping ankles, or would taping a shoulder be too different for Emily to have an advantage?

Although it is evident through Emily's sustained improvement that she has learned how to properly tape an ankle, motor learning is not always so transparent. Instructors may have only limited time with their learners, making it especially challenging to assess the amount of motor learning that has occurred. Physical educators and health professionals are an essential component of childhood and adolescent motor development. Teachers, physical therapists, and coaches engage their students in fitness activities, sports, games, and other activities, teaching fundamental motor skills that are critical to motor development. Practitioners may assist delayed infants in learning to crawl; they may help children learn how to throw a ball, young athletes to serve a volleyball, or adults to bench press properly. It is important not only to properly instruct motor skills, but also to appropriately measure and assess learners' movement patterns.

Understanding how to tape an ankle will likely benefit Emily when she is learning how to tape other joints. Previous movement experiences can greatly influence the performance of similar movement patterns—some in positive ways (positive transfer) and some in negative ways (negative transfer). This chapter discusses transfer of learning, including the types of transfer and how to foster positive transfer, in addition to how to assess motor learning and retention.

We can take many performance characteristics into consideration to determine whether students are learning motor skills, such as improved coordination patterns, increased consistency, and reduced mental and physical effort, to name a few. These are all important in assessing performance, but the key to determining the level of learning attained is to assess the permanency of the motor skill. Think about an occupational therapist who is teaching a stroke patient how to brush her teeth or write her name again, or a physical therapist who is teaching a victim of a car accident how to walk again. What char-

acteristics of the learner's performance assure the instructor that the learner is actually learning the movement and not simply showing improved performance? Just as math, science, and language teachers assess learning through examinations that cover the material, practitioners must administer retention tests to assess the learning of motor skills. Physical educators and movement clinicians assume that their students and clients have learned the material when they can perform at or near the same level as their previous performance following a break.

Indicators of Motor Skill Learning

Learning takes time, and practitioners must understand and accept this fact. Classrooms are based on the premise that the learning of some basic concepts will adequately prepare students for the next step in their careers, be that university or a first professional job. Physical education classrooms assume that practicing basic movement patterns will transfer to other, more complex activities; sporting practices are centered on the assumption that drills will positively influence game day performances; and therapists assume that exercises performed in the clinic will transfer to real-world settings. However, many factors must be addressed to ensure skill transfer. Motor learning is defined as a relatively permanent change in the capability to execute a motor skill as a result of practice or experience. This section discusses how motor learning is assessed and how to facilitate positive transfer and prolonged retention. The following are some movement characteristics that can indicate that motor learning has occurred:

- Performance improvement: Are observable performance changes shown across practice?
- Consistency or stability: Can the learner sustain a higher level of performance over time?

- Persistence: Can the learner perform the motor skill proficiently following a break in practice or performance?
- Effort: Is the learner performing with less physical or mental effort across practice?
- Attention: Does the learner require less attention to perform the motor skill?
- Adaptability: Can the learner adapt to changing environments or conditions with increased motor skill proficiency?

Performance Improvement

The most intuitive behavioral characteristic of learning a motor skill is **performance improvement**, which is defined as an overall increase in the performance outcome. Consider the discussion of performance and learning in chapter 1. Performance is the act of executing a motor skill at a particular time. Learning is the result of *permanent* changes, whereas performance is a temporary, *nonpermanent* change. Performance is observable, whereas learning is a construct. We can assume that someone has learned only after monitoring performance changes over a period of time.

Performance improvement is the most common indicator of learning simply because it is the most obvious. We make inferences every day based on our observations; for example, we look for signs of a person's mood in his face. People often assume that someone is in a good mood because he is smiling, even though he may actually be sad or angry and smiling to hide his true feelings.

Although performance measures do not necessarily indicate motor learning at any particular point in time, assessing performance provides a good indicator of learning if it occurs across an extended period of time and the results are combined with other factors, such as consistency, persistence, and coordination stability. Depending on the performance measure, improvement may be marked by a decrease, as with error or speed. It is often assumed (although sometimes incorrectly) that people have learned when they exhibit significant performance gains. To assess whether motor learning has occurred, however, one must assess performance following a break in practice.

Improved performance may also result from the acquisition of bad habits. Learners can adopt bad habits when they are focusing on the outcome or product of the movement as opposed to the coordination patterns involved in moving skillfully. For example, when learning how to throw the discus, athletes must learn some movements that may feel unnatural to them until they become proficient. They must learn the rhythm of the throw, how to turn the lower body in a whipping motion with a relaxed upper body and with the lower body trailing. They must also keep their heels off the ground throughout the movement. It is important to note that, as with all motor skills, the precise technique and style of the throwing pattern is unique to every thrower, based on individual structural and functional constraints. Novices who are learning the throwing pattern may have a tendency to tighten the upper body, which initially may allow them to throw farther because of the increased power behind the throw; but ultimately, this movement will prevent them from reaching their full potential. The more they practice this incorrect throwing pattern, the more difficulty they will have developing proper technique. A similar problem could result from continuing practice when ill or fatigued.

Because humans are competitive by nature, practitioners should eliminate movement outcomes when teaching novices the basic movement patterns. This will help prevent them from adopting unorthodox movement patterns, or bad habits. To prevent a thrower from focusing on the outcome of her throw, such as the distance the object traveled, a practitioner could have her throw into a net. Basketball players could take practice shots on

Exercise 5.1

Refer to the Performance Improvement section.

1. Name one of the bad habits of the novice discus thrower in the text example.
2. Explain why this habit was bad and needed to be overcome.
3. Have you ever learned a bad habit that you had to later overcome to move more proficiently? Explain what the bad habit was and how you overcame it.
4. How long did it take you to eliminate the bad habit and move more proficiently?

the wall, so they are focused on their form and not on whether they made the shot. Avoiding the formation of a bad habit is important, because, once formed, it can be very challenging to overcome. Using dynamic systems terminology (see chapter 3), bad habits result when the individual becomes trapped in a very deep and stable attractor state that has enabled the person to perform at an adequate level, even though other, more effective states should be found.

Performance Curves

Practitioners need to not only evaluate learners' progress through subjective evaluations, but also obtain and record objective performance measures over time. When deciding to quantify performance, the practitioner must first choose a performance measure that would be most appropriate to record. This decision is completely task dependent and may be driven by the resources available. For quantifying many motor skills, a measure of performance magnitude may be most appropriate, such as the distance of a throw, the height of a high jump, or the amount of weight benched. Error is a good performance measure for motor skills in which the objective is accuracy. Instructors who have access to more technology may be interested in quantifying the kinematics of the movement—for example, by measuring joint angle changes using high-speed video

cameras and motion detectors. To assess the amount of effort required to perform the task, measuring heart rates throughout the performance may be useful. By quantifying performance, instructors can document performance changes over time and examine the effectiveness of their instructional techniques or strategies.

Performance curves can be generated by collecting a performance measure across a period of time—for instance, the number of catches made each day in juggling or the number of foul shots made in each practice session. Figure 5.1 illustrates the maximal distance jumped per week for a long jumper. The distance jumped in feet is plotted on the y axis, and the weeks are plotted on the x axis. This allows the performer and instructor to see the gradual progress across the season.

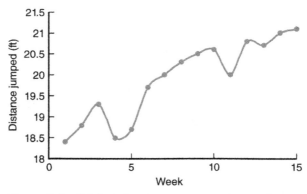

Figure 5.1 Fabricated performance curve of mean distance jumped in the long jump per week across 15 weeks.

Types of Performance Curves

There are four main types of performance curves (see figure 5.2). The most common, known as the **negatively accelerating curve**, illustrates a very rapid initial rate of improvement followed by a gradual reduction in the rate of improvement. This rate of change is so common that it has been assigned a mathematical law known as the **power law of practice** (Newell & Rosenbloom, 1981; Snoddy, 1926). Negatively accelerating curves are common because performance gains occur much more rapidly during early practice when a learner is essentially starting a motor skill from scratch. Initially, the learner experiences rapid improvements because there is much room for improvement; however, this rate of improvement is impossible to maintain. As the learner continues practicing, the room for improvement decreases, and further improvement becomes increasingly difficult to obtain.

A **positively accelerating curve** is illustrated by small initial gains, but this rate of improvement increases with every practice session. Learners may exhibit a positively accelerating curve when performing a challenging task such as juggling. Initially, learners may have difficulty improving, making only two to four catches per attempt. At some point, the learner will figure out the task and experience rapid gains in improvement. A **linear curve** indicates that there is a direct relationship between the performance measure and time. A perfectly linear curve would be found for someone who shows the same gain in performance with every practice session or performance attempt. For example, a juggler makes one

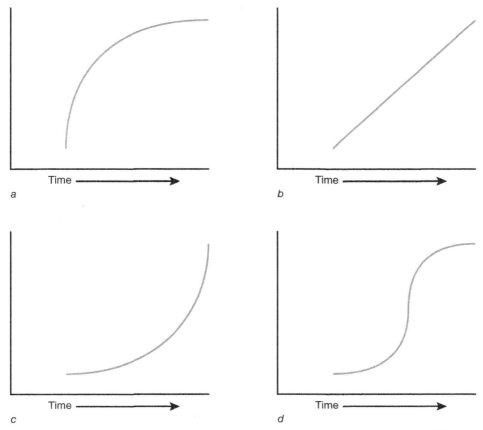

Figure 5.2 Performance curves: *(a)* negatively accelerating, *(b)* linear, *(c)* positively accelerating, and *(d)* S-shaped.

Checkmate!

Many studies have exhibited the power law of practice; however, the generality of the power law of practice to complex skills has been in question (Howard, 2014). To address this, the power law's generality was examined over the development of a complex task, chess playing, over a period of 27 years among 387 participants, most of whom became grandmasters at some point during this time. The objective of the study was to examine performance based on the amount of practice. Typically, practice is defined as actually performing a task. For this study, however, practice was considered playing Fédération Internationale des Échecs (FIDE)–rated games. FIDE-rated games are internationally rated chess games. Players increase their rating by defeating a player of higher ranking, but can lose their rating when losing points. A FIDE rating is considered reliable after 25 games. The results revealed that the power law of practice was found for group data, but not for individual data, meaning that the power law was only found when the results were averaged across all individuals. This is likely due to the high variability across the skill level of the participants. When examining individual data, there was an effect for skill level. The higher-skilled chess players improved with the power law; however, the lower-skilled players did not. It is possible that the results did not follow the power law of practice for all participants because of the complexity of the game of chess. Complex skills may develop on different time scales (Newell, Liu, & Mayer-Kress, 2006), and learning curves may vary across skills and individuals, such as in learning how to juggle (Haibach, Daniels, & Newell, 2004).

catch on day 1, two catches on day 2, three catches on day 3, and so on. This juggler improves at the same rate every day. On average, a person following a linear curve performs proportionately better each week. Finally, the **S-shaped curve** combines the rates of improvement found in the positively and negatively shaped curves. The learner initially takes some time to learn the motor skill. After a period of time, the learner experiences an "aha" moment and can perform the movement pattern much more successfully, similar to the positively accelerating curve. Performance then follows a gradual decline in the rate of improvement, similar to the negatively accelerating curve.

Keep in mind that the direction of the performance curve depends on the performance variable being measured. A thrower would be concerned with *increasing* the distance of the throw, but a sprinter would be concerned with *decreasing* the duration of the sprint. In the latter case, the performance curve would illustrate a downward trend. The same would be expected for a target shooter who is measuring error.

Limitations of Performance Curves

Although performance curves are a very useful objective method of measuring and assessing performance, it is important to understand that performance curves represent only temporary effects. Because performance does not always indicate that learning has occurred, assessing learning through performance curves may falsely imply that someone has learned, even if the effects are not permanent. Performance curves may also mask learning effects when there are no observable performance changes but the learner has gained some learning. For example, if several people are learning to juggle, some may progress very rapidly, some may progress slowly at first, and others may not ever show observable improvements. Those who are still averaging only two or three catches per attempt in juggling after many practice sessions may have learned the overall movement pattern of the hands in relation to the balls, or a better technique to toss the balls through trial and error and observation, or both, even though their performance does not illustrate such learning. These people may have poorer eye–hand coordination, which would make the motor skill more challenging for them. They have gained some learning even though their performance curves are flat.

Performance curves also provide only a limited perspective. For example, when averaging across participants, individual trends are often lost. An averaged performance curve may indicate that participants have learned a motor skill very quickly, when only one person may have learned very quickly while the others showed a very small amount of improvement. Figure 5.3a shows a performance graph of the performances for four jugglers across 10 practice sessions. Juggler 1 progressed very quickly, whereas jugglers 2, 3, and 4 progressed at a much slower rate (and none of these three performed at nearly as high a level as juggler 1). It is difficult to even notice that juggler 4 became proficient with cascade juggling, averaging 15 catches by practice session 10. Although juggler 4's score doesn't com-

pare to 250 catches, it does show that the juggler has acquired the basic coordination pattern of this complex motor skill. Examining figure 5.3a, we may infer that only one juggler learned the motor skill of juggling. Now take a look at figure 5.3b, which exhibits the mean performance across the four jugglers. If we examined only figure 5.3b, it would appear that all jugglers most likely learned cascade juggling because the rates of learning are lost when performances are averaged across participants.

There are also limitations to averaging across trials for an individual's data. A graph that depicts only the average performance per session, as in figure 5.3a, does not provide any information about the consistency of an individual's performance. The consistency of an individual's performance provides important information regarding the learning process. As discussed in chapter 4, learners in the cognitive stage are inconsistent in comparison to learners in the associative and autonomous stages. Analyzing individual trials can also provide information regarding the effects of a warm-up decrement. A **warm-up decrement** is a reduction in performance as a result of a period of inactivity. These effects are generally short in duration. It is important to assess the amount of performance that is generally lost as a result of the warm-up decrement and the length of time or number of attempts required to overcome the

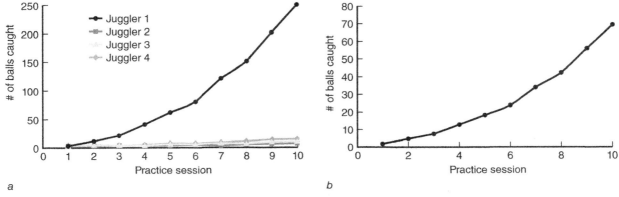

Figure 5.3 Performance curves: *(a)* individual performance curves for four jugglers and *(b)* mean performance across the four jugglers.

warm-up decrement. This can be valuable information when people are preparing for a competition or event.

Consistency

The consistency of performance is another important indicator of motor skill learning. A consistent performer is capable of sustaining a higher level of performance over time. Although it is often assumed that consistency implies learning, this is not always the case. Let's refer back to the definition of motor learning. Motor learning has been defined as the relatively permanent change in the learner's capability to execute a motor skill as a result of practice. Although the performance appears permanent because it is consistent, instructors must be careful not to use this as the only measure of motor learning. This is because it does not necessarily mean that the motor skill has actually been learned.

The consistency of a movement pattern from the dynamic systems perspective indicates the stability of the movement pattern—in other words, the depth of the attractor well. Again, it is possible that the learner has adopted a bad habit and is consistently performing less skillfully because she has become trapped in a strong attractor state. Sometimes these attractor states can become *too* stable, making it very difficult to change a movement pattern. At this point, it is best for the instructor to force the learner out of the stable pattern. It will take time for the learner to become consistent with the new movement pattern; however, it is better to be inconsistently producing the desirable movement pattern than consistently performing the flawed movement pattern. Learners may feel uncomfortable producing a new movement pattern for a while, but it is important to encourage them to continue pushing through this potentially awkward stage. For example, body posture is a very important element in ballroom dance, and many dancers have poor body postures such as curved shoulders or a forward head position. The more a ball-room dancer has practiced with these bad habits, the more challenging they are to overcome. It is easy for dancers to focus on the steps and forget about maintaining their posture. When they are focusing on maintaining their posture, they are likely to mess up their steps or make some other errors. Over time, the bad habit will be eliminated without detriment to the overall performance.

Persistence

Learning can also be measured by increased persistence in the performance of a motor skill. With practice, the learner will be able to perform following longer and longer durations of time without practice, as reflected in the saying *It's like learning to ride a bike*. When initially learning a motor skill, people need to practice regularly; however, with increased practice, skill proficiency is maintained for longer periods of time, extending from days and weeks to months and even years. Of course, some losses can be expected as a result of forgetting or undergoing physical changes over time, but a sustained relative permanency should be present. This performance characteristic is central to the definition of motor learning (a relatively *permanent* change in the capability to perform a motor skill).

Effort

Another method of measuring performance or learning changes is by assessing effort. Experts perform challenging feats effortlessly. BMX bikers can complete phenomenal jumps; outfielders can leap into the air to make amazing catches; and dancers can complete incredible lifts in what appear to be effortless, seamless movements. Novice performers, on the other hand, can expend a lot of mental and physical effort to perform just a simple version of the coordination pattern. Many learners expend a great deal of energy producing an inefficient movement pattern because they have not learned the

---

RESEARCH NOTES

Improving With Less Energy Requirements in Racewalking

To examine energy expenditures and perceived exertion when learning a new motor skill, researchers had seven participants engage in seven racewalking learning sessions on a motorized treadmill (Majed, Heugas, Chamon, & Siegler, 2012). Racewalking was chosen because it demands a lot of energy and is biomechanically constrained. Throughout the practice sessions, the speed of the treadmill was increased until the goal of a performance speed of 10 km/h (6.3 mph) was reached. With practice, a reorganization of the movement patterns resulted in the racewalkers walking with progressively less variability across the practice sessions. These changes continued through the fourth practice session; however, improvements in energy expenditures and perceived exertion occurred throughout all of the practice sessions. The authors suggested that the trend of less energy expenditures occurred concurrently with a reorganization of the movement patterns.

---

correct muscles to activate, or the correct sequence for activating the muscles, or both. This causes them to exert much more effort than necessary to perform the task. Learners can become quickly fatigued and frustrated through this process.

Novice swimmers, young and old, initially keep the body in a more vertical position, which is very inefficient for swimming yet seemingly more comfortable for the inexperienced swimmer. This vertical positioning forces the swimmer to expend much energy to produce little if any forward propulsion. This can lead to frustration, and in an attempt to increase forward propulsion, the swimmer will kick harder and use more arm motion. He exerts a great deal of effort but only tires himself out without gaining much forward motion, which frustrates him even more. With practice, swimmers become increasingly comfortable in the water, and their body positions gradually become more horizontal. This change enables them to produce more fluid motions with less overall energy expended.

Attention

The amount of conscious attention required to perform a motor skill decreases significantly with practice and skill level. Novices

require focused attention on the overall mechanics of the movement. Because they are so focused on the coordination patterns of producing the movement, they cannot attend to game-playing strategies. Instead, they are focused on the technical components of the movement. With the development of skill, the learners attend to the specifics of the movement pattern less and less. If they practice long enough to reach the autonomous stage, they can perform the skill with essentially no conscious attention devoted to the production of the movement pattern. This is termed **automaticity**. The following are the primary criteria of automaticity: (a) No processing capacity is required for the task; (b) the task is performed independently or without the performer's intentional control (involuntarily); and (c) the movement is not produced with consciousness or introspection (Neumann, 1984).

Because novices cannot perform the movement pattern efficiently and require much conscious attention when performing, their movements appear deliberate and choppy. Not only can experts produce the movement fluidly, but also their attentional resources are freed up, allowing them to focus on strategic elements of the game or task. For instance, a skilled soccer player does not have to focus on foot position and ball control; instead she can focus on the positions of teammates and defenders as well as on strategies and game plays. By attending to these other game elements, the soccer player can respond quickly to changing environmental conditions.

Once automaticity is achieved, attention to the production of the movement pattern can have a negative impact on performance. Attention directed toward the production of a well-learned performance may interfere with the processes that have become automatic in a skilled performer, disrupting the production of the skilled movement (Beilock, Bertenthal, McCoy, & Carr, 2004). Skilled performance is unconsciously controlled (Anderson, 1993; Fitts & Posner, 1967), whereas novice performances are produced with a focus on declarative knowledge and the production of the coordination patterns. Drawing attention to the production of the movement pattern distracts an expert, disrupting the skillful performance. This may also explain why some skilled athletes choke under pressure. They may be able to perform very skillfully under most conditions, but under intense pressure they may shift their attention to the production of the movement, which distracts them just enough to degrade their performances.

Adaptability

Another method of assessing performance is to measure adaptability. **Adaptability** is the ability to make movement adjustments to fit the changing demands of the task and environmental conditions. The adaptability required for a particular movement is situation and skill dependent. For example, the catching ability of an outfielder will likely extend to catching other objects besides baseballs. A tennis player's experience with striking a ball with a racket will increase her ability to play other racket sports. Adaptability is especially critical for open skills, which test people's ability to adapt to constantly changing environmental demands, such as returning the ball with a forehand or backhand, at various positions on the court, with variable force, or some combination of these. Although closed skills do not require split-second adjustments necessarily, performers need to be adaptable in closed skills because every movement is variable. There are always at least some changes in the environment, the context of the movement itself (individual constraints), or the task.

People become increasingly adaptable with increased motor skill proficiency. The reason is that they are now comfort-

TRY THIS

Can You Multitask?

Exercise 5.2

We do many activities without thinking, such as walking, taking a shower, and locking the door. You are probably also capable of doing some skillful activities automatically, such as typing on a keyboard, throwing a ball, or riding a bicycle. If you are a skilled typist, try typing while paying more attention to exactly what you're typing. It is likely that when you attended to your typing, you slowed down. Even breathing rate can be altered by focusing on breathing. Try counting your breaths. Did you feel as though you were controlling your breathing rate? Do you think you may have slowed down or sped up your breathing rate?

On the other hand, the benefit of performing a motor skill with little attention is that you can focus on other things; for example, you can talk while you are walking. What are some other examples of activities you can perform along with another functional task (i.e., multitasking)? Provide some sport-related examples.

able with the movement pattern and are no longer required to focus on internal processes. They can alter their strategies for changing weather conditions, plays, or stressors such as the importance of a game or situation.

Performance and Learning Tests

Performance curves can provide a means to evaluate changes in performance measures over time. A simple method of measuring performance changes is to compare performance on a **pretest** (conducted prior to the practice session) with that on a **posttest** (conducted at the end of the practice session). This allows inferences of learning, but does not reveal the persistence of the improved performance (i.e., retention). To assess the persistent capability to perform a motor skill, a retention test must be administered. A **retention test** is given following a break from practice. It allows the practitioner to determine whether the change in skill level is temporary (performance) or permanent (learning). Effects that are temporary are unlikely to be reproduced following the **retention interval** (the amount of time between the last practice session or posttest and the retention test). The appropriate length of the retention interval depends on the duration and complexity of the motor skill and how often the motor skill is practiced. A motor skill that is practiced regularly, such as every day or even multiple times per day, could be assessed following a retention interval of only a day

or two. A motor skill that is practiced less frequently will require a longer retention interval for adequate assessment of persistence.

It is important to understand the difference between learning and retention. Measures of performance during the acquisition phase allow inferences about learning, such as the mechanics, processes, and outcomes of learning (Rose & Christina, 2006). Measures of performance following a retention interval allow practitioners to make inferences about remembering and forgetting processes by assessing what was maintained or lost following the retention interval.

Another test that examines the permanence of motor skill acquisition is a transfer test. The difference between a transfer test and a retention test is that a retention test assesses performance on the same task following the break, whereas a transfer test assesses performance on a similar, but different task following the break. **Transfer tests** measure the adaptability from the experience of one motor skill to a novel, related motor skill or performance situation. For example, a transfer test could examine how the experience of snowboarding in the winter affects wakeboarding performance in the summer. A retention test would simply examine the person's snowboarding performance following a retention interval, but a transfer test would measure the performance on a similar motor skill (wakeboarding) following the retention interval. Table 5.1 provides a breakdown of the types of performance and learning tests.

Table 5.1 Performance and Learning Tests

Type of test	Definition	Measurement
Pretest	Test prior to practice of a motor skill	
Posttest	Test following practice of a motor skill	Performance (may or may not reveal learning)
Retention	Test following a retention interval; conditions are the same as in acquisition	Retention (remembering and forgetting)
Transfer	Test following a retention interval; conditions are different from but also similar to those in acquisition	Adaptability

Measuring Retention

The simplest way to measure retention is to measure **absolute retention**—that is, the learner's performance immediately following the retention interval. This value is limited and does not provide information about how the learner did in comparison to prior performance levels.

Two other basic methods of measuring retention provide a comparative measure relative to performance during the original learning period. There are two main types of relative retention. The first is the difference score. To calculate the **difference score**, subtract the absolute retention score from the last score during the acquisition phase (original learning). This score is the change in performance following the retention interval. It represents the amount of performance that was lost during the break. This score is somewhat limited because it does not reveal how much was lost relative to the change in the original learning. The **percentage score**, the most informative measure of retention, represents the percentage of performance that was lost (or gained) following the retention interval. To calculate the percentage score, divide the difference score by the change in original learning and then multiply by 100 percent. To calculate the change in original learning, subtract the performance on the first session (or trial) from the performance on the last session (or trial) of the original learning trials. In the pursuit rotor example in figure 5.4, the participant is timed on how long he can track the movement. In this example, the absolute retention is 60 seconds because the learner's time on target was 60 seconds during the first trial following the retention interval of one week. To calculate the difference score (40 seconds), the absolute score (60 seconds) was subtracted from the last score of the original session (100 seconds). To calculate the percentage score, the difference score (40 seconds) was divided by the change in original learning (100 seconds – 30 seconds) and multiplied by 100 percent. The percentage score is calculated as 57.14 percent, which can be interpreted to mean that 57.14 percent of the original improvement was lost over the retention interval, or conversely, 42.86 percent was retained.

Another useful retention measure is the **retention savings score**, which reflects how much time is required to return to the same level of performance as compared to the time required to reach this level during the original practice sessions (see figure 5.4). During the original sessions, the learner took 10 sessions to reach a peak of 100 seconds. However, following the retention interval, the learner reached this same level in only three practice sessions. The retention savings score is the difference between these two values, so seven sessions were saved in reaching the

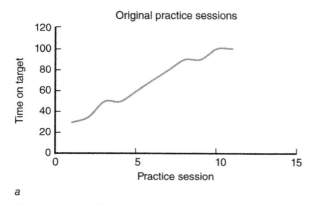

a

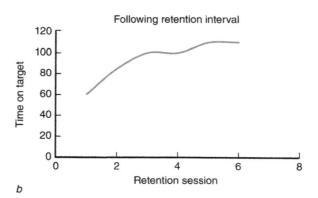

b

Figure 5.4   *(a)* Time on target was measured across 11 sessions. The goal of the task was to stay on target for as long as possible. *(b)* Following 11 sessions, the learner took one week off (retention interval) and then practiced for an additional six sessions.

WHAT DO YOU THINK?

Exercise 5.3

The data shown in this exercise are from a patient undergoing active rehabilitation of an injured rotator cuff. The main goal of the rehabilitation is to increase the patient's range of motion. The patient began physical therapy immediately following the injury. The original data are from the first three months of physical therapy. The patient then traveled for two weeks (retention interval) and returned to physical therapy.

1. What is the absolute retention value?
2. Calculate the difference score.
3. Calculate the percentage score.
4. Calculate the retention savings score.
5. Interpret the results.

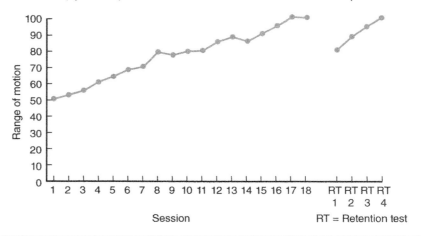

Types of Transfer

Previous movement experiences influence the ability to perform a new motor skill. This is referred to as **transfer of learning**. The three types of transfer are positive, negative, and zero; the type depends on the direction of the transfer.

Positive transfer occurs when the learning of a previous motor skill enhances the performance of another motor skill. You may have experienced positive transfer if you were experienced with one racket sport and then tried to play a new racket sport. A tennis player will likely experience an advantage when learning how to play racquetball because of the similarities in contacting a ball with a racket. Positive transfer generally occurs only in beginners to a sport or activity.

When a previous movement experience hinders performance, **negative transfer** has occurred. Players who switch from baseball to softball can experience negative transfer because of the differences in tracking the ball following the pitch. In baseball, the ball is released high and then moves down because it is pitched overhand; in softball, pitchers use an underhand pitch, causing the ball to approach the plate from a low-to-high position (Coker, 2013). This previous experience could cause temporary negative transfer with batting when the player switches from softball back to baseball.

When the previous movement experience does not change performance, then **zero transfer** has occurred. This happens when the two motor skills are unrelated, such as hurdling and fencing, or punting in American football and the backstroke in swimming.

Practitioners should be aware of learners' previous movement experiences because initial poor performance may be caused by negative transfer from prior experience in a similar skill. Luckily, when negative transfer does occur, as in batting in softball after prior experience with batting in baseball,

same level of performance following the retention interval.

RESEARCH NOTES

Does Cascade Juggling Transfer to Bounce Juggling?

A research group investigated the transfer effects of cascade juggling experience (the typical figure-eight pattern of juggling in which the balls are tossed up in the air) on learning bounce juggling (in which the ball is bounced on the floor rather than thrown in the air) (Bebko, Demark, Im-Bolter, & MacKewn, 2005). Four experienced cascade jugglers and five novice jugglers learned to bounce juggle for a period of five weeks. The experienced jugglers had an initial advantage of approximately seven days over the novice jugglers at the start of the study, and by the end of the study, they were about 10 days ahead of the novice jugglers. The lag in the novice jugglers' performances was not the result of not performing well or not acquiring the task of bounce juggling, since each was able to make at least 20 consecutive catches by the end of the practice sessions. Instead, it appears that previous cascade juggling experience provided positive transfer to bounce juggling, enabling the experienced jugglers to pick up the skill of bounce juggling faster and improve further than the novice jugglers did.

---

it is generally temporary. On the other hand, learners often capitalize on previous movement experiences that provide positive transfer. In general, most transfer effects are small and positive. The more movement experiences people have, the more likely they are to pick up new motor skills quickly.

Some of the strongest evidence for the persistence of negative transfer is found when learning a second language (Asher, 1964; Figueredo, 2006). The production of speech sounds necessary for speaking a particular language strongly influences how the person will produce the speech sounds for another language. This is why German and Chinese natives have very different accents in English. The negative transfer is causing nonnative speakers to have difficulty pronouncing certain sounds. For example, native Japanese speakers confuse the letter *l* with the letter *r*, so they often pronounce *salary* as *sarary* (Cook, 1997). French speakers have difficulty pronouncing *h*, saying *ouse* for *house* (Morris, 2001). These accents are so persistent that it is generally easy to determine the nationality of speakers simply from hearing their pronunciations. People who learn a second language can spend years or even decades speaking it while being immersed in the newer culture but still maintain their very distinct accents.

Transfer Tests

Sometimes practitioners want to assess the performer's adaptability of a motor skill. The ability to adapt quickly to unpredictable changes in the environment is especially important when performing open skills. Transfer tests (a method of assessing adaptability) are very similar to retention tests; however, rather than assessing performance on the same motor skill, they assess performance on a similar skill or a variation of the same skill following the retention interval. Examples are examining performance at different positions for a soccer player, such as playing midfield, defender, or forward, or learning to throw a different pitch in baseball. Transfer tests could also examine performance in an entirely new but similar sport, such as a learner who played racquetball for several months and then was tested on squash. Both are racket sports played inside a court with four walls and a ceiling. The main difference between the two is the size and elasticity of the balls and

WHAT DO YOU THINK?

Exercise 5.4

1. Choose a motor skill and then identify a different motor skill that you would expect to do the following:
   a. Cause positive transfer to that motor skill.
   b. Cause negative transfer to that motor skill.
   c. Produce zero transfer to that motor skill.
2. Explain why you chose each skill.
3. Explain how you could reduce or eliminate the effects of negative transfer in your example.

rackets. Squash balls are much smaller and less bouncy than racquetballs. When switching from racquetball to squash, racquetball players are generally quite surprised to find that they must move to the ball because it is not going to bounce to them.

Practitioners often make context changes in transfer tests rather than assessing different sports or games. For instance, a regulatory condition that can vary in some activities is the surface, as in American football (grass or AstroTurf) or tennis (grass, clay, acrylic, or asphalt). Other regulatory conditions remain constant from location to location, such as the size of the field or court and the height and length of the net. A transfer test could assess tennis performance on a different surface. A transfer test could also assess performance under varying nonregulatory conditions, such as changing the importance of the situation. For instance, an athlete who is preparing for a competition should be tested while she is under increased emotional stress.

It is useful to assess performance with varying regulatory and nonregulatory conditions. This enables the practitioner to assess not only the adaptability of the learner, but also the stability of the performance. A learner should not be limited to performing skillfully during controlled conditions, but should be able to adapt to changing situations and environmental conditions. This is important not only in physical education classes and sport, but also in rehabilitation. The role of rehabilitation is to prepare patients to function outside of the rehabilitation clinic. Rehabilitation specialists design movement activities with the expectation that they will help the person produce functional movement patterns. For example, when treating stroke patients with hemiplegia (paralysis on one half of the body), specialists should have the patients practice moving the paralyzed leg with many repetitions and a focus on task-relevant movements that include problem solving (Forrester, Wheaton, & Luft, 2008). The movements should be generalizable to real-world environments by making them long lasting and meaningful in regard to gait function.

Movements practiced diagonally are very beneficial for moving in everyday life and in sports (Voss, Ionta, & Myers, 1985). This is because diagonal movements are commonly produced to avoid obstacles. Although diagonal limb patterns may be beneficial, they are not used often in rehabilitation because it is simply more convenient for specialists to manipulate the limbs in a supine or sitting position (Mount, 1996). It is always important when designing an activity either for a sporting drill or for rehabilitation to focus on the similarities between the tasks. Tasks must be very similar to produce positive transfer.

Transfer of Throwing Positions

Mount (1996) investigated the effect of transfer between throwing while sitting versus throwing while reclining. The task was to throw a dart to a target with a fixed elbow in an extended position. The prediction was that participants who practiced throwing the dart in one position would perform the skill in the same position better than those who practiced in a different position.

Forty right-handed female participants aged 20 to 34 participated in the study. The two conditions were sitting on a Balans chair and reclining on a table at a 45-degree angle. Participants were randomly separated into four groups: Control group 1 used the chair during both the practice and transfer sessions; control group 2 used the table during both sessions; experimental group 1 practiced with the chair and tested with the table; and experimental group 2 practiced with the table and tested with the chair. Participants practiced four sets of five throws. Following the practice session, participants were given a five-minute break before completing four sets of five throws for the test.

Negative transfer occurred between the two positional conditions even though the task was the same. Mount's interpretation was that this negative transfer occurred because of a strong linkage between the first position learned and the movement of the arm. When the participants then switched positions, they had to adjust to the new body position. These results indicate the importance of taking body position into consideration prior to practicing a motor skill to avoid bad habits resulting in prolonged learning periods and poorer performances.

Theories of Transfer

The **identical elements theory** asserts that the amount and direction of transfer depend on the number of identical elements between two motor skills (Thorndike, 1914). It would be expected, then, that transfer would occur if two motor skills involved similar equipment and movements, such as the example at the beginning of this chapter of the aspiring athletic trainer, Emily, learning how to tape different joints. Movements in board sports, such as snowboarding, wakeboarding, surfing, and skateboarding would be expected to transfer, whereas sports and games with similar strategies but very different movement patterns, such as American football and ultimate, would be expected to have zero transfer. Ultimate and American football are both outdoor sports played on a rectangular field with

two end zones. The object is to keep passing the ball or disc until it gets into the end zone. In both sports, play begins with two teams lined up opposite each other. One main difference between the two sports is that in ultimate, the players may not run.

Although the movement patterns necessary to throw and catch a disc versus a football are very different, there are many similarities in the strategies and conceptual aspects of the two sports. According to the **transfer-appropriate processing theory**, movements or games that require similar cognitive processing can positively transfer (Bransford, Franks, Morris, & Stein, 1979). Activities that require learners to engage in similar problem-solving strategies promote positive transfer. For instance, the strategy of faking an opponent is employed in many sports, such as basketball, hockey, and American football. A skilled basketball player will be much better at reading an opponent's intentions even in a different sport, such as hockey, than someone who has not had experiences with opponents, such as a gymnast or diver.

One common method of implementing transfer into instruction is to simplify the task using progressions; the expectation is that the simpler version will transfer to the more complex motor skill. For instance, preschoolers often first learn how to bat by using a tee. This allows them to learn the fundamental movement pattern without the temporal component of making contact with a moving ball, changing the motor skill from externally paced to self-paced. The spatial component of the motor skill is also less challenging because the ball is stationary, which changes the initiation of the skill to self-paced. Learners may then progress to batting a ball that is hung from a string, then a balloon or a large, light ball that is pitched, and finally a regular ball. It is expected that positive transfer occurs during each transition, enabling the child to learn how to bat quickly and safely. Skill progressions are often used for complex or activities that carry a risk of injury.

Games Classification for Promoting Transfer

Given the vast number of sporting activities, classification schemes are necessary to generalize similarities across games, thus increasing opportunities for positive transfer across games from the same classification. Physical educators do not have enough time to adequately teach all games, and they cannot offer an extensive variety of games. Also, students do not have enough time to become skillful in all activities. By classifying games, teachers can introduce one game from the classification group and then build on the students' understanding by adding a second game from the same classification. They can then compare and contrast the two games while also improving proficiency on similar skills (Werner & Almond, 1990).

A **game** is "any form of playful competition whose outcome is determined by physical skill, strategy or chance employed singly or in a combination" (Loy, 1968, p. 1). It is important to note from this definition that games arise out of play, are competitive, and require physical skill, strategy, or chance (Siedentop, 2012). Each game has its own defining set of rules and strategies. The rules that characterize the play of the game and how the game is won are the **primary rules** (Almond, 1986). Games can be modified to be developmentally appropriate. Rules that can be modified without changing the nature of the game are termed **secondary rules**. For example, National Basketball Association (NBA) regulations have extended the 3-point shot from 19 feet 9 inches (6 m) to 23 feet 6 inches (7.2 m). Changing this regulation has not changed the play of the game. However, it has made it more challenging for

WHAT DO YOU THINK?

Exercise 5.5

1. Provide some examples of games in which you have modified the secondary rules. What did you modify and why?

2. Choose a game and discuss how you could modify it for one of the following:

   a. An elderly person with some shoulder and wrist arthritis

   b. A child with a sensory impairment (such as a visual or hearing impairment)

   c. An elite athlete

professional basketball players to score a 3-point basket. Other secondary rules in basketball include the size of the ball (women vs. men), the 3-second zone rule, and the 10-second half-court rule.

Classifying games became popular in the 1970s and 1980s, providing instructors with a framework for a more balanced curriculum based on the tactics of the games (Hopper & Bell, 1999). A problem-solving theme was employed that used six criteria: the purpose of the game, the initiation of the game, the conclusion of the game, game play rules, skill requirements, and game scoring (see table 5.2). In this section, we discuss games using Thorpe,

Bunker, and Almond's (1986) games classification system. The five game categories are target games, in which the goal is accuracy (e.g., golf and archery); fielding and run-scoring games with the essential skills of throwing, striking, and receiving the ball (e.g., cricket and baseball); net and wall games, with the essential skills of striking and controlling the placement of the ball (e.g., tennis and volleyball); invasion games, which require sending away, retrieving, and retaining the ball (e.g., basketball and American football); and personal performance games, which are self-contests (e.g., track and field and gymnastics) (see table 5.3).

Table 5.2 Classification Scheme for Game Categories

	Purpose	Start of game	End of game	Rules	Skills	Scoring
Invasion	Invade the opposing team's territory and score points.	Players on one's own half of the field; play begins with players moving to the opponent's side.	A certain period of time has elapsed.	Include restrictions on body contact and ball handling.	Offensive skills and defensive skills.	Points scored by invading the other team's territory and scoring (shots, goals, touchdowns).
Net or wall	Keep the ball in play and outsmart the opponent by positioning the ball such that it cannot be returned.	One player serves the ball either across a net or at a wall.	A certain score has been achieved by one team.	Include contact with the net and boundary and serving violations.	Accuracy and control of the ball.	Points are scored when the serving team prevents opponents from returning the serve or hits.
Target	Be the individual or team able to perform more accurately than the opponent(s).	One player or team initiates; then play occurs alternately from one side to the other.	All performers have had an equal number of attempts.	Regulate where and how the object is propelled and what defines accuracy.	Accuracy and control of the object.	Determined by a measure of accuracy.
Fielding	The batting team's aim is to score runs; the fielding team tries to get the batter out.	Opening pitch.	Each team has had a certain number of opportunities to score runs.	Include boundary restrictions on ball trajectory, batting, and pitching.	Temporal and spatial; fielding, catching, and throwing.	Number of runs.
Personal performance	Often a self-contest in which the performer competes alone, striving for peak performance.	Initiated by the performer or by an external stimulus (e.g., starter's gun).	All performers have completed the activity.	Regulate the movement type and equipment used.	Specific skills for each activity, which requires specific equipment.	Each performance is ranked after the performer completes the activity.

Adapted from Werner and Almond 1990.

Table 5.3 Sports for Each Games Classification System Category and Type

Category	Type and examples
Invasion	Focused target • Basketball • Lacrosse • Ice hockey • Field hockey • Soccer • Water polo
	Open end target • Ultimate • American Football • Rugby • Speedball
Net or wall	Divided court (net) • Volleyball • Tennis • Badminton • Table tennis
	Shared court (wall) • Racquetball • Handball • Squash
Target	Opposed • Croquet • Horseshoes • Shuffleboard
	Indirectly opposed • Archery • Bowling • Golf • Billiards
Fielding	Striking • Baseball • Cricket • Rounders • Softball
	Kicking • Kickball
Personal performance	Racing • Cycling • Track and field • Swimming
	Combative • Wrestling • Judo • Boxing
	Subjective performance • Gymnastics • Diving • X sports

Invasion Games

In **invasion games**, players are divided into two opposing teams separated by sides on the playing field. During the game, the teams invade each other's territory. Invasion games can be subdivided into games that have a focused target, such as basketball and soccer, and games in which a line must be crossed to score (open end target), such as American football and ultimate (Thorpe, Bunker, & Almond, 1986). The offensive goal of invasion games is to maintain possession of the ball and score, whereas the defensive objective is to obtain possession of the ball and defend the goal area to stop the other team from scoring. Taking the ball from the opponent serves two purposes: preventing the opponent from scoring and taking possession of the ball, thus giving the team a chance to score. Play is broken down into timed segments. Invasion games are won by the team with the higher score at the conclusion of a set time period. The final score indicates the team that was more successful at invading the opposing team's territory and scoring. These games have similar tactical problems; however, they differ in the task constraints imposed, including rules, equipment, and goals, as well as environmental regulations (e.g., terrain, weather, indoor vs. outdoor play).

Net or Wall Games

Net or wall games are games in which the object of play is to serve or return the ball strategically so that the opponent is unable to sustain the play of the ball. These games separate opposing players by a net, or may use a wall, and players alternate hitting. Players gain points each time they serve the ball and prevent their opponent from returning it. The contest ends when a certain number of points have been achieved by one player or team. One key component in skill proficiency in net or wall games is accuracy. The player must manipulate the speed and angle of the hit to control the ball position and the pace of the game. The ball must land within designated lines. Tactical understanding in net and wall games is to outsmart the opponent by placing shots where they cannot be returned, and the rules are geared toward boundary restrictions and serving. Most net and wall games use an implement to strike the ball (e.g., table tennis, badminton, racquetball); however, some require use of the hand (e.g., volleyball, handball).

Target Games

Target games include activities during which performers compete without direct body contact or physical confrontation. The main goal of target games is accuracy. During target games, competitors wait until the activity has been completed by other performers before beginning their attempts (e.g., golf, archery, billiards). The focus of target games is self-testing. The winner is generally the performer with the highest score (except in golf).

Fielding Games

Fielding games are team games in which the contest begins with one team occupying positions throughout the field (the fielders) or with one player who throws the ball (pitcher) toward a player on the opposing team. Examples of fielding sports are softball, baseball, rounders, cricket, and kickball. All fielding games use a striking implement except for kickball. Players score points for their team by running counterclockwise around bases when batting or kicking. The offensive team strikes the ball into the defensive team's territory. The defensive team fields, throws, and catches the ball in an effort to prevent the offensive team from scoring runs. Generally, fielding games have no time restrictions. Instead, each team has a set number of opportunities to bat or kick and score runs. The team with the most runs wins the contest.

Personal Performance Games

There are many games in which participants attempt to outperform their opponents, exceed their personal best performance measures, or both. **Personal performance games** include racing activities such as cycling, running, and swimming; combative activities such as wrestling, judo, and boxing; and games with subjective performance measures such as diving and gymnastics. In recent decades many new performance games have emerged that are often referred to as X games (e.g., snowboarding and BMX biking) because of their extreme nature. Each requires unique skills and equipment, in addition to much intrinsic motivation and drive, because the games challenge participants to compete not only against competitors but also against their own records.

Teaching Games for Transfer

When teaching games, the instructor should emphasize movement concepts, principles, and strategies that will transfer from one game to another in the same classification. Movement concepts are cognitive ideas, such as a particular pattern of movement (Rink, 1998). The concept of the overhand throwing pattern would be expected to transfer to some extent to throwing other implements (e.g., a javelin) or to performing an overhand serve. When teaching a movement concept, the instructor should focus on key action words that can transfer from one situation to another. When teaching learners how to strike, an instructor can provide many opportunities for striking an object, as well as focus on where to apply the force on the object and how this affects the trajectory. Learners should be able to apply the information learned from one experience (e.g., striking a ball with a bat) to another (e.g., striking a ball with a racket).

Movement skills can also transfer from one game to another in the same games classification. Movement tactics include stealing the ball in defensive play in invasion games and controlling the ball in net or wall games. Movement strategies—defined as how movement is used in cooperative and competitive relationships with others (Rink, 1998)—such as offensively faking defensive players to gain an advantage are similar in basketball and hockey. Zone defensives are similar for many invasion games as well. Movement concepts, tactics, and strategies transfer best when they are clearly explained and learners are given a wide array of opportunities to apply them.

Promoting Positive Transfer for Any Motor Skill

The first step in promoting positive transfer is to analyze the transfer task. A good practitioner analyzes skills when designing drills and activities. Positive transfer depends on the similarities between the two tasks. These similarities can be either in the fundamental movement pattern, as proposed by the identical elements theory, or in the strategies and concepts of the tasks, as asserted by the transfer-appropriate processing theory. Skills that involve striking have similar fundamental movement patterns. Someone who has experience with cricket will have an advantage in playing softball or baseball. Both skills have temporal and spatial elements. The bat must make contact with the ball at a specific time and position.

The strategic and conceptual components of the skills can also provide positive transfer. For instance, the fundamental movement patterns in kickball and baseball are very different and even require the use of different limbs. However, the strategies of the games are similar. In both, one team has possession of the ball (the fielding team) while the other team (the batting or kicking team) attempts to hit or kick it. Each side has a role that does not change until one team has acquired a certain number of outs. As noted earlier, games are classified according to similar strategies and concepts, so positive transfer would be expected for those who play multiple games in the same classification.

Knowing how to analyze motor skills effectively not only is important in designing practices, but also can assist in maximizing positive transfer based on the learners' past experiences. Learners understand new skills more quickly when comparisons are made with skills they are familiar with. For instance, baseball and cricket have a similar defensive component that occurs in parallel with the offensive component of scoring runs. In baseball, the batter defends the strike zone, whereas in cricket, the batsman defends the wicket. Highlighting the differences can be just as beneficial to learners as pointing out the similarities. Some of the many differences between cricket and baseball include the terminology for similar positions such as bowler versus pitcher, wicket-keeper versus catcher, and batsman versus batter. Another big difference between cricket and baseball is the batting stance. In cricket, the handle of the bat is held vertically with the end of the bat toward the ground; in baseball, the bat is held upward and cocked behind the head.

Comparing two motor skills or pointing out analogies between them can be helpful to learners. For example, when teaching how to swing a bat, an instructor can compare the lead arm position to that in throwing a disc. The back arm moves right through the movement with the elbow in, similar to the action of skipping a rock across a pond. The instructor must be sure that the learner has experience with the skill being compared to the new skill; if not, the comparison could be ineffective or even confuse the learner further.

Another factor that should be considered in promoting positive transfer is the learner's skill level. Novices gain more benefit from transfer than those at higher skill levels. For example, someone learning to play racquetball will gain more advantages from previous tennis experience than an experienced tennis player would from playing racquetball in the off-season. Learners in the associative or the autonomous stage benefit much less because they can produce the fundamental movement pattern and are now focusing on much more specific movements involved in the given motor skill. In these cases, some negative transfer may occur for higher-level players if the previous movement experiences alter some of their techniques.

Before incorporating progressions or drills into a practice design, practitioners should examine the cost–benefit trade-off. This requires assessing how much practice is necessary to obtain positive transfer. The amount of practice that the transfer group required to gain the initial advantage should also be taken into consideration. If more practice was required for the transfer task than for the primary task alone, then the cost would outweigh the benefit.

Summary

This chapter discussed how to measure and assess motor learning. The indicators of motor learning include consistency of performance, permanence of movement production, decreased effort, reduced attentional demands, and increased adaptability. Learners who have acquired the capability to perform a motor skill can consistently perform at a higher level. Their performance is also sustainable and permanent over long periods of time. Skilled learners can also perform the motor skill with less cognitive and physical effort than they could when they were initially learning the motor skill. They also need to devote less attention to the movement production, allowing them to focus on strategies rather than on producing the coordination pattern. Finally, improved performance can be measured by the adaptability of the learner, meaning that learners can perform similar and related motor skills at a higher level as a result of their experience with another task.

The true test of motor learning is sustained performance following a period away from regular practice, also known as a retention interval. Motor learning is a permanent change in the ability to produce a skilled movement; so if learners lose their ability to produce a particular movement pattern following the passage of time, the motor skill has not been learned. In this case, only performance (temporary) changes have occurred.

The chapter also discussed transfer of learning. Understanding transfer, including the types of transfer, how to measure transfer, and how to foster positive transfer, is of critical importance to practitioners in school, athletic, and rehabilitation settings. Educators in school settings must design activities that promote both the transfer and the retention of fundamental movement skills and sport-specific skills. Coaches must focus on drills that will positively transfer to the sport, preparing the athletes for competitive situations. Structuring the environment and the task so that they are as realistic as possible is critical for promoting transfer from the rehabilitation setting to patients' homes. The key points to take away about transfer are as follows:

- Transfer is generally small and positive.
- Transfer depends on the number of similarities between the two motor skills.
- Negative transfer is generally temporary.
- Previous movement experiences often provide some transfer.
- Most positive transfer effects are found in early acquisition.

ONLINE LEARNING

Visit the web resource at www.HumanKinetics.com/MotorLearningAndDevelopment for an accompanying lab activity and exercises from the chapter.

LEARNING AIDS

Supplemental Activities

1. Choose a motor skill that requires you to produce a movement pattern that you have not produced before (e.g., juggling, unicycling, speed stacking, standing on an exercise ball, Hacky Sack, handstand).
    a. Practice the skill every day for 10 days for a set period of time (e.g., five minutes per day). Record your performances every day.
    b. Following 10 days of practice, wait for a week (one-week retention interval) and then perform a retention test. Record your performance on the retention test.
    c. Make a performance curve exhibiting your performance changes across the 10-day practice sessions.
    d. What type of performance curve is this graph?
    e. Calculate your retention scores, including absolute retention, the difference score, the percentage score, and the retention savings score.
    f. Did you learn the motor skill?

2. Using the following chart, list all of the games you have participated in for each of the classifications.

    a. Count the number of games you have participated in under each classification and write the number in the "Number of games" row. Divide these numbers by the total number of games in all columns and multiply by 100 percent. Write these percentages in the percentage row.

    b. Do you participate in one classification of games more than the others? If yes, what in particular interests you about these games?

    c. Which categories have you avoided to some extent? Why do you think you have avoided activities in these categories?

	Invasion	Net or wall	Target	Fielding	Personal performance
Number of games					
Percentage					

From P.S. Haibach-Beach, G.W. Reid, and D.H. Collier, 2018, *Motor learning and development*, 2nd ed. (Champaign, IL: Human Kinetics).

Glossary

absolute retention—The learner's performance immediately following the retention interval.

adaptability—The ability to make movement adjustments to fit the changing demands of the task and environmental conditions.

automaticity—The ability to perform a skill with essentially no conscious attention devoted to the production of the movement pattern.

difference score—A measure of relative retention calculated by subtracting the absolute retention score from the last score during the acquisition phase (original learning).

fielding games—Team games in which the contest begins with one team occupying positions throughout the field (the fielders), with one player who throws the ball (pitcher) toward a player on the opposing team.

game—Any form of playful competition whose outcome is determined by physical skill, strategy, or chance, employed singly or in combination.

identical elements theory—A theory on transfer that asserts that the amount and direction of transfer depend on the number of identical elements between two motor skills.

invasion games—Games in which players are divided into two opposing teams separated by sides on the playing field.

linear curve—A performance curve that indicates a direct relationship between the performance measure and time.

negatively accelerating curve—A performance curve that illustrates a very rapid initial rate of improvement followed by a gradual reduction in the rate of improvement.

negative transfer—Interference of previous experience on the performance of another motor skill.

net or wall games—Games in which the object of play is to serve or return the ball strategically so that the opponent is unable to sustain the play of the ball.

percentage score—A measure of relative retention calculated by dividing the difference score by the change in the original learning and then multiplying by 100 percent. This score is interpreted as the percentage of performance that was lost (or gained) following the retention interval.

performance improvement—An increase in the overall performance outcome.

personal performance games—Games in which individuals attempt to outperform their opponents, their personal best performance measures, or both.

positively accelerating curve—A performance curve that illustrates only small gains initially but an increasing rate of improvement with every practice session.

positive transfer—Enhanced learning of a motor skill because of the performance of another motor skill.

posttest—A test conducted at the end of the practice sessions.

power law of practice—A mathematical law describing a negatively accelerating rate of performance improvement.

pretest—A test conducted prior to the practice sessions.

primary rules—The rules that characterize the play of the game and how the game is won.

retention interval—The amount of time between the last practice session or posttest and the retention test.

retention savings score—A measurement of the amount of time required to return to a given level of performance as compared to the time required to reach this level during the original practice sessions.

retention test—A performance test given following a break from practice.

secondary rules—Rules that can be modified without changing the nature of the game.

S-shaped curve—A performance curve indicating that initial learning occurred at a positively accelerating rate for a period of time and then continued to increase at a negatively accelerating rate.

target games—Games in which performers compete without direct body contact or physical confrontation.

transfer-appropriate processing theory—A theory on transfer asserting that movements or games requiring similar cognitive processing can positively transfer.

transfer of learning—The effect of a previous movement experience on performance in another task.

transfer tests—Tests that measure the adaptability between the practiced motor skill and a different, but related, motor skill or performance situation.

warm-up decrement—A reduction in performance as a result of a period of inactivity.

zero transfer—The lack of effect of a previous movement experience on performance in another task.

Life Span Physical Activity and Movement

Part II presents an overview of physical activity and movement changes across the life span. Part I addressed some of the basic principles, terminology, and theoretical approaches in motor behavior; this part expands on this knowledge with a focus on growth and development. The discussion begins in chapter 6, which examines the reflexive behavior and spontaneous movements present during infancy. In the first year, the infant advances through a series of motor milestones from holding the head up to sitting up to creeping and eventually walking, to name a few. Because the way and the time infants progress through these motor milestones vary greatly, this chapter addresses both typical and atypical development. Chapter 7 offers an extensive discussion of the fundamental movement skills that appear and are refined between the ages of two and six. The emphasis is on fundamental movement skills because they are essential to the healthy development of children in all domains. Practitioners need a solid understanding of how and when these fundamentals are achieved.

The developmental discussion then moves to the movement and physical activity of adults in chapter 8, from young to older adulthood. Also addressed are factors that affect adults' participation in physical activity. The exercise–aging cycle illustrates the detrimental effects of a sedentary lifestyle. Olympic and masters athletes' performances offer a window into how peak performance declines with advancing age, because performance changes in this demographic are less likely to be affected by chronic disease or long periods of physical inactivity and disuse. The chapter concludes with a summary of movement patterns in older adulthood, including locomotor patterns, fundamental movement patterns, and movements during functional activities.

INFANT MOTOR DEVELOPMENT

After reading this chapter, you should be able to do the following:

- Define the terms *neural plasticity* and *teratogens*.
- Identify healthy behaviors in pregnancy.
- Understand prenatal development and the factors that positively and negatively affect it.
- Explain the factors that interfere with early movements.
- Understand the important interactions of motor development, cognitive development, and affective development.
- Identify developmental disorders in infants.
- Appreciate how researchers and clinicians assess infant motor development.

That's Our Little Girl!

When Lauren was a newborn, her parents were tremendously excited—but more than a little nervous and apprehensive. She was so tiny and seemed to have trouble not only seeing things but maintaining any control over her body at all. They'd read a lot (as well as seen other newborns), but with Lauren lying beside them, this was a whole new level of awareness. However, over her first year of life, Lauren underwent a stunning transformation. She changed from being a dependent infant who struggled to maintain her balance (much less move around her environment) to a child who could locate a partially hidden toy in the corner of the room, trot right over (while avoiding the dog and dealing with the slippery floor), and smoothly and confidently grasp the item—and then put it in her pocket! How and at what point, and to what degree, these impressive perceptual and motor skills emerge during infancy is the focus of this chapter.

How developing infants move from a limited repertoire of motor behaviors to efficiently solving a vast number of movement tasks is becoming increasingly clear. This knowledge base is available to both scientists and practitioners as research tools (including, but not limited to, the ability to look deeply into the developing brain with precise imaging tools) become more and more advanced.

The development of motor skill in infancy has been answered historically from the vantage point of the maturation of the central nervous system (CNS; Gessell, 1946; McGraw, 1943; Shirley, 1931). Using a longitudinal approach (that is, observing an individual or group of individuals on multiple occasions over an extended period of time), these investigators were able to precisely catalog the appearance of phylogenetic movement skills common in developing children. Phylogenetic movement skills are those common to our species and, generally, are performed all over the world by people from all different cultures. Examples include walking, jumping, reaching, and grasping. These researchers assumed that the emerging skill set of the developing infant is tightly controlled by CNS maturation. Although this neuromaturational perspective of motor development continues to influence both scientific inquiry and clinical intervention, the theoretical approach referred to in this text as the dynamic systems approach moves away from the unicausal (the CNS) perspective of the neuromaturationists in explaining development. Instead of considering the brain, as interesting and important as it is, as the controller of development, proponents of this new approach believe that new and increasingly complex forms come from multiple developing subsystems that act within a specific physical and social context (Thelen, 1992). Thus, the quality of the emotional and physical environment is of great importance to optimizing development—motoric and otherwise.

Robust and varied early movement experiences in rich environments are crucial for healthy physical, cognitive, and affective development. Strongly related to the need for appropriate movement experiences is the important concept of **neural plasticity** (Sporns & Edelman, 1993), which posits that long-lasting, functional changes in the brain (primarily the neuronal pathways) are largely due to experience. Although this plasticity is present throughout the life span, it is particularly evident during infancy. This adaptive neural substrate changes based on not only novel, sustained experience, but also individual adaptation (e.g., disease, trauma, injury).

These research-based observations regarding neuroplasticity point to the need for rich early movement experiences for all infants—those who are typically developing and, maybe more important, those with identifiable disabilities. Unfortunately, vast inequities in many societies put infants at great risk. These risks are both intrinsic/genetic (such as having Down syndrome) and extrinsic/environmental (such as being exposed to cocaine prenatally or to lead-based paint as a toddler). Nutritional, movement-related, and linguistic inequities also abound. This chapter examines in some depth both the why and the when of infant development, for children who are typically developing and those who are at risk of having a developmental disability.

Prenatal Development

At birth, an infant has already gone through an incredible amount of growth in a very short period. Although prenatal growth and development may be taken for granted, it is important to understand the many changes that occur and how this period of growth provides critical building blocks for normal development after birth. Prenatal age, often referred to as **gestational age**, begins the first day after the mother's last menstrual period. It may be confusing that conceptual age is actually only 38 weeks because the gestational age begins two weeks prior to conception. Due dates are typically estimated as 40 weeks after the gestational age begins.

Prenatal development begins with the fertilization of the female egg (ovum) by the male sperm (spermatozoon). At this point, the 23 chromosomes from the father combine with the 23 chromosomes from the mother to form a new cell with 46 chromosomes. The first prenatal period is referred to as the **germinal period**, which lasts approximately two weeks. During this period, the fertilized ovum (zygote) migrates along the fallopian tube into the uterus, which it reaches in three to four days. Throughout this migration, the number of cells increases rapidly. By 9 to 12 days from fertilization, the mass of cells (blastocyst) embeds itself into the endometrium in the wall of the uterus.

The second stage, known as the **embryonic period**, lasts for approximately six weeks. During this very critical period, cells that make up organs are defined through a process known as **organogenesis**. At around week 3, the central nervous system is one of the first systems to develop, with the heart following shortly behind. Movement begins after the heart starts beating at a conceptual age of about four weeks. Other organs that develop during the embryonic stage include the limbs, eyes, ears, and palate. Around the end of the embryonic period, the embryo exhibits **myogenic movements**, which are not generated by the central nervous system or external stimulation.

The final stage of prenatal development is the **fetal period**, which begins at the completion of organ differentiation around week 8 and lasts until birth. During this period, the fetus continues to grow rapidly, and **neurogenic movements** appear at approximately 20 weeks postconception. Neurogenic movements are generated by the central nervous system. Exposure to environmental factors such as teratogens (discussed next) is less critical during the fetal stage because most of the major

organs have differentiated and as such are not as susceptible to functional defects and minor congenital anomalies.

Teratogens

Prenatal development is a precarious period during which the fetus is influenced by both extrinsic and intrinsic factors experienced by the mother. The mother's nutrients, or lack thereof, physical activities, and the external environment (e.g., pollutants) all influence the growing fetus. At critical time periods of embryonic and fetal development, exposure to a **teratogen** (any agent that can cause defects or deformities) can be particularly harmful. Development is most vulnerable during the embryonic period; exposure to teratogens at this time can be harmful to the developing organ(s). Before examining specific teratogens, we want to clarify the difference between genetic abnormalities and environmental causes of congenital disorders. Genetic abnormalities are not the result of the environment; rather, they often result from chromosomal abnormalities, such as phenylketonuria, the product of an abnormal recessive autosomal gene (Piek, 2006).

A pregnant woman should avoid many environmental substances and events to limit any harmful exposure to her child. The more obvious harmful substances are illegal drugs and cigarettes, but prescription medications should not be overlooked. A pregnant mom should discuss with her doctor both the risks of medications to her fetus and the risks to her of stopping any medication during the pregnancy. At times the risks to the mother from stopping a medication are greater than the risks to the fetus. Certain antidepressants increase the risk of developing heart defects, especially when taken during the first trimester. Antiepileptics increase the risk of neural tube defects, and antibiotics increase the risk of developing heart abnormalities (Lynch & Abel, 2015). In addition, pregestational diabetes

(diabetes that develops in the mother prior to pregnancy) is linked to congenital heart disease (CHD) when birth occurs when the mother's glycemic control is poor (Jenkins et al., 2007).

Cigarette smoking during pregnancy can cause intrauterine growth restriction, preterm birth (Robinson et al., 2000), and health problems in childhood including short stature and obesity. This prevalence increases with the number of cigarettes smoked daily (Koshy, Delpisheh, & Brabin, 2010). In addition to cigarette smoking, oxygen deprivation or exposure to other harmful events can cause embryonic or fetal damage, which is related to preterm birth. Infectious maternal diseases, such as rubella, syphilis, HIV, and AIDS can cause anything from minor congenital abnormalities to spontaneous abortions (Piek, 2006).

Experts widely accept that alcohol is a teratogen that can cause fetal alcohol syndrome. Fetal alcohol syndrome is considered the leading preventable cause of birth defects and intellectual disability. Although alcohol ingested during pregnancy is considered a teratogen, there is considerable confusion about the amount that is acceptable. As a result, many researchers suggest that the only safe amount of alcohol during pregnancy is no alcohol (Tracy, 2013).

Healthy Pregnancy

A pregnant woman must make many positive behavioral choices because her behavior affects not only her body, but also, even more directly, the growing fetus inside of her. Poor choices may have a profound effect on the areas currently developing in the fetus. In addition to avoiding teratogens, pregnant women must also eat well, including taking vitamins A, B_3, B_6, C, D, and folic acid, and maintain a physically active lifestyle throughout pregnancy.

To have a healthy pregnancy, a woman should have a healthy prepregnancy weight and gain weight appropriately throughout the pregnancy. Energy needs for a pregnant woman should be the same as her prepregnancy needs during the first trimester and should increase by 340 kcal and 452 kcal during the second and third trimesters, respectively. Physical activity should include either 150 minutes of moderate-intensity aerobic activity throughout the week or 30 minutes of moderate-intensity exercise most days of the week (Kaiser & Campbell, 2014).

Sensory Capabilities

The sensory capabilities of newborns have been widely studied; researchers have examined both the limitations and capabilities exhibited in this early period. The development of sensory capabilities during infancy greatly affects the child's movements and motor development. This section provides a brief description of vision, hearing, and proprioception from birth throughout infancy.

Vision

Although the visual system holds 70 percent of all sensory receptors, vision is the last sense to develop in infancy (Mercer, 1998). Structurally, the eye is completely intact at birth; however, all visual structures change following birth (Gabbard, 2011). The eye of a newborn is not smaller in overall size than the eye of an adult, but the depth is shorter and the distance between the retina and the lens is less, causing farsightedness (difficulty seeing close objects). The structure of the retina changes rapidly over the first year. Retinas in newborns are thicker and the foveae are not well formed, making it difficult for them to see images clearly (Gabbard, 2011). Infants also have difficulty focusing on objects (astigmatisms) as a result of their weaker ciliary muscles.

At birth, infants can perceive color, and newborns as young as two days old can distinguish form (Frantz, 1963). Previous to this research, many believed that new-

Exercise 6.1

Devise a list of teratogens, including some from the chapter and others not mentioned in the chapter. For each one, identify the potential effects on the fetus. Alcohol is provided as an example.

Teratogen	Effects
Alcohol	Birth defects, intellectual disability

Devise a list of healthy behaviors for pregnant woman. Do a web search to find some not mentioned in the chapter. An example has been provided.

Healthy behavior	Benefits
400 mcg of folic acid daily	Helps to prevent birth defects of the brain and spinal cord

borns several weeks or even months old did not have pattern vision. Infants can perceive depth around two to three months of age, but depth perception continues to improve throughout early childhood. Visual acuity slowly develops and improves across infancy and childhood beginning at around 20/400 at birth (Haywood & Getchell, 2014). This means that a newborn sees at 20 feet (6 m) approximately what someone with 20/20 vision can see at 400 feet (122 m).

What Can Infants Really See?

Examining vision capability in infants can be tricky. Clearly, they cannot respond verbally or explain what they can see. Thus, vision is often assessed by acclimating infants to visual scenes. The assumption is that spending more time gazing at one scene than at another indicates that they find it novel or interesting. Once infants have habituated to something, they will not gaze at it for very long. For example, to assess pattern vision, infants' length of gaze was examined for black and white patterns in comparison to plain colored surfaces. Infants two days old or older spend approximately twice as much time gazing at the patterns than at the plain surfaces (Frantz, 1963).

Hearing

Infants have acute hearing, which begins prior to birth (Piek, 2006). By birth, most of the ear structures are developed (Timiras, 1972), with the exception of the drum membrane, the ear canal, and the Eustachian tube. Infants can hear prior to and following birth and often turn their heads in the direction of sound. Infants under four months of age can differentiate both nonspeech sounds (Vouloumanos & Werker, 2004) and speech sounds (Eimas, 1975). By six months of age, infants can differentiate their native language from nonnative languages (Kuhl, Williams, Lacerda, Stevens, & Lindblom, 1992) and become increasingly interested in listening to their native language as they are beginning to understand that the sounds are associated with meaning.

Proprioception

Proprioception includes tactile, vestibular, and kinesthetic sensory information (Abernathy, Kippers, Mackinnon, Neal, & Hanrahan, 1996). Newborns have a highly developed sense of touch (Piek, 2006). It is also assumed that they can sense pain and temperature at least to some degree based on their responsiveness to medical procedures around the time of birth. The vestibular system, which is located in the inner ear, is one of the most highly developed systems in newborns (Carmichael,

1946). The vestibular system assists in maintaining equilibrium by providing information about head position and movement. Little is known, however, about kinesthetic sense because of the difficulty of measuring this sense in infants. Kinesthetic sense includes body and spatial awareness.

Early Movements

During the exciting and rapidly changing time of infancy, three relatively distinct types of movements occur. Although authors may use slightly different terminology, these movement types are (a) reflexive (some reflexes have been observed as early as the second or third month of fetal life until 4 months of age); (b) spontaneous, also referred to as rhythmical stereotypies (from 4 to 10 months of age, peaking between 6 and 10 months); and (c) voluntary (motor milestones), which appear and are generally refined between birth and 2 years of age.

Reflexive Movements

Reflexive movements (also called reflexive behaviors or reflexes) are thought to be automatic, involuntary responses to stimuli that are controlled at a subcortical level. That is, the higher brain centers are not involved in these movements. Generally, reflexive behaviors are broken down into three categories: primitive reflexes, postural reactions, and locomotor reflexes. It is hypothesized that **primitive reflexes** serve the functions of protection (e.g., the startle reflex) (see figure 6.1*a*) and securing nourishment (e.g., the sucking reflex) and disappear within a specific time frame. For example, the sucking reflex is present from birth to three months of age (see figure 6.1*b*). A particular reflex that is present beyond the typical point of disappearance may indicate an underlying neurological problem. **Postural reactions** (e.g., the parachute reflex) serve to automatically maintain the appropriate pos-

ture in a changing environment (Haywood & Getchell, 2014). The parachute reflex is an example of a postural reaction (see figure 6.1*c*). It is elicited when the infant is held in a vertical position and then suddenly lowered forward. The infant reacts by extending the arms and hands forward in a protective manner. **Locomotor reflexes** (e.g., the stepping reflex) are thought by some theorists (Thelen, 1995; Ulrich, Ulrich, & Collier, 1992) (see figure 6.1*d*) to be precursors to voluntary locomotion and serve, at some level, as practice for these later motor milestones. Reflexive behaviors are not voluntary but are critical to the

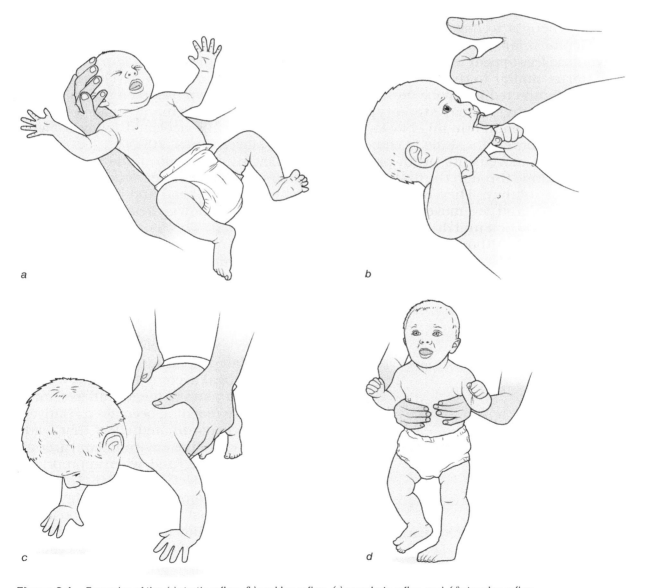

a

b

c

d

Figure 6.1   Examples of the *(a)* startle reflex, *(b)* sucking reflex, *(c)* parachute reflex, and *(d)* stepping reflex.

initial survival and later development of the infant.

Spontaneous Movements

Although less often discussed than the earlier reflexive movements and the exciting motor milestones to come, spontaneous movements (rhythmical stereotypies) are frequently exhibited and are of great importance to the developing infant (see figure 6.2). If you've ever watched an infant kick his legs rhythmically, thrust his arms into the air, or extend his fingers, you have observed spontaneous movements. Although they do not appear to be goal directed, these seemingly random movements are thought to have a purpose for the developing infant. These movements of the arms and legs appear to have coordination patterns similar to those of later voluntary, goal-directed behavior. Research suggests that rhythmical stereotypies could be fundamental building blocks for the voluntary movement skills to come.

Spontaneous movements begin prenatally and continue through the first couple of months of infancy. They are characterized by arm and leg movements that vary in both direction and duration (Hadders-Algra, 2000). Although limited variability in spontaneous movements might indicate a neurological deficit (Karch et al., 2012), the opposite holds true for voluntary, goal-directed movements. For these movements, reduced variation indicates good neurological function (Piek, 2002).

Voluntary (Goal-Directed) Movements

Early voluntary movement skills are the motor milestones that mothers and fathers look forward to with great anticipation. Although it is quite exciting for parents to see their infant sit up unassisted for the first time, it is even more exciting to see her take her first steps. These cortically controlled movements (contrasted with the subcortically controlled reflexes) follow a fairly predictable sequence, although people may vary widely in terms of when a given skill will appear. Figure 6.3 shows the normative order in development and has been redrawn based on seminal work that was published many decades ago and is still generally accepted today (Newell, Liu, & Mayer-Kress, 2003).

Following a cephalocaudal direction, in terms of movement development, infants first control the head and then the upper body, which allows them, over time, to sit unassisted. This is followed by independent standing as well as exploration of the environment through a variety of ambulatory patterns that include crawling, creeping, cruising, and walking. Development also takes place in a proximodistal direction, where control of the center of the body precedes control of more distant body parts. Relatedly, hand and arm control are also critical accomplishments; during the first two years of life, undifferentiated and reflexive reaching becomes a relatively smooth and coordinated effort that leads to exploration of the environment through reaching, grasping, and, when appropriate, releasing the object of interest. To attain these critical motor milestones, the developing infant must have adequate postural control. The following sections address the development of important motor milestones, including balance and stability.

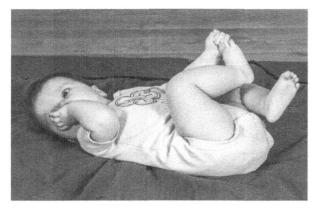

Figure 6.2 Early rhythmic behavior is demonstrated by an infant (approximately five months of age) kicking in a supine position.

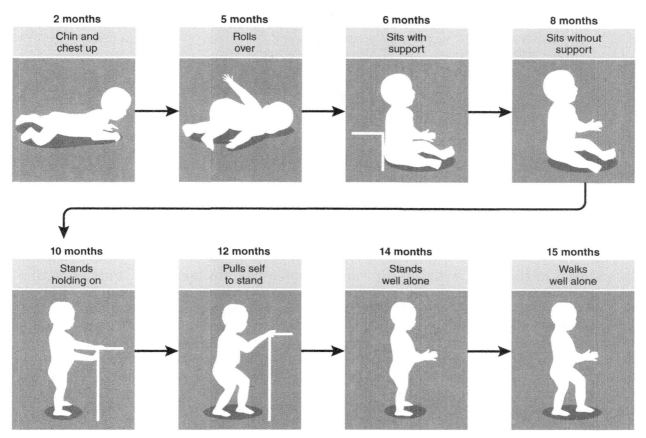

Figure 6.3 Infant motor milestone sequence.
Based on Shirley 1931.

Voluntary Head and Body Control

Although not frequently thought of as a motor milestone, adequate postural control of the head and trunk is fundamental to the attainment of an array of movement skills including, but not limited to, head control, sitting, standing, and a variety of locomotor patterns (crawling, creeping, cruising, and walking). With progressively more refined control of the body comes an improved ability to navigate and explore physical and social environments. Body control during infancy occurs sequentially, directionally, and cumulatively. This means that each movement is a building block to subsequent movements. As previously mentioned, development occurs in a cephalocaudal direction.

One of the first motor milestones to develop is the ability to lift the head while in a prone position. When considering the relatively large size of the infant's head in comparison to the body, one can appreciate the neck strength and coordination necessary to accomplish this task. An infant's head is approximately one fourth the size of the entire body. This is illustrated in figure 9.3 in chapter 9. Infants typically begin to lift the head while prone at around two months, but they cannot extend the neck while prone until three months. The ability to extend the neck enables the infant to visually scan the room, further advancing perceptual–motor development. It is not until approximately five months of age that an infant is able to raise the head while in a supine position (see figure 6.4).

The ability to control body movements continues to follow the cephalocaudal direction as the infant learns to control the upper body by first elevating the chest

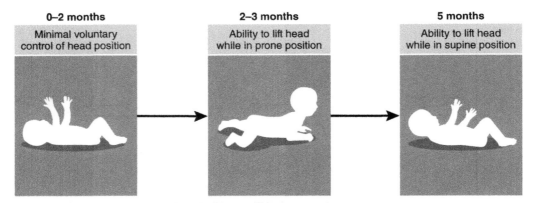

Figure 6.4 The typical progression of voluntary head control in early infancy.

in addition to the head while in a prone position. This further increases the ability to view the world in a different way, while also increasing strength and coordination in the arms and chest and preparing the infant for future locomotor patterns. Young infants use this arm control to roll from a supine to a prone position, setting themselves up for crawling. Early rolling is more of a reflexive movement, rather than a sign of advanced motor development. Controlled rolling isn't typical until around six months of age. At this point, most infants can only roll from supine to prone and not prone to supine, which is generally acquired by around eight months.

Infants can sit with assistance at around the age of three months. They generally have enough neck and head control to remain in a supported sitting position. At this time, because lumbar control is quite weak, they require additional support on the back and abdomen. Pillows have been developed to support young infants with sitting; however, if left alone, the infant may slide forward or sideways. Infants progress to being able to sit alone by holding something to support themselves at around five months and can sit with no support at around eight months.

Reaching and Grasping

A whole new world opens to an infant who can sit upright independently. Now her hands are free, enabling her to reach and grasp for objects. Once sitting, the infant has a new vantage point and can manipulate objects much more easily. Although reaching and grasping may not appear to be as monumental a motor milestone as creeping or walking, these skills are challenging because they require incorporating haptic (exploration through touch) and visual perception with the motor control and coordination of the arms, wrists, and hands. In addition, these perceptual–motor experiences are also greatly affected by memory. Let's say that you reach for a large empty pot with two hands. When you grasp it, you realize that it is plastic rather than ceramic and requires only one hand to lift. You will likely then free up the other hand to grab something else. Following this experience, you remember that the empty pot is light and does not require two hands. Children and adults have many years of experience with a large variety of objects and can fairly accurately prejudge the requirements necessary to grasp each object (e.g., one hand, two hands, different grasps).

Many studies have been conducted to better understand how infants change and improve their reaching and grasping as well as how they use visual and haptic information. Reaching and grasping emerge as a confluence of both intrinsic factors (i.e., the infant's age, experience, level of postural control, and exposure to risk conditions) and extrinsic factors (i.e., body position, physical properties of objects, spatial orientation of the object, speed of the object, and any additional load to the infant's arm or arms) (Campos, Rocha, & Savelsbergh, 2009). Through experience, infants learn to adjust their reach and grasp relative to the environmental properties. They learn how to preplan their reach and grasp including deciding when to use one hand versus two hands and how to adjust their grasp based on the object's size and shape (Gibson & Pick, 2000). Postural control is considered a particularly important rate limiter for reaching because infants have been found to reach and grasp at much earlier ages when placed in an appropriate posture.

Reaching and grasping develops fairly rapidly over the course of the first eight months. Newborns have poor coordination and control in their arms and hands as well as poor visual acuity. They typically bring their hands toward objects with very jerky prereaching movements (Campos et al., 2008). Prereaching movements often appear as movements toward an object without a successful grasp. Prior to four months, infants tend to move their hands closer to an object when they are visually fixated on the object than when they are not focusing on it (Von Hofsten, 1984). Often, they reach with clenched fists because they cannot open them. Typically, infants do not begin reaching with an open hand until four months. Prior to four months is considered phase I reaching, which is characterized by an inability to reach and grasp for objects.

Successful reaching generally begins to occur around the age of three to four months; it is defined at this point as being able to control the hand in such a way as to make contact with an object. Early "successful" reaching (referred to as phase II reaching) is characterized by much variation in movement velocity, amplitude, and duration. The next several months demonstrate improvement in reaching through progressively increased movement velocity and reduced corrections in movement kinematics (Hadders-Algra, 2013). At these early ages, vision plays a minimal role in reaching. After six months, the ability to reach improves at a slower pace, but is marked by progressively straighter movement trajectories. However, infants as young as five to six months of age can differentiate their grip configurations based on the object's size relative to the size of their fingers and hands (Newell, McDonald, & Baillargeon, 1993).

Think about the importance of manual dexterity in tasks such as writing, using hand tools, sewing, and cutting with scissors. These fine motor skills are quite difficult to acquire. Infants typically cannot use a **precision grip** (finger and thumb grasp) until they are closer to one year of age. Prior to that they use what is termed a **power grip**, in which they grasp an object by supporting it with the palm of the hand and the undersurface of the fingers. Infants begin making contact with objects and grasping them at around five or six months with this type of grip, but they have little control or ability to manipulate the object. As adults, we use visual information and memories from many previous experiences of manipulating objects to anticipate the type of grasp necessary prior to reaching for the object. We may need all of our fingers and thumb if the object is large or awkward to pick up, but we use a precision grip for smaller objects. Likewise, we use one hand rather than two hands if the object is light enough. A timeline showing the development of grasping over the course of the first year of life is shown in figure 6.5.

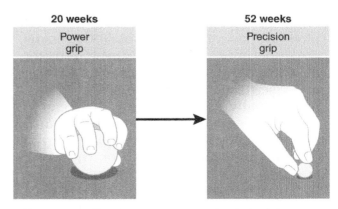

Figure 6.5 The development of grasping during infancy.

TRY THIS

Acquiring Manual Dexterity

Exercise 6.2

Lay out a few common objects that you have with you right now (e.g., a pencil, quarter, water bottle, textbook, laptop computer) and pick them up one at a time. Describe the grip you used for each, and explain why you chose the grip you did for each object.

- Pencil
- Quarter
- Water bottle
- Textbook
- Laptop computer

Now, describe how you would expect an eight-month-old infant to pick up each item. What rate limiters do you think would affect an eight-month-old who is picking up these objects?

The Three Cs of Locomotion

Locomotion is perhaps the most celebrated early motor milestones in infancy. Locomotor patterns in infancy typically begin with crawling; however, there is considerable variation in how and when infants crawl. Although many people refer to crawling as any movement in which an infant locomotes on all fours, **crawling** includes only the prone progression in which the infant pulls the trunk forward by extending and flexing the forearms while the legs extend symmetrically and are passively dragged forward (Gesell & Ames, 1940). **Creeping** is forward progression on all fours with the belly off the ground. Indeed, *creeping* and *crawling* are frequently confused, and in general conversation (and even in some physical education textbooks), the terms are sometimes reversed. However, as motor developmentalists, we should be aware of, and use, the correct terminology. Crawling typically occurs around 34 weeks of age and progresses to an alternating arm motion. Parents tend to refer to this type of crawling as commando or the army crawl. Initially, crawling involves minimal leg involvement. Infants pull themselves forward in a sliding motion, and some push themselves backward. Some infants skip this milestone entirely and begin with creeping, which includes moving on all fours alternately with the belly and chest lifted off the ground. Creeping is typically exhibited by infants after nine months. Figure 6.6 shows the difference.

Many infants begin crawling or creeping using a homolateral pattern, meaning that the limbs on the same side move either forward or backward together. Infants that skip crawling may begin with contralateral creeping, in which the limbs on each side oppose one another (Piek, 2006). Keep in mind that there is much variability in crawling and creeping; some infants skip crawling altogether, and a small percentage skip creeping. Although crawling and creeping are considered motor milestones, skipping one or the other is not an indication of abnormal development.

The third C is **cruising** (moving laterally while upright, using both arms for support) leading to the ultimate method of locomotion—walking. This tremendously exciting—and important—motor milestone is discussed in depth in chapter 7.

Although the order and approximate timing of these milestones has been carefully cataloged since the early 1900s

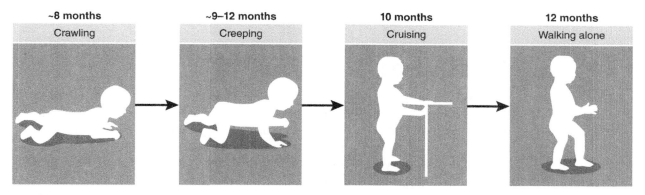

| ~8 months | ~9–12 months | 10 months | 12 months |
| Crawling | Creeping | Cruising | Walking alone |

Figure 6.6   The typical early motor milestone locomotor progression for infants.

(Gesell, 1946; McGraw, 1943), *how* the developing infant learns to control a rapidly changing body while learning new movement skills—in varied and often unpredictable environments—has been less examined. Adolph (2008) referred to this conundrum as a "learning to learn" issue. Based on work by Harlow (1949), Adolph posited that each new motor milestone (unassisted sitting, creeping on hands and knees, reaching and grasping, or walking) presents its own unique movement challenges for the infant to solve. Furthermore, these new challenges (often occurring in less predictable or novel environments) take place as the infant's body is undergoing rapid neurological and morphological change. And so, as infants grow and simultaneously get more practice at a given skill (say, walking), they become more adept.

Interestingly, Adolph and Berger's research (2006) provides evidence that knowledge and ability gained in one posture do not transfer to a second. Briefly stated, they contended that because motor milestones such as independent sitting, crawling, creeping, and walking have different motoric and perceptual requirements, learning is specific to each milestone. This speaks against the widely held neuromaturational perspective (e.g., Gesell, 1946; Shirley, 1931) that each new motor milestone builds on the previous one—that is, what an infant learns while sitting transfers to crawling. In an investigation into how infants learn to navigate

slopes, Adolph (1997) concluded that the strategies that infants honed over time that were effective for creeping did not transfer to walking. That is, when learning this new locomotor pattern, the infant generally had to start from scratch. "In other words, *each* problem space [in this example, creeping and walking] has its own set of information-generating behaviors and its own learning curve" (Adolph, 2008, p. 214). Thus, as previously noted, the breadth, depth, and variety of movement experiences available to an infant—for each motor milestone—influence the rate and quality of motor development (Cintas, 1995).

Although appropriate motor experiences are important for all developing infants, it is intuitively evident that they are crucial to infants who are at risk (Maitre, Slaughter, & Aschner, 2013). These include, but are not limited to, infants who come from low socioeconomic backgrounds as well as those with identifiable disabilities such as Down syndrome, cerebral palsy, autistic spectrum disorder, and developmental coordination disorder. Seminal work by Thelen and colleagues (Thelen, 1985; Thelen, Corbetta, & Spencer, 1996; Thelen & Ulrich, 1991) has emphasized the individuality of motor development. That is, as practitioners and researchers, we should attend to how individual babies solve individual movement problems "in their own unique ways" (Spencer et al., 2006, p. 1533). Tying this idea to the depth and variety of movement experiences

RESEARCH NOTES

How Should Babies Sleep?

A wide-ranging societal change with significant (and unexpected) negative ramifications for motor development involved American Academy of Pediatrics (AAP) guidelines issued in 1992. In this brief, it was strongly suggested that parents have their infants sleep in a supine, as opposed to prone, position to reduce the incidence of sudden infant death syndrome (SIDS). This position statement was very effective in reducing the number of infant deaths; however, an unintended negative consequence was that, while awake, infants who slept in a supine position were placed in a prone position very infrequently (Monson, Deitz, & Kartin, 2003; Salls, Silverman, & Garry, 2002). The result of infants being predominantly in a supine position while awake has been a decrement in upper-body (particularly the shoulder girdle) strength resulting in a delay in motor milestones that require upper-body strength (rolling from prone to supine, tripod sitting, crawling, creeping, and pulling to stand). Because of a reduced ability to navigate and explore their environment, these delays are thought to have a deleterious effect on infants' intellectual and social development.

previously mentioned, individual learners bring their own unique sets of skills to problems they are solving in real and changing environments.

Postural Control

Of course, environments grow and change in many important ways as infants become capable of observing from different heights and angles, reaching and grasping items of interest, and, before we know it, locomoting smoothly. As noted by Haywood and Getchell (2014), postural control (along with balance) is an excellent example of action systems and perceptual systems working in concert. Specifically, the visual and kinesthetic senses (with input from both the vestibular and proprioceptive systems) supply the sensory inputs required by the developing, active infant.

It is important to note that the term *postural control* is not universally understood or defined consistently (Pollock, Durward, Rowe, & Paul, 2000). We need a broadly accepted definition to understand the development and maintenance of postural control over the life span, as well as to determine whether developmental problems are the result of an identifiable disability (e.g., cerebral palsy or Down syndrome) or acquired through injury or disease. For our purposes, postural control involves (a) the ability to maintain the correct relationship between body segments and the environment or a specific task, or both; (b) the maintenance of stability, specifically, keeping the center of mass (center of gravity) within the person's base of support; (c) predictive (anticipatory) strategies that potentially involve an increase in muscular activity or a specific, voluntary movement prior to a predicted disturbance; and (d) reactive (compensatory) strategies, again potentially involving increased muscular activity or a voluntary movement (or both) in response to an unanticipated disturbance (also referred to as a perturbation).

As discussed earlier in the chapter, Thelen's developmental work within a dynamic systems context stressed the importance of individual differences with regard to solv-

Exercise 6.3

1. What rate limiters do you think are holding back an infant from progressing to creeping from crawling?

2. What rate limiters are holding back an infant who can pull to a standing position with the assistance of a couch but cannot stand or walk independently?

3. What control parameters can help a toddler progress from walking with a wide stance to walking with a narrow stance?

4. Order the following motor milestones in a typical developmental order:
   a. Standing independently
   b. Holding the head up
   c. Creeping
   d. Crawling
   e. Pulling to stand
   f. Rolling over
   g. Sitting independently

ing movement problems in ever-changing environments. In the same vein, Thelen, as well as her colleagues (Spencer et al., 2006; Ulrich & Ulrich, 1993), examined variability in motor responses both in a given infant (intraindividual differences) and between individuals (interindividual differences). That is, across trials by a specific infant, one could expect, especially early in development, that the responses would be different. Given innate and acquired differences between infants, we would expect different solutions to the same movement problem depending on each infant's very personal characteristics. These empirically derived hypotheses apply to the development of movement abilities, including, of course, postural control. Dusing and Harbourne (2010) outlined a number of principles that address the complexity of developing postural control that are in accord with the dynamic systems perspective.

To summarize, although the route taken by a given infant may differ from that of the infant's peers, over the course of the first year, a number of significant postural achievements have taken place. Although newborns do not appear to have much in the way of postural control, and their actions seem to be excessive, random, and nonfunctional, even at this point they are exploring movement possibilities and developing strategies that support looking around, reaching, and moving through their environments. Perception and action are working together in a bidirectional manner in which each informs the other. This allows developing infants to use visual, vestibular, and somatosensory information to adjust their rapidly changing bodies over a dynamic base of support that changes position frequently. As do all behaviors, the development of postural control results from the interaction of rapidly changing organismic constraints, the more or less dynamic physical and emotional environment in which the child resides, and the movement task to be accomplished (Newell, 1986).

Infants At Risk

Although differing one from another, infants who are at risk frequently have characteristics that significantly hinder the quality, quantity, and emergence of their movement skills. Interacting with the environment reflexively, using spontaneous movements, maintaining balance, reaching and grasping, and moving through space are not only important for their own sake. They also directly affect learning in the social and intellectual domains. Therefore, the early and accurate identification of infants at risk for movement problems is of great importance. With the exception of infants with Down syndrome (who are often identified at birth and sometimes in utero), only infants who are severely affected are accurately diagnosed early in their lives. Thus, a large number of at-risk infants are undiagnosed until they are much older, leading to a delay in the presentation of well-designed early intervention programs.

A particularly important reason for the early identification and, relatedly, early start to rehabilitative interventions concerns infants' neural plasticity, as previously discussed in this chapter. Because neural plasticity is greatest during infancy and early childhood, this is the time frame during which therapeutic interventions are most likely to reap long-term developmental benefits (Maitre, Slaughter, & Aschner, 2013). Although, as noted, many disabling conditions and environments negatively affect the development of movement skills, the following section briefly examines three prevalent conditions: prematurity, cerebral palsy, and Down syndrome. Although the underlying etiologies (causes) of these three conditions generally differ, the principles underlying the interventions have much in common.

Prematurity

Prematurity (or being born preterm) is defined as being born at least three weeks before the due date, or before the start of the 37th week. Because the important growth and development of vital organ systems that takes place over the last weeks (and months) of pregnancy take place outside the womb (in the extrauterine environment), prematurity often results in serious health complications as well as being the leading cause of infant death (Piek, 2006). Infants born prematurely have significantly higher rates of respiratory problems, feeding difficulties, hearing and vision impairments, developmental delays, and cerebral palsy than do those who are born full term. In general, the more immature the preterm infant is, the more acute the problems will be. How an infant's organ systems respond to the extrauterine environment, along with the level of immediate medical care provided (generally, this occurs in a neonatal intensive care unit), has a significant influence on both short- and long-term health outcomes. Important secondary factors that influence the development of the infant born preterm include socioeconomic status and the educational, physical, and social environments within which the infant develops.

One might assume that given improved medical care, particularly in developed countries, the incidence of premature births would decrease. However, as a result of a considerably higher survival rate for very low-birth-weight infants, the rate of preterm infants has, in fact, increased. As noted, the earlier the birth is, relative to full term, the more serious the health concerns will be. The terminology used when categorizing preterm births is as follows:

- Late preterm: Born between 34 and 36 weeks of pregnancy
- Moderately preterm: Born between 32 and 34 weeks of pregnancy
- Very preterm: Born at less than 32 weeks of pregnancy
- Extremely preterm: Born at or before 25 weeks of pregnancy

It should be noted that the vast majority of preterm births are late preterm.

Clearly, reducing premature births is of paramount importance. The causes of prematurity and how these causes may intersect remain poorly understood. However, suggestions (Moore, 2003) have included poor nutrition, stress, hypoxia, fetal stress, changes in the mother's hormonal levels, and problems associated with upper genital tract infection. Although some risk factors are not changeable, interventions are possible with others. The movement abilities of infants born prematurely are often compromised, and more severe impairments are evident in those of lower birth weight or more pronounced prematurity, or both. Table 6.1 lists premature infant risk factors and prevention strategies.

Developmental differences in the movement domain associated with prematurity include hypotonia (low active and passive muscle tone), predominant extensor muscle tone resulting in difficulty acting against gravity, and reduced variability in spontaneous movements (Lenke, 2003). With regard to reflexive movements, primitive reflexes such as the asymmetrical

tonic neck reflex, moro reflex, and palmar grasp reflex may be entirely absent or persist longer than normal. Along with frequently severe medical complications and reduced opportunities to move (given a severely restricted environment), movement abilities are compromised as a result of often extended time spent in the hospital (Lenke, 2003). This protracted time in the hospital results, not infrequently, in gross motor delays in head and trunk control.

Researchers have noted that a single delay or abnormal sign is not necessarily indicative of a significant movement or cognitive impairment; however, early assessment and careful observation are warranted. To a significant degree, the rate and quality of development is unpredictable (developmental lags and then catch-up periods are evident). Finally, when assessing motor development (including, but not limited to, motor milestones), parents and professionals must keep in mind the infant's corrected age (chronological age minus the number of weeks the infant was preterm). "Early [motor] differences may not always be indicative of an emerging deficit and may resolve, although some

Table 6.1   Risk Factors for Premature Birth and Prevention Strategies

Premature infant risk factor	Prevention strategies
Unplanned pregnancy	Family planning education Provision of appropriate contraception
Number of embryos implanted in assisted reproduction	Discussion between physician and families contemplating assisted reproduction
Young age at pregnancy	Comprehensive family planning education at community, state, and national levels
Weight at time of pregnancy	Encouragement and education regarding appropriate weight for height at every doctor's visit
General health status (hypertension, diabetes mellitus, clotting disorders, anemia)	Treatment to ensure best health status prior to pregnancy Under certain circumstances, consideration of pregnancy avoidance
Uterine fibroids	Treatment prior to pregnancy
Low income, life stress	Individual support Advocacy for education, employment, and community improvements
Cigarette smoking	Assessment at every health visit Referral for smoking cessation
Other substance abuse	Referral for substance abuse assistance

are associated with long-term problems and should be closely monitored" (Lenke, 2003, p. 105).

Cerebral Palsy

Of babies born prematurely, a considerable percentage (14.7 percent of infants born before 28 weeks of age; 6.2 percent of children born between 28 and 31 weeks of age) present with **cerebral palsy (CP)**, a serious neurodevelopmental condition. CP has been referred to as "a group of permanent disorders of the development of movement and posture, causing activity limitation, that are attributed to nonprogressive disturbances that occurred in the developing fetal or infant brain" (Rosenbaum et al., 2007, p. 9). Although experts in the field (Rosenbaum et al., 2007) have maintained that motor dysfunction is a critical and necessary feature of CP, they have argued persuasively that problems related to perception, sensation, communication, cognition, and behavior are often present. It is important to recognize that CP isn't a single disability but rather a group of neurodevelopmental disorders that, based on the severity, location, and timing of the insult to the brain, present somewhat unique obstacles and challenges to different people. Furthermore, these challenges (motoric, cognitive, perceptual, communicative, etc.) may be more significant during one period of life than another.

Although CP does originate with some type of prenatal or perinatal insult, it is clear that the environment (including, but not limited to, early intervention and familial support) plays a large role in the person's development. Each infant (given that CP is generally identified before 18 months of age) requires individualized, multidimensional attention from a trained team of professionals (that should, of course, include the parents and, when appropriate, siblings). As noted, the underlying cause or set of causes (etiology) of CP varies; thus, it is important that approaches to remediation and education be determined based on the functional limitations (as well as strengths) of the infant as opposed to the medical diagnosis. This is not to say that certain empirically determined best practices for those who present with, for example, spasticity can't be very similar from one infant to another. However, professionals and parents should keep in mind the unique characteristics of the child (referred to, from a dynamic systems perspective, as intrinsic dynamics) as well as the unique environment when determining an intervention. The type of intervention, as well as the people who administer it, will also likely change over time because the needs of the individual are not static. Although CP is a nonprogressive disorder of the brain, clear functional changes (in all the aforementioned domains) resulting from aging, learning activities, therapeutic intervention, and movement opportunities, among others, will occur.

The extent and accuracy of information available to accurately classify children thought to have CP vary significantly across the life span as well as geographic areas (for example, the availability of neuroimaging equipment, diagnostic specialists, and biochemical laboratories—as well as accurate historical data on the course of the pregnancy—may be unavailable). Nonetheless, it is critical that classification information include, at the least, the age of the child, whatever historical information is available (e.g., maternal recall, systematic observation, clinical notes), and whether neuroimaging or metabolic testing occurred.

The emphasis throughout this chapter has been on the individuality of developmental trajectories (i.e., the path a people take as they develop over the course of their lives). However, people with a particular classification of CP demonstrate, in general, particular motor patterns and deficits. The severity, as well as the specific limbs involved, differs depending on the motor pathways affected by the lesion. Motor deficits have been categorized based on (a) movement type (spasticity, ataxia, dyskinesia, and hypotonia; Evans & Alberman, 1985) and (b) the affected body part (Aicardi & Bax, 1992).

Regardless of the etiology or classification, it is essential to identify an infant as having CP as early as possible in order to begin the appropriate intervention(s). As noted earlier in this chapter, the developing brain is at its most malleable (that is, neural plasticity is most evident) early in life. Because of this neural plasticity, interventions begun at younger ages are more effective than those begun later. As we know, improved motor function has far-reaching, positive developmental consequences.

Down Syndrome

Down syndrome (DS), given its clear and unambiguous etiology, is one of the very few genetic disabilities that is identified soon after birth and results in moderate to severe intellectual disability (specifically, significant delays in speech, language production, auditory short-term memory, and nonverbal cognitive development) as well as delays in the onset of motor milestones and atypical motor skill acquisition (Angulo-Barroso, Burghardt, Lloyd,

& Ulrich, 2007). DS is the most common organic cause of intellectual disability: approximately one in every 800 births in the United States.

Understanding the course of motor development as well as how infants with DS acquire stable and efficient basic movement skills not only lays the foundation for the more complex and socially valued movement abilities to follow but also enables developing infants to interact meaningfully with their environments. These movement skills have, as with all infants with and without identifiable disabilities, an important role in the affective, intellectual, and communicative development of infants with DS. Although research with infants who develop atypically has been largely descriptive, chronicling behavioral differences and similarities with peers who develop normally (Henderson, 1985), more recent work from a dynamic systems perspective has rigorously examined atypical developmental using sophisticated quantitative and qualitative tools, at both individual and group levels of analysis.

Earlier researchers (Carr, 1970; Hogg & Moss, 1983) postulated that infants with DS acquire physical skills in the same sequence as their typically developing peers, albeit in a more extended fashion. However, evidence has been accumulating that suggests that infants with DS develop not only more slowly, but also in a qualitatively distinct fashion (Henderson, 1986; Lloyd, Burghardt, Ulrich & Angulo-Barroso, 2010; Ulrich, Ulrich, Collier & Cole, 1993). An example of unique movement solutions comes from Lydic and Steele's (1979) investigation, during which they queried parents about their infants' movement patterns. The results of the questionnaire confirmed the authors' observation that excessive external rotation and abduction of the hips resulted in the following atypical sitting and walking patterns: (a) when sitting, the infant's legs were frequently spread out at an extreme angle; (b) achievement of the sitting position from prone was accomplished by spreading the legs close to 180 degrees apart and then pushing up with the arms or head; and (c) walking was performed with a waddling gait and a wide base of support (a variety of arm movements were used in place of alternating swinging).

Subsequent research has identified a litany of qualitative and quantitative motor deficiencies in children with DS, including less frequent self-generated spontaneous movements, less frequent and lengthy general movements (e.g., gross movements involving the whole body), more low-intensity movement, and atypical gait (walking only emerging at approximately two years of age). Physiological characteristics that would negatively affect motor development in infants (and young children) with DS include poor postural control and balance, low muscle tone and ligamentous laxity, lower cardiorespiratory fitness, a higher percentage of body fat, and a lower maximal heart rate (Angulo-Barroso et al., 2007; Lloyd et al., 2010). The physiological, sensory, cognitive, and morphological reasons for these significant barriers to skilled and frequent movement include a less efficient nervous system, smaller cerebellum, reduced hand size, visual and hearing problems, and reduced kinesthesia.

Some have suggested that increasing the activity level of self-generated spontaneous movements and general movements in children with DS would likely improve strength, endurance, and coordination and thus have a positive impact on the acquisition of motor milestones. Ulrich and Ulrich (1993) compared the spontaneous movements of typically developing infants with infants with DS and found that the quantity of spontaneous movements (particularly supine kicking) was significantly less in infants with DS than in their typically developing peers. Relatedly, a relative absence of these self-generated movements was discussed by Henderson in a 1985 review of movement skill development in infants with DS. She suggested that the

delayed and abnormal trajectory regarding movement skills may be closely related to diminished exploratory behavior. She went on to suggest that a "form of self-perpetuating sensory-motor deprivation" occurs (Henderson, 1986, p.74), resulting from this lack of exploratory behavior.

Interventions

We end this section with a critically important question that applies to all infants who are at risk of some kind of developmental delay including, but not limited to, those who are born prematurely, are at risk for CP, or have DS. Simply put, are there interventions that have proven efficacy? That is, how do we know they work? This is particularly challenging given the limited amount of research and the heterogeneity of the infants we're considering. Specific issues include identifying important outcomes; identifying the tools needed to accurately assess these outcomes; deciding (beyond choosing an appropriate theory-driven, data-based approach) how intense and frequent the sessions should be, who will carry out the interventions, and how those people will be trained; and finally, ensuring that the interventions are carried out effectively and consistently. Because it is impossible to find a generic patient, and given that infants, regardless of their diagnoses, vary along the dimensions of intellect, attention, sensory impairment, and behavior, can we identify one intervention that can apply to all infants?

Cesar Torres (personal communication, February 12, 2015) noted that what are considered best practices do not always align with research-based practices. Over the past 25 years, Thelen and colleagues (Angulo-Barroso et al., 2006; Lloyd et al., 2010; Ulrich, Ulrich, & Collier, 1993) have used a dynamic systems approach to inform therapeutic practice. A particular tenet of the dynamic systems approach posits that behavior is "softly assembled." That is, the developing infant uses what is maturationally available at a given point in time, in a particular environment, to solve a specific movement task. By *maturationally available*, we are referring to individual characteristics (intrinsic dynamics).

Because behavior is thought to be determined by the status of all of the underlying systems (for walking, these would include muscular strength, dynamic balance, and motivation), if one or more of these systems is compromised, the appearance or the quality (or both) of a given movement (in our example, walking) would be affected. Therefore, therapeutic interventions should be individually tailored to improve the functioning of one or more systems, should a given system prove to be ineffective. For example, if a child with CP solves the movement task of walking across the room with an awkward, inefficient gait that requires a lot of energy, this might be (probably would be) the best way for her to get from one place to another. Therefore, a targeted therapeutic intervention would identify the rate limiter(s) (what, specifically, was hindering her) and work specifically on the issue at hand. Here, the intervention might involve increasing range of motion and muscular strength, leading to a more efficient gait pattern. We would, of course, keep a good eye on the program, collecting formative and summative data that would indicate whether the child is improving. If the answer is no, the next question would address whether we have the correct approach but are not implementing it properly, or whether we're barking up the wrong therapeutic tree (i.e., not using the correct approach). At all times, our intervention must be individually tailored, thoughtful, and based on, to the extent possible, scientific findings.

Assessment

As we've discussed at some length in this chapter, movement allows developing infants to explore and engage with their expanding worlds, thereby increasing their social, language, and learning skills. The fact that approximately one in six children who visit the pediatrician's office has an identifiable disability speaks to the tremendous need for practical, accurate, and reliable assessment tools.

A growing body of evidence points to the importance of early intervention for infants at risk for developmental delays, an important reason to accurately assess. However, Palfrey, Singer, Walker, and Butler (1986) and others make the point that pediatricians infrequently screen for developmental delays; instead, they often rely on clinical judgment along with a review of the attainment of motor milestones. Unfortunately, these clinical judgments have been found to be frequently inaccurate. The fallout from relying on this clinical judgment approach has been that a significant number of children who should have been identified as eligible for early intervention (under U.S. federal law) were not. Although the conditions we have discussed (prematurity, low birth weight, cerebral palsy, and Down syndrome) are recognizable, other, more subtle developmental delays such as learning disabilities and cognitive impairments are more difficult to identify. Even if a more easily recognized condition (such as Down syndrome) is identified (through clinical observation), a more accurate assessment would provide more precise information about the person's status. As mentioned earlier in this chapter, the developmental course (developmental trajectory) of individual children, even given the same diagnosis, may vary widely.

Although accurately assessing to provide appropriate early intervention is of tremendous importance, it is not the only reason to assess. Burton and Miller (1998) discussed assessment as a means to identify (i.e., diagnose) movement problems and then to further categorize a given individual's skill level. If a particular movement problem is precisely identified, there is, clearly, a better chance that the appropriate interventions will ensue.

Motor assessment in infancy provides information about a variety of movement categories that include the quality and quantity of reflexive behavior, spontaneous movements, muscle tone, and how and when motor milestones are achieved. Although the time frame varies, depending on the motor area examined, it is particularly important to assess over time—that is, to examine an infant's progress or change on multiple occasions. This allows the parents and professionals to carefully observe not only the child's development, but also the effectiveness of the chosen intervention(s).

Currently, there are two broad approaches to infant motor assessment: (1) examiner-administered assessments and (2) parent-report measures. Examiner-administered assessments are valid, objective, and repeatable (reliable) measures that, when competently done, reveal an infant's movement capabilities at that particular point in time. The examiner-administered tests most frequently used (Libertus & Landa, 2013) are the Bayley Scales of Infant Development (BSID-III; Bayley, 2006) and the Mullen Scales of Early Learning (MSEL; Mullen, 1995). However, there are several limitations to examiner-administered assessments. Test administration by a trained practitioner is often both time consuming and costly. Additionally, long assessments may tire the infant, result-

ing in scores that may not be accurate. In the same vein, if rapport between the examiner and the infant has not been established, one must doubt the veracity of the test scores (Libertus & Landa, 2013). Parent-report measures provide a cost effective and relatively quick alternative to examiner-administered assessments. Indeed, Libertus & Landa (2013) have noted that if parent-completed developmental questionnaires (PCDQs) are used, the extensive knowledge that a parent has about their child can be put to good use. Although concerns remain regarding the validity of this approach (parents may under or overestimate their child's skills), researchers are optimistic that reliable and valid questionnaires are on the horizon (Johnson & Marlow, 2006). PCDQs that examine motor development over the first two years include The Minnesota Infant Development Inventory (MIDI; Creighton & Sauve, 1988; Ireton & Thwing, 1980) and the Ages & Stages Questionnaire (ASQ; Squires, Bricker, & Potter, 1997).

Summary

Infant development is a period of immense change. Newborns have minimal volitional control and quickly grow and develop to being able to manipulate objects with their hands and even locomote by the end of the first year. This chapter began by discussing the importance of healthy pregnancies and detailed the development of the embryo and fetus. Many factors affect development during the critical months in the womb. Pregnant women must avoid harmful substances and potentially dangerous situations that may have dramatic and lasting effects on their unborn children.

Infants change in how they respond to the environment as they progress from making mostly spontaneous and reflexive movements to making controlled volitional movements. Their senses improve dramatically throughout the first year; improved vision, hearing, and somatosensation enable them to respond to the environment in increasingly more meaningful ways. Infants can more efficiently reach and grasp objects as a result of improved vision and increased experiences. They learn when it is appropriate to use one hand versus two hands and begin to be able to use a precision grip for smaller objects. This grip becomes increasingly more important as they grow older and learn how to use crayons and later to write.

During the first year, the infant advances through a series of motor milestones from holding up the head to sitting up to creeping and eventually walking, to name a few. The way and the time in which each infant progresses through these motor milestones vary greatly. Most infants follow the progression discussed in this chapter; however, some advance more quickly than others. Slower progression through the motor milestones does not necessarily indicate developmental delays. The onset of motor milestones occurs as a result of both genetic and environmental factors. For example, infants who live in homes with slippery floors may learn to walk later, and those who are carried a lot are more likely to locomote at a later age. Infant personalities can also drive some of these changes. A particularly curious infant or an infant who has older siblings running around may be motivated to locomote earlier to be able to explore more of the environment.

This chapter also discussed infants who are at risk, including preterm infants and those with the identifiable disabilities of cerebral palsy and Down syndrome. Early identification of these disabilities is crucial to ensure an early start to rehabilitative interventions. Because neural plasticity is greatest during infancy and early childhood, therapeutic interventions undertaken at this time would be most likely to reap long-term benefits for the developing infant.

ONLINE LEARNING

Visit the web resource at www.HumanKinetics.com/MotorLearningAndDevelopment for an accompanying lab activity, video clips, and exercises from the chapter.

LEARNING AIDS

Supplemental Activities

1. Develop an advertisement (brochure), front and back, providing prenatal information to pregnant women. Be sure to format it so that it folds like a brochure. You are free to choose any issue related to pregnancy and prenatal development for the brochure; anything from fetal alcohol syndrome to exercise and pregnancy is appropriate. Make the brochure appealing to the eye to catch people's attention, and provide as much pertinent information as you can.

2. Interview someone close to you about his or her child's development as an infant.

    a. Describe who you interviewed as well as the child. Did this child go through all the motor milestones? At what ages did the child go through each milestone? If the child did not go through all of the milestones, what milestones were missed?

    b. If an infant skips a motor milestone, what might this tell us about how individual, environmental, and task constraints interact? Look up information on the Internet with regards to the skipping of motor milestones. Please cite your sources.

Glossary

cerebral palsy (CP)—A neuromuscular disorder that negatively affects coordination; typically, it is caused by external factors that prevent optimal brain development.

crawling—A prone progression in which the infant pulls the trunk forward by extending and flexing the forearms while the legs extend symmetrically and are passively dragged forward.

creeping—Forward progression on all fours with the belly off the ground.

cruising—Moving laterally while upright, using both arms and a stable object for support.

embryonic period—The second prenatal period, which lasts for the first six weeks.

fetal period—The final stage of prenatal development, which begins at the completion of organ differentiation at around week 8 and lasts until birth.

germinal period—The first prenatal period following conception, which lasts approximately two weeks.

gestational age—The prenatal age that begins the first day after the mother's last menstrual period.

locomotor reflexes—Reflexes that are thought to be precursors to voluntary locomotion and serve at some level as practice for these later motor milestones.

myogenic movements—Movements that are not generated by the central nervous system.

neural plasticity—The ability of the brain to change function as a result of either damage or experience.

neurogenic movements—Movements generated by the central nervous system.

organogenesis—The process by which cells are defined to make up organs.

postural reactions—Reflexes that automatically maintain the appropriate posture in a changing environment.

power grip—An early form of grasping in which the object is supported with the palm of the hand and the undersurface of the fingers.

precision grip—A finger and thumb grasp that is generally acquired around age 1.

primitive reflexes—Reflexes that serve the functions of protection and securing nourishment.

teratogen—Any agent that can cause defects or deformities in the fetus.

FUNDAMENTAL SKILLS IN CHILDHOOD

Chapter Objectives

After reading this chapter, you should be able to do the following:

- Define the term *fundamental movement skills*.
- Identify levels of competency in selected fundamental movement skills.
- List factors that facilitate the acquisition of fundamental movement skills.
- List factors that interfere with the development of fundamental movement skills.
- Understand the important interactions of motor development, cognitive development, and affective development.
- Appreciate how researchers study the emergence of fundamental movement skills.
- Distinguish between the whole-body and component approaches to the development of fundamental movement skills.

Ayisha in Physical Education Class

Ayisha and her family had just arrived in the United States from Saudi Arabia, and she was getting used to many new experiences. As she walked around her new neighborhood, she noticed both boys and girls playing an exciting game together. That they played together was something new to see, and it looked like they really enjoyed the running, catching, turning, twisting, and throwing that went on in the game. Although some of the children were quicker than others, others seemed to be able to catch and throw more skillfully. Ayisha found it interesting that being pretty good at one movement skill didn't mean that a person was also good at a different movement skill. Also, no one really cared whether the people they teamed up with were excellent or not. They said nice things whether someone caught the ball or missed the ball. Although she'd had very few opportunities to run, catch, and throw in the past, she was looking forward to doing it a lot in the future.

As children begin to spend more time in school settings, moving well and playing competently, both independently and with their peers, becomes tremendously important. Indeed, having successful early experiences, experiences that Ayisha hadn't had up until this point, is very important to promote involvement in physical activity over the life span. As well, there are many ancillary cognitive and social benefits to being a skilled mover, especially in the United States, where physical skill is often rewarded. This chapter discusses the important fundamental movement skills that emerge over the first six years of life, as well as how and why they emerge. It also addresses how skilled (and less skilled) movement affects a child's development in the cognitive and social–affective domains.

Fundamental Movement Skills

During the first two years of life, amazing motor skills emerge, allowing children to interact with their environments in meaningful ways. They are now able to explore somewhat capably and to act on their environments by walking around objects and by reaching for, grasping, manipulating, and then—if they feel like it—releasing items. No longer are they prisoners of gravity; rather, they can maintain and change their postures while lying, sitting, standing, and moving. Although no one would argue that typically developing children two years of age or younger are necessarily *skillful* movers, they have progressed systematically at a tremendously rapid rate and have developed an important array of rudimentary movement abilities. At the age of two, they are acting on (and are acted on by) their physical and emotional worlds in such a way that the amount they are learning is truly amazing. This time of rapid and observable motor development is studied extensively. Researchers interested in early, preverbal cognitive,

and affective development conduct elegant experiments that make use of observable motor acts as a window into their areas of interest (Hayne & Findlay, 1995; Kretch & Adolph, 2015; Soska, Adolph & Johnson, 2010; Yoshida & Smith, 2008). As we know, a picture—or in this case, an action—is worth a thousand words.

Recent decades have seen a rekindling of interest in the underlying processes that lead to developmental change in the motor domain. This renewed interest coincides with the advent of the ecological approach (Adolph, 2008; Cole, Chan, Vereijken, Beatrix, & Adolph, 2013; Gibson, 1977; Newell, 1986) and the dynamic systems (Spencer, Perone, & Buss, 2011; Thelen, 1985; Thelen & Ulrich, 1991; Ulrich, 2010) approach to how perception and action develop (and influence each other) over time. These related approaches to development have been discussed extensively in earlier chapters and provide the theoretical underpinnings as we explore the development of fundamental skills in early childhood. To recap briefly, from the ecological and dynamic systems perspectives, movement skill emerges and becomes refined over time through changes in individual constraints as well as environmental and task-related constraints "imposed on the organism-environment system" (Savelsbergh, Davids, van der Kamp, & Bennett, 2003, p. 6). One or more of these constraints—at a particular point in developmental time—may act in a *rate-limiting* capacity, potentially inhibiting the emergence of new skills, slowing the development of existing skills, or even causing the person to regress (i.e., to return to a less skillful level). An example of regression due to individual constraints was seen in the world-class gymnast Aurelia Dobre. Before she turned 15, Dobre was the world gymnastics champion, but she was unable to retain that incredibly high level of performance because of a combination of growth spurts and injury. She retired from international competition before she turned 19.

Exercise 7.1

Can you identify two highly skilled athletes who, because of changes in rate limiters, regressed or became less skillful (that is, experienced a phase shift to a less competent level)? This regression could be due to injury, changes in body type (morphology), or changes in movement pattern (either planned or unplanned).

Athlete	Rate limiter	Phase shift

With respect to motor development, what goes on during that interesting period following infancy that we refer to as early childhood? It has been noted (Whitall, 2003) that regarding movement skill, the primary goal during early childhood changes from acquiring movement skills to becoming an adept and proficient mover. Into and during adulthood, people's developmental goals change to maintaining skills and finally to creating functional adaptations to the aging process. In a nutshell, between the ages of two and six, some new and important movement abilities appear while existing skills become more refined, flexible, and functional. Preservice physical education teachers (i.e., those still doing their postsecondary prep), physical therapists, and movement scientists must be knowledgeable about (a) the fundamental movement skills that emerge during this period, (b) how researchers study these skills, (c) the factors that lead to skilled movement, (d) the factors that interfere with the development of skilled movement, (e) how to facilitate skill acquisition, and finally, (f) why we should care.

Breakdown of Fundamental Movement Skills

To best understand how, between two and six years of age, **fundamental movement skills** develop and why they are so important to the developing child, we must first be clear about what skills we are talking about. Referred to at times as the movement foundation (Gabbard, 2012) because of their importance in the subsequent development of more complex skill combinations used in sport, gymnastics, and dance, fundamental movement skills can be divided into three general groupings: **stability skills** (also referred to as nonlocomotor skills), **locomotor skills**, and **manipulative skills** (also referred to as **object control skills**).

The term *stability skills* refers to axial movements—that is, movements around the axis of the body such as bending, stretching, swinging, swaying, pushing, pulling, turning, and twisting. These movements are performed with little or no movement of the base of support.

Locomotor skills, in contrast, transport a person from one place to another. Although human beings most commonly move by walking or running, locomotor activities also include jumping, hopping, galloping, and skipping. These less common ways to move are nevertheless often used in sporting events (e.g., gymnastics, track and field, fencing, court games, and combative activities) and in dance as children get older.

The third grouping, manipulative skills, includes an array of abilities: overarm and underarm throwing, rolling, strik-

WHAT DO YOU THINK?

Exercise 7.2

As children (and adults) become more skilled, they combine fundamental movement skills while engaging in sporting activities. For example, while fielding a ground ball during a softball game, a right-handed player has to slide to her right (locomotor skill), bend and turn her body as she prepares to field the ball (axial movements), field the ball with a backhand motion (absorptive manipulative skill, using an implement), and then throw the ball to first base (propulsive manipulative skill). Identify two motor skills that involve axial, locomotor, and manipulative skills. These combinations could be used within a game context (e.g., a team game or a racket sport) or an individual pursuit (e.g., cycling or rock climbing).

Motor skill	Axial skill(s) involved	Locomotor skill(s) involved	Manipulative skill(s) involved

ing, heading, kicking, punting, catching, and trapping. If we examine manipulative skills more closely, a number of issues become apparent. First, they can involve, primarily, either the upper body (arms or head) or the lower body; second, they can also involve either imparting force to an object and moving it *away* from the body or positioning a part of the body in front of an oncoming object to deflect or stop it. Gallahue and Ozmun (2005) referred to these actions as propulsive and absorptive, respectively. A third issue involves the use of an implement to either impart force to an object or absorb the force of an object. Examples of implements are rackets, bats, and gloves. Obviously, implements may or may not be used depending on the person's skill level, the rules of the game, or both.

A later section of the chapter revisits some of these locomotor and manipulative skills and examines what research and practice have shown about how children become competent in their execution over developmental and chronological time. At this point we consider why it is important for prospective teachers and therapists to understand the development of fundamental movement skills.

Importance of Understanding Fundamental Movement Skills

Researchers and practitioners, as well as social critics, have addressed why the timely acquisition of fundamental movement skills is crucial to the development of young children. From a scientific vantage point, Whitall (2003), as noted earlier, suggested that careful study of motoric skillfulness in young children offers a window into the development of perceptual, cognitive, and affective processes. There are also clinical reasons for careful study, given that a significant number of young children struggle with movement skills. An understanding of both the level of movement skill development that should be expected of children of a given chrono-

logical age and individual differences in how a given skill is performed (keeping in mind functional and structural constraints) helps us to develop individualized educative programs for students who struggle with movement skills.

Across all societal groups, people have become more sedentary over the past two decades, with a concomitant increase in obesity and the host of health risks that accompany obesity (Owen, Healy, Matthews, & Dunstan, 2010). Teasing out the relative contributions and interactions of diet and physical inactivity, as well as genetic predispositions to obesity, remains challenging; however, it is clear that physical inactivity plays a significant role in reducing healthy living. An important task, therefore, is to identify the factors that are likely to maintain appropriate physical activity levels throughout the life span. An array of motor developmentalists (Gallahue, Ozmun, & Goodway, 2012; Haywood & Getchell, 2014; Payne & Isaacs, 2012) have argued strongly that competence in fundamental motor skills is essential to remaining active over the course of our lives. Regarding the importance of establishing strong foundational skills, Clark and Metcalfe (2002) noted that an inability to perform fundamental locomotor and object control (manipulative) skills results in limited opportunities for physical activity as children age, because prerequisite skills are not adequately developed.

Young learners with poorly developed stability, locomotor, or manipulative skills are clearly at a disadvantage when it comes to taking part in games and movement activities. Before too long, the requirements of play become more demanding. Movements have to be done more quickly; decisions regarding which pattern to use become more complicated; and the consequences of making the wrong play, or choosing the right play but making an error, become more important. It is little wonder that so many children stop moving.

They see no reason to participate in activities that they are not good at and that lead to derision from peers, often in very public ways. As Ted Wall (personal communication, September 15, 1973) pointed out, when a student struggles with reading, a good teacher likely will not embarrass him by having him read aloud to his classmates. When it comes to physical activities, there often is no choice. In a high-stakes game of kickball at recess, when the ball comes to a child and bounces off her hands (likely not for the first time), the result is public humiliation. The child sees no reason to endure this if she does not have to. Clark and Metcalfe (2002) noted that the acquisition of a solid base of fundamental movement skills is a prerequisite to enjoying the multiple benefits of sport and lifetime activities. In essence, for physical activity to become an integral part of life—with the concomitant physical and psychological health benefits—people need a solid base of fundamental movement skills. This is in addition to the more general but still tremendously important benefits of movement in terms of acquiring cognitive and affective information about one's place in the environment and how one relates to that place.

Gabbard (2012) noted that *how* children acquire and develop fundamental motor skills has likely been the most carefully studied area in motor development. Indeed, beginning with Wild's seminal work on overarm throwing (Wild, 1938), researchers and practitioners have been intrigued with the apparent age-related changes in fundamental motor skills, as well as the components that make up particular skills. Whereas much of the earlier work focused on cataloging age-related (as well as sex-related) changes in fundamental movement skills from a **quantitative**, or *product*, perspective (that is, how fast, how far, or how high), more recent work has attended to the **qualitative**, or *process*-related, changes in fundamental movement skills over time. It should be intuitively clear that if a child's form (i.e.,

WHAT DO YOU THINK?

Exercise 7.3

Consider a soccer player who is just learning the game. Imagine him standing in front of the goalie trying to score on a penalty kick. What does the kick look like? Now imagine the legendary Lionel Messi or some other soccer superstar. What does his penalty kick look like? In the following table, describe in a qualitative manner what each kick looks like. Describe the kick as a whole, but keep in mind all parts of the body—legs, torso, arms, and head.

	Qualitative description of a penalty kick
Novice kicker	
Expert kicker	

mechanics) is closer to a mature level of execution, the outcome will be better. As an example, if Juan is in right field and takes a long contralateral step, pointing his toe at his target, he will likely throw the baseball farther and more accurately than if he did not take a step. The stepping action is considered to be at a mature level, whereas not stepping is considered to be at the initial stage. If, on the other hand, Juan were playing darts, taking a contralateral step would hinder his performance; he would be much better off taking a small step, if any, with the leg on his throwing side (an ipsilateral step). Gallahue and Cleland Donnelly (2003) suggested that practitioners use a three-tiered system to classify the level of development for a given fundamental motor skill; the tiers are initial, elementary, and mature. As discussed later, the way researchers and practitioners examine qualitative changes in movement skills has been an area of debate over the past five decades.

Whole-Body Approach Versus Component Approach

When Wild (1938) did her classic cross-sectional research on the overarm throw for force, she concluded that children move through relatively invariant stages of development for the entire body. In the preceding example of Juan, if he were at an unskilled (initial) stage with regard to his foot (stepping) action, he would also be at the initial stage with regard to all of the other body components involved in the throw. These would include the trunk (pelvis and spine), upper arm (humerus), and forearm. As Juan's performance improved qualitatively in one component, it would improve in all of the other components. Roberton and colleagues (Roberton, 1977; Roberton & Konczak, 2001), however, took issue with the **whole-body approach** to the development of fundamental movement skills. Their longitudinal and cross-sectional research indicated that rather than all components becoming qualitatively more advanced (that is, moving toward the mature form) at more or less the same time, different components improved at different times. Roberton referred to this perspective as the **component approach**. In this view, Juan's foot action might be at a mature level with the long contralateral step, whereas his trunk action, with a forward–backward movement, might be at the initial level, often referred to by practitioners as an immature level.

Fundamental Locomotor and Manipulative Skills

As discussed earlier in the chapter, the development of fundamental movement skills allows children to explore and act on the environment in a progressively more adept fashion. At the same time, this steady improvement results in concomitant gains in the intellectual and social arenas. This section examines the development of fundamental locomotor and manipulative skills. The locomotor skills discussed are walking, running, jumping, and hopping; the manipulative skills are overarm throwing, kicking, and striking. A considerable body of research has been devoted to understanding and accurately assessing the development of fundamental movement skills; knowledge of this area helps practitioners develop the tools necessary to work effectively with young children in the motor arena.

Locomotor Skills

Although locomotor skills have been described simply as movements that transport people from one physical location to another, and although their development seems to be relatively automatic, they received considerable attention over the course of the 20th century. That this attention came from fields as diverse

WHAT DO YOU THINK?

Exercise 7.4

Take a moment and think back to when you were developing fundamental movement skills. For some of them (e.g., running), it may be difficult to remember how and when you realized, *Hey, I'm pretty good at this!* But for others, such as catching a ball, you might have a stronger memory. As you look back, think about (a) how you knew you had mastered the skill and (b) how you arrived at that point. For example, was it by playing around with your friends in the driveway? Practicing with your mom? Playing on a travel team? Or was it through some other avenue?

as biomechanics, physical therapy, and medicine suggests that efficiently moving through space may be a more complex undertaking than meets the eye. The truth is that the developing child must commandeer a dizzying array of body systems (many that are changing rapidly) and use them in a controlled and coordinated way to navigate through changing physical environments. Four-year-old Marty might be walking along a level and firm pathway and suddenly come across a steeply angled dip; to make things even more challenging, the ground has also become spongier and less firm. If he doesn't speed up—that is, run downhill—he'll land flat on his face. Suddenly, he has to deal with a change in angle and surface characteristics, and all at once there is a need for a new locomotor pattern, from a calm walk to a somewhat frenzied run. Flexibility is needed because Marty has to solve specific movement tasks that often require an array of skills. At one point he might be running downhill, and at another he might be playing a tag game and need to look out for others as he moves while also quickly changing direction.

When examined in more depth, the requirements for Marty to efficiently navigate from point A to point B seem quite remarkable. As noted earlier, the development of efficient and effective locomotor skills takes place as a variety of constraints interact. A child's weight and height, as well as arm and leg length, are undergoing radical changes, and at the same time, societal values influence how motivated a child might be (e.g., boys don't skip). Thus, in dynamic systems terms, children develop a variety of forms of locomotion while also dealing with physical and cultural constraints that are often changing and constantly interacting.

The following sections address the locomotor skills of walking, running, jumping, and hopping. Although jumping and hopping have not received the empirical attention that walking and running have, these movements have been carefully examined by researchers, therapists, and physical education teachers. We focus here on the development of these skills during childhood.

Walking

More than three quarters of a century ago, the eminent developmentalist Mary Shirley (1931) suggested that the emergence of independent walking was the most important, and certainly the most impressive, of the developmental milestones. Few parents who delight at their children's first uncertain steps would disagree. Although up to now, the child has been able to locomote through the environment by crawling (moving on hands and stomach), creeping (moving on hands and knees), and cruising (moving sideways so both hands and feet can be used to aid balance), the arrival of independent walking frees up the hands to further explore the changing environment. Although we often think of walking as a highly automatic skill that, once learned, changes little over the course of our lives, this is not necessarily true. As people's physical abilities change (e.g., with arthritis) or their confidence wavers (e.g., after a serious fall), their technique might change. Environmental variables might also play a role. Vacationers walking on a sandy beach are likely to slow their pace. People who encounter heavy snow or slick ice will likely modify their cadence, their trunk angle, and the amount of force used. Logic would suggest that 36-year-old Dan, dealing with early-onset arthritis of the hip and navigating an icy parking lot, would walk in a very different way than his cousin, 29-year-old Louis, who is enjoying perfect health and walking his dog in 75-degree Fahrenheit (24 degrees Celsius) weather. Other factors that can influence walking patterns are (a) moving while handling an object (e.g., dribbling a basketball); (b) performing activities that require a great deal of balance and stability (e.g., traversing a balance beam); and (c) walking with an external load (e.g., carrying a backpack) (Payne & Isaacs, 2008).

A number of motor developmentalists (Haywood & Getchell, 2014; Wickstrom, 1983) have noted, with reference to walking, that what does remain constant over the life span is the underlying timing of the act. During walking, weight shifts from the left to the right foot, and one foot is in contact with the ground at all times. Generally, the initial contact of the foot occurs halfway through the gait cycle. This is referred to as a 50 percent phasing between the legs. A gait cycle (also referred to as a walking cycle) is made up of a support phase and a swing phase. The swing phase begins when the toes of one foot (or the whole foot) leave the ground and ends when the heel of that foot (or the whole foot) returns to the ground. The support phase of the gait cycle takes place when one foot is in contact with the ground. Therefore,

when one foot is in the swing phase, the other is in the support phase. When both feet are in contact with the ground, the walker is in the double-support phase. Although early walking has been called a "precarious adventure" (Wickstrom, 1983) featuring frequent falls, the young walker over the next two to six years becomes an accomplished mover whose gait resembles that of a mature adult. Figures 7.1 through 7.3 outline the whole-body approach for walking (Gabbard, 2012; Gallahue et al., 2012; Haywood & Getchell, 2014; Payne & Issacs, 2012; Wickstrom, 1983).

Although the ability to perform an alternating movement pattern is present from birth (Thelen, Ulrich, & Jenson, 1989), the beginning walker must deal with the rate limiters of balance and strength. To move around the environment without falling too often, the developing walker must take short "baby" steps while using a wide stance with the toes pointing slightly outward. With the hands held in a high guard position to protect against falls, the beginning walker moves tentatively with little trunk rotation and lands on a flat foot. The pelvis tilts slightly, and the ankles are pretty well locked. Although this walking pattern is, at one level of analysis, immature, it allows for relatively stable ambulation. What it does not allow for is efficient movement with the ability to change direction smoothly and quickly. Haywood and Getchell (2005) observed that proficient walking involves the person's "exploiting biomechanical principles as body dimensions change" (p. 87). As a more mature gait gradually emerges (generally by age 4 or 5), the following characteristics are seen (Gabbard, 2012; Haywood & Getchell, 2014):

• *Base of support and foot angle.* The dynamic base of support (i.e., the base of support during moving) is reduced to approximately the width of the person's trunk. This narrowing generally takes place four and a half months after

FIGURE 7.1

FIGURE 7.1

Whole-Body Approach for Walking—Initial Stage

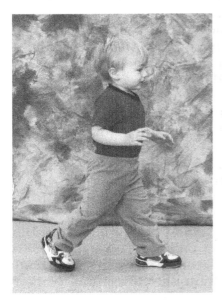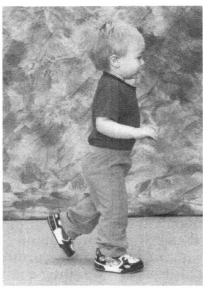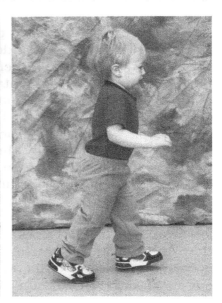

- Base of support is wide.
- Contact is flat footed.
- Toes point outward.
- Steps are short, quick, and rigid.
- No trunk rotation occurs.
- Single-knee lock pattern is used.

- Knee flexes at contact followed by rapid knee extension.
- Hip flexion is significant.
- Pelvis tilts forward slightly.
- Arms are in high guard position.
- Arms are rigid with little or no movement.

independent walking begins, allowing for more efficient movement. With regard to foot angle, the beginning walker tends to move with the toes out (toeing out). This pattern disappears at approximately the same time the base of support narrows, with the foot becoming aligned in a straight fore–aft position. Both the narrowing of the base of support and the disappearance of toeing out result in the application of forces in a forward–backward plane (Haywood & Getchell, 2014), a significantly more efficient movement pattern. In-toeing (commonly referred to as a pigeon-toed gait)

is not a normal pattern and is seen only infrequently.

- *Foot contact.* As walkers develop, they move from the flat footfall to a heel–toe pattern, resulting in an increased range of motion. Toe walking is often seen in young children and is not a cause for concern; however, if it persists beyond three years of age, it should be examined.

- *Step and stride length.* Between ages one and seven, step and stride length almost double. This is due, for the most part, to significant increases in force and

FIGURE 7.2

Whole-Body Approach for Walking—Elementary Stage

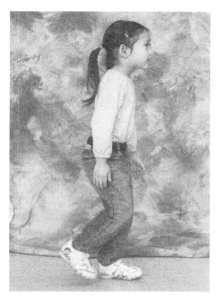 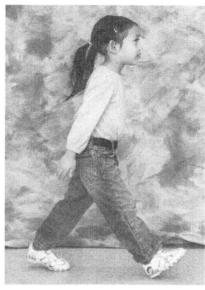 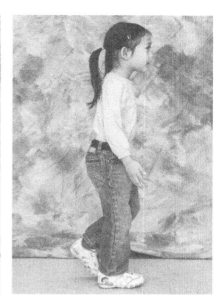

- Base of support is narrower.
- Out-toeing occurs less frequently.
- Pelvic rotation is increased.
- Heel strike becomes apparent.

- Stride length is increased.
- Hip flexion is reduced.
- Forward pelvic tilt is reduced.

leg extension at push-off. Secondarily, children's stride length increases because of increased leg length.

- *Walking speed and step frequency.* As walking develops, speed increases while step frequency (steps per minute) decreases. Sutherland (1997) hypothesized that increased neuromuscular control in older walkers is primarily responsible for the decreased step frequency. Fundamentally, younger walkers lack the postural control to increase speed through longer strides and thus must take more frequent steps.

- *Double-knee lock.* As walking improves, children increase their range of motion through the double-knee lock pattern. The knee is extended at heel strike, flexed slightly as body weight shifts over the support leg, and extended once more at push-off.

- *Pelvic rotation.* By 14 months of age, pelvic rotation is apparent, allowing for full range of motion as well as oppositional movements of the upper and lower bodies.

- *Oppositional arm swing.* As noted earlier, beginning walkers have their arms in a high guard position with elbows slightly flexed and abducted. Over the ensuing months, this position is gradually replaced by a mechanically efficient oppositional arm swing. Initially, the arm swing may

FIGURE 7.3

Whole-Body Approach for Walking—Mature Stage

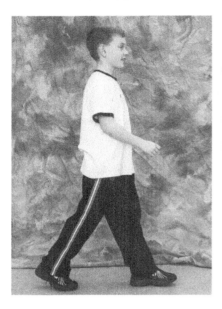 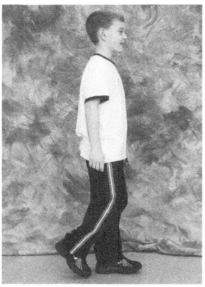 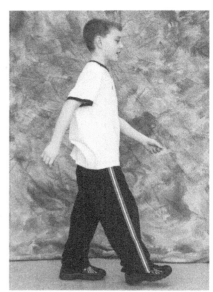

- Base of support is significantly narrower.
- Foot contact becomes heel–toe as opposed to flat footed.
- Single-knee lock pattern is replaced by double-knee lock pattern.

- Step and stride lengths are increased.
- Walking speed and step frequency are increased.
- Oppositional arm swing is apparent.

not be coordinated; the arms may sometimes come forward in unison. Over time, oppositional arm swing becomes established, and the opposite arm and leg move forward and backward at the same time. As this reciprocal movement is refined, the arm swing becomes relaxed, with slight movement at both the shoulder and the elbow.

As noted previously, the development of proficient walking not only allows children to explore their environment capably but also provides a stable and effective base for more advanced locomotor skills.

Running

Twelve-year-old Randy looked down at his watch and realized that dinner would be on the table in six minutes and he had a long way to go before he got home. Walking would not get him there on time, and a light jog wouldn't do it either. Even though the terrain was uneven, he launched into a smooth run. Randy made it to the dinner table with minutes to spare. Running has been characterized as an extension of walking, and certainly the two forms of locomotion have much in common—the reciprocal arm and leg action as well as the alternating leg action. However, there are clear differences; primary among these is that running does not have a double-support phase. Instead there is a flight phase during which neither foot is in contact with the ground.

Randy's running wasn't always as smooth as on that evening. When he began to run (approximately seven months after beginning to walk independently), he had to develop enough strength to become airborne, as well as the balance to catch himself on one leg and maintain balance on that leg while moving forward. Thus, developing adequate strength and balance is imperative, and these factors may act as *rate limiters* for the developing runner. Figures 7.4 through 7.6 present a hypothesized developmental sequence for running, including both leg and arm action (Gabbard, 2012; Gallahue et al., 2012; Haywood & Getchell, 2014; Payne & Issacs, 2012; Wickstrom, 1983).

As children mature physically (specifically, gain in body size and strength as well as coordination) and get more practice, they show concomitant improvements in both process and product measures related to running. With regard to product measures, they run more quickly and increase the amount of time spent in the flight phase. With respect to the running

FIGURE 7.4

Whole-Body Approach for Running—Initial Stage

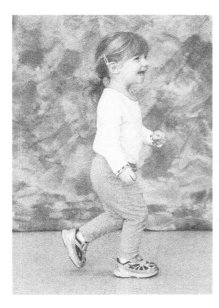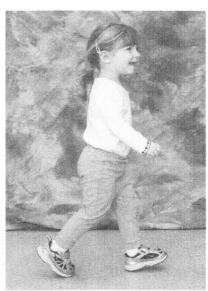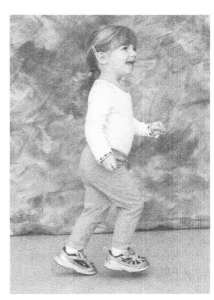

- Movements of legs and feet are exaggerated.
- Flight period is minimal.
- Contact is generally flat footed (although some children run on tiptoes).

- Base of support is wide.
- Arms are held in either a middle or high guard position.
- Arms move to the sides as opposed to back and forth.

FIGURE 7.5

Whole-Body Approach for Running—Elementary Stage

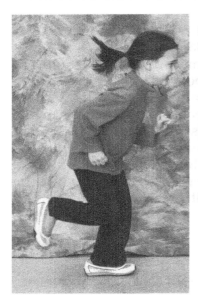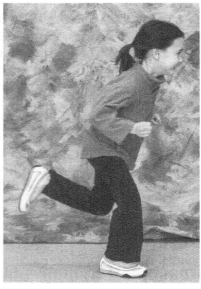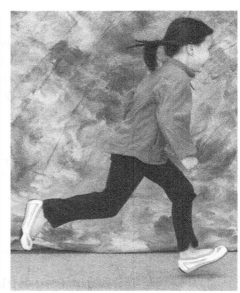

- Hip, knee, and ankle extension is increased at takeoff.
- Height of the forward knee is increased at takeoff.
- Length of the running stride is increased.

- Speed of running is increased.
- Flight period is increased.
- Horizontal arm swing is increased.

---

process, the following positive changes take place over developmental time, resulting in a mature running pattern (Haywood & Getchell, 2014; Wickstrom, 1983):

- A slight forward lean is maintained throughout the stride.
- The arms swing in a synchronized pattern in opposition to the leg pattern, with the elbows held at approximately 90 degrees.
- The support foot makes contact with the ground approximately under the center of gravity in a flat-footed fashion.
- The knee of the support leg bends slightly after the foot contacts the ground.
- The body moves forward and upward (into the nonsupport phase) through

forceful extension of the support leg at the ankle, knee, and hip.

- The recovery knee moves forcefully to a high knee raise, while the lower leg simultaneously flexes, bringing the heel close to the buttock.
- Out-toeing is eliminated and the base of support is narrowed.
- Trunk rotation increases, leading to greater stride length as well as improved arm–leg opposition.

In typically developing children, learning to run proficiently occurs fairly automatically. However, when they are learning advanced maneuvers (e.g., chasing, fleeing, changing direction quickly) or trying to increase speed, instructors should use techniques based on their developmental age.

FIGURE 7.6

Whole-Body Approach for Running—Mature Stage

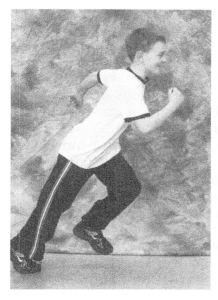 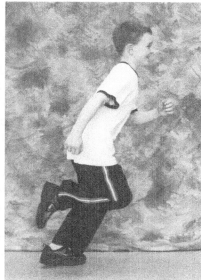 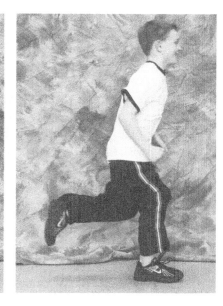

- Base of support is narrow.
- Length of running stride is increased further.
- Application of force is greater.
- Trunk leans forward slightly.
- Arms move in a large arc, in opposition to the leg movements.

- Arms are bent at the elbows at approximately 90 degrees.
- Recovery knee is raised high and swings forward quickly.
- Support leg bends slightly at contact and subsequently extends quickly and completely.

Jumping

A child who can run has the essential ingredients needed to be a jumper; and from the age of two, children begin to explore and develop ways of moving other than walking and running. The family of jumps is a large one and is made up of leaping (a one-foot takeoff followed by a landing on the opposite foot), hopping (jumping from one foot to the same foot rhythmically), the vertical jump for height (a two-foot takeoff with a two-foot landing), and the standing long jump or horizontal jump for distance (a two-foot takeoff with a two-foot landing).

Developing proficiency in this assortment of jumps allowed Randy in our example not only to speed along quickly and fluidly but also to keep his brand-new shoes dry by jumping over a narrow stream. As he got closer to home and knew that he had time to spare, Randy gathered himself, jumped high in the air, and grabbed an apple from a tree. As Randy became older, all the jumping skills he had developed helped him with the activities he liked—hitting a volleyball, making a layup, and running the steeplechase.

Jumping is the fundamental movement skill of projecting the body into the air by the force generated by either one or both legs, and then landing on one or both feet. Jumping can be done in a forward, backward, or sideways direction. Although related to walking and running (the leap is actually an exaggerated running step), jumping is a more challenging movement skill for children to master. They need adequate strength to get the body into the air, postural control and coordination while in the air, and balance on landing. Strength is particularly important in hopping because the one-foot-to-one-foot pattern is done repeatedly. Wickstrom (1983) observed that, beyond the significant physical requirements of jumping, there are confidence requirements. Jumping from heights, in particular, requires a certain level of bravery. In an early investigation, Gutteridge (1939) noted that when children had to jump from an increased height or were introduced to a new, challenging type of jump, they reverted to an earlier form of jumping.

Gutteridge's (1939) and Wickstrom's (1983) observations lead to an interesting question that motor developmentalists must answer, regardless of the skill being considered: How do we measure improvement or regression? Haywood and Getchell (2005) suggested the following three methods:

1. Age norms: Comparing when the person acquired a skill to when most people acquire the skill

2. Quantitative measures: Determining how much of something is present; for jumping, determining the height or the distance of the jump

3. Qualitative measures: Observing the pattern or form of the movement

Along with these three methods, Wickstrom's (1983) perspective regarding courage or confidence should be considered. Although this is more difficult to evaluate objectively, how confident a child is of her skill level has a considerable bearing on how well she performs.

With respect to the age at which preschool children typically learn types of jumps, early scholars in the area of motor development (Bayley, 1935; McCaskill & Wellman, 1938) assigned approximate ages (e.g., jump from a 12 ft [3.7 m] height with one foot ahead: 24 months; jump from a 12 ft [3.7 m] height with both feet: 34 months; jump over a rope 2 to 8 inches [5 to 20 cm] high with both feet: 41.5 months). Wickstrom (1983) stressed that these are approximate because of the wide range of scores observed. Given that people of all ages have changed in size and strength over the past century (referred to as a *secular trend*), children born in the 21st century will very likely achieve these jumping landmarks at somewhat younger ages.

Skill development in children involves the gradual refinement of movement abilities over time. Indeed, researchers examining the acquisition of movement skill from a dynamic systems perspective have noted that children who refine their movement patterns appear better able to take advantage of the principles of motion. These observations clearly apply to the acquisition of jumping skill. With respect to the refinement of movement abilities over chronological time, Haywood and Getchell (2012) noted that even if beginning jumpers intend to perform a long jump, because of limitations in their form (the qualitative components of the jump), they end up doing a vertical jump. This is largely a result of posture that is too erect. By three years of age, however, the developing child can modify the trunk angle to perform either a vertical or a horizontal jump as desired (Clark, Phillips, & Peterson, 1989).

Early jumps, for either height or distance, are characterized by a shallow preparatory crouch. That is, the hip, knees, and ankles are not flexed enough to generate a significant amount of force. Additionally, the legs remain slightly flexed at takeoff. Beginning jumpers often use a one-foot takeoff (also referred to as a stepout), as well as a landing during which one foot touches down before the other. Because of the one-foot takeoff, the legs are frequently asymmetrical during flight. Adopting a two-foot takeoff, with an appropriate body lean, generally keeps the legs symmetrical and thus more aerodynamic during flight.

To this point, the discussion has concentrated on the lower body; however, the way the arms are used can help or hinder jumping. Beginning jumpers often demonstrate arm actions that are not beneficial for a long jump or vertical jump. These jumpers may use the arms asymmetrically, hold them stationary (at the sides), or hold them in a high guard position for protection in case of a fall.

Despite these inauspicious beginnings, most children learn to jump effectively by the time they begin school. Movement toward the mature jumps outlined earlier depends on the opportunity to practice in varied environments as well as normal growth in size and strength. Although consistent quantitative changes in jump distance (average increases of 3 to 5 inches [7.6 to 12.7 cm] a year during the elementary years) and jump height (average increases of 2 in. [5 cm] per year during the elementary ages) have been cataloged (DeOreo & Keogh, 1980), qualitative changes are more varied (Haywood & Getchell, 2014).

As discussed earlier, and demonstrated for the skill of running in figures 7.4 through 7.6, researchers have presented changes in movement skill as developmental sequences that capture the qualitative changes in the critical features of a skill. Both the whole-body approach and the component approach identify the steps children go through as they move from inefficient movements to more skillful patterns. Figures 7.7 through 7.9 present

FIGURE 7.7

Whole-Body Approach for the Standing Long Jump—Initial Stage

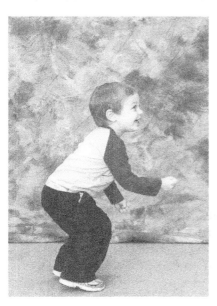 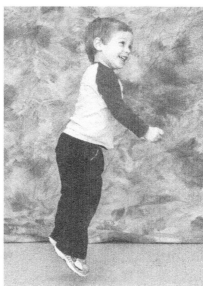 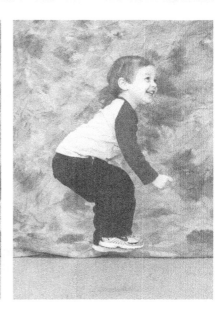

- Preparatory crouch is limited and inconsistent.
- Trunk lean is less than 30 degrees.
- Extension of the hips and knees at takeoff and during flight is minimal.
- Arm swing is minimal and ineffective (arms are held rigidly at the sides with elbows flexed or arms held in winged position).
- Legs are positioned asymmetrically during flight.
- Vertical force is generally greater than horizontal force, leading to an upward rather than a forward jump.
- An inability to flex the hips and knees during the jump leads to an abrupt landing.

FIGURE 7.8

Whole-Body Approach for the Standing Long Jump—Elementary Stage

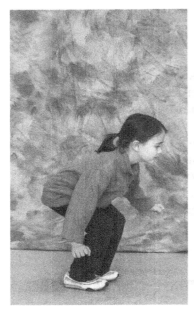 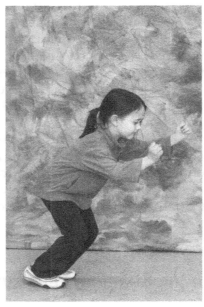 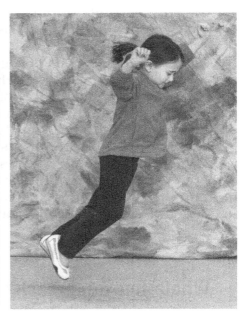

- Preparatory crouch becomes deeper and more consistent.
- Extension of hips and knees is increased.
- Forward swing of arms (in the anteroposterior plane) is increased.

- Total-body extension at takeoff is increased.
- Thigh flexion during flight is increased.

developmental characteristics of the standing long jump, and figures 7.10 through 7.12 present developmental characteristics of the vertical jump, using the whole-body approach (Gabbard, 2012; Gallahue et al., 2012; Haywood & Getchell, 2014; Payne & Issacs, 2012; Wickstrom, 1983).

The standing long jump (also referred to as the horizontal jump or broad jump) and the vertical jump have much in common.

Both have easily identifiable preparatory, takeoff, flight, and landing phases, and the takeoffs and landings are two footed. However, the standing long jump presents more movement challenges than the vertical jump does. Because the jumper is moving the body both upward and outward, the center of gravity must be slightly in front of the base of support at takeoff. Proficient jumping requires a takeoff angle

FIGURE 7.9

Whole-Body Approach for the Standing Long Jump—Mature Stage

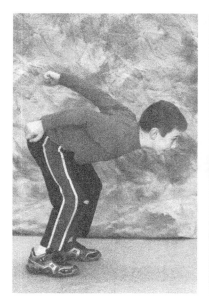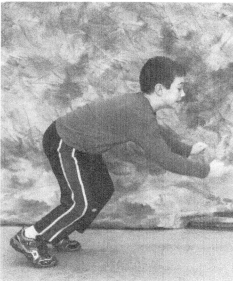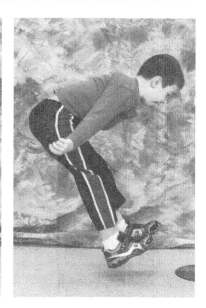

- Preparatory crouch is deep with flexion of the hips, knees, and ankles.
- Trunk lean is at least 30 degrees.
- Arms are swung backward simultaneously in a smooth fashion.
- Heels come off the ground before knee extension.
- There is a rapid and vigorous extension at takeoff of the hips and knees in the direction of travel.

- Arms vigorously swing forward and upward.
- Both knees are flexed, and the thighs are brought forward, parallel to the ground, during flight.
- Lower legs swing forward for a two-foot landing.

of approximately 45 degrees. Because this is a challenge for developing jumpers, they frequently step out to maintain their balance. A second significant movement challenge for long jumpers is swinging their legs from behind the center of gravity (at takeoff) forward and under the trunk in preparation for landing. Because the vertical jump does not require the body to tip forward or the legs to swing forward, it is an easier jump to perform and master than the long jump.

FIGURE 7.10

Whole-Body Approach for Vertical Jumping—Initial Stage

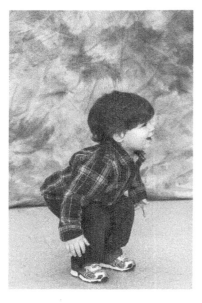 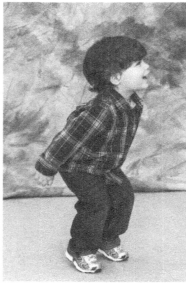 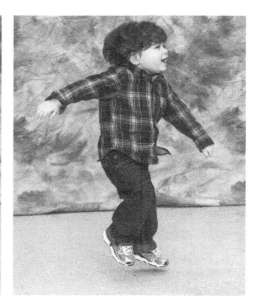

- Form is variable and unpredictable.
- Preparatory crouch is limited and inconsistent.
- Legs are not fully extended at take-off.

- There is very quick flexion of hips and knees (the legs are tucked under the body).
- Arms and shoulders are elevated sideways.
- Head flexes forward.

FIGURE 7.11

Whole-Body Approach for Vertical Jumping—Elementary Stage

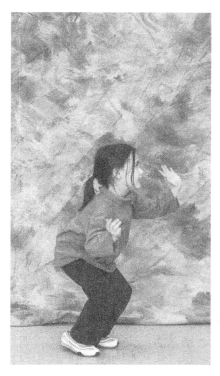 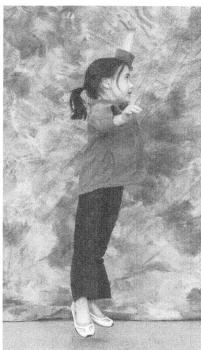 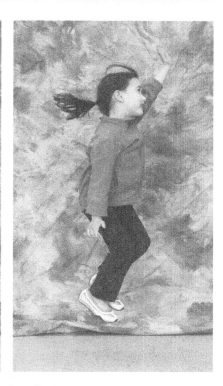

- Form becomes less variable and more predictable.
- Preparatory crouch becomes deeper (with increased knee bend).

- A two-foot takeoff takes place.
- Arms are used to aid in flight and balance, but often unequally.
- Body does not extend completely during flight.

FIGURE 7.12

Whole-Body Approach for Vertical Jumping—Mature Stage

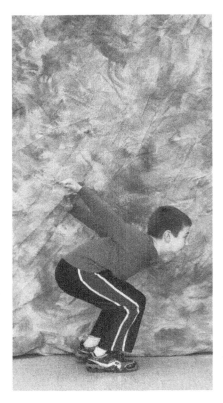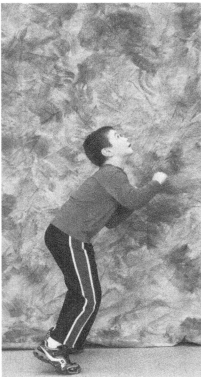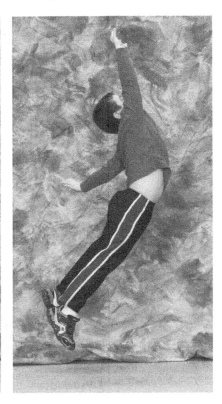

- There is a deep preparatory crouch with flexion of the hips, knees, and ankles.
- Hips, knees, and ankles extend completely upon takeoff.
- There is very quick flexion of the hips and knees (the legs are tucked under the body).
- Arms are swung forward and upward.

- One hand continues up while the other comes down, resulting in an effective tipping of the shoulder girdle near the peak of the jump.
- Head flexes backward.
- Trunk extends at the crest of the reach.
- Landing is on the balls of the feet with the hips and knees flexed.

Hopping

A hop is defined as taking off and landing on the same foot. As discussed earlier, this movement requires considerable strength and balance. The proficient hopper demonstrates the following characteristics (Haywood & Getchell, 2014, p. 145):

- The swing leg leads the hip.
- The support leg extends fully.
- The arms move in opposition to the legs.

- The support leg flexes at landing to absorb the force of the landing and to prepare for extension at the next takeoff.

Both a component developmental sequence (Halverson & Williams, 1985) and a whole-body developmental sequence (Gallahue et al., 2012) have been developed for the hop. Figures 7.13 through 7.15 present a whole-body sequence (Gabbard, 2012; Gallahue et al., 2012; Haywood & Getchell, 2014; Payne & Issacs, 2012; Wickstrom, 1983).

FIGURE 7.13

Whole-Body Approach for Hopping—Initial Stage

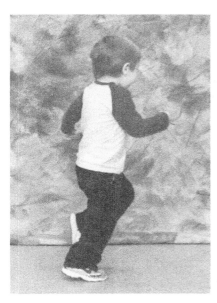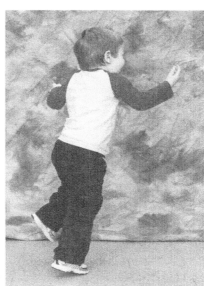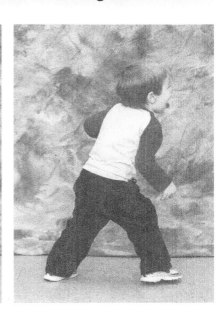

- Forward movement is minimal.
- Elevation is minimal.
- Movement is jerky.
- Support leg is lifted by flexion rather than by forceful extension.
- Nonsupport (swing) leg is generally held high and is largely inactive.

- Arm action is minimal or inconsistent.
- Arms are held in the high guard position and to the sides for balance.
- Landings are flat footed.

FIGURE 7.14

Whole-Body Approach for Hopping—Elementary Stage

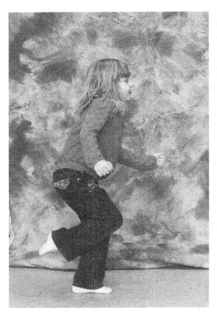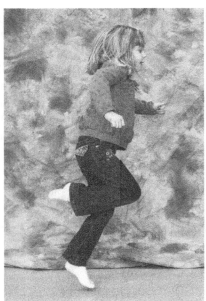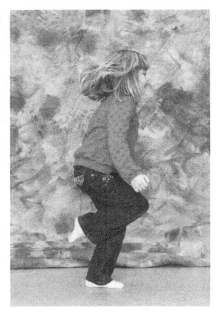

- Forward movement is increased.
- Elevation is increased.
- Support leg is lifted by minimal knee and ankle extension because of slight body lean.

- Nonsupport (swing) leg moves forward and upward.
- Arms begin to be used (bilaterally) for thrust rather than for balance.

FIGURE 7.15

Whole-Body Approach for Hopping—Mature Stage

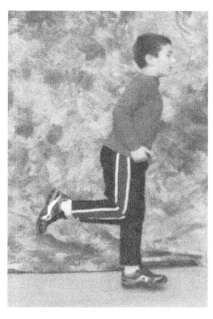 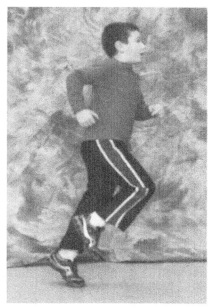 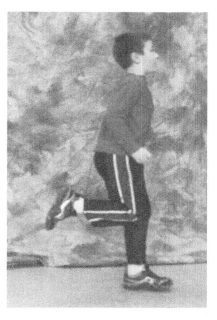

- Weight is transferred smoothly, upon landing, to the ball of the foot of the support leg before the ankle and knee extend.
- Support leg reaches almost full extension upon takeoff.
- Swing leg leads the movement, pumping up and down.
- Pumping action of the swing leg increases such that, when viewed from the side, it passes behind the support leg.

- Arm opposite the swing leg moves upward and forward in synchrony with the upward and forward movement of the swing leg.
- Other arm moves in a direction opposite that of the swing leg.
- Vigorous swinging action may not be present unless there are speed or distance requirements, or both.

Manipulative Skills

When children are able to walk in and around the immediate environment independently and with some fluidity, their hands (and feet) are suddenly available to explore even more thoroughly. All of a sudden, they can impart force to an object and watch it move through the environment. They can also receive objects projected toward them. Manipulative skills (also referred to as object control skills) generally involve a combination of at least two movements and are performed in concert with other types of movements. For example, in striking a ball with a bat, stepping, turning, swinging, and stretching occur. Fundamental manipulative skills include overarm throwing, catching with one or both hands, and kicking and striking objects (with or without an implement). This section discusses the development of the ballistic skills of overarm throwing, kicking, and striking.

Overarm Throwing

Objects can be thrown in a variety of ways including, but not limited to, underhand, sidearm, and overarm (also referred to as overhand). The pattern chosen has much to do with the task to be performed; that is, (a) what the thrower hopes to accomplish and (b) specific constraints of the task as defined by the size, shape, and weight of the implement to be thrown (e.g., a regulation-size American football versus a basketball) as well as the rules of the game. From a biomechanical (technique) perspective, the three throws have much in common. In this section we concentrate on the overarm throw because it is frequently used in sports (e.g., softball, European handball, American football) and has been extensively studied over the past 80 years (Halverson, Roberton, & Langendorfer, 1982; Jones-Petranek, & Barton, 2011; Lorson, Stodden, & Goodway, 2013; Rober-ton & Konczak, 2001; Thomas, Alderson, Thomas, Campbell, & Elliott, 2010; Wild, 1938).

As with all fundamental motor skills, overarm throwing can be examined in a number of ways. Researchers who use a quantitative or product approach focus on such outcomes as ball velocity, distance thrown, and accuracy. Since Wild's initial work in 1938, researchers have also looked at throwing using a qualitative or process approach. Haywood and Getchell (2014) persuasively argued for the usefulness of rigorously examining the quality of the movement. Coaches, parents, and physical education teachers will be of most use to developing throwers by becoming skilled at (a) assessing *how* they throw and (b) setting up tasks and environments that engage and excite them (thereby increasing the likelihood that throwing improves).

Children first demonstrate a rudimentary overarm throw when they are approximately six months of age and in a sitting position (Eckert, 1987). Although a majority of children demonstrate a mature overarm throwing pattern by six years of age, a significant number remain unskilled into adulthood (this is particularly true of girls, an observation that has garnered a large amount of research attention over the past four decades).

A study by Halverson and colleagues (1982) supports observations that many children remain unskilled throwers well into their middle school years, and that many more girls remain unskilled when compared to boys. The authors observed the development of overarm throwing in a sample of both boys and girls from kindergarten through grade 7. Using this longitudinal approach, the authors noted that by the seventh grade, 80 percent of males had reached the mature level of upper arm action, whereas only 29 percent of females had done so.

Other studies (see, for example, Leme & Shambes, 1978) indicate that many women never achieve a mature throw. Indeed, it has been repeatedly demonstrated that men outperform women in overarm throwing at all ages (Butterfield & Loovis, 1993; Halverson et al., 1982; Rehling, 1996). However, in a 2013 study, Lorson and colleagues noted that the gap between the sexes narrowed during adulthood. In their cross-sectional investigation, the authors found that while qualitative and quantitative aspects of overarm throwing regressed for males during adulthood, they remained consistent, in most regards, for females. However, it should be noted that although the gap narrowed slightly, males continued to outperform females, and did so throughout the time periods examined: middle adolescence (14-17 years), young adolescence (18-25 years), and adulthood (35-55 years). The decrease in throwing skill observed in males between young adulthood and adulthood was hypothesized to occur as a result of rate limiters such as decreased overall flexibility and decreased shoulder strength and flexibility, reduced motivation to practice, and decreased opportunities to engage in forceful overarm throwing. The finding that women in the study did not demonstrate a regression in skill at any of the three age groupings was thought to relate to the fact that women, generally, do not ever attain the most advanced level of throwing, regardless of age.

Some hypothesized that with the advent of Title IX law in the United States, the gap between boys and girls would narrow; however, work by Runion, Roberton, and Langendorfer (2003) on throw velocity suggests that qualitative and quantitative differences between the sexes remain. Title IX has, however, led to significant increases in female sport participation, and thus opportunities to practice overarm throwing. In an investigation done in 2011, Jones-Petranek and Barton examined the overarm throwing patterns of 13- and 14-year-old female softball players who took part in highly competitive play. As would be expected, they were significantly more skilled than girls who were not engaged in high-level, organized athletics. However, the authors found that despite frequent practice in overarm throwing, boys (from Germany and the United States) who had not engaged in systematic throwing practice were still better than their female counterparts, using both qualitative and quantitative measures. The authors suggested that, "practice when combined with genetics and evolution may afford boys the ability to exhibit more advanced throwing patterns with greater ball velocities than girls" (p. 227). It was further suggested that the precise spatial and temporal qualities of advanced throwers should be further examined, along with the quality of the throwing practice and the specific training approaches used in baseball and softball.

Irrespective of sex differences, the route to a mature throwing pattern appears to be a circuitous one, and considerable variability in movement patterns is a consistent observation. By being aware of the elements involved in a proficient throw, practitioners and parents can become more attuned to what is missing in more immature attempts. As presented earlier in this chapter, changes in throwing proficiency can be cataloged using either a component or a whole-body approach. Both approaches precisely delineate changes in competency as the developing child moves toward throwing proficiency. Figures 7.16 through 7.18 present the hypothesized whole-body developmental sequence for the overarm throw for distance (Gabbard, 2012; Gallahue et al., 2012; Haywood & Getchell, 2014; Payne & Issacs, 2012; Wickstrom, 1983).

FIGURE 7.16

Whole Body Approach for the Overarm Throw for Distance— Initial Stage

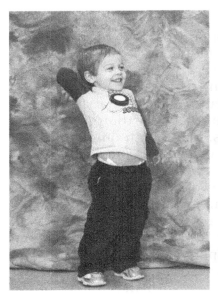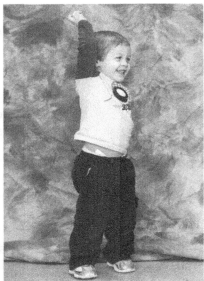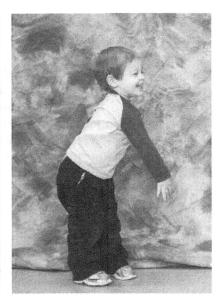

- Throw tends to result from arm action only.
- No preparatory backswing occurs; rather, the hand is brought back with the elbow up.
- Throw is completed by releasing the ball following elbow extension.
- Follow-through occurs in a forward direction, if present.

- There is either little or no trunk action; if trunk action takes place, it does so in a forward–backward direction.
- Body weight may shift slightly to the rear to maintain balance.
- No step is taken.

FIGURE 7.17

Whole Body Approach for the Overarm Throw for Distance— Elementary Stage

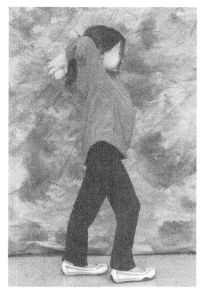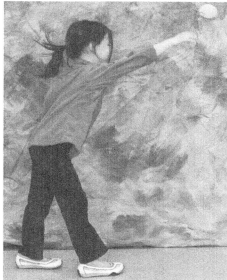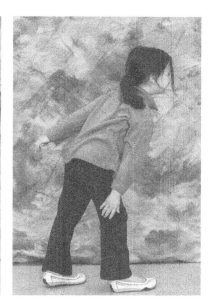

- Trunk and shoulders rotate toward the throwing side to prepare for the throw.
- Sideward and backward swing of the arm then brings the ball to a position behind the head with the elbow flexed.
- Arm is swung forward, high over the shoulder.

- Forearm extends before the ball is released.
- Forward shift in body weight is evident.
- Ipsilateral (same-side) step is taken during the throw.

Taking a Look at the Quality of Your Throwing

Exercise 7.5

Stand 20 feet (6 m) from a target located at head height. Using an overarm technique, throw a tennis ball at the target 10 times with your dominant hand, keeping track of the number of times you hit the target. Think about how you're throwing—that is, the quality of the throw. Now, throw the tennis ball 10 times with your nondominant hand, again keeping track of how many times you hit the target and the quality of the throw. Then write down the differences you experienced both quantitatively (how many times you hit the target) and qualitatively. After having done this exercise yourself, have a partner observe you doing it. Compare your partner's qualitative observations with your own. Which observations would you consider more accurate, and why?

FIGURE 7.18

Whole-Body Approach for the Overarm Throw for Distance— Mature Stage

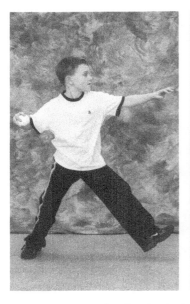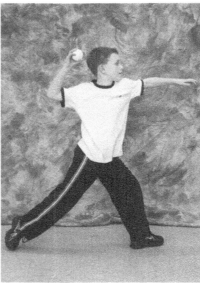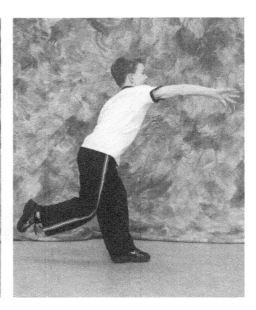

- Body pivots to the throwing side with the weight on the foot of the throwing side.
- Throwing arm swings back in a circular, downward direction.
- Elbow of the nonthrowing arm is raised for balance.
- Elbow of the throwing arm is bent at approximately a right angle.
- Long contralateral (opposite-side) step is taken in the direction of the target.
- There is differentiated trunk rotation; that is, the pelvis begins to rotate before the upper spine in the initiation of trunk rotation.
- Throwing elbow moves forward horizontally as it extends.
- Forearm lags behind at the moment the shoulders are front facing.
- Ball is released just forward of the head; at this point, the arm is extended at the elbow.
- Arm follows through across the body after ball release.

Can the Throwing Gap Be Narrowed?

That most girls throw, well, like girls has been an insult thrown around (pun intended) for many years. Generally speaking, regardless of whether researchers have focused on distance and velocity (Atwater, 1979; Thomas & French, 1985) or the biomechanical properties of the throw (Atwater, 1979; Thomas & Marzke, 1992), females have lagged way behind their male counterparts. These stark differences are evident long before puberty, when physiological differences between the sexes are much less pronounced. So, this begs the question, Why such a big difference? and secondly, Can the throwing gap between the sexes be narrowed?

Thomas and colleagues (2010) hypothesized that the very different cultural expectations of men and women—over the centuries—have contributed significantly to differences in throwing ability. Specifically, men have been the hunter-gatherers, while women have been the primary food producers. Thus, men had to be able to throw weapons of one sort or another, whereas women didn't. This is an interesting hypothesis, but difficult to prove. However, if the researchers could locate a culture in which both men and women were responsible for hunting, they could, to a degree, test this hypothesis. Aboriginal Australians fit this description: the historical record suggested that women, historically, threw for defense and hunting alongside the men (Clarke, 2003). Thomas and colleagues (2010) found that aboriginal boys tested on the overarm throw had velocities and biomechanical properties that were similar to their counterparts in the United States, Germany, Japan, and Thailand (where the previous research had been done). However, the aboriginal girls threw with significantly greater velocity than girls in the United States, Germany, Japan, and Thailand. Additionally, aboriginal boys and girls were more similar with respect to the velocity and biomechanical properties of their throws compared to children from the United States. None of the aboriginal boys and girls received any special training, and yet the girls were more skilled than their peers in other countries. Could the results be due to somewhat different societal expectations, or is there another explanation (maybe one that could lead to the phrase *throwing like a girl* being considered a compliment)?

Kicking

Like throwing, kicking imparts force to an object. However, the kicker strikes the object as opposed to hurling it. To kick proficiently, a person must have adequate perceptual abilities along with eye–foot coordination. As with throwing, children kick in a number of ways. Gallahue and colleagues (2012) postulated that the kick is chosen based on the desired trajectory and how high the ball is when contacted. These authors also noted that the type of kick chosen is influenced by the force of the ball as it comes to her when she receives a pass and (as frequently noted in this text) the desired outcome; that is, the task at hand. Another consideration in the playing of a sport, as mentioned with reference to the throw, is the techniques the rules allow. For example, in soccer, the goaltender may hold the ball in the hands, drop it, and then kick it; other players may not contact the ball with the hands, which means that a different type of kicking technique is necessary.

As with the other fundamental movement skills, an advanced kick has certain critical features. In this section we consider the place kick, a kick that is performed when the ball is either on the ground or on a kicking tee.

As in throwing, immature kickers do not sequence their actions; rather, the kick is a single action, and the force imparted to the ball is inadequate. The action is more of a push, with the kicking leg often remaining bent on contact. The development of kicking skill has not been carefully examined with regard to the qualitative changes needed for proficiency. Given that only 10 percent of the 7.5- to 9.0-year-olds studied by Haubenstricker, Seefeldt, and Branta (1983) were proficient kickers, it appears that a more careful examination of developmental changes in this fundamental movement skill is imperative. Initial work has been done on the validation of a whole-body developmental sequence for place kicking (Seefeldt & Haubenstricker, 1975). Figures 7.19 through 7.21 show the hypothesized whole-body developmental sequence for place kicking (Gabbard, 2012; Gallahue et al., 2012; Haywood & Getchell, 2014; Payne & Issacs, 2012; Wickstrom, 1983).

FIGURE 7.19

Whole-Body Approach for Place Kicking—Initial Stage

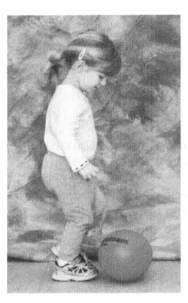 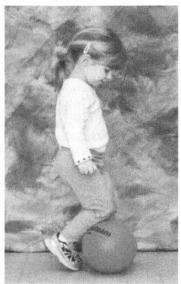 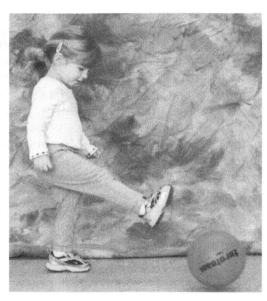

- Action is a simple pushing of the ball with the foot.
- Motion of the kicking leg is straight and perpendicular.
- Range of motion is very limited; backswing and follow-through are minimal.
- Nonkicking leg does not step forward.

- Trunk remains upright with no rotation present; there is very limited movement of the upper body.
- Knee of the kicking leg is often bent at contact.
- Arms are held out to the sides to aid in the maintenance of balance.

FIGURE 7.20

Whole-Body Approach for Place Kicking—Elementary Stage

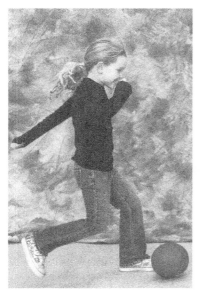
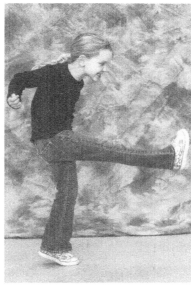
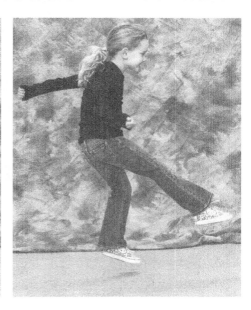

- Range of motion of the kicking leg (backswing and follow-through) increases at the hip and knee.
- Kicker takes one or more deliberate steps while approaching the ball.
- Kicker tends to start farther behind the ball and move the body forward into the kick.

- Support leg is placed slightly to the side of the ball.
- Kicking leg is in a cocked position and tends to remain bent throughout the kick.
- Kicking leg often retracts after completing the kick; that is, follow-through is minimal.
- Compensatory trunk lean and arm opposition increase.

TRY THIS

Do You Have What It Takes to Kick Like a Pro?

Exercise 7.6

As you did with throwing, stand 20 feet (6 m) from a target located at head height. Kick a soccer ball with your dominant leg at the target 10 times, keeping track of the number of times you hit the target. Think about how you're kicking; that is, the quality of the kick. Now, kick the soccer ball 10 times with your nondominant leg, again keeping track of how many times you hit the target and the quality of the kick. Then write down the differences you experienced both quantitatively and qualitatively. Have a partner observe you doing the same thing. Compare your partner's qualitative observations with your own. Which observations would you consider more accurate, and why?

FIGURE 7.21
Whole-Body Approach for Place Kicking—Mature Stage

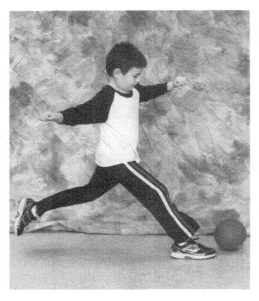
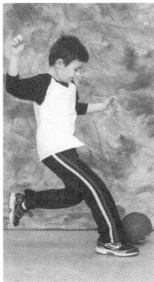
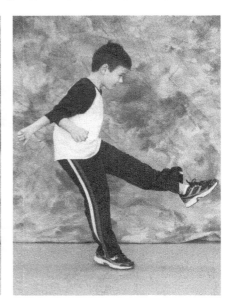

- Following one or more deliberate steps, the kicker becomes airborne immediately before contacting the ball, allowing appropriate hip hyperextension and knee flexion.
- Trunk is rotated to the side, and the knee of the kicking leg is flexed.
- Knee of the kicking leg extends rapidly just prior to contacting the ball.

- Arms are used in opposition to the legs during the kick.
- Trunk bends at the waist during follow-through.
- Forward momentum is sufficient; the kicker either hops on the support leg or scissors the legs while in the air, thus allowing a landing on the kicking foot.

Striking

Striking, a skill used in many sporting activities, has many configurations. It can be done with an implement (e.g., bat, racket, golf club) or with a body part (e.g., head, hand, foot). It can be performed in a variety of orientations—swinging a bat sidearm, spiking a volleyball overhand, or driving a golf ball underhand. Striking can also be done with either one or two hands (e.g., one-handed backhand or two-handed backhand in tennis). With such an array of orientations, implements, and sporting activities, one would think that this fundamental motor skill would have been studied extensively. It has not.

Haywood and Getchell (2014) suggested that the relative lack of research may be a result of the difficulty of the task. Indeed, the perceptual judgments needed to make effective contact with a projectile, often a moving one, are tremendously complex. As many frustrated golfers know, even making contact with a ball that isn't moving at all can be more than a little difficult.

Nevertheless, because the developing child generally lacks the ability to strike a moving object, teachers and researchers adapt the task by making the ball stationary. As the child becomes more adept, a slowly moving ball with a smooth trajectory can be used. The size and shape of the object to be struck can be modified, as can the length and weight of the striking implement. As with jumping for height and jumping for distance, different configurations for striking (e.g., overarm, sidearm) have certain features in common such as using an upward or downward chopping motion for early strikers (as opposed to striking in a more horizontal plane as seen in more accomplished strikers). With increased practice, the swing usually becomes more fluid as learners incorporate more degrees of freedom into their movement patterns. This more accomplished movement pattern may include taking a contralateral step, adding a backswing, rotating the hips and trunk, and developing a coordinated wrist snap (Payne & Isaacs, 2012).

Although the research base for striking is sparse, Seefeldt and Haubenstricker (1975) hypothesized a whole-body developmental sequence for striking with a bat. This sequence, although not validated, provides practitioners with fundamental and important information regarding the development of mature striking. Figures 7.22 through 7.24 present a hypothesized

---

FIGURE 7.22

Whole-Body Approach for Sidearm Striking—Initial Stage

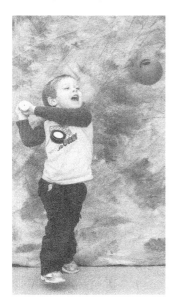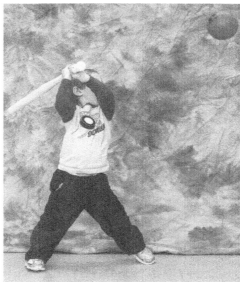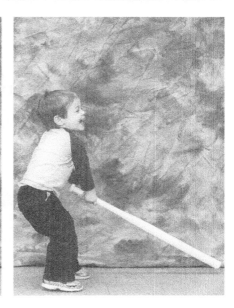

- Early attempts to strike are similar to the immature throwing motion; the bat (or other implement, such as a racket) is swung using a vertical (chopping) motion.
- Motion is from back to front with a slight bend at the waist.
- Striker flexes and extends the forearm to chop at the ball, while the trunk directly faces the direction of the tossed ball.
- Trunk and legs are minimally involved, and the feet are generally stationary.
- There is minimal or no weight transfer.
- Arms are held rigidly, with little or no wrist snap.

FIGURE 7.23

Whole-Body Approach for Sidearm Striking—Elementary Stage

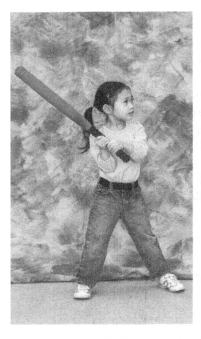
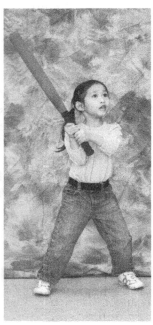
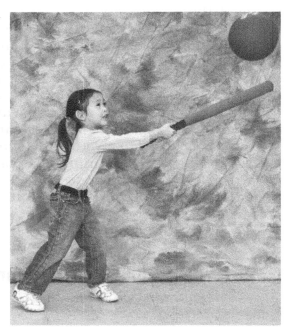

- Striker stands sideways to the ball.
- Striker transfers weight from the rear foot to the front foot by taking a step forward.
- Differentiated (hip, then shoulder) rotation is apparent.

- Plane of the swing changes from vertical (a chop) to oblique to horizontal.
- Elbows are held away from the sides, allowing for extension of the arms before contact, which results in increased force production.

FIGURE 7.24

Whole-Body Approach for Sidearm Striking—Mature Stage

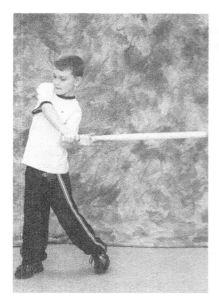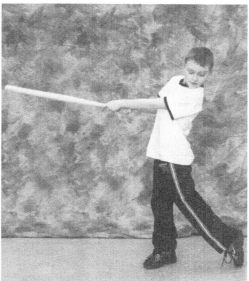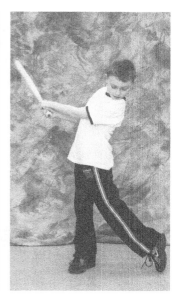

- Trunk is turned to the side in antici-pation of a thrown ball.
- Weight is shifted to the back foot, and the trunk and hips subse-quently rotate before ball contact.

- Striker uses a full range of motion and strikes the ball in the horizontal plane.
- Weight shifts to the forward foot at contact.
- Arms are relaxed.

whole-body developmental sequence for sidearm striking (Gabbard, 2012; Gallahue et al., 2012; Haywood & Getchell, 2014; Payne & Issacs, 2012; Wickstrom, 1983).

Summary

Acquiring fundamental movement skills is essential to the healthy development of children. Children given a strong move-ment foundation will have the skill set—and the confidence—to be physically active on their own, with their families, and with their peers. Whether the child ultimately decides to participate in more formalized athletic events or is content to play more recreationally is of course up to the child. What is evident, though, is that carefully designed movement environments and progressive educational experiences that are well thought through are essential to ensure early and sustained success. This chapter laid a solid foundation for under-standing how and when these fundamen-tals are achieved. Practitioners can take the concepts presented and build on them through practical experiences, focused research, or a combination of the two.

ONLINE LEARNING

Visit the web resource at www.HumanKinetics.com/MotorLearningAndDevelopment for an accom-panying lab activity, video clips, and exercises from the chapter.

LEARNING AIDS

Supplemental Activities

1. It is imperative that you be able to accurately and qualitatively assess how skillfully a given person moves through space. Accurate assessment requires frequent well-thought-out observations. From the Internet (YouTube or another video-sharing website), access video clips of novice and expert runners (one of each) and assess their proficiency. Watch each video clip at least five times. Use the following checklist in completing the assignment.

	Novice Age: Gender:	Expert Age: Gender:
Base of support		
Length of running stride		
Application of force by support leg		
Arms held in middle guard position		
Arms are swung backward and forward together (bilateral arm swing)		
Arms are swung forward and back in an opposition pattern		

From P.S. Haibach-Beach, G.D. Reid, and D.H. Collier, 2018, *Motor learning and development*, 2nd ed. (Champaign, IL: Human Kinetics).

   a. Were some components more difficult to observe than others?
   b. Did the observations become easier the more you viewed the video clip?
   c. Was it easier to rate the expert runner? Why or why not?

2. For this activity, you will watch 11- or 12-year-old students playing either soccer or softball. Having received the permissions necessary, go to a local sports complex, recreational facility, or school. Choose two male players and two female players and watch them throughout the contest. Using the whole-body approach as outlined in this chapter, assess the proficiency level of the four players you chose. If you are watching soccer, assess kicking; if you are watching softball, assess the overarm throw. As best you can, choose a boy and a girl who are relatively unskilled and a boy and a girl who are relatively skilled.

   a. Did you observe differences in the proficiency levels between boys and girls?
   b. If so, why do you think this was the case? If there were no sex differences, why not?
   c. Do you feel you became more proficient at assessing kicking or throwing as you had more experience observing?

Glossary

component approach—The perspective that learners' component body parts move toward the advanced form at potentially different times.

locomotor skills—Skills that involve moving from one place to the next.

manipulative skills—Skills that involve controlling implements and objects such as balls, hoops, bats, and ribbons by hand, by foot, or with any other part of the body.

qualitative changes—Process-related changes in skills over time.

quantitative changes—Product-related changes in skill over time.

secular trend—A change in an ability or skill over successive generations.

stability skills—Movements around the axis of the body (e.g., bending, stretching, swinging, swaying, pushing, pulling, turning, twisting) that are done with little or no movement of the base of support.

whole-body approach—The perspective that learners move through relatively invariant stages of movement skill development in which all body components move toward the advanced form at more or less the same time.

MOVEMENT IN ADULTHOOD

After reading this chapter, you should be able to do the following:

- Define aging, contrasting biological and chronological aging.
- Explain the exercise–aging cycle.
- Compare peak athletic performance for various sports and activities.
- Discuss how peak performance changes from young to older adulthood.
- Describe how movement patterns change from young to older adulthood in locomotor movements, fundamental movement patterns, and functional activities.

Never Limit Yourself

Martina Navratilova has marveled the world with her remarkable tennis skills and ability to seemingly defy not only aging but also cancer. At almost 50 years old, Martina won the U.S. Open mixed doubles championship and won the senior doubles Wimbledon title only days after completing radiation treatment for breast cancer at the age of 53. She was quoted as saying to ESPN, "You can do great things regardless of your age if you just believe and, you know, go for it," when she won the U.S. Open. She also said: "Don't get limited by people that say, 'No, you can't do that because you're too old or because you're heavy or you're not an athlete.' Whatever your limitations might be, don't let them define you. I didn't let it define me" (DeSimone, 2006). Being able to stay at the top of her game at an age at which most people consider themselves decades past their prime, Martina is a true testament of successful aging.

Adults advance through many stages throughout life, and these stages affect not only the activities they are involved in but also how they move. Young adults are considered to be at their physical peak, yet some avoid an active lifestyle for various reasons. Older adults, on the other hand, can avoid many age-related declines by maintaining a healthy and active lifestyle.

Some older adults are becoming increasingly physically active, participating in physical recreation activities, fitness activities, and even competitive sports. Every year, more seniors, both male and female, compete in races and triathlons, play golf and tennis, and join gyms and fitness groups. Some older adults are going extreme, competing in marathons and even Ironman triathlons. The Ironman is an ultimate testament to physical human capabilities, with a 2.4-mile (3.9 km) swim, a 112-mile (180 km) bike ride, and a 26.2-mile (42 km) run. In a period of 10 years, the number of Ironman competitors at Kona (on the Big Island of Hawaii) over the age of 70 increased threefold, from only 11 in 1997 to 37 in 2007. Now, more than ever, adults are aware of the importance of physical activity and the role fitness plays in their lives. With today's medical advances, changing technology, and increased focus on the benefits of good nutrition and physical activity, we can only expect this trend to continue.

This chapter discusses movement from young adulthood through older adulthood. Peak athletic performance is discussed for both younger and older adults, as are changing movement patterns in the areas of locomotor skills, fundamental motor skills, and functional activities.

Aging

In the minds of many, the term *aging* refers to declining physical function. Aging is generally thought of as something that occurs in older adulthood. However, in its simplest terms, aging can be defined as the number of time units over which an organism has existed following birth (Spirduso, Francis, & MacRae, 2005). When aging is defined this way, it becomes synonymous with time. The biological changes associated with infancy and childhood are referred to as developmental, whereas the changes that occur as a result of declining functional systems are referred to as aging (Spirduso et al., 2005). Because aging does not have a definitive onset, it is helpful to define **aging** as a process or group of processes occurring in living organisms that with the passage of time lead to a loss of adaptability and functional impairment, and eventually death (Spirduso et al., 2005).

Although we all age, we do not all age in the same way. We age differently and at varying rates. Functional impairments cannot be predicted because so many factors affect how we age, such as environmental, lifestyle, and cultural factors, as well as heredity. Individual differences are even greater for older adults than they are for young adults or children, allowing for wide variability. Older adults range from the frail elderly to masters athletes competing in marathons. An impressive example is Fauja Singh who, at the age of 81, became serious about running and began running marathons at the age of 89. At the age of 94, he had run seven marathons and was picked up by the Adidas "Impossible Is Nothing" campaign, along with David Beckham (retired soccer player who played for the England National team, Manchester United, England, Real Madrid, and the L.A. Galaxy) and Jonny Wilkinson (retired English rugby player known as one of the world's best).

In general, when we refer to a person's age, we are referring to **chronological age**. This is simply the number of years the person has been alive. This age does not take into account any biological or health factors, such as the person's overall well-being, fitness level, or health. **Biological aging** refers to the physiological adaptations that occur within the body as a result of the passage of time. Chronological age is one of the most important risk factors for morbidity, yet people at the same chronological age often have markedly different biological aging states. For example, a very active, healthy man may have a very low biological age in comparison to his chronological age. The situation could be the opposite in an overweight sedentary person who smokes and drinks.

The abundant literature on assessing biological age reveals a debate about how to most accurately assess it. Assessments of biological age include those that focus on one measure or score, such as metabolic age based on urinary metabolics (Hertel et al., 2016) or the degree of gray or white hairs as a risk factor for coronary artery disease (Kocaman, Cetin, Durakoglugil, Erdogan, Canga, & Cicek, 2012). Other assessments of biological age are rather complicated because biological systems age at different rates. For example, Comfort's biological age index (1979) includes anthropometric measures (e.g., body mass, graying of hair), physiological scores (e.g., vital capacity, tidal volume, blood volume, heart size, grip strength), bone and connective tissue integrity (e.g., skin elasticity, nail calcium, osteoporotic index), sensory tests (e.g., audiometry, visual acuity), biochemical data (e.g., serum cholesterol, copper, albumin, elastase, RNAase), cellular characteristics, intelligence tests, and psychomotor tests (e.g., reaction time and light extinction tests).

Although a thorough biological aging examination is complex, one should take biological age, rather than chronological age, into consideration when assessing a person's fitness, whether the purpose relates to fitness for a job, an exercise program, or skill learning (Shephard, 2008). Active older adults have been found to outperform sedentary young adults on many fitness tests. Let's take the incredible fitness level of Jack LaLanne, the well-known father of fitness who died in 2011 at the age of 96. At age 90, Jack still performed better than an average 30-year-old on

physical fitness tests (he was three times older than young adults who should be in their prime). Jack's enthusiasm for fitness and his incredible athleticism across his long life are a testament to the possibility of really pushing the aging envelope, enabling people to maintain their fitness levels decades past young adulthood.

Physical Activity

Note in table 1.2 in chapter 1 that young adulthood generally includes the period from the early third decade to the beginning of the fifth decade (ages 21-40). Middle adulthood is classified as the fifth through sixth decades (approximately 41-60 years). It is during young adulthood and halfway through adulthood that both biological function and physical performance are at their peak (Shephard, 2008). Unfortunately, a sedentary lifestyle remains common for older adults (Agency for Healthcare Research and Quality and the Centers for Disease Control and Prevention, 2002).

Although there is general agreement that physical activity is important for adults of all ages, it is not quite as clear how active older adults need to be, what types of activity are most important as people age, and how to encourage older adults to become or continue to be physically active. (Macera, Cavanaugh, & Bellettiere, 2015)

During middle-aged adulthood (ages 41-60), physical activity levels tend to decline further in most people as women go through menopause and men experience a reduction in sex hormones (Shephard, 1998). Physically active adults in the United States over the age of 55 most commonly participate in walking, gardening, cycling, golf, and aerobics (DiPietro, Williamson, Caspersen, & Eaker, 1993). Not until adults reach retirement age (young-old adults, ages 61-74) is there is an increase in physical activity; most people that increase their physical activity at this point take up walking, swimming, cycling, and dancing (Stephens & Craig, 1990). However, according to the 2007 Behavioral Risk Factor Surveillance System of the U.S. Centers for Disease Control and Prevention, Americans over the age of 65 have the highest prevalence of physical inactivity; 23.7 percent are "inactive," and 32.7 percent take part in no "leisure-time physical activity" (Centers for Disease Control and Prevention, 2009).

Physical activity levels decline again during old adulthood (ages 75-99) and beyond as many adults develop physical disabilities. Approximately 35 percent of males and 45 percent of females have two or more chronic diseases between the ages of 60 and 69. By the age of 80, approximately 53 percent of males and 70 percent of females have two or more chronic diseases (Guralnik & Simonsick, 1993).

Barriers to Physical Activity

Although in some Eastern cultures aging is revered, in the Western Hemisphere, aging is often associated with many negative stereotypes. Stereotyping people based on aging has become so common that it is referred to as **ageism**. Like racism (stereotyping based on a person's race) and sexism (stereotyping associated with a person's sex), ageism can have a severely negative impact on people. Older adults can be discriminated against for jobs and social activities. Ageism can also have a negative effect on older adults' participation in physical activities, because they are assumed to be less fit than younger adults and less able to perform physical activities. In light of these attitudes, it is not surprising that many adults progressively limit their physical activity levels. When adults buy into these negative attitudes, they often decrease their involvement in physical activity, and the attitudes turn into a self-fulfilling prophecy (Berger & McInman, 1993). Decreasing physical

activity levels based on age is referred to as **age grading**.

Participation in physical activity often begins to decline as young adults approach middle adulthood and face increasing responsibilities with finances and growing families (Payne & Isaacs, 2016). Single parents find it particularly difficult to fit exercise into their schedules. Retired adults have more free time but often limit participation in physical activity because of reduced financial means, limited means of transportation, and an apprehension about starting after so many years of not participating.

As adults age, many further decrease their involvement in exercise-related activities. These changes affect their body composition and athletic abilities. Poor physical health is considered the most common reason for lack of participation in physical activity in older adults (Baert, Gorus, Mets, Geerts, & Bautmans, 2011). In 2012, 35.9 percent of older Americans reported a disability, and 23.1 percent reported difficulty with walking or climbing stairs, or both (U.S. Department of Health and Human Services, Administration for Community Living, 2015). Common disabilities affecting physical activity participation are reduced mobility, pain, sensory deficits, cognitive impairments, and other medical problems (Macera et al., 2015). Approximately 25 to 50 percent of community-dwelling older adults and up to 80 percent of nursing home residents in the United States experience physical disability which is either caused by or results in pain (AGS Panel on Persistent Pain in Older Persons, 2002). Adults often find dealing with their changing bodies and abilities emotionally difficult, which affects their self-esteem and increases anxiety and stress. These changes cause people to become even less interested in physical activity, which in turn further impairs them physiologically. This phenomenon is known as the **exercise–aging cycle** (Berger & Hecht, 1989) (see figure 8.1).

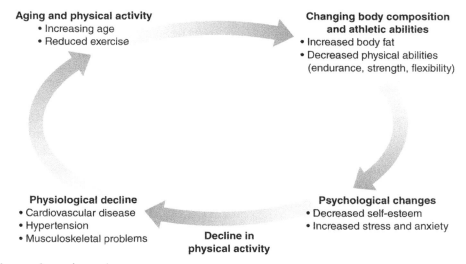

Figure 8.1   The exercise–aging cycle.

Adapted from Berger and Hecht 1989.

Physical Activity Recommendations

The current public health recommendation in the United States is to participate in moderate-intensity aerobic physical activity for at least 150 minutes per week or vigorous-intensity physical activity for 75 minutes per week. For additional benefits, adults should engage in physical activity beyond these minimums and incorporate muscle-strengthening activities that are moderate or high in intensity, involving all major muscle groups, two or more days per week (U.S. Department of Health and Human Services, 2008). According to the 2008 U.S. Department of Health and Human Services physical activity guidelines, older adults can do three things to improve their physical activity levels: increase aerobic activity, increase muscle-strengthening activity, and reduce sedentary, or sitting, behavior (Macera et al., 2015).

Approximately one in five (21.3 percent) American adults over the age of 18 met the current and age-adjusted U.S. federal physical activity guidelines for aerobic and resistance activities in 2014 (National Health Interview [NHIS]). Figure 8.2 illustrates the percentage of adults over the age

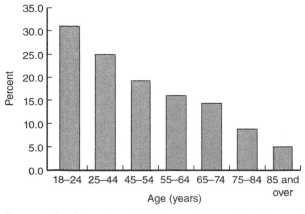

Figure 8.2   Percentage of adults over the age of 18 who meet the U.S. federal physical activity guidelines.

Data from Centers for Disease Control and Prevention/National Center for Health Statistics, 2014, *National Health Interview* [NHIS].

of 18 who meet the U.S. federal physical activity guidelines. Furthermore, the percentage of adults over the age of 25 who met the physical activity guideline levels was proportional to their levels of education. Only 6.9 percent had less than a high school education, 12.9 percent had a high school diploma or equivalent, 19.8 percent had some university, 20.1 percent had an associate's degree, 29.1 percent had a four-year university degree, and 31.3 percent had an advanced degree.

Peak Athletic Performance

One of the most intriguing issues in human motor development is the connection between chronological age and physical performance. In general, research on highly skilled athletes indicates that peak athletic performance occurs between the ages of 25 and 35 (Gabbard, 2012). It is certainly rare for a 12-year-old to achieve a world record, and a 75-year-old who breaks a world record would perhaps be even less expected. The main limiting factor for the 12-year-old or the 75-year-old is not motivation or behavior; rather, it is biological (Schultz & Curnow, 1988). During adolescence, many growth and developmental changes are still occurring, and the systems are not capable of working together for maximal function until early adulthood. On the other end of the spectrum, the biological capacity of older adults is declining, limiting their physiological capacity and peak performance.

The simplest way to measure the age of peak athletic performance in humans is to compare the ages of world record holders (Hill, 1925). Most sport records (e.g., in running, swimming, cycling, and weightlifting) are achieved by people in their late 20s or early 30s (Kenney, Wilmore, & Costill, 2015). This suggests that humans are in their physical prime during this age range.

TRY THIS

Peak Performance

Exercise 8.1

Work in a small group of two to four. Divide up the following sports yourselves: gymnastics, swimming, running, baseball, wrestling, boxing, tennis, and golf. Search for the peak performance age for each sport for both males and females. You can further divide up the sports (e.g., divide running into sprinting and long distance running) or add to this list. Write the sport in the appropriate box for age and sex. Shot put and diving are included as examples.

Age	Male	Female
17		
18		
19		
20		
21		Diving
22	Diving	
23		
24		
25		
26		Shot put
27		
28		
29	Shot put	
30		
31		

The age of peak athletic performance depends on the most important physiological element of the sport (Shephard, 2008). In gymnastics, the key element is the ratio of strength to body mass. This becomes a large structural constraint for females when they become young adults, because they gain fat in the breasts and hips. This may explain in part why so many female gymnasts reach their peak prior to puberty. In aerobic activities, such as swimming and running, the average velocities for 100-meter and 10-kilometer runs and the 100-meter front crawl decrease by a rate of about 1 percent per year after the age of 25. The rates of decline are approximately the same for both sprints and distance performances. Muscular strength generally increases up to approximately age 25 to 35, and decreases by a rate of about 1.8 percent per year thereafter.

Performances in Olympic Events

The ages of peak athletic performances in track and field events range in the lower to mid-20s; women reach their peak approximately one year sooner than men in most events (Schultz & Curnow, 1988). For the running events, the average age for peak athletic performance tends to depend on the distance of the run. The mean ages for sprints are younger than those for distance running, ranging from a mean age of 22 for the 100- and 200-meter sprints to 27 for the 5,000 and 10,000 meter and marathon. Interestingly, this trend was not observed in swimming events. The mean age for peak athletic performance was 20 for men and 18 for women. The age remained the same for men regardless of the swimming event. For women, the age was younger for longer distances, which is opposite the trend for running events. This is well illustrated by the world record–breaking performances in 1987 by Janet Evans at the age of 15 in the 400-, 800-, and 1,500-meter freestyle.

Surprisingly, the age of peak athletic performances from the standpoint of gold medals and world records changed very little across a period of 90 years (Schulz & Curnow, 1988), even though the performances themselves improved quite dramatically. For example, the age of the 1,500-meter gold medalist in 1896 was 22, and 90 years later the gold medalist was 24 years old, yet a 37.8 percent improvement was seen in the men's marathon record times over this 90-year period. In 1896, the fastest marathon time was 2:58.50; it decreased dramatically to 2:11:03 in 1980. The greatest percentage of improvement was found in the men's shot put—an increase of 90 percent! Although there were huge improvements across this period, performances have stabilized in more recent years.

WHAT DO YOU THINK?

Exercise 8.2

Given that the age of peak athletic performance remained consistent over a period of 90 years, even though performance improved substantially (sometimes as much as 90 percent), we can conclude that there are biological limitations to performing at a peak level. Using this information for a sport of your interest, answer the following questions:

1. How could you use this information to maximize the performance of an athlete who is above the mean age for peak athletic performance for this sport?
2. Would you use this information to help you identify talent (i.e., would you use age as a factor when selecting your team and athletes)? Why or why not?

With the vast improvements in training programs, equipment, technology, diet, and other factors, it is not surprising that elite performance has improved quite significantly. Yet it is surprising that the age at which elite peak performance occurs has not changed. The simple fact that the age of peak athletic performance remained consistent over a century regardless of all of these large scientific advancements leads to the assumption that the major factor affecting age at peak athletic performance is biological. The only exception to the stability of age at optimal performance is golf. Schulz and Curnow (1988) suggested that the higher age variability at elite levels seen in complex tasks is affected by variables additional to the biological factors that strongly affect motor skills and that rely heavily on endurance, strength, or both. Biological developmental factors do not seem to affect skills with a higher cognitive component. World chess champions tend to be significantly older than track and field athletes, with a mean age of 38. Similarly, productivity in the arts and sciences does not peak until the late 30s to early 40s (Belsky, 1984).

Performances in Selected Sports

Assessing the age of peak athletic performance in a sport such as baseball is more complicated than it is in track and field or swimming because of the complexity of the game and the large number of performance measurements compiled. To assess the age of peak athletic performance in baseball, Schulz and Curnow (1988) analyzed 10 categories for nonpitchers (runs, hits, doubles, triples, home runs, RBIs, walks, strikeouts, stolen bases, and batting average) and six categories for pitchers (wins, win–loss percentage, strikeouts, earned run average, shutouts, and saves). Although many categories were assessed, the mean age of peak athletic performance remained very consistent at age 27 to 28.

To examine the age at peak athletic performance for two other complex games, tennis and golf, the age of the number one–ranking athlete per year was recorded. In tennis, the mean age was 25 for men and 24 for women. Mean ages for golfers were significantly higher, at approximately 33; women averaged one year younger than men. A trend toward younger golf champions began in the late 1960s and certainly continues with golf sensation Tiger Woods. In 1997, at the age of 21, Woods became the youngest Masters winner, won three other PGA events, and achieved the number-one world ranking all within 42 weeks of becoming a pro. Rory McIlroy is another golf champion, along with Jack Nicklaus and Tiger Woods, to win three majors by the age of 25.

Performance Changes in Older Adults

In general, regardless of sport or activity, performance declines tend to occur at a fairly slow to moderate rate between 30 and 50 years of age, followed by a steeper performance decline from 50 to 60 years. After age 70, the reduction in performance is significant (Bernard, Sultana, Lepers, Hauss-wirth, & Brisswalter, 2009; Reider, 2008). A sharp decline in athletic performance at the age of 70 has been found in masters athletes in running events, both sprints and endurance (Wright & Perricelli, 2008), weightlifting (Meltzer, 1994), and swimming (Donato, Tench, Glueck, Seals, Eskurza, & Tanaka, 2003). These trends are found with most performances with few exceptions. One of the rare exceptions is the ultra marathon (100 km), in which race times actually continue to decrease (i.e., better performances) until age 30; the record times do not increase (i.e., slower times) again until age 49 for men and age 54 for women (Knechtle, Rüst, Rosemann, & Lepers, 2012).

After ages 60 or 70, people find it significantly more difficult to perform at the levels they have previously. It is as if these older adults are pushing a boulder up a hill that is getting steeper and steeper (Reider, 2008) as they fight with age-related physiological changes such as decreasing muscle mass, reduced size of type II muscle fibers,

RESEARCH NOTES

Senior Athletic Track and Field Performances

To examine age-related changes in peak athletic performance among elite senior athletes, researchers looked at track and field Olympians over the age of 50 who participated in the 2001 National Senior Olympic Games (Wright & Perricelli, 2008). Examining elite athletes provides a clearer picture of age-related peak performance changes because these are less likely to be affected by chronic disease or long periods of physical inactivity and disuse. Age-related changes were determined from the mean winning performance times in various track and field events, and age and sex differences were compared. Performance times significantly increased for both sprints and endurance events for both males and females. Performances declined slowly until the age of 75, and then declined dramatically. Men declined at a similar rate in both sprints and endurance events, whereas women declined at a higher rate in sprints than in endurance events.

Senior elite athletes provide an excellent example of what the aging human body can achieve. They demonstrate that aging alone should not prevent people from participating in physical activity or from competing in high-level contests. Even though significant declines in peak athletic performance occur, most notably beyond the age of 75, these athletes are delaying the onset of chronic disease and are maintaining a high sense of both physical and mental well-being.

lower maximal oxygen volumes and heart rates, and stiffening connective tissues. It is important for rehabilitation specialists and geriatric instructors to be aware of this sharp decline in elderly adults. Although the decline is inevitable, interventions such as endurance training and strength training can help elderly adults maximize their functional potential.

Movement Patterns

Age-related declines in strength, flexibility, and processing speed all contribute to changing movement patterns in older adults. Older adults are also much more likely to have secondary factors such as disease or injury that can compound age-related movement changes. This section focuses on the factors affecting healthy aging in relation to locomotor skills (running and jumping), fundamental motor skills (throwing and striking), and functional activities (driving, handwriting, and typing).

Changes in Locomotion

Changes in gait have been associated with the aging process. Reduced gait speed is one of the most significant changes seen in healthy older adults, who walk on average 20 percent more slowly than young adults (Spirduso et al., 2005). The reduction in gait speed is surprisingly not the result of decreased stride frequency (the number of strides per unit of time). Rather, it is largely the result of reduced stride length (the distance traveled between right-foot contacts). A reduced stride length negatively affects many other aspects of the gait, resulting in reduced joint rotation in the lower extremities, increased double-support time (time during which both feet are in contact with the ground), reduced arm swing, and a more flat-footed contact with the ground (Elble, 1997). Older adults have also been found to have less push-off power than young adults have (Winter, Patla, Frank, & Walt, 1990) and increased out-toeing (Murray, Kory, & Sepic, 1970). Out-toeing is a strategy used to improve lateral stability (Gabbard, 2012).

Recently, researchers have questioned some of the age-related findings in regard to locomotor patterns after comparing gait in a laboratory setting to gait in real-world settings. When assessed in the lab, older adults' step duration was longer, their angular limb excursion (lower limb joint angles) was smaller, and they had higher gait variability. However, when assessed in real-world settings, they exhibited variability only in angular limb excursions (Bock & Beurskens, 2010). In this study the lab setting appeared to destabilize the older adults more than real-world settings did.

Locomotion becomes even more challenging when older adults are faced with obstacles, as when they have to step up over a curb or step around a chair (Steffen, Hacker, & Mollinger, 2002). Every day we avoid many obstacles without even noticing ourselves doing it. However, the ability to negotiate many different obstacles while traveling from point A to point B is an important component of independent living.

Age-related changes in gait occur as a result of many factors, including muscular weakness in the hip abductors, hip extensors, knee extensors, plantarflexors, and dorsiflexors, as well as sensory impairments in the visual, somatosensory, and vestibular systems. Spirduso and colleagues (2005) found 10 age-related gait changes:

TRY THIS

Mall Walkers

Exercise 8.3

Take a trip to a mall or other location where many people are walking around in a leisurely fashion. Notice the kinematic, temporal, and distance variables of the people walking. Compare two adults in each of the following age groups: young adults, middle-aged adults, and older adults. Use the chart to take notes on gait-related variables to describe each of their walking patterns.

	Young adults		Middle-aged adults		Older adults	
	1	2	1	2	1	2
Velocity						
Step length (distance traveled of alternate feet)						
Step frequency (walking cadence)						
Stride length (distance traveled of same foot)						
Stride width (distance between the two feet)						
Time in double support (time when both feet are in contact with the ground)						
Arm swing						
Other observations						

What variables other than age may cause some of the differences in gait that you observed?

Temporal and Distance Variables

- Decreased velocity
- Decreased step length (distance traveled of alternate feet)
- Decreased step frequency (walking cadence)
- Decreased stride length (distance traveled of same foot)
- Increased stride width (distance between the two feet)
- Increased stance phase (begins when the first foot contacts the ground)
- Increased time in double support (time when both feet are in contact with the ground)
- Decreased time in swing phase (begins as the foot leaves the ground)

Kinematic Variables

- Flatter foot–floor pattern
- Reduced arm swing

The causes of gait changes may not be limited to physiological age-related changes. Evidence supports the possibility that many older adults alter their gait because they are afraid of falling. Older adults adopt a "safer" gait by taking shorter steps, with more time in double stance, to decrease their risk of falling. Willmott (1986) proposed this after finding that older adults walked significantly faster on carpet than on vinyl flooring.

Running

The movement pattern characteristics (kinematics) of older adults up to age 80 have been found to be the same as those of female university track athletes (Adrian & Cooper, 1995). On the other hand, few similarities were seen in the sprinting kinematics of older females and young athletes. Young athletes use longer strides and generate more force through greater flexion and extension. This enables them to take fewer strides. It is also not surprising that older adults show a steady decline in both jogging and running speeds in comparison to young adults (Nelson, 1981).

Jumping

Research on jumping has revealed age-related differences in the kinematics of vertical jumping. Young adult males (18-year-olds) were compared with males in their mid-60s on vertical jumping (Wang, 2008). The older men had significantly less strength in the knee and hip, which can affect the ability to perform other activities of daily living. During the jump, the older men exhibited less hip flexion and extension than the young men, but had no difference in their knees. The decreased hip joint angles enabled them to maintain hip angular stiffness. Hip angular stiffness is important because it increases joint stability by resisting sudden angular displacements of the hip (Flanagan & Harrison, 2007), which can cause damage to the cartilage and ligaments (Butler, Crowell, & Davis, 2003).

Changes in Fundamental Movement Patterns

Unfortunately, studies on movement patterns in adults are limited (Lorson, Stodden, Langendorfer, & Goodway, 2013; Williams, Haywood, & VanSant, 1998). Most research studies have instead focused on functional activities such as walking, running, and rising from a seated to a standing position. Research on movements using maximal force is also quite limited; most studies have focused on performing the movements at preferred speeds. Although research is limited in this area, this section discusses fundamental movement patterns in older adulthood for throwing and striking.

Throwing

A hypothetical life span developmental trajectory was developed for the progression of throwing patterns from middle adolescence to young adulthood, and then the regression to middle-aged adulthood (Lorson et al., 2013). Researchers used the developmental sequence for the overarm throw for force divided into categories for each of four body segment actions: trunk, humerus, forearm, and foot action (Roberton & Halverson, 1984). Age-related differences are more pronounced in males than females, but this gap decreases with age. This sex-related difference is likely attributable to larger developmental improvements in males than females (Lorson et al., 2013).

A further regression was found in adults over the age of 70 using less mature throwing patterns (Williams et al., 1990, 1991). Very few older adults threw with developmentally advanced actions for any of the body segments. Older adults also threw with reduced range of motion and took smaller steps. Only 11.4 percent of participants were in the most advanced stage of humerus action (humerus lag), and none of the participants were in the most advanced stage of the forearm action (delayed forearm lag). Similar results were found in the advanced stage of the trunk action component (0 percent of the older adults exhibited differentiated trunk rotation), and only 3.5 percent of participants were in the advanced stage of the foot action (contralateral long step). Sex differences were reported: women threw with significantly fewer developmentally advanced actions of the forearm and humerus than men did (Williams et al., 1991).

When the throwing velocities of the older adults were compared with those of children and adolescents by Halverson, Rober-ton, and Langendorfer (1982), the older adults' speeds were comparable to those of 8- and 9-year-old children (see figure 8.3). Throwing velocities were higher for males than for females in all age groups, which is likely due to the more advanced movement patterns produced by the males. The developmental level of movement patterns has been found to predict ball velocities in children (Roberton & Konczak, 2001).

Striking

The fundamental movement pattern of striking is a coincident timing skill that requires a person to make contact with a ball by manipulating an object such as a racket, bat, or club. Striking skills can vary quite considerably. The planes of motion—overhand (e.g., tennis serve), sidearm (e.g., batting), and underhand (e.g., golf, hockey)—vary from sport to sport, as do the size and elasticity of the ball and the implement (e.g., tennis racket, baseball bat, golf club).

Slower extension velocities have been found in the striking patterns of the tennis backhand and batting in older adults (Klinger, Masataka, Adrian, & Smith, 1980), but not in the golf swing for a short shot (Jagacinski, Greenberg, & Liao, 1997). Although no differences were found between young and older adults in the tempo of the golf swing or the overall speed of the swing, marked group differences were observed in the rhythm of

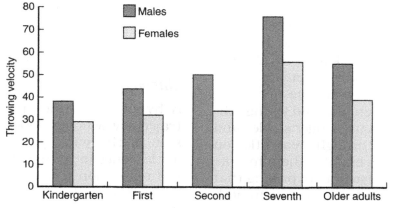

Figure 8.3 Overhand throwing velocities (feet per second) for 5- to 12-year-olds and older adults.
Data from Williams, Haywood, and VanSant 1991.

Maybe Older Adults Aren't So Bad at Throwing

Williams, Haywood, and VanSant (1998) conducted a longitudinal study on overhand throwing in adults between the ages of 62 and 77. Over a period of seven years, eight older adults were videotaped from the sagittal plane (side view) as they threw a tennis ball. The results indicated that many of the age-related differences found in older adults may actually be the result of the study design, because previous studies on overarm throwing were cohort studies, comparing people of different ages rather than the same people across time. The developmental levels were the same across the seven years 90 percent of the time, which indicates that only small changes in the coordination patterns occurred in the participants during this period. The older adults coordinated their movements similarly to younger throwers with the exception of the control of the overarm throw, the amount of trunk rotation, and the range of shoulder motion. The changes seen in movement control are likely the result of factors such as chronic disuse (Spirduso et al., 2005), osteoarthritis, and losses in balance (Thapa, Gideon, Fought, Kormicki, & Ray, 1994).

The researchers also found that older adults coordinated their backswings differently than younger throwers did. Because of the different movement patterns performed by the older adults during the backswing, two new steps were added to the developmental sequence (levels 3 and 5):

Level 1: No backswing

Level 2: Elbow and humeral flexion

Level 3: Humeral lateral rotation

Level 4: Circular, upward backswing

Level 5: Shortcut circular, downward backswing

Level 6: Circular, downward backswing

The older adults threw using these two new steps more than any other preparatory backswing step. These movements are likely adaptations resulting from changes in the range of motion at the shoulder.

the swing, or the speeding up and slowing down within a shot. The older adults actually reached their peak downswing force earlier than the young adults did. Young adults reached this peak just prior to making contact with the ball. These results may indicate that older adults have reduced control during the swing compared to young adults. The older adults also exerted more effort, although most of them performed as well as the young adults.

Age-related effects on movement performances have been shown to be reduced in active adults (Klinger et al., 1980). In general, active older adults can maintain their movement patterns at a level similar to that achieved during young adulthood. Movement speed and range of motion are affected to a lesser degree in active adults than in inactive adults.

Changes in Functional Activities

Given the many physical changes that accompany aging, it is important to understand how these changes affect older adults' abilities to perform functional tasks such as driving, handwriting, and typing. These activities are very important for quality of life and independence. Older adults who lose the ability to drive become dependent on either public transportation or friends and family for transportation. Public transportation can be limited for adults who do not live in metropolitan areas, forcing them to rely on others to drive them. Handwriting and typing are also important everyday functional tasks and are strong indicators of cognitive and physical declines.

Driving

The primary mode of transportation for older adults in the United States is driving (Jette & Branch, 1992). Driving provides an increased quality of life for many adults, allowing them to pursue activities they could not if they were not permitted to drive. Policy makers often suggest public transportation as the solution. However, older adults do not perceive public transportation as a viable alternative to driving. Some do not have access to public transportation, some don't like using it, and some cannot physically walk the distance necessary to access the system (Donorfio, Mohyde, Coughlin, & D'Ambrosio, 2008).

The number of drivers over the age of 60 is increasing as the baby boomer generation joins this age group and as people are living longer. And not only are there more drivers over the age of 70, but it is expected that the older drivers will dramatically increase their driving miles (Castro, Martínez, & Tornay, 2005). With the growing older population and increased mileage, the number of vehicle fatalities in adults over 70 years in the United States increased 10 percent from 1990 to 2000 and is expected to increase 25 percent by 2030 (National Highway Traffic Safety Administration, 2000). In general, older adults are safer drivers and are less likely to be involved in accidents than younger adults are. Yet because of their physical declines, older adults involved in accidents are much more likely to sustain serious injuries or die (Braver & Trempel, 2003).

Older adults are generally aware of their functional declines, both physical (i.e., eyesight, hearing, reflexes, neck or shoulder mobility) and psychological (i.e., confidence, enjoyment, ability to concentrate, trust of other drivers, independence, and ability to drive in stressful environments). Because of this heightened awareness in relation to driving abilities, they tend to compensate with strategies such as an increased awareness of their performance, the driving behaviors of other drivers, their vehicle, and road rules (Donorfio et al., 2008). Driving shifts from an activity that is largely automatic to a chore, requiring more planning and increased concentration and cautiousness.

Policy making for older adults is challenging. Older drivers often have physical declines, but positive alterations in their driving behaviors allow them to drive more safely than younger adults do. Older adults are also quite variable, so rating driving ability solely on the basis of age would not be fair. Some older adults can drive competently in their 90s, whereas others show significant impairment in their 60s or 70s.

Medical conditions that are more prevalent in older adults have been associated with increased accident risk (Marshall, 2008). Cardiovascular disease, cerebrovascular disease, depression, diabetes, medication use, musculoskeletal disorders, and visual deficit have been shown to cause a slight to moderate increase in crash risk. Alcohol abuse and dependence, dementia, epilepsy, schizophrenia, and sleep apnea, on the other hand, are associated with a moderate to high increase in crash risk. The accident risk fluctuates according to the severity of the condition, which varies considerably across individuals.

One factor that may be as important, or even more important, to driving safety than these medical conditions, sensory limitations, and cognitive declines is the ability to self-assess changes affecting driving skills (Meng & Sirin, 2012). Older adults who are more cognizant of these changes are more likely to compensate for them by either stopping night driving,

Exercise 8.4

What are the implications of aging for driving? What declines could affect driving ability? Do you believe that drivers should be assessed or lose their driving privileges (or both) after they reach a certain age? If so, at what age? If not, why not? Weigh the pros and cons of implementing a policy on the cessation of driving in older adults. Think about the physical, psychological, and cognitive changes in older adults. Also think about the effects that driving cessation can have (e.g., emotional effects, impact on social life).

driving more slowly, or not driving long distances. In addition, many advances have been made to cars including backup cameras, adaptive headlights, and even auto-pilot, which help older adults in particular to continue driving.

Handwriting and Typing

Handwriting is one of the most common daily activities. It is necessary for not only professional activities, but also leisure activities. Handwriting is a complex activity involving eye–hand coordination, dexterity, motor planning, visual and kinesthetic perception, and manual skills (Tseng & Cermak, 1993). Moreover, many years are needed to acquire the skill. Hand function has been found to decrease with increasing age as a result of reduced physical activity levels and neuromuscular decline in hand strength, speed, and coordination (Cole, Rotella, & Harper, 1999).

Older adults often report having no impairment in handwriting, but research has shown that they write significantly more slowly and with less pressure than young adults do (Rosenblum & Werner, 2005). The decreased pressure is likely due to decreased hand strength (Fried, Storer, King, & Lodder, 1991), including reduced finger-pinch strength (Ranganathan, Siemionow, Sahgal, Liu, & Yue, 2001). Decreased handwriting speed was not simply the result of slower movements; also noted was increased air time—the time during writing in which the pen or pencil is not making marks on the paper (Rosenblum & Werner, 2005). Unlike for

other tasks requiring muscular strength, no sex differences were found with age for handwriting (Rosenblum & Werner, 2005).

In today's digital age, communication consists largely of typing on computers or small screens such as phones and tablets. Currently, there is not a lot of research examining the effect of age on the ability to type. One study compared young adults (21-31 years) to older adults (65-83 years) on typing measures such as speed and self-corrections. The younger adults spent less time typing and used the delete keys more often than the older adults did. The number of typing errors increased in the older adults as they increased their speed. It was perhaps even more interesting that the older adults spent more of their total time typing (70 percent compared to 50 percent in younger adults) and less time editing and correcting. These results may be due to a cohort effect, in that they grew up in era when much more time was spent writing than typing. On the other hand, these results could be due to age-related changes such as a decline in motor skills, timing, or sequencing, or a combination of both a cohort and an aging effect (Kalman, Kavé, & Umanski, 2015).

Summary

Aging refers to the physical changes that occur across time. Chronological age is the most commonly used indicator of age; however, this age marker is limiting, because adults can vary markedly in physiological adaptations and physical function. Two people can be the same chronological age but decades apart in biological age. On the other hand, there is a strong connection between chronological age and peak athletic performance. The age of peak athletic performance is between 25 and 35 with very few exceptions. Even following vast improvements in technology, training programs, and nutrition that have resulted in dramatically improved performances in all sports, the age at which elite performances are achieved has not changed. Performance declines can be minimized by continuing to practice the sport, although large performance declines tend to occur after the age of 75 regardless of the sport or activity.

Current public health recommendations in the United States are for adults to maintain moderate- to vigorous-intensity physical activity for a minimum of 30 minutes per day, five days per week, yet many adults are insufficiently physically active. Aging stereotypes and age grading contribute to negative stereotypes of older adults and seriously affect physical activity participation. This often leads to the exercise–aging cycle of decreased function as a result of decreased physical activity, leading to further decreased function, and so on. Adults who continue to be physically active have been found to maintain many of their physical capabilities, including physical performance, functional activities, and independence.

ONLINE LEARNING

Visit the web resource at www.HumanKinetics.com/MotorLearningAndDevelopment for an accompanying lab activity and exercises from the chapter.

LEARNING AIDS

Supplemental Activities

1. How much time have you spent with an older adult—not your grandmother, grandfather, or another older relative, but an unrelated older adult? Unless you work with older adults, you likely haven't often had an extended conversation with one. For this supplemental activity, visit a senior center or an assisted-living facility and spend some time with an older adult. Ask about the physical activities the person participated in as a child, an adolescent, a young adult, a middle-aged adult, and an old adult. Ask why the person participated in those activities and why he or she may have dropped out of certain activities or taken up different activities as an older person.

2. Choose a sport.
   a. Search for the record performances in that sport across time (e.g., the records for the sport in the 1930s, 1950s, 1970s, 1990s, and today).
      1. How have records changed?
      2. Did they change significantly more during one period of time than during others?
      3. What may have caused this more significant change in this sport?
      4. Why do you think performances are better now than they were in previous decades (e.g., new techniques, technological advances, diet changes)?
   b. Now search for record performance times across ages (e.g., 20s, 30s, 40s, 50s, 60s, 70s). Graph the performance changes across these ages. Discuss your findings.

Glossary

age grading—Decreasing physical activity levels based on age.

ageism—Stereotyping someone on the basis of age.

aging—A process or group of processes occurring in living organisms that with the passage of time lead to a loss of adaptability, functional impairment, and eventually death.

biological aging—The physiological adaptations that occur within the body as a result of the passage of time.

chronological age—The number of years a person has been alive.

exercise–aging cycle—The downward cycle that occurs when older adults decrease their physical activity participation due to physical and psychological changes, which in turn worsens their physical and psychological states. This causes a cycle of further reduction in physical activity and state of health.

PART III

Functional and Structural Constraints

Part III emphasizes structural and functional constraints across the life span. Structural constraints—physical growth and the changing dynamics of the body systems—are explored in chapters 9 and 10. The focus in chapter 9 is on structural factors that constrain, or promote or limit, the acquisition and performance of both fundamental and skillful movements, providing knowledge of how structural constraints may interact with functional factors, tasks, and the environment. We then turn to age-related changes in the body systems during adulthood in chapter 10, with a primary focus on normal age-related changes; we also include a discussion of secondary aging.

To many people, the term *aging* is synonymous with time, but even though everyone does age, we do not age the same. Environmental factors and behavioral lifestyle factors play a large role in our health and well-being, and these effects compound every year. Because people age so differently, assumptions about an individual's physiological function based solely on a simple measure of age with respect to time, or chronological age, are not very accurate. Because of this high variability in motor behavior across adulthood, this part of the book focuses on primary aging—that is, age-related changes that are not due to disease or poor behavioral practices such as obesity, smoking, and sedentary lifestyles.

The discussion then turns to functional constraints. Chapters 11 and 12 focus on the development of functional constraints during childhood and adolescence—those that influence motor learning and performance. The first of these chapters addresses cognitive development, knowledge, and the changing dynamics of attention and memory; the second addresses psychosocial and social–affective development. Learners have different abilities with regard to cognition, knowledge, personal skills, attention, and memory—abilities that affect them in motor learning and performance situations. The powerful impact of self-esteem, motivation, and emotion on learning and performance cannot be overstated.

We then extend the examination of functional constraints to adulthood in chapter 13, including psychosocial factors and changing cognitive function across adulthood. It is important to distinguish psychosocial factors in adulthood from those in childhood and adolescence, because they can differ quite considerably. Adults show wider variability than do children and adolescents, and this variability increases with age. Because of the combination of experiences and age-related structural and functional changes, adults become increasingly unique with age. A strong knowledge base with regard to the structural and functional constraints that affect movement and how they change across the life span will help readers appreciate the individual differences in a class of children or adolescents or when working with adults, better enabling them to design developmentally appropriate programs as discussed in part IV.

PHYSICAL DEVELOPMENT

After reading this chapter, you should be able to do the following:

- Explain the role of genes and the environment in motor learning and development.
- Discuss distance and velocity curves as well as relative growth.
- Discuss key developmental changes in the skeletal, nervous, endocrine, and adipose systems.
- Understand the developmental changes in three sensory systems.

Systems, Many Systems!

Chelsea is a preschool teacher and a young mom of a four-year-old daughter. She has an education degree and this year is responsible for 6 little ones, including her daughter, at the preschool. Even among the 6 four-year-olds, she has noticed a remarkable difference in height and weight. Chelsea did not expect all the children to be the same size, but one of the girls towers over all the other youngsters. This is a preschool, so she has had to lift them from time to time, but she did not anticipate the weight differences in the group. She wonders whether the tallest and heaviest children will become the biggest teenagers. There are certainly some differences in strength, if opening jars is any indication. One of the boys wears glasses; that was not expected at four years of age. As the children play and interact, Chelsea realizes, just as her university professors said, that the human body is a wonderful combination of many interacting systems, and each plays a role in development, sometimes exerting more influence at specific times.

As the dynamic systems and ecological approaches predict, intrinsic dynamics are constraints that affect observable motor patterns and the learning or refinement of motor skills. We hinted in chapter 1 that a person's size and shape are important constraints, but we did not explain developmental changes in height, weight, or physique—nor did we describe other structural differences such as bone growth and development, muscular development, and sensory changes such as in vision and spatial awareness. This chapter explains how both genetic and environmental factors may affect motor learning and development. It then deals with the important and fascinating growth changes in height and weight and outlines the developmental changes in systems—the skeletal, nervous, endocrine, and adipose systems as well as the sensory systems of vision, audition, and kinesthesis. All of these systems can function as constraints to learning and development. Chapters 11 and 12 deal with the functional constraints of learners that would further help Chelsea understand the vast differences in her group of four-year-olds.

Have you ever seen a young child with a basketball in hand, looking up, up, up at a distant hoop? There is motivation to throw that basketball, but also the realization that size and strength are not quite there for a successful toss. Growth in height and gains in strength are important structural constraints in children and adolescents. Other examples of structural constraints are spinal cord damage that restricts or eliminates lower limb movement, and hearing and visual problems. People with these constraints can be very independent, but they perform tasks in unique ways, with wheelchairs, hearing aids or sign language, and canes or a guide dog, respectively.

Nature and Nurture

We are amazed by truly exceptional performances, whether it is Beethoven or Mozart in music or Usain Bolt, Serena Williams, or Sidney Crosby in sport. Because their brilliance seems to defy the notion that their achievements are the result of practice and learning, we often explain their excellence as the result of some inborn talent or gift. Recent research identifying specific genes in DNA may have resulted in the illusion that it is only a matter of time before one or more genes are linked to exceptionality. Ericsson (2007) suggested that the complete genetic account of superior abilities is exceedingly complex and that an environmental perspective of extensive practice is better able to account for exceptional abilities. The relative contribution of genes (nature) and environment (nurture) to individual differences that we observe in everyday life has been the topic of one of the most energetic scientific debates for over 140 years (Baker & Davids, 2007).

There is much to be learned about the role of genetic constraints in living organisms. Genetic factors are almost the sole determinant of characteristics such as height, blood type, and hair color in humans. Genes largely control the timing of growth, such as the onset of the adolescent growth spurt and loss of muscular strength later in life. However, growth can be significantly affected by extrinsic factors; poor prenatal nutrition, ingestion of the wrong drugs, or exposure to X-rays can negatively affect the growing embryo or fetus. Good nutrition and exercise, on the other hand, can positively affect growth and development across the life span. Therefore, motor learning and development most certainly are affected by both genetic and environmental constraints, but the precise manner of their interplay is not well known. More often than not, we simply read about the interaction of genes and experience as contributing to sport performance or academic learning, as if this fully explains the relationship. There is some truth to this idea, but the interaction is exceedingly complex and influenced by one's theoretical viewpoint of genetic action (Davids & Baker, 2007).

The impact of genes and extrinsic influences on human behavior is often studied with **monozygotic** and **dizygotic twins** (Klissouras, Geladas, & Koskolou, 2007). Human beings receive genes randomly from both parents, which results in a unique genetic makeup, or genotype. Monozygotic (identical) twins have identical genotypes, whereas dizygotic (fraternal) twins share half their genes like ordinary siblings. Occasionally, twin research provides one of the monozygotic twins with some special treatment to determine the impact of heredity or environment in producing the phenotype—that is, an observable characteristic or behavior such as height, personality, or fitness. Because these twins are genetically identical, a positive impact from the special treatment suggests that the characteristic or phenotype is modifiable by the environment (e.g., gain in $\dot{V}O_2$max or motor skills). Thus, the characteristic or phenotype is not completely determined by the genotype. Twin studies also include situations in which monozygotic twins are reared apart. In this case it is assumed that the life experiences of the two twins are different. If they have a similar phenotype after many years apart, it is usually concluded that the phenotype was largely determined by genes rather than environment.

Nature–nurture research attempts to explain differences in individuals in a population as a function of genetics, extrinsic factors, or both; it cannot explain how much of your weight is controlled by your genes or your exercise and your eating habits, nor can it predict how much improvement you might expect as a function of training or practice. It can only explain differences in a group of people. Suppose a group of 40 were requested to practice a juggling task until each person reached a criterion of 10 consecutive tosses without dropping a ball. Assume that 200 trials (on average) were required to reach that criterion. The quickest individual in the group needed 150 trials, and the slowest needed 250.

Genetic research attempts to explain how much of the 100-trial difference in the group of 40 is due to genetic factors. A statistic called **heritability** can be calculated (see Klissouras et al., 2007, for more details and other estimates of genetic influence). A heritability score closer to 1 is interpreted as a strong genetic influence in producing differences between individuals, but it has no meaning for the abilities of an individual. A high heritability score of 0.9 does not mean that an individual's $\dot{V}O_2$max score is due to 90 percent genetic and 10 percent training factors. Nor should such a high score be interpreted as suggesting that the environment has almost no impact. The 0.9 does mean that "after individuals have reached the upper limits of their $\dot{V}O_2$max, with appropriate training, there will still be wide interindividual variability which is genetic in origin" (Klissouras et al., 2007, p. 52).

Heritability scores are often quite high for physical fitness measures, body mass index, physique, height, and somatotype, as well as personality and cognitive abilities (Klissouras et al., 2007). Investigations have explored individual differences in motor learning, but the studies are fewer and the overall findings remain mixed. Fox, Hershberger, and Bouchard (1996) used both monozygotic and dizygotic twins reared apart to investigate individual differences in motor performance in a pursuit rotor tracking task for 75 trials. They concluded that performance differences between individuals did reflect genetic influence. It is important to remember that the authors did not discount the role of practice; they asserted simply that there is a significant genetic impact on the outcome of practice. Marisi (1977) also used the pursuit rotor task with twins, but found that the genetic influence diminished over trials. Generally, these findings support the impact of genetic factors on motor learning and are consistent with the views of Klissouras, Bouchard, and their colleagues (Bouchard et al., 1999; Klissouras et al., 2007).

A Classic Nature–Nurture Study in Motor Development

McGraw (1935) conducted an early and classic longitudinal study on the impact of environment on the acquisition of motor skills—specifically, to determine whether a stimulating and challenging movement environment would alter motor development. Twins Johnny and Jimmy were involved in the research for several years. McGraw began observing them soon after birth, but Johnny began receiving stimulation and practice on several motor activities at about one year that were not offered to Jimmy. At various times Johnny was exposed to climbing, jumping, riding a tricycle, swimming, jumping, and roller skating. If motor development is fixed and determined largely by the maturation of the central nervous system, as most theorists at that time believed, the extra exposure and practice received by Johnny should not have had any positive influence on his acquisition of motor skills. Nature would have scored a point over nurture. Support for the impact of nurturing by practice in a stimulating environment would have resulted if Johnny's motor development had exceeded that of Jimmy. Unfortunately, the results of the study were equivocal. In some movement skills, such as climbing, Johnny demonstrated superiority over Jimmy, which supported the nurture perspective. In other activities there seemed to be no difference between the twins, supporting a nature explanation. Of course, this type of twin research requires monozygotic twins, which unfortunately was not the case, because it was later revealed that Johnny and Jimmy were dizygotic twins. This fact may have influenced the results of McGraw's research.

In the domain of musical talent, Howe, Davidson, and Sloboda (1998) concluded that "individual differences in some special abilities may indeed have partly genetic origins" (p. 407). Thus, they accepted the notion that genetic endowment can constrain ultimate skill level, acting as a ceiling of performance. Geladas, Koskolou, and Klissouras (2007) stated: "It seems that training will never erase individual differences that are due to innate abilities. Training can exert its . . . profound effect only within the fixed limits of heredity" (p. 125). Thus training and practice, true environmental factors, are considered critical even if genetics determines a ceiling of performance. It is important to remember that these statements say nothing about the extent of improvement or the ultimate level of performance for a specific individual. Parents, teachers, and therapists can justifiably remain optimistic about the motor learning of each child and adolescent.

Ericsson (2003, 2007, 2013, 2016) advanced an opposing viewpoint of expert performance. He acknowledged that genes are important in developing physiological adaptations of the body and nervous system, but maintained that they place no limits on the performance of healthy people. He argued that genetic differences in innate talent cannot explain the remarkable improvement of individuals in training research because "the DNA stored in the nucleus of each cell of a person is the same before and after training" (Ericsson, 2007, p. 6).

Deliberate practice is a proposed theoretic explanation. Deliberate practice is specific practice requiring much effort without an immediate reward; performance improvement is the motivation, and it is not necessarily enjoyable. Through the lengthy process of deliberate practice and the accompanying changes in cognitive activity, any healthy person can become an expert. To state this differently, deliberate practice, rather than genetic endowment, can explain differences between individuals who have access to the instruction, training, and social support necessary to reach high levels of achievement. Most people do not become experts in part because they cannot sustain the intensity and effort of the required practice. The only exceptions to the deliberate practice hypothesis acknowledged by Ericsson are height and body size. Neither has been shown to be influenced by training and practice. These can be viewed therefore as influenced primarily by genes. The deliberate practice account of expertise, including what constitutes practice and how to measure it, is an issue of some current debate (e.g. Ericsson, 2013, 2016; Macnamara, Moreau, & Hambrick, 2016; Tucker & Collins, 2012).

Galton made the distinction between nature and nurture in 1874 as an explanation for individual differences. Thus began the nature–nurture debate in science. Much of the debate has centered on which one is more important for a specific domain, such as movements skills. Some scientists have expressed frustration over this debate because the two are inextricably linked so that it is impossible to distinguish what is nature and what is nurture (Baker & Davids, 2007).

Kimble (1993, as cited by Baker & Davids, 2007) suggested that trying to determine whether individual differences in behavior are caused by heredity or environment is like asking whether the area of a rectangle is determined more by its width or its length. Genetic and environmental forces influence each other, are interactive in producing behavior, and must be studied together to understand human development (Kail & Cavanaugh, 2016; Shulman, 2016). Although the precise impact of genes and environment on skill acquisition is not clear, there is certainly no evidence of a physical skill acquisition gene (Davids & Baker, 2007). Individual differences in motor learning and development are no doubt influenced by many genes interacting with many extrinsic factors, from types of practice, to amount of practice, to social support mechanisms, to motivation, to personal value beliefs, to cultural influences.

Although many current theories of development and learning adopt a genetic–environment interaction perspective, the dynamic systems approach minimizes the privileged status of genetic influence on conceptual grounds (Thelen & Smith, 1994). According to this argument, a key issue in development is the respective impact of many systems, and genes are only one system. The continued search for the genetic impact may be slowing the search for more important explanations of development.

Does Athleticism Run in a Family?

Exercise 9.1

Let's look at the complexity of heritability a bit further. Find a person in your class (maybe yourself) who has achieved a reasonably high level of athletic success (e.g., university or high school varsity). Was this person's mom or dad athletic at a young age? Or perhaps an aunt or uncle? Was it in the same sport as the person? Are physical characteristics such as height important in this sport?

Exercise 9.2

1. Has the previous section of the chapter challenged your views of instruction in physical education? Is it fair to view students as naturally talented? Explain.
2. Pick two sports. Describe how students' ability to play these sports may be influenced by both nature and nurture.

Physical Growth and Maturation

The size and shape of children and adolescents change as they grow, and these structural realities affect how they coordinate their movements and learn motor skills. Most certainly, a small child will throw a 7-inch (18 cm) playground ball with two hands because the ball is almost impossible to balance on one hand, whereas a teenager (with a larger hand) may use a one-handed throw. Older adults might change how they perform physical skills because of loss of strength or arthritis. Thus, motor performance and learning are affected by changes during growth and aging in the skeletal, muscular, and nervous systems (Haywood & Getchell, 2014).

The rate of physical growth in the first year of life is remarkable. A newborn who is 7.5 pounds and 20 inches long (3.4 kg and 51 cm) at birth may grow to be 22.5 pounds and 30 inches long (10.2 kg and 76 cm) by her first birthday. This represents a 200 percent gain in weight and a 50 percent gain in height. Never again does the body change so much in a year. In fact, if the **rate of change** in the first year after birth continued until age 20, this person would be 1,150 feet tall (350 m) and weigh nearly 50 million pounds (22.7 million kg) (Krogman, 1972). Many new motor skills are acquired in the first year of life, such as sitting, standing, crawling, and walking, and the child must coordinate his rapidly growing body with the changing tasks and environmental constraints he faces.

Growth Curves

Stature (height) growth curves for males and females are shown in figure 9.1, a and b. Other common body size measures in growth research are weight; sitting height; leg length; limb and head circumferences; and breadth of shoulders, hips, and knees (Malina, Bouchard, & Bar-Or, 2004). The pattern of change for height and weight is called a **sigmoid curve** after the Greek letter for s. The rapid change after birth and again at adolescence make the sigmoid shape curvilinear rather than straight. Because the values on the y axis are accumulated heights, this type of curve is also called a **distance curve**. These curves also include **percentile** rankings. The 50th percentile is the average for the age group; half the children score above this height or weight and half score below it. A child who falls at the 75th percentile is taller at this age than 75 percent of his chronological-age peers.

These growth charts show whether a particular person is short, tall, light, or heavy for his age. A group of adolescents of the same age can vary greatly in height and weight. A parent may be concerned if a child is at the 50th percentile for height but at the 80th percentile for weight, suggesting extra weight for that height. Pediatricians monitor the extremes of stature and weight as possible indicators of growth pathology.

A youngster could be relatively short for her age because of genetic factors or a growth problem. Additional assessment would be required to determine the reason.

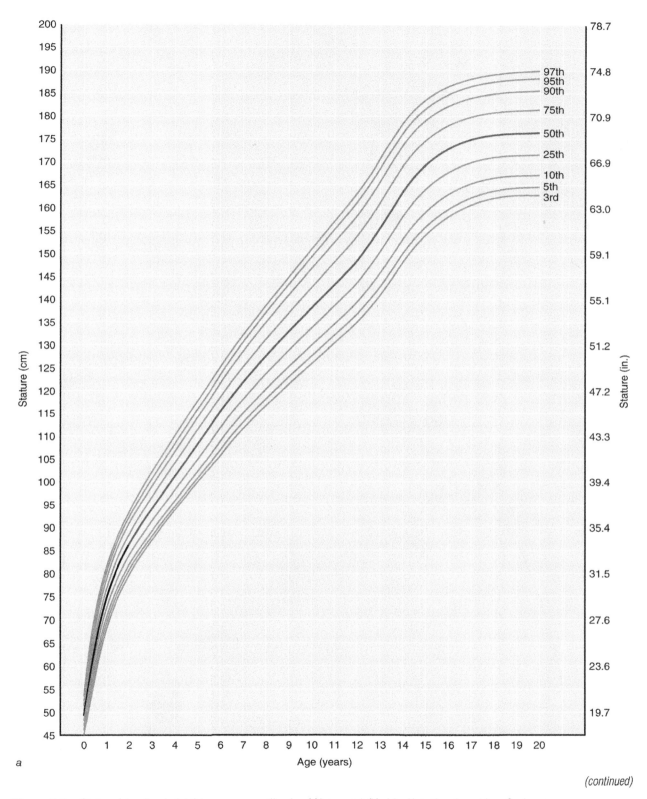

a

(continued)

Figure 9.1 Stature (standing height) by age percentiles for *(a)* boys and *(b)* girls. Note the sigmoid, or S-shape, curves.

Data from the National Center for Health Statistics in collaboration with the National Center for Chronic Disease Prevention and Health Promotion 2000. Adapted from www.cdc.gov/nchs/about/major/nhanes/growthcharts.clinical_charts.htm

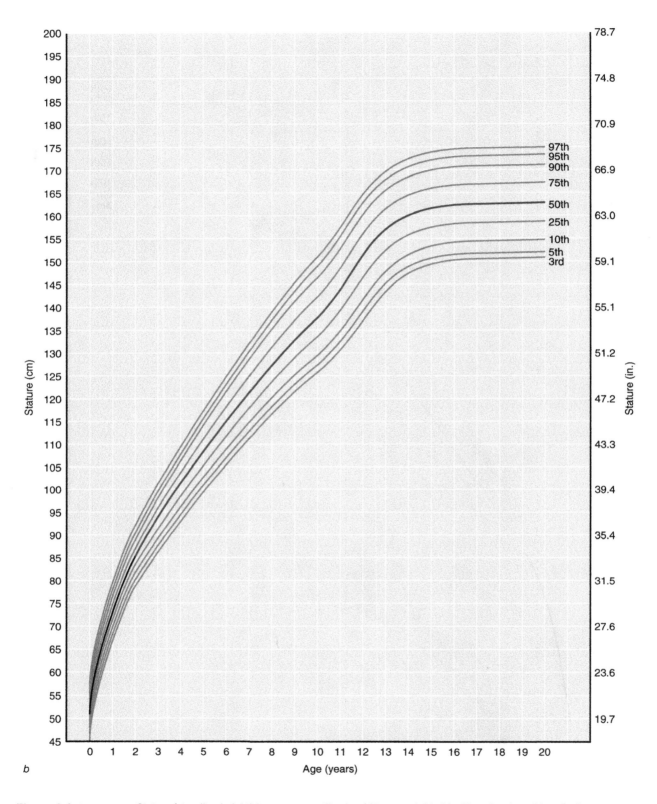

Figure 9.1 *(continued)* Stature (standing height) by age percentiles for *(a)* boys and *(b)* girls. Note the sigmoid, or S-shape, curves.

Data from the National Center for Health Statistics in collaboration with the National Center for Chronic Disease Prevention and Health Promotion 2000. Adapted from www.cdc.gov/nchs/about/major/nhanes/growthcharts.clinical_charts.htm

Much to the disappointment of parents of a big newborn child, perhaps, size at birth is not an accurate predictor of final height or weight. By age 2 or 3, children tend to remain in their percentile position compared to others (Haywood & Getchell, 2014; Malina et al., 2004). Thus, a boy at four years of age who is at the 90th percentile for height (taller than 90 percent of the four-year-old boys) is likely to be a tall adult, and a boy at the 30th percentile will likely be shorter than the typical adult male. This relative stability in growth can be used for clinical evaluation, because a child would not be expected to be at the 80th percentile at one age and the 30th at a subsequent age. Such dramatic changes might indicate unhealthy growth and be cause to seek further assessment.

Distance curves show only the extent of growth and hide whether children are growing fast one year and slower the next. The sigmoid distance curves are created by averaging the heights of many children, and they also hide the dramatic changes that can occur in an individual. Notice that the **velocity curve** for height shown in figure 9.2 looks very different from the distance curve for height. A velocity curve describes *change* in height (centimeters per year) over 18 years. Think of centimeters per year like miles per hour. A change from 60 to 40 miles per hour is described as decelerating, or slowing down. Forward movement is still occurring, just more slowly. The same thing happens in height over the first five years; each year less height is gained compared to the previous year, and therefore the velocity of height gain is *decelerating*. The person is getting taller each year, just not as fast as the previous year.

Figure 9.2 shows that height velocity continues to slow slightly from age five until the initiation of the adolescent growth spurt, at which time height gain accelerates for about two years. Notice that the **peak height velocity** is the time when gain in height is the fastest since the first year of life. The peak height velocity corresponds to the dramatic change in stature that most adolescents experience. For females this may be 3.4 inches (8.6 cm) per year; for males, 3.9 inches (10 cm) per year. It is small wonder that some children experience some awkwardness as they attempt to incorporate rapidly growing limbs into their movements. The velocity curves also demonstrate that girls enter the adolescent growth spurt and puberty about two years before boys do—9 and 11 years, respectively. As shown in figure 9.2, girls also stop growing two years before boys do. The difference in adult height between the sexes is largely due to females' lower peak height velocity and their cessation of growth two years prior to males (Haywood & Getchell, 2014; Malina et al., 2004).

The motor learning of children and adolescents is affected not only by changes in overall stature and weight, but also by changes in **body proportions** or form. Figure 9.3 demonstrates postnatal changes in body proportions, a phenomenon called relative growth (Haywood &

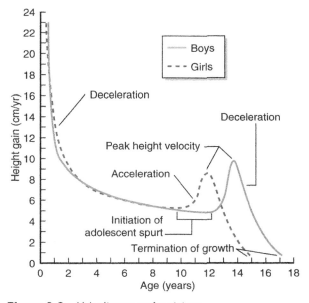

Figure 9.2   Velocity curves for stature.

Reprinted, by permission, from K.M. Haywood and N. Getchell, 2005, *Life span motor development*, 4th ed. (Champaign, IL: Human Kinetics), 39. Adapted from J.M. Tanner, R.H. Whitehouse, and M. Takaishi, 1966, "Standards from birth to maturity for height, weight, height velocity, and weight velocity: British children, 1965, part II," *Archives of Disease in Childhood* 41(220): 613-635.

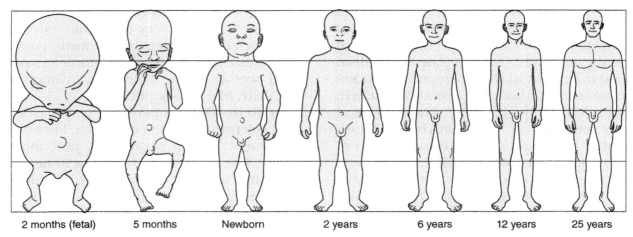

| 2 months (fetal) | 5 months | Newborn | 2 years | 6 years | 12 years | 25 years |

Figure 9.3 Changes in body form: relative growth.

RESEARCH NOTES

Environmental Constraints Can Affect Height

Did you know that the tallest people in the world are the Dutch? How they became the tallest is an interesting story of human plasticity over many generations (Bogin, 1998). In the mid-1800s, Americans were the tallest males in the world at an average 5 feet 6 inches (168 cm), whereas the Dutch stood at 5 feet 4 inches (163 cm). At the turn of the 21st century, Dutch men averaged 5 feet 10 inches (178 cm), whereas the typical American man was 5 feet 8 inches (173 cm). Bogin argued that over the last 150 years, the Dutch profited in stature from societal changes that include purifying drinking water, installing sewer systems, regulating the safety of food, and providing public health care and diets to children. The Dutch children responded to the changing environment by growing taller. Although these changes are available to many Americans, those who are poor often lack adequate housing, sanitation, and health care. This scenario demonstrates the plasticity of stature over generations if people's life conditions improve, showing that height, although influenced almost completely by the genes inherited from parents, can change over generations.

Getchell, 2014). In essence, body parts and tissues have different rates of growth. The head grows more than the legs during prenatal months. At birth, the head is about one fourth of the infant's length, but it contributes only one eighth to the height of an adult. It is clear that a child is not a miniature adult. One of the movement problems of the first year of life is how to balance a large head on a relatively small body. The legs are about three eighths of height at birth and one half when growth terminates. In other words, from birth to adulthood, the legs grow faster than the head.

Thus, although obviously taller than young children, adults have a distinctly different form. Newell (1984) argued that

TRY THIS

The Early Maturer

Exercise 9.3

Assume that a female is 59.1 inches (150 cm) tall. Look at figure 9.1*b*. How old is the girl if 59.1 (150 cm) inches places her at the 90th percentile? How old is she if 59.1 inches (150 cm) places her at the 50th percentile? How about the 5th percentile? Those three ages represent quite a wide range. Which of the ages leads you to believe she is an early maturer? What other information is necessary to support your prediction?

these changes are biomechanical constraints that affect coordination. As children grow, their movement patterns must include a constantly changing body shape. In some cases, performance is affected. For example, as elite female gymnasts progress through puberty, they may not maintain sufficient strength to compensate for their longer and heavier limbs, resulting in a decline in skill.

Limitations to Growth Curves

Distance and velocity curves describe average patterns of change, but individuals have very unique timing of these events. This is illustrated clearly by those who mature early and late. The initiation of the adolescent growth spurt may differ by several years. An early-maturing male may begin to accelerate in growth at 9 years of age, while his late-maturing counterpart may be delayed until age 15. Peak strength velocity follows within a year of peak height

velocity, and therefore it is not surprising that the early maturer will be taller and stronger than most of his peers for a few years despite being the same chronological age. Because stature and strength are structural constraints, the early maturer may be more coordinated than her same-aged peers and hence enjoy an athletic advantage. Early-maturing adolescents may ultimately be shorter than their later-maturing peers if they terminate growth earlier and therefore do not grow for as many years. It is not uncommon for athletically talented children who mature early to be very successful as a 12-year-old (girl) or 14-year-old (boy), yet lose relative placement in their peer group when peers mature. Early maturers do not suddenly become poorly coordinated or uninterested; the later-maturing athletes simply catch up and possibly surpass them in size and strength. In this adolescent period of rapid change in size and strength, predicting future athletic success is difficult.

WHAT DO YOU THINK?

Exercise 9.4

1. How will the age at which a person experiences a growth spurt influence his performance in sport? What other factors (e.g., social) must be considered?
2. Describe growth differences and similarities between the sexes from birth to adulthood.

Body System Constraints

Motor learning and development can theoretically be constrained by any body system. The systems that most affect movement and performance are the skeletal, muscular, cardiovascular, nervous, endocrine, adipose, and sensory systems. Just as with relative growth as shown in figure 9.3, these systems do not change at a constant rate. The developing child and adolescent must learn to incorporate changing limb size, muscle mass, and visual capabilities into new and old movement patterns. Once again, the changes described next underscore the notion that children are not miniature adults.

Skeletal System

The skeleton is the structural support system of the body and provides a lever for muscles, enabling movement. Large developmental changes occur in bone size and structure from birth through adolescence, as previously discussed. Bone changes do not end following the cessation of growth during late adolescence. Bone is a living and growing tissue. Old bone is removed (resorption) while new bone is continually being formed. Through this process termed remodeling, an entire skeleton is replaced every 10 years. During childhood, bone building occurs at a much faster rate than bone resorption, allowing for increases in bone size to occur.

Our previous discussion of stature dealt with the typical development of the skeletal system, but difficulties with skeletal growth can occur. **Osgood-Schlatter dis-** **ease** is a painful disruption in the growth of the upper shinbone where the patellar tendon attaches. **Legg-Calvé-Perthes disease** is an irritation of the femur where it inserts into the hip. These are childhood problems that restrict weight-bearing activities and make movement painful. People who have limb amputations perform some movements in unique ways to compensate for the loss of the limb.

Muscular System

The muscular system follows a sigmoid growth curve similar to that for weight (Haywood & Getchell, 2014). Muscle mass becomes a relatively larger component of overall body weight with development. It is about 25 percent of total body weight at birth, but 54 percent for men and 45 percent for women at maturity. It has been suggested that a critical level of strength is an important rate limiter for independent walking (Ulrich, Ulrich, Angulo-Kinzler, & Yun, 2001). This helps explain why heavier babies might not walk as early as leaner babies (more strength is needed to move a larger mass). Strength is important for many motor skills and is influenced by the amount of muscle mass, maturation, and the recruitment of muscle fibers, as well as extrinsic factors such as nutrition and exercise.

Strength

A growth in muscle mass can occur through an increase in the number of muscle fibers (**hyperplasia**) or through an increase in the relative size, or volume, of the muscle fibers (**hypertrophy**). Muscle

WHAT DO YOU THINK?

Exercise 9.5

Provide an example of how strength can be a rate limiter for the following.

- A four-month-old infant learning to crawl
- An eight-year-old baseball batter

fibers increase by both hyperplasia and hypertrophy prenatally and for a short time postnatally. Then, muscle mass can be increased only by hypertrophy. Sex differences in muscle mass are small until adolescence, when both sexes experience a rapid gain in muscle mass. However, the spurt in muscle mass continues in girls only until age 13, whereas in boys the rapid increase continues until age 17 (Malina, 1978). Following maturity, muscle mass can be changed only through hypertrophy (increase in size of muscle fibers) or through atrophy (decrease in size of muscle fibers) (Gollnick, Timson, Moore, & Riedy, 1981). Muscle fibers increase in both diameter and length during growth and development. Increases in muscle length occur in conjunction with increases in bone length, whereas increases in the diameter of a muscle fiber result from physical activity (Malina & Bouchard, 1991).

Flexibility

Flexibility is the ability to move body parts through a range of motion without strain (Gabbard, 2012). Flexibility is necessary to perform well athletically and prevent muscular injury, as well as to perform activities of daily living from dressing oneself to climbing in and out of a car (Shephard, 1998). The sit and reach test is one of the most commonly used measures of flexibility. This test assesses the flexibility of the hamstrings, low back, and hip flexors.

Sex differences exist in flexibility: females tend to be more flexible than males. Flexibility increases in both males and females until approximately the age of 10 for males and 12 for females (Clarke, 1975). Females tend to be more flexible than males from the age of 5 through adulthood (Haubenstricker, Wisner, Seefeldt, & Branta, 1997). The sex differences have been attributed to body size and composition, hormone levels, and physical activities (Gabbard, 2012). People with larger body sizes generally have poorer flexibility. Females also participate in physical activities that promote increased range of motion (e.g., dance and gymnastics) more often than males do. Flexibility changes occur at specific joints rather than across the body as a whole and are greatly affected by physical activity.

Cardiovascular System

The simplest cardiovascular measure is of heart rate. Heart rate is a convenient measure of cardiac effort at rest, during moderate exercise (submaximal heart rate), and during maximal effort (maximal heart rate) (Gabbard, 2012). Heart rate provides an indicator of both cardiac output (amount of blood pumped) and maximal oxygen consumption. On average, resting heart rate decreases with age (Lowrey, 1986). At birth, resting heart rate is very high, averaging 140 beats per minute. By age 2, it has decreased to about 105 beats per minute, and by age 20, it is approximately 66 beats per minute. The increase in heart rate in infancy and childhood is a physiological compensation for a smaller heart size. With a smaller heart, the stroke volume (volume of blood pumped during each contraction) is decreased. To compensate, the heart rate increases. For this same reason, females average about five beats per minute more than males.

WHAT DO YOU THINK?

Exercise 9.6

Females participate in physical activities that promote flexibility more often than males do. Why do you think that is? List ways to encourage male students (of all ages) to increase their flexibility.

$\dot{V}O_2$max is considered the best measure of aerobic capacity and cardiorespiratory fitness. $\dot{V}O_2$max is the maximal amount of oxygen that can be transported and used during exercise. Endurance performance and $\dot{V}O_2$max are highly correlated (Joyner, 1993); however, this does not mean that a person's $\dot{V}O_2$max is set. $\dot{V}O_2$max can be greatly increased with endurance training. Athletes' $\dot{V}O_2$max increases as they are able to run farther and faster because $\dot{V}O_2$max is determined by the maximal amount of oxygen that is required. Someone who is running fast requires more oxygen than someone who is running more slowly. This increase continues until the runner cannot run any faster. Some highly trained competitive athletes have reached as much as 8 liters per minute. In general, $\dot{V}O_2$max increases for both boys and girls at the same rate throughout childhood. At the age of 12, boys and girls have similar $\dot{V}O_2$max measures. Girls continue to increase their $\dot{V}O_2$max until about the age of 14, and boys continue to increase their $\dot{V}O_2$max until age 18 (Gabbard, 2012). The increase in $\dot{V}O_2$max in boys is a result of continued growth through a later age.

Nervous System

The nervous system undergoes change throughout life. As many as 100 billion neurons are formed, most by the third or fourth prenatal week. Later in the prenatal period and early in the first postnatal year, the neurons fire and establish **synapses** (connections) with other neurons. At birth the brain is 25 percent of its adult weight, and by five years of age, it is 90 percent (Keogh & Sugden, 1985; Piek, 2006). Beyond the rapid development of the number of neurons, which may continue until age 6 (Piek, 2006), learning and life experiences alter the nervous system throughout life. Motor learning produces synapses between motor and sensory neurons. In fact, one account of motor control proposed that muscle synergies (the synchrony of motor neurons) produce coordinated movement patterns. Practicing new motor skills results in hundreds of thousands of new groups of synapses. Neuromotor difficulties can severely affect coordination, for example, in someone with cerebral palsy. In this case, an extrinsic factor such as loss of oxygen to the developing brain, prenatally or during birth, may damage brain tissue needed in coordination. Severe malnutrition can also keep the brain from functioning optimally.

Endocrine System

The **endocrine system** controls the hormones in body tissue. For example, **pituitary** growth hormones and **thyroid** hormones are largely responsible for skeletal growth. In some cases, shorter stature may be related to a deficiency of these hormones and may be a structural constraint. Hormones from the testicles or ovaries and adrenal glands, primarily estrogen and androgens (e.g., testosterone), are responsible for the growth spurt and for epiphyseal fusion of the long bones, which terminates growth.

Adipose System

The age-related changes in fat-free mass resemble the sigmoid curves of height and weight. Adipose tissue develops rapidly in the last three months of pregnancy. Babies born prematurely often have a skinny appearance because they have not remained long enough in the womb during this important period of adipose tissue formation. As figure 9.4 demonstrates, adipose tissue continues to develop rapidly during the first 6 to 12 postnatal months (Malina et al., 2004), when fat constitutes as much as 30 percent of body weight. When adipose tissue is expressed as a percentage of body weight, there is a decline in both sexes after a peak at about age 1, until the adolescent growth spurt. However, if body fat is expressed as an absolute value in pounds or kilograms, adipose tissue continues to develop from

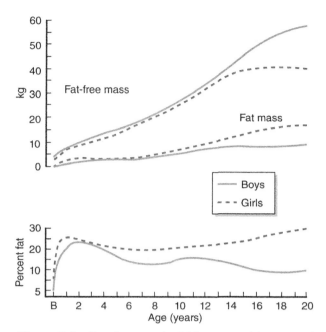

Figure 9.4 Growth curves for fat-free mass, fat mass, and relative fatness derived from measurements of total body water.

Reprinted, by permission, from R.M. Malina, C. Bouchard, and O. Bar-Or, 2004, *Growth, maturation, and physical activity*, 2nd ed. (Champaign, IL: Human Kinetics), 113. Data from Malina 1989, Malina, Bouchard, and Beunen 1988.

12 months to 20 years. The absolute amount of adiposity increases during childhood and adolescence, like skeletal or muscular tissue, but this is simply due to the fact that children and adolescents are still growing. Compare a 50-pound (23 kg) child to one at 100 pounds (45 kg). We would expect the 100-pound child to have more adipose tissue than the 50-pound child because of the difference in weight. The average adult female possesses about 70 percent of the fat-free mass of her male counterpart, largely because males at adulthood are taller than females and gained more muscle mass during adolescence than females did.

At least since 1990, there has been an epidemic of childhood obesity in developed and developing countries caused in part by inactivity. Obesity is associated with many health issues, but is also a structural constraint during performance because greater energy expenditure is necessary to move the additional weight. Obesity is associated with sedentary behaviors, and

perhaps not surprisingly, there is evidence that obesity is associated with poor motor skills (Marshall & Bouffard, 1994, 1997). Malina and colleagues (2004) concluded that after six years of age, the fattest children have a higher risk of remaining fat until adolescence and adulthood than their peers. Variation is large, and some people are fat as children and not as adults, whereas some lean children become fat in adolescence or adulthood. It appears that professionals and parents should be very concerned with children after six years of age who carry too much body fat.

Sensory Systems

Many developmental changes occur in the sensory systems. Sensory system development is of particular importance to motor development and motor learning, because it has many implications for skillful performance. Movement depends on and is intricately related to perception. Our movements are based on what we see, hear, and feel. A child's sensory development can greatly affect how she performs. Practitioners should take developmental changes in vision, audition, and kinesthesis into consideration when designing programs. Equipment and tasks should be modified according to not only the physical capabilities of children or adolescents, but also their perceptual capabilities.

Vision

Among the many visual functions, we focus only on those of particular importance to moving skillfully: visual acuity (see chapter 2 for more detail), visuomotor coordination, depth perception, and figure–ground perception. Visual acuity is the sharpness of vision. Visual acuity allows us to see an image clearly, such as a face or words on a page. There are two types of visual acuity, static and dynamic. Static visual acuity is the ability to clearly see an image that is stationary; it is most commonly assessed using the Snellen eye chart. Normal vision is considered 20/20, meaning that the image can be clearly seen from 20 feet (6 m) away. At birth, visual acuity is approximately 20/400, meaning that the newborn can distinguish at 20 feet (6 m) what people with normal vision can see at 400 feet (122 m). Newborns can clearly see images only if they are less than 1.5 feet (46 cm) away (Kellman & Arterberry, 1998). Visual acuity improves rapidly throughout the first year and then continues to improve at a slower rate to a 20/20 rating by the age of 10 (Williams, 1983).

The perception of motion is a particularly important factor in motor development and motor learning. Infants can visually perceive motion at birth, but they cannot perceive the direction of motion until approximately eight weeks of age (Wattam-Bell, 1996). **Visuomotor coordination**, the ability to visually track a moving object and guide the body or limbs (or both) to intercept the object, improves with the infant's active exploration of the environment (e.g., playing with the hands and toys, and eventually throwing). One of the reasons young children have difficulty catching is underdeveloped visuomotor coordination. Children cannot accurately track a moving object, such as a tossed ball, until the age of five or six (Morris, 1980). Parents often throw balls with a high arc to children to give them more time to prepare for a catch; however, it is even more challenging for children to catch a ball thrown in a high arc because they cannot visually track objects in two planes until they are eight or nine years old. Movement perception continues to develop until approximately age 12 (Williams, 1983).

These are only a few of the developmental changes in vision. It is also important to consider that children have difficulty separating an object from the background. The ability to do this is referred to as **figure–ground perception**. Figure–ground perception improves through childhood and adolescence until approximately age 18. The ability to distinguish the object from its surroundings is of critical importance to many sports and activities. A ball that is not easily discernible apart from the environment is much less likely to be caught or struck. **Depth perception**, the ability to see in three dimensions, is also a critical component in intercepting an object. Depth perception arises partly from the **retinal disparity** of the two eyes. Because the eyes are in different locations, they see images at different visual angles. The development of depth perception is affected by the development of visual acuity because depth perception depends on the clarity of the image to each eye, allowing a better comparison. Many factors affect the perception of the depth of an approaching ball, such as the ball's size, color, speed, and trajectory (Payne & Isaacs, 2008). A child must be able to clearly distinguish the ball from the background and use all depth cues to make a catch.

Audition

Children can locate sound effectively by the age of three years. The ability to localize sound continues to improve through the teens. The ability to localize sounds is especially important in sporting contexts, such as knowing the location of an oncom-

---

WHAT DO YOU THINK?

Exercise 9.7

Provide an example of how vision can be a rate limiter for the following populations based on visual development.

- A four-month-old infant learning to crawl
- An eight-year-old male baseball batter

Exercise 9.8

Choose two activities. As an instructor, how would you include auditory information to enhance learning? Would this change if you were instructing children versus adolescents? Explain.

ing ball based on the sound it made when hitting a wall in racquetball or the position of other players relative to one another in invasion sports. Localizing sound is also very important for driving; it allows drivers to react after hearing sirens, horns, or other sounds.

Young children can differentiate similar speech sounds, such as *b* and *d*. Differentiating *b* and *d* becomes quite important when learning to read and write. A child who cannot discern the difference will have difficulty spelling or pronouncing words with these letters because they cannot hear the difference. The ability to differentiate similar sounds amid noisy background sounds is particularly challenging for children. Improvements in the ability to discriminate speech sounds in noisy environments continue through late childhood (Neuman & Hochberg, 1983). The ability to ignore background noise while attending to particular sounds is called **auditory figure–ground perception**. Although some children appear to have more difficulty with figure–ground perception than others do, it is not well known how figure–ground perception changes during childhood because research in this area has been minimal.

Proprioception

The kinesthetic system provides us with our sense of proprioception and is supported by muscles, tendons, joints, and skin receptors as well as the inner ear and eyes. Proprioceptively, some of the most important aspects to develop are body awareness and spatial awareness.

Body awareness is an individual's sense of the body, such as knowledge of the different body parts, and body image.

Body awareness includes being able to locate body parts, knowing the movement of the body parts, and knowing how to efficiently move the body parts (Gallahue & Ozmun, 2005). The development of body awareness begins at birth and continues through childhood. Infants are born with an unconscious sense that enables them to orient themselves toward pleasant sensory experiences. The initial discovery of their own hands can be very exciting. Infants often spend much time simply staring at their hands, opening them and closing them and watching them move closer and farther away. This discovery becomes even more exciting when they shake a rattle. They are beginning to understand the relationship of their movements to other objects, as well as the placement of their body parts with respect to other body parts. Through active exploration, older infants learn how to propel themselves by understanding the relationship between their feet and leg movements and the ground. Preschoolers (three- to four-year-olds) continue to develop their body awareness through active experiences in relation to their own bodies, as seen in the following story.

While they are eating a snack together, four-year-old Joseph's teacher says to him, "You have the longest eyelashes!" Looking straight ahead, Joseph asks, "Do they reach all the way out to the juice pitcher?" The teacher laughs and replies, "Not that far." Curious, Joseph wonders aloud, "Then how far?" Spontaneously, he holds up his finger and moves it slowly toward his eye until he feels it gently touch his lashes. Delighted with his experiment,

Exercise 9.9

Describe activities that could help children develop kinesthetic perception.

---

he shares, "Now I can see and feel how far!" Later, Joseph and his friends have more fun checking out their eyelash lengths in a mirror. (Poole, Miller, & Booth Church, 2006)

Joseph not only further developed his body awareness, but also gained a better sense of distance and size. By comparing the feeling of his eyelashes with the image he saw in the mirror, he also gained a better understanding of the link between visual and kinesthetic perception. When instructing young children, practitioners should help them become more aware of their bodies by asking them where their body parts are and what their body parts do.

Spatial awareness is the awareness of the size of the body and the position of the body in relation to people and objects. Toddlers are very interested in spatial concepts. A favorite activity of toddlers is to place small objects into containers and take them out again. They learn about size and dimensions by filling open containers with smaller objects. Toddlers are also gaining a sense of **object permanence**, which is the concept that an object still exists even if it can no longer be seen. They learn that the ball they put in a box is still inside the box even if the lid has been placed on top. Because children learn spatial awareness through active exploration, they need a wide variety of experiences in manipulating objects and interacting with other children and adults. Preschoolers relate the positioning of objects to their own personal space. At this age, children are very **egocentric**, meaning that they perceive the world only in terms of themselves. By age 5 or 6, children learn spatial

orientation and the words associated with orientation, such as *near* and *far, left* and *right,* and *front* and *back* (Poole, Miller, & Booth Church, 2006). Children learn much better through active experiences than through observation or verbal instruction. By the age of six, children are less egocentric and their spatial awareness is much more established. They also have a stronger sense of personal space and are able to locate objects relative to other objects and general space (Gallahue & Ozmun, 2005). Activities that encourage various movements through space, such as obstacle courses, are especially helpful for young children.

Summary

Chapter 7 outlined changes in movement skills during childhood and adolescence. Most of us go through these changes if exposed to experiences and environments that encourage motor development (Clark, 2007). This chapter explored some of the structural factors that constrain (i.e., promote or limit) the acquisition of and forms of these movements. With this information, Chelsea (the mother and preschool teacher from the chapter-opening scenario) can appreciate the vast range of structural differences in her group of preschoolers. Parents, therapists, and leaders such as Chelsea need to understand how structural constraints may interact with functional factors (the focus of chapters 11 and 12), tasks, and the environment. For example, we can understand the difficulty many youngsters have with catching if we know that tracking and movement perception are rather late to develop.

The structural systems we have described change at very different rates; for example, the rapid growth in stature during the first year of life decelerates in subsequent years until the growth spurt of puberty. The endocrine system is rather quiet until puberty, when its influence on skeletal and muscle tissue becomes dramatic. Although systems change at different rates, change among individuals is extremely variable as well. Our discussion of early and late maturers underscores this fact. The discussion of relative growth (both in stature and percentage of muscle mass) from birth to adolescence reminds us that structural changes provide challenges and new opportunities for coordination, and that children are not miniature adults. Finally, differences in structure between the sexes are generally minimal until puberty. Thus, motor development and learning differences between girls and boys prior to adolescence are likely influenced largely by environment constraints.

ONLINE LEARNING

Visit the web resource at www.HumanKinetics.com/MotorLearningAndDevelopment for an accompanying lab activity and exercises from the chapter.

LEARNING AIDS

Supplemental Activities

1. It seems that almost weekly we read about a new research study that indicates that more and more children are becoming obese. This is a significant challenge for our society and for the professions associated with kinesiology and physical education. A good professional should keep up-to-date on statistics such as those on obesity. Search the website of the U.S. Centers for Disease Control in Atlanta to find the most recent statistics and recommendations for practice.

2. Are athletic injuries in developing children and adolescents detrimental to growth? Are some sports (e.g., American football and long-distance running) associated with injuries to such an extent that parents or professionals should restrict kids from playing them? Search the Internet for information on this topic.

Glossary

auditory figure–ground perception—The ability to ignore background noise while attending to particular sounds (e.g., in a conversation).

body awareness—A sense of the body in space, including the ability to locate body parts, knowing the movement of body parts, and knowing how to efficiently move body parts.

body proportions—The relationships of body parts in terms of size.

depth perception—The ability to see in three dimensions.

distance curve—The extent of growth in terms of height and weight.

dizygotic twins—Twins who develop from two separate ova and therefore share no more genes than typical siblings do.

egocentric—The inability to view the world from a perspective other than one's own.

endocrine system—The body system that controls the hormones of body tissue.

figure–ground perception—The ability to distinguish an object from its surroundings.

heritability—A statistic that can be calculated to estimate genetic influences in producing differences in individuals.

hyperplasia—An increase in the number of muscle units such as muscle fibers or neurons.

hypertrophy—An increase in the relative size or volume of muscle fibers or neurons.

Legg-Calvé-Perthes disease—An irritation of the femur where it inserts into the hip.

monozygotic twins—Twins who develop from a single fertilized ovum and therefore have identical genotypes.

object permanence—An awareness that an object exists even if removed from vision.

Osgood-Schlatter disease—A disruption in growth of the upper shinbone where the patellar tendon attaches.

peak height velocity—The period during adolescence in which height gain is fastest.

percentile—A relative rank or position on a scale; the percentage of a distribution that is equal to or below that position.

pituitary—A gland that secretes the hormones responsible for skeletal growth.

rate of change—The speed at which a variable changes over time.

retinal disparity—Differences in the two retinal images produced by the eyes as a result of the different positions of the eyes in the head.

sigmoid curve—An S-shaped pattern of change—for example, for height and weight.

spatial awareness—Awareness of the size of the body and the position of the body in relationship to people and objects.

synapses—Gaps between two nerve cells in which a nerve impulse is transmitted.

thyroid—A gland that secretes the hormones responsible for skeletal growth.

velocity curve—A curve that describes change per unit of time, such as height in centimeters per year.

visuomotor coordination—The ability to visually track a moving object and guide the body, the limbs, or both, to intercept the object.

PHYSICAL AGING

After reading this chapter, you should be able to do the following:

- Describe peak physiological function.
- Explain age-related changes in the skeletal, muscular, nervous, cardiovascular, and sensory systems.
- Compare the effects of a physically active lifestyle and a sedentary lifestyle in each of these systems.
- Understand the effects of normal aging on aerobic capacity and body composition, as well as any benefits of a physically active lifestyle on each.

Where Did I Put Those Keys?

Priya was headed to the grocery store but was delayed because she could not remember where she had put her keys. She looked in the usual places—her purse, the key holder, coat pockets, counters. It turns out they were upstairs on her nightstand. She must have absentmindedly carried them upstairs. When Priya arrived at the grocery store, she ran into a familiar face. They carried on a conversation, but Priya could not remember the man's name or how she knew him. While shopping, Priya could not remember some of the items she intended to purchase. Were these memory lapses signs of dementia, or simply age related? Priya was starting to become concerned. Her mother had had dementia, and the thought of that happening to her terrified her.

Experiences of occasional short-term memory loss can occur at any age. You have likely had one or even all of the experiences mentioned—not remembering where you put an object, not recognizing an acquaintance, or forgetting what you intended to purchase at the grocery store. These experiences are certainly irritating, but how does age affect memory? Should we expect to forget more and more, or is this a sign of something more, such as dementia?

With old age, humans experience many declines, including in cognitive function, cardiorespiratory function, muscular strength, and behavioral speed, to name a few. This chapter discusses these as well as other age-related body system changes, including those of the skeletal, muscular, cardiovascular, nervous, endocrine, and sensory systems. Although many age-related declines are associated with aging (**primary aging**), older adults have discovered that by maintaining an active and healthy lifestyle, they are able to not only avoid some secondary aging changes, but also reduce many age-related declines. **Secondary aging** refers to changes that are the result of disease or environmental effects. Although primary aging changes can be expected in everyone as a function of age, secondary aging is not inevitable. Examples of primary aging are mild memory losses and slower central nervous system responses; an example of secondary aging is Alzheimer's disease.

Much research indicates that physically active older adults can maintain much of their function for years longer than their sedentary counterparts, allowing them to experience a higher quality of life into old adulthood, with reduced secondary diseases and improved physical and cognitive function. All practitioners who work with older adults should understand these aging effects on the physiological systems, the impact they have on movement, and the effects of physically active lifestyles on physiological systems.

Human peak physiological function occurs between the ages of 25 and 30 (McArdle, Katch, & Katch, 2001). It is during these years of peak physiological function that the greatest sex differences are found. Women mature earlier and reach their peak physiological function between 'the ages of 22 and 25; men mature later, reaching their peak between the ages of 28 and 30 (Gabbard, 2012). Peak athletic performance parallels peak physiological function, because muscular strength, cardiorespiratory efficiency, and reaction time are at their maximum.

How people move or learn motor skills is greatly affected by the changes occurring in their body systems. Chapter 9 discussed the development of body systems from birth through adolescence. Changes in body systems do not cease following growth and maturation. Profound age-related changes occur in the body systems across the life span. When aging is combined with environmental and behavioral factors, such as diet and physical activity, even more variability is found across individuals of the same age and sex. Structural constraints are among the most important factors to consider when designing programs. Practitioners must understand how aging affects both these systems and movement. They must also understand the wide variability across adults. Because adults vary considerably more than children and adolescents do, individualizing their programs is essential.

Skeletal System

Peak bone mass occurs around the age of 30 in both males and females (Spirduso, Francis, & MacRae, 2005). Physical activities undertaken during adolescence and young adulthood help determine the size and strength of bones. Those who participate in more resistance training activities or activities that require much physical stress and load (e.g., weightlifters and powerlifters) develop stronger and thicker bones than endurance athletes (e.g., runners and cyclists) do. Increased bone density has been found in those who take part in all types of resistance training (Bemben & Bemben, 2011). Because swimming is not a weight-bearing activity, swimmers often have weaker, less dense bones than runners do (Nillsson & Westlin, 1971). Bone health acquired during youth and young adulthood provide lifelong benefits. It has been suggested that denser bones may delay the onset of microfractures in older adulthood (Schultheis, 1991). Bone health in adulthood is determined by **peak bone mass** (the highest bone mass acquired before the age of 30) and the age-related rate of bone loss (Spirduso et al., 2005).

Osteoporosis

Bone tissue is eventually lost in older adulthood, causing bones to become so weak that they may fracture from mild falls or even coughing (Shephard, 1998). Fractures, especially hip fractures, in adulthood can seriously hamper an independent lifestyle. The threat of bone fractures increases even further in those with **osteoporosis**, a crippling disease resulting from low bone mass and poor structural bone quality. From a structural viewpoint, the vertebrae may be damaged, resulting in a stooped posture that affects the execution of well-learned skills. Motivationally, a person with osteoporosis may be reluctant to learn new motor skills or use former motor skills for fear of falling and fracturing a limb.

The risk of osteoporosis increases with age, but the disease can occur at any age (Spirduso et al., 2005). As a result of decreased peak bone mass and an increased rate of bone loss, women are at a much higher risk of osteoporosis than men are. One out of three women over 50 years of age and one in five men over 50 years of age, worldwide, will experience a fracture as a result of osteoporosis (Kanis, Johnell, Oden, et al., 2000). Thin-framed women and women under 127 pounds (58 kg) are at an increased risk of osteoporosis. Ethnicity has also been linked to osteoporosis risk; Caucasian and Asian women are at highest risk, and African American women are at lowest risk (Finkelstein et al., 2002).

Women have a higher risk of microfractures and osteoporosis than men because they generally attain a peak bone mass that is 10 percent below men's peak bone mass (Shephard, 1998). The most important risk factor for bone loss in women is menopause; however, there is much variability across women. Rate of bone loss can vary greatly across individuals with some experiencing very rapid bone loss (Reeve et al., 1999). Bone loss is also much higher in women during menopause; it increases from an average of 0.7 to 1 percent loss per year to between 2 and 3 percent loss per year after menopause over a 5- to 10-year period. During menopause, women can lose between 30 and 50 percent of their bone mineral density. Bone loss then increases in both men and women during old adulthood, between the 9th and 10th decades (Spirduso et al., 2005).

Many of the risk factors for osteoporosis are modifiable, although some are not.

Nonmodifiable Risk Factors for Osteoporosis

- Sex: Women have a higher risk.
- Age: Bones become thinner and weaker with age.
- Body size: Thin-framed women are at highest risk.
- Ethnicity: Caucasian and Asian women are at highest risk.
- Family history: Heredity can increase risk.

Modifiable Risk Factors for Osteoporosis

- Lifestyle: Increased weight-bearing physical activity decreases risk.
- Calcium and vitamin D: Increased calcium and vitamin D intake decreases risk.
- Sex hormones: Low estrogen or low testosterone levels can increase risk.
- Medications: Glucocorticoids and some anticonvulsants can lead to loss of bone density.
- Anorexia: Serious reductions in food intake and body weight increase risk.
- Cigarette smoking: Smoking increases risk.
- Excessive alcohol intake: Alcohol consumption increases risk.

Adapted from National Institutes of Health, Osteoporosis and Related Bone Diseases National Resource Center, 2010, *Osteoporosis overview*. Available: www.niams.nih.gov/Health_Info/Bone/Osteoporosis/overview.asp#c

Participating in regular load-bearing exercise such as resistance training and running can decrease or even reverse bone mineral loss even throughout older adulthood (Shephard, 1998). Increasing calcium intake to 1,500 milligrams per day can also help decrease bone loss.

Body Stature

With age, there is a general trend toward a decrease in standing height (Shephard, 1997), starting around the age of 40. Women lose height at a faster rate than men do. A cross-sectional study (i.e., a study of different people at different ages) showed that men aged 80 and older were on average 1.1 inches (2.8 cm) shorter, and women over 80 were about 2.8 inches (7.2 cm) shorter than young adults (U.S. National Center for Health Statistics, 2007-2010). Losses in height accelerate after age 70, to an average of under 1/10 of an inch (2 mm) per year in both sexes (Svänborg, Eden, & Mellstrom, 1991). Decreases in height largely result from a progressive compression of the intervertebral discs (Shephard, 1997). This compression shortens the spine and can cause **kyphosis**, which is a curvature of the upper spine (see figure 10.1). Kyphosis can also be the result of years of poor posture, weak back muscles, senile osteoporosis, and osteoarthritis of the vertebrae. **Osteoarthritis** is a degenerative joint disease that can affect any joint but most often affects the hips, vertebrae, feet, and knees. Arthritis crip-

ples millions of Americans, impairing their ability to move fluidly and comfortably and affects 49.6 percent of adults over the age of 65 years (Barbour, Helmick, Boring, & Brady, 2017). Fortunately, many of the symptoms of arthritis can be controlled

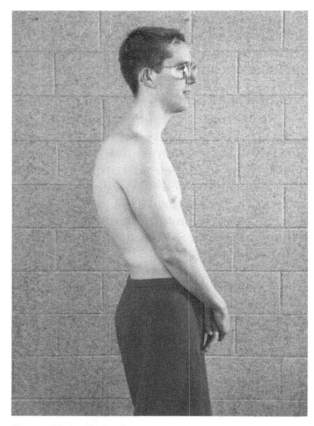

Figure 10.1 Kyphosis.

WHAT DO YOU THINK?

Exercise 10.1

You are an instructor or clinician working with an 82-year-old woman who has osteoporosis. She is frail and relatively sedentary.

1. What exercises might you prescribe? Explain why you chose these exercises. What exercises should this woman avoid? What are some warnings (signs and symptoms) for a frail woman with osteoporosis?

2. What activities would you prescribe for her if she also had osteoarthritis in her knees and ankles? What activities should a person with arthritis avoid? Explain why developing a program for someone with both osteoporosis and osteoarthritis would be particularly challenging.

through non-weight-bearing exercise such as swimming and cycling, flexibility training, and light resistance training (Van Norman, 1995).

Muscular System

The muscular system works in concert with the skeletal system to allow the body to move. Large changes in body composition occur in adulthood, resulting in a progressive loss of lean body mass. The loss of lean body mass results more from an increase in body fat than from a reduction in muscle mass (Haywood & Getchell, 2014). Losses in muscle mass are small until around the age of 50, after which they accelerate. People can avoid much of this loss in muscle mass by maintaining moderate to high physical activity levels and good nutrition (Shephard, 1998).

Strength

Maximal strength correlates with muscular cross-sectional area, which is largest during the 20s and plateaus until the age of 35 to 40 (Shephard, 1998). Strength declines generally begin at the age of 40 but can begin earlier in sedentary people. A loss of between 30 and 50 percent of skeletal muscle mass occurs between the ages of 40 and 80, thus contributing to a decline in motor performance (Akima et al., 2001). Subsequent declines in strength and power generally parallel, but are often greater than, the rate of skeletal muscle mass decline (Bassey, Fiatarone, O'Neill, Kelly, Evans, & Lipsitz, 1992; Goodpaster et al., 2006). Increases in muscle weakness and fatigability also result from decreased muscle mass (Faulkner & Brooks, 1995). Declines in maximal strength are greater in the legs than in the arms (Shephard, 1998). This may be attributed to reduced use of the legs with age.

Most adults experience a reduction in muscle mass as a result of heredity, intergenerational lifestyle, nutrition, socioeconomic factors, and other factors (Lazarus & Harridge, 2010), but the biggest factor is lack of adequate physical activity or inactivity (Blair, 2009). Because the number of muscle fibers decreases around the age of 50, losses in muscle mass at younger ages occur as a result of a sedentary lifestyle (Faulkner, Larkin, Claflin, & Brooks, 2007).

The changes in muscle mass occur as a function of muscle fiber types. There appears to be an age-related decline in fast-twitch, or Type II, fibers, whereas slow-twitch, Type I fibers can be maintained with a physically active lifestyle even through old age (Lexell, Taylor, & Sjostrom, 1988). **Slow-twitch fibers** have a slower contraction–relaxation cycle than fast-twitch fibers do and are best suited for endurance activities; **fast-twitch fibers**, with their much quicker contraction–relaxation cycle, are better suited for short-duration, high-intensity activities such as sprinting and powerlifting. Although a loss of fast-twitch fibers appears inevitable, the amount and rate of decline are greatly affected by the frequency and intensity of physical activity. Older adults can not only reduce this rate of decline, but also experience hypertrophy in the muscle fibers that remain (Lexell, 1995). The Type II fibers tend to decrease, while the Type I fibers are maintained. This tendency remains even with frequent and intense physical activity (Shephard, 1998).

The loss of muscular strength in older adults can be quite significant, affecting their ability to maintain independence. Activities many people take for granted such as carrying a bag of groceries, climbing steps, or even opening a medicine bottle can be very challenging for an older adult with significant losses in strength (Shephard, 1991). Losses in muscular strength are exacerbated by long-term physical inactivity, which leads to frailty. **Frailty** is characterized by severe limitations in mobility, strength, balance, and endurance, resulting from weak and highly fatigable muscles; it is often due to a long-term inactive lifestyle (Faulkner et al., 2007). Reversing this condition is often difficult. A long-term inactive lifestyle combined with genetic factors, disease, injury, or aging (or some combination of these) causes muscular atrophy, decreased strength, and increased fatigability, leading to frailty (see figure 10.2). Frail people experience impaired mobility and balance and are at an increased risk of falls. With declining fitness, health, and quality of life, the frail elderly often spiral downward, participating in less physical activity. This further reduces their strength and mobility, continually worsening their condition by limiting their physical activity and activities of daily living (ADLs) even more. By further limiting their physical activity, they experience more muscle wasting (atrophy), resulting in a worsening condition.

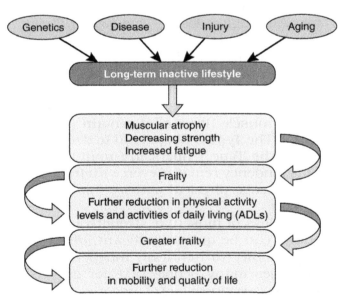

Figure 10.2 Downward spiral of physical inactivity leading to frailty and reduced mobility.

Flexibility

The elasticity of the tendons and ligaments and the condition of the synovial fluid enable smooth body and limb movements (Gabbard, 2012). With age, flexibility decreases as cross-linkages between collagen fibrils develop and synovial fluid degrades. The cross-linkages reduce the elasticity of the tendons, ligaments, and joint capsules (Shephard, 1998). Females experience a more gradual per year decline in flexibility than men do (0.6 vs. 0.8 percent) (Baptista de Oliveira Medeiros, Sardinha Mendes Soares de Araújo, & Gil Soares de Araújo, 2013). Declines in flexibility accelerate at a faster rate following middle age; adults lose approximately 3 to 4 inches (8 to 10 cm) of flexibility of the low back, hips, and hamstring as assessed by the sit and reach test (Shephard, 2008). Declines in flexibility are joint specific; shoulder and trunk flexibility declines at a faster rate than knee and elbow flexibility. These differences may be attributed to individualistic activity patterns (Baptista de Oliveira Medeiros et al., 2013). To mitigate the aging effects on flexibility, the joints must be taken through their full range of motion. Stretching exercises done when muscles are warm and yoga are beneficial in maintaining flexibility and reducing the effects of aging.

Aerobic Capacity

A progressive age-related decline in aerobic capacity is found in adults from age 25 to 65 (Shephard, 1997). Similar to losses in strength, age-related losses in aerobic capacity accelerate at the age of 70 and over (Shephard, 1998). It is difficult to separate age-related losses in function from changes due to other factors such as reduced regular physical activity and the intensity of physical activity bouts. Although some research has suggested that aerobic capacity can be maintained with regular intense training (Kasch, Wallace, Van Camp, & Verity, 1988), most research has found this to be only a short-lived training response. Following the initial training response, the rate of age-related declines in aerobic power follows a pattern similar to that in nontraining people (Shephard, 1998). Some of the factors of an age-related decline in aerobic power are maximal aerobic capacity, lactate threshold, and exercise economy.

Maximal Aerobic Capacity

Maximal aerobic capacity, often referred to as $\dot{V}O_2$max, begins to decline following young adulthood. Although $\dot{V}O_2$max is highly correlated with endurance, the decline in $\dot{V}O_2$max throughout adulthood tends to be greater than performance declines. Endurance training can increase $\dot{V}O_2$max by 5 to 20 percent in children and adults (Gabbard, 2012). One would expect endurance-trained older athletes to experience a decreased rate of decline compared to sedentary people, yet recent studies have not found this to be true. Longitudinal studies have indicated that endurance-trained older women decline at twice the rate of sedentary women (Eskurza, Donato, Moreau, Seals, & Tanaka, 2002), but endurance-trained and sedentary men decline at the same rate (Wilson & Tanaka, 2000). Greater declines in endurance-trained men than in sedentary men have been found but have been related to a reduction in training (Pimentel, Gentile, Tanaka, Seals, & Gates, 2003). Keep in mind that these comparisons are with individuals' $\dot{V}O_2$max at an earlier age, not with that of the average younger adult, so the endurance-trained adults had more $\dot{V}O_2$max to lose than sedentary adults because of their higher initial levels. Also, many of the older women had significantly reduced their training volume, which would decrease their $\dot{V}O_2$max. Declines in the rate of $\dot{V}O_2$max are similar in endurance-trained and sedentary adults, but the endurance-trained adults have a much higher $\dot{V}O_2$max because they start at a much higher level.

Sex differences in the $\dot{V}O_2$max of adults are quite large, due to lean body mass and overall body weight differences across the sexes. Men generally have a $\dot{V}O_2$max that is 40 to 60 percent greater than that of women (Hyde & Gengenbach, 2007). An untrained male averages approximately 3.5 liters per minute, whereas an untrained female averages 2 liters per minute.

Lactate Threshold

Aerobic performance can also be determined by **lactate threshold**, which occurs at the exercise intensity at which blood lactate begins to accumulate significantly above baseline levels in the bloodstream (Tanaka & Seals, 2003). Lactate threshold declines with increasing age, resulting in reduced overall performance. Although reductions in endurance performance are largely affected by declining lactate threshold in young and middle-aged adults, reduced endurance performance is more affected by reductions in $\dot{V}O_2$max in older adulthood (Evans, Davy, Stevenson, & Seals, 1995).

Exercise Economy

The oxygen cost of exercise at a particular velocity is known as **exercise economy** (Tanaka & Seals, 2003). Exercise economy is a strong indicator of endurance ability (Morgan & Craig, 1992). Although only a few studies have addressed the effects of age on exercise economy, aging does not appear to have such an effect. Thus, the reductions in endurance performance

WHAT DO YOU THINK?

Exercise 10.2

1. Define maximal aerobic capacity, lactate threshold, and exercise economy.
2. Which is the strongest indicator of endurance ability?
3. Which is most affected by aging?
4. What types of activities increase aerobic capacity?

found with aging are likely largely the result of declines in $\dot{V}O_2$max and lactate threshold.

Cardiovascular System

The cardiovascular system declines by approximately 30 percent between the ages of 30 and 70 (Spirduso et al., 2005). Heart rate, most notably heart rate during maximal exertion (maximal heart rate), decreases across the lifetime. Declines in stroke volume are also seen with aging. Increases in arteriovenous oxygen difference occur in older adults, although little difference is found in older adults who exercise regularly. Furthermore, blood pressure tends to increase in older adults. Note that these changes occur in healthy adults. Some people may exhibit some form of cardiovascular disease resulting from heredity and lifestyle behaviors. It is important to evaluate cardiorespiratory fitness level prior to involvement in a fitness program or teaching a motor skill, because it will greatly affect the person's ability to perform aerobic exercise.

Heart Rate

Heart rate is one of the most commonly used measures of response to exercise because of the relative ease of measuring it. Heart rate is particularly important because it is a major determinant in cardiac output and maximal oxygen consumption (Gabbard, 2012). Measurements can be taken at various points from resting heart rate to maximal heart rate (taken when people are exerting themselves to their maximal oxygen uptake).

Resting heart rate exhibits only small changes with age throughout adulthood (Fagard, Thijs, & Amery, 1993). Heart rates during submaximal exercise, however, tend to be lower in older adults than in young adults (Sachs, Hamberger, & Kaijser, 1985). This is because heart rates not only increase at a faster rate in young adults, but also continue to increase to higher levels than in older adults during submaximal exercise (Paterson, Cunningham, & Babcock, 1989). The largest age-related change in heart rates is found during maximal physical effort. A simple and common formula for computing maximal heart rate is to subtract a person's age in years from 220 beats per minute. For instance, a 50-year-old's maximal heart rate would be 170 beats per minute. Although a maximal heart rate of around 190 beats per minute would be expected for a 30-year-old, this formula does not always hold for fit and healthy older adults. Some older adults have been found to reach maximal heart rates 20 beats per minute higher than would be expected based on the formula (Dempsey & Seals, 1995).

Stroke Volume

Stroke volume is the amount of blood pumped through one ventricle of the heart during one contraction. Not all of the blood is pumped out during a contraction. Approximately one third of the blood remains in the left ventricle. Stroke volume depends on the size of the heart, the duration of the contraction, preload (the amount of ventricle stretching prior to the contraction), and afterload (aortic pressure during the contraction). In general, men tend to have higher stroke volumes than women because their hearts are larger. Stroke volume can be increased through aerobic training, which can also result in lower resting heart rates.

The human heart is quite flexible, enabling heart volume to be well maintained until very old ages (Shephard, 1997). Older adults can have higher stroke volumes than younger adults during submaximal exercise; however, increased stroke volume is difficult for older adults to maintain even when exercise intensity nears maximal effort (Niinimaa & Shephard, 1978). As older adults approach maximal effort, many actually exhibit declines in stroke volume, whereas young adults exhibit a gradual increase in stroke volume when approaching maximal effort (Tate, Hyek, & Taffet, 1994).

Arteriovenous Oxygen Difference

The **arteriovenous oxygen difference** is the difference in oxygen content between arterial and venous blood. The mean arteriovenous oxygen difference determines the volume of oxygen that is transported to the tissues following a contraction (Shephard, 1997). Physically active men can sustain the arteriovenous oxygen difference during rest and submaximal exercise, whereas the largest arteriovenous oxygen differences are found in sedentary women, up to 50 milliliters per liter greater than their physically active counterparts (Dempsey & Seals, 1995). In very healthy and fit older adults, the maximal arteriovenous oxygen difference can remain the same, but it generally decreases by approximately 20 milliliters per liter (Shephard, 1998). This change is due in part to a larger distribution of the cardiac output to regions, such as the skin and internal organs, with age (Shephard, 1993).

Blood Pressure

A blood pressure reading is a combination of the pressure from the contraction of the left ventricle forcing blood into the aorta (systolic) and the brief relaxation of the ventricle that follows (diastolic). A healthy blood pressure for a young or middle-aged adult is typically 120/80 (Saxon, Etten, & Perkins, 2010). It should be understood that blood pressure fluctuates throughout the day as a result of physiological and psychological changes. High blood pressure is considered a systolic reading of over 140 mmHg (millimeters of mercury) or a diastolic reading of 90 mmHg or higher. Recommendations may vary for people with different conditions; however, changes are common with age (see figure 10.3). Early treatment of prehypertension

is highly recommended to prevent serious health complications (Hernandez, 2008).

Older adults are more prone to both orthostatic hypotension (postural low blood pressure) (Shephard, 1997). This is due in part to the fact that older adults are less able to respond to changes in body position or heat than young adults are. Sharp drops in blood pressure can occur when an older adult moves from a lying position to standing or when stepping out of a swimming pool. These drops in blood pressure may also occur following an exercise bout. Orthostatic hypotension induces dizziness, confusion, and sometimes fainting (Fagard et al., 1993).

The following recommendations for the general population are from the U.S. National Institutes of Health (2014):

- Recommendation 1: Treat adults over the age of 60 who have a systolic blood pressure of 150 mmHg or higher or a diastolic blood pressure of 90 mmHg or higher.
- Recommendations 2 and 3: Treat adults under the age of 60 who have a systolic blood pressure of 140 mmHg or higher or a diastolic blood pressure of 90 mmHg or higher.

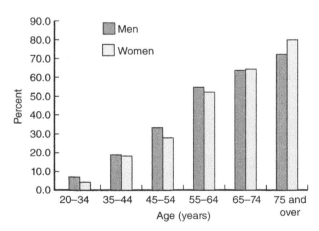

Figure 10.3 Rates of hypertension in men and women over the age of 20 in the United States, 2011-2014.

Data from National Center for Health Statistics, 2015, *Health, United States, 2015: Health risk factors.* Available: http://www.cdc.gov/nchs/hus/healthrisk.htm#high

Clinical hypertension affects two thirds of adults over the age of 65 (Yen, 2004). Blood pressure can rise as much as 35 mmHg or more across a life span (Kannel, Sorlie, & Gordon, 1980). This rise is generally found in people living in developed countries; indigenous community dwellers show little to no increase in hypertension across age (DeStefano, Coulehan, & Wiant, 1979). This cultural change is largely attributed to lifestyle differences between urban community dwellers and many indigenous people, such as the Navajo and the Pacific Islanders. Some behavioral factors have been found to increase blood pressure such as sedentary lifestyles, excessive body weight, and sodium intake, whereas others can decrease blood pressure, including the intake of omega-3 fatty acids (Saxon et al., 2010). The following are lists of both nonmodifiable and modifiable risk factors for high blood pressure and the development of cardiovascular disease.

Nonmodifiable Risk Factors for High Blood Pressure

- Gender: Men are at higher risk in young and middle adulthood; women have a higher risk after age 55.
- Age: Blood pressure increases with age.
- Ethnicity: African Americans have the highest incidence.
- Family history: Heredity can increase risk.
- Diabetes: This poses a higher risk.

Modifiable Risk Factors for High Blood Pressure

- Lifestyle: Regular exercise reduces risk.
- Sodium intake: Excessive sodium intake increases risk.
- Obesity: Maintaining a healthy weight reduces risk.
- Lipids and cholesterol: Reducing lipids and cholesterol in the diet reduces risk.
- Stress: Stress reduction is beneficial.
- Cigarette smoking: Smoking increases risk.
- Alcohol intake: Excessive alcohol consumption increases risk.

Adapted from Saxon et al. 2010.

Blood pressure tends to increase during physical exercise regardless of age. These increases are even larger for people with higher resting blood pressures (Zerzawy, 1987). Elderly men have averaged 37 mmHg higher than young adults, and elderly women have averaged 26 mmHg higher (Shephard, 1997). Continued regular or vigorous exercise (or both) can decrease resting, submaximal, and maximal blood pressure in young and older adults, bringing them down to a level similar to that of young adults over time.

People with hypertension should not participate in high-intensity exercise, because it will increase blood pressure and place them at risk for cardiac problems

WHAT DO YOU THINK?

Exercise 10.3

You are an instructor or clinician working with a 72-year-old hypertensive man with arthritis in his knees and hips. Your client was an athlete as a young adult but did not continue a physically active lifestyle beyond his 30s. He held a sedentary job for 40 years and has been obese for about 30 years.

What exercises might you prescribe for this man? Explain why you chose these exercises. What exercises should he avoid? What are some warnings (signs and symptoms) for an obese hypertensive older adult with arthritis?

(Hagberg, 1988). Regular systematic exercise can reduce blood pressure, decrease the risk of developing cardiovascular disease, and lower weight (Bradley, 2007). Low- to moderate-intensity exercise (40 to 65 percent of maximum) is quite beneficial and can actually decrease blood pressure. Weight training is also favorable; however, high resistance with low repetitions should be replaced with lower resistance and higher repetitions. Because some people tend to hold their breath during weight training, it is very important to encourage breathing during the movements to avoid further increases in blood pressure (Van Norman, 1995).

Nervous System

The central nervous system is composed of the brain and the spinal cord. There are approximately 100 billion neurons in the brain, giving rise to a very complex neuronal network. The neuron consists of the cell body, axon, and dendrite. With age, the dendrites and axons gradually wither away. The brain also experiences a gradual loss in the number of neurons (thousands each day). These changes contribute to the reduced size and weight of the brain. Even though the structure of the brain undergoes substantial losses, generally only small functional losses result.

RESEARCH NOTES

An Idle Mind Is the Devil's Plaything

The benefits of neural plasticity may be best evidenced by a longitudinal study on the effects of aging and brain health conducted on a group of 678 nuns in Mankato, Minnesota, in the United States (Snowdon, 2003). Snowdon studied nuns because they are a much more homogeneous population than the general population. They have very little to no drug or alcohol use, live in similar environments, and have similar reproductive histories. This group is also particularly interesting because, on average, they live much longer than the general population, many into their 90s and 100s. Not only do the nuns live longer, but they also suffer dementia at a much lower rate; those who do suffer dementia generally have milder cases than the average population. **Dementia** is defined as a substantial loss in cognitive ability above normal age-related declines.

After following these nuns for years, Snowdon believed that the reason for their prolonged length and quality of life was their belief that "an idle mind is the devil's plaything" (Ratey, 2001). The nuns continued to challenge themselves mentally even in their 90s and beyond, keeping their minds actively engaged with puzzles, debates, weekly seminars, vocabulary quizzes, and daily journal writing; some even continued working in their late 90s. Sister Matthia, featured in *National Geographic* at the age of 103, was one of the first nuns to participate in the study and became a model for healthy aging. Her postmortem neuropathological evaluation revealed that she had no signs of brain pathologies, which is very rare for someone over the age of 90 (Snowdon, 2003).

The education level of the nuns and the jobs they held greatly affected both their brain health and their length of life. The nuns with university degrees who continued to challenge themselves lived longer and had less dementia than the nuns who held more mundane positions such as housecleaning and food preparation. Those who continually challenged themselves mentally had more neural connections, enabling them to recover from disease and stay healthier and active longer (Ratey, 2001).

The brain can recover from much of these losses through a process called neural plasticity. Plasticity refers to the brain's ability to actually rewire itself to compensate for such changes (also discussed in chapter 6). The brain restructures itself based on past experiences and what it learns. Neuronal connections increase in areas of the brain that receive information more frequently than areas of the brain that are used less frequently. For instance, a soccer player would have more of the cortex devoted to the feet, and a violinist would have more devoted to the fingers. Neural plasticity can occur at any age but is most adaptable during childhood. The incredible ability of the brain to adapt does decline with age, but it can be strengthened through both cognitive and physical activity.

Aging is associated with an increase in abnormal formations such as neurofibrillary tangles and senile plaques. **Neurofibrillary tangles** occur when the fibers of a neuron become twisted with one another. These tangles can lead to the death of the neuron and are thought to contribute to the slowing of central nervous system responsiveness (Gallahue & Ozmun, 2012). **Senile plaques** form on the outside of neurons and have been related to memory loss. Plaques and tangles are found, to some degree, in the majority of adults over the

TRY THIS

Brain Exercises

Exercise 10.4

Performing simple activities that cause a mental conflict or require the opposing sides of the body to perform opposite or different activities is mentally challenging. The following are exercises designed to integrate both sides of the brain while providing challenging movements for the whole body. With practice, they become easier. Try each of these activities seated or standing.

1. Repeatedly say the word *yes* while turning your head back and forth from left to right (as if you were saying no).
2. Say the word *no* while nodding your head up and down.
3. Swing your arms up and down while at the same time shaking your head no and saying the word *yes.*
4. Move your arms forward and backward while nodding your head up and down and saying the word *no.*
5. Move one of your shoulders up and down while moving the other one forward and backward.
6. Move your shoulders in circles going in opposite directions.
7. Move one shoulder in a circle while moving the other shoulder forward and backward.
8. Do regular jumping jacks; then switch to jumping with the feet apart and the arms together.
9. Try alternating from feet apart and arms together to feet together and arms together.

Were you surprised at the difficulty of some of these simple activities? You probably required more time to adjust to each change. Can you think of other activities that would challenge the brain?

age of 80 (Saxon et al., 2010), and many are found in adults with dementia.

Older adults require more time to learn motor skills than young adults do. This could partly be the result of memory losses associated with aging (Shephard, 1997). Losses occur in both long-term and short-term memory in older adults (Lee, 2010). People can slow many age-related cognitive losses by maintaining moderate physical activity levels and keeping the mind sharp through mental activities such as word puzzles, reading, and writing.

Brain games have become a popular tool in recent years; advertising particularly targets young children and older adults. Although there is some research to support the benefits of brain games (Nouchi et al., 2012), others claim that the benefit is merely a placebo effect (Foroughi, Monfort, Paczynski, McKnight, & Greenwood, 2016). Although some companies are facing federal regulations regarding the efficacy of their products, brain games continue to be quite popular. Although not as catchy, there are many brain game activities that people can do without having to purchase products (see the activities in exercise 10.4).

Endocrine System

The endocrine system plays an important role in maintaining homeostasis by signaling hormones through an integrated system of organs including the pineal gland, pituitary gland, thyroid gland, thymus, adrenal gland, pancreas, ovary, and testes. Much like the nervous system, the endocrine system is an information signaling system. The endocrine system influences metabolism, tissue function, growth, and mood regulation. The endocrine system also affects energy production and mental activity. These functions undergo changes during the aging process; however, the endocrine system also adapts to these changes as they occur (Hashizume, Suzuki, Takeda, Shigematsu, Ichikawa, & Koizumi, 2006).

Age-related changes in the endocrine system include declining thyroid function, decreasing gonadal hormone levels, and declining neural and hormonal control systems (Shephard, 1997). The thyroid hormone has a role in increasing basal metabolic rate and thermoregulation in extended cold exposure. Changes in basal metabolic rate across a lifetime are more greatly affected by a decrease in lean body mass than by changes in the thyroid. Gonadal hormone changes can increase muscular atrophy and osteoporosis. Hormonal regulatory systems also play an important role in the maintenance of homeostasis during exercise. Hormones are particularly important during vigorous exercise, affecting cardiovascular regulation in warm environments, fuel mobilization, and the synthesis of new protein (Shephard, 1997). The role of the endocrine system during aging has been studied extensively because it affects so many other systems and aspects related to quality of life. Some genetic factors have been associated with longevity; they have also been found to protect against age-dependent diseases and promote exceptional health in later years (Barzilai & Gabriely, 2010).

Body Composition

Body weight tends to increase in adults until the age of 60 and decrease thereafter. In the United States, the mean weight of women in their 60s (the age at which they are at peak weight) is 4.3 pounds (2 kg) greater than that of women in their 20s; men in their 50s (the age at which they are at peak weight) are 5.8 pounds (2.6 kg) heavier than men in their 20s (U.S. National Center for Health Statistics, 2007-2010). The increase in body weight is largely due to an increase in fat mass (FM). In conjunction with the increase in FM with age is a redistribution of body fat. With age, body fat tends to be redistributed from the limbs to the abdominal area (Spirduso et al., 2005). Intra-abdominal fat accumulation begins in the 20s and increases through the 60s (Schwartz, 1990). Abdominal obesity, which is associated with an apple-shaped body, is associated with a high risk for cardiovascular disease.

While FM increases with age, fat-free mass (FFM) decreases with age. Fat-free mass, including the nonfat components of the body such as organs, muscle, bone, and skin, peaks in the 20s and 30s and then gradually declines. The decline in FFM is largely attributed to muscle atrophy, or wasting of the muscle. Decreases in FFM are a result of reduced physical activity, osteopenia (bone loss), hormonal changes, and diet changes (Spirduso et al., 2005).

Exercise is the best defense against age-related changes in body composition. Physical activity can increase muscle mass while decreasing FM, increase resting metabolism, and improve mood state. Although dieting in addition to physical activity is preferred, replacing physical activity with dieting alone is detrimental. Dieting alone often leads to a loss in body mass as a result of decreased muscle mass, a reduction in resting metabolism, and a depressed mood state (Shephard, 1997).

Sensory Systems

Movement is profoundly affected by the ability to receive and interpret sensory information. How we move is determined by our response to the sensory information we receive. Infants who are blind take significantly longer to crawl, stand, and walk because they lack the incentive that infants with vision are provided (Fazzi et al., 2002). Similarly, older adults who have progressive vision loss tend to walk with slower, more deliberate steps. Sensory losses begin in the 30s. These losses generally do not affect everyday function until older adulthood, but they do affect athletic performances in many sports. Although we receive sensory information

from the senses of smell and taste, it is vision, audition, and proprioception (kinesthetic perception) that are essential in motor performance.

Visual System

With age, many anatomical and physiological changes occur in the visual system. Age-related changes, some of which begin in the 20s, result in reduced function, which can greatly affect skillful performance and learning new motor skills. It can even have an impact on independent living in older adults. Older adults have increased difficulty with visual cues, which affects driving ability and walking across the street without assistance.

Physiological and Anatomical Changes

The many age-related physiological and anatomical changes in vision include changes in the cornea, iris, lens, and retina. With age, the cornea increases in thickness, resulting in decreased corneal sensitivity (Millodot, 1977). The iris also undergoes many changes, including decreased thickness, increased rigidity, and reduced pigmentation, causing a degraded retinal image as a result of an increased amount of stray light (Weale, 1963). The pupil begins decreasing in size in the teens. The lens grows throughout life and begins to become less compliant in adulthood. Changes in the lens reduce visual accommodation and the ability to focus clearly on close objects. **Accommodation** is the process that enables the eye to adjust and focus to produce a clear image. The retina also increases in thickness, affecting **peripheral vision** (vision outside of the center of gaze). The rods and cones experience age-related changes that affect vision in light and darkness, as well as color sensitivity. Changes also occur in the primary visual cortex, the area of the brain responsible for interpreting visual images. Table 10.1 lists age-related structural and functional changes in several of the main structures of the eye.

Table 10.1 Age-Related Changes in Vision

Eye structure	Structural changes	Functional changes
Cornea	Thicker and less curved	Increased sensitivity to glare; reduced refractive ability and more prone to astigmatism
Anterior chamber	Decreased size	Can lead to glaucoma
Iris	Pigmentation changes	Faded eye color
Pupil	Decreased diameter	Sensitivity
Lens	Thicker, denser, and less elastic	Impaired refractive ability and changes in color vision; cataracts can develop
Retina	Loss of rods and cones	Reduced adaptation to light and dark

Functional Changes

Functional changes result from the many anatomical and physiological age-related changes in the eye. Young adults are quite good at discriminating colors; they can see differences in up to 100,000 colors (Garzia & Trick, 1992). With age, color and brightness sensitivity declines, affecting the eye's ability to adapt to changing levels of light and dark. Older adults may find it particularly challenging to find open seats in a dark theater because it takes longer for their eyes to adjust.

One of the most common measures of vision is the Snellen chart, which is used to assess visual acuity (the sharpness of vision) by having people identify high-contrast letters. Visual acuity decreases with advanced age (Saxon et al., 2010). Although visual acuity is the most common method of assessing vision, contrast sensitivity provides a better overall assessment (Garzia & Trick, 1992). **Contrast sensitivity** is the amount of contrast necessary to discriminate between an image and its background. Contrast sensitivity, which peaks at age 20 and declines thereafter, is an important factor in many motor skills. A person who needs a lot of time to detect the position of a ball will likely not make contact with it.

Eye movement control also declines with age, causing further difficulty with tracking moving objects and **visual search** (the act of directing attention toward important cues in the environment). Visual search is an important factor in moving skill-fully. Skilled performers' decision-making abilities and reaction times depend on their visual search strategies. Effective visual search strategies can be developed. Instruction and feedback should direct the learner to the most important cues. For example, experts tend to fix their visual gaze on the most important aspect of the movement, whereas novices tend to alter their visual gaze. **Fixation** is the focusing of visual attention on an object (Coker, 2013). By looking at unimportant cues, people often miss important information. Shank and Haywood (1987) found that during the windup of a baseball pitch, skilled baseball batters fixated on the release point, whereas novice batters alternated between the release point and the pitcher's head. Skilled batters were able to identify the correct pitch nearly 100 percent of the time, whereas novice batters identified the correct pitch only 60 percent of the time. It is important to focus on the critical cues, such as the release point, but just as important to ignore irrelevant cues such as the head (Coker, 2013). With age, visual search can become increasingly difficult, not only compromising skillful performance, but also affecting everyday activities such as identifying street signs and locating house numbers.

Older adults begin to experience difficulty with driving and mobility. Driving at night can be particularly challenging for an older adult because of increased problems with glare and night vision. The issue of driving in old adulthood has evoked a lot of controversy, given that driving provides the

Vision Screening

Exercise 10.5

The Amsler grid screening test is used to detect diseases of the retina such as macular degeneration. Macular degeneration causes a loss of vision in the central visual field as a result of damage to the retina. This loss can make facial recognition or reading nearly impossible. When taking the following test, wear glasses or contacts if you typically wear them.

1. Perform an Internet search for the Amsler grid screening test and print out a copy of the grid. Hold the grid at eye level approximately 15 inches (38 cm) away.
2. Look at the dot in the center of the grid.
3. While maintaining your gaze, cover your right eye and continue to look at the dot.
4. Repeat this test covering the left eye.

Did you notice any changes, such as the dot disappearing or the squares blurring or changing shape? A yes answer to any of these questions would indicate damage to the retina and possible macular degeneration. Macular degeneration is a serious condition that could result in legal blindness if not treated.

primary mode of transportation for most Americans. Although driving ability is a complex motor skill dependent on many factors including attentional focus, coordination, reaction time, processing speed, and sensory information, vision is one of the most important factors affecting driving performance. Loss of peripheral vision is particularly important (Linton, 2007) because research has revealed that twice as many older drivers with peripheral deficits experienced accidents and conviction rates than did older drivers without peripheral field deficits. Dynamic visual acuity (clearly seeing an object while it is moving) is also a risk factor for driving accidents in older adults (Owsley & Ball, 1993).

Auditory System

Hearing losses generally begin in the mid-30s but can occur earlier or be exacerbated by an overexposure to noise. Hearing loss that occurs from noise is called noise-induced hearing loss (NIHL). Losses of higher-pitch tones are very common and begin to occur in adults as early as age 18. This loss, termed **presbycusis**, occurs as a result of hardening auditory nerve cells. High-pitched ring tones, such as the mosquito ring tone Teen Buzz, have been designed specifically for teenagers, and most adults over the age of 20 (including their teachers) cannot hear them.

Females tend to have markedly better hearing than males beginning at the age of 40 (Schieber, 1992). This difference may be due in part to increased environmental noise in many male-dominated occupations. Hearing loss continues in both males and females throughout middle and older adulthood. Many older adults experience an inability to hear not only high-pitch tones but also some lower-pitch tones, making it increasingly difficult to maintain conversations in noisy environments. Although age-related hearing losses are not life-threatening, they do negatively affect quality of life. Hearing impairments can affect the ability to respond to auditory signals of danger, but more frequently affect daily communication with family members, friends, and coworkers. Older adults with hearing impairments are sometimes even treated as if they are mentally incompetent or have early signs of dementia (Saxon et al., 2010). When communicating with someone with a hearing impairment, at any age, speak face-to-face so that the person can clearly see you; speak slowly and enunciate; do not shout; and if you have a high-pitched voice, try to lower the pitch of your voice.

Kinesthetic Perception

Unlike with the visual system, knowledge of the extent of age-related changes in kinesthetic perception is limited. Evidence of the changes in body and spatial awareness with age is conflicting; some reports show age-related declines, and others do not (Gabbard, 2012). One common change in kinesthetic perception is a reduction in tactile sensitivity. The lower extremities tend to be more affected than the upper extremities (Corso, 1987); however, reduced sensitivity in the lower extremities may be attributed to other factors such diabetes, circulatory issues, or injuries (Gabbard, 2012). The loss of tactile sensitivity is due to an age-related decline in the number of touch receptors in the skin. A progressive loss of sensitivity to pain and temperature also occurs with age (Kenshalo, 1977). Reduced vestibular function, which negatively affects balance, begins in the 30s. The vestibular system, located in the middle ear, provides information regarding head position and movement. Deficits in the vestibular system can cause dizziness and **vertigo**, a balance disorder with signs and symptoms that can vary from dizziness and vomiting to difficulty standing and walking.

Summary

Aging is a unique experience for everyone. It is affected by genetic factors, behavioral lifestyle, and past experiences. These factors interact, causing us all to age at different rates. Not only do adults age differently from one another, but their physiological systems age at different rates, too. For example, some people may experience faster rates of decline in the cardiovascular system than in the endocrine or nervous system.

This chapter outlined age-related changes in the skeletal, muscular, cardiovascular, nervous, endocrine, and sensory systems. These physiological changes are due to healthy aging (primary aging) and are not the result of disease or the effects of the environment (secondary aging). Although a physically active lifestyle can slow or delay many of these age-related declines, they are inevitable. The rate of decline in many areas increases at the age of 75. Healthy, physically active adults experience similar rates of decline beyond this age in most areas; however, they are starting at higher levels, which enables them to maintain their physical function much longer than their sedentary peers.

Maintaining a physically active lifestyle is a key ingredient in sustaining a high quality of life. Regardless of age, a physically active lifestyle reduces the risk of many secondary diseases, decreases the symptoms of secondary diseases, and improves physical and cognitive function. Clinicians, physical educators, fitness instructors, and coaches who work with older adults must understand the effects of aging on the physiological systems and the impact these changes have on movement. Because variability across individuals in older populations is much higher than in children and adolescents, it is perhaps even more important to individualize programs for older than it is for younger adults.

ONLINE LEARNING

Visit the web resource at www.HumanKinetics.com/MotorLearningAndDevelopment for an accompanying lab activity and exercises from the chapter.

LEARNING AIDS

Supplemental Activities

1. Primary aging includes age-related declines as a function of healthy aging, whereas secondary aging is the result of disease or environmental effects. For each of the systems discussed in this chapter, list several examples of primary aging and secondary aging.

	Primary aging	Secondary aging
Skeletal system		
Muscular system		
Cardiovascular system		
Nervous system		
Endocrine system		
Sensory system		

From P.S. Haibach-Beach, G.D. Reid, and D.H. Collier, 2018, *Motor learning and development*, 2nd ed. (Champaign, IL: Human Kinetics).

2. Research one of the following conditions: osteoporosis, arthritis, cardiovascular disease, hypertension, or stroke. In an essay, describe this condition and how it differs from primary aging (age-related changes that are not due to disease or poor behavioral practices such as smoking, a sedentary lifestyle, or obesity). Explain whether and how this condition could be prevented through behavioral changes.

Glossary

accommodation—Related to vision, the process that enables the eye to adjust and focus, producing a clearer image.

arteriovenous oxygen difference—The difference in oxygen content between arterial and venous blood.

contrast sensitivity—The amount of contrast necessary to discriminate between an image and its background.

dementia—A substantial loss in cognitive ability above normal age-related declines.

exercise economy—The oxygen cost of exercising at a particular velocity.

fast-twitch fibers—Muscle fibers that have a quick contraction–relaxation cycle and are well suited for short-duration, high-intensity activities such as sprinting and powerlifting.

fixation—The focusing of visual attention on an object.

frailty—A condition in which a person exhibits severe limitations in mobility, strength, balance, and endurance, resulting from weak and highly fatigable muscles following a long-term inactive lifestyle.

kyphosis—Curvature of the upper spine; can be the result of years of poor posture, weak back muscles, senile osteoporosis, or osteoarthritis of the vertebrae.

lactate threshold—The exercise intensity at which blood lactate begins to accumulate significantly above the baseline levels in the bloodstream.

neurofibrillary tangles—Neural fibers that are twisted together.

osteoarthritis—A degenerative joint disease that affects approximately 80 percent of adults over the age of 65; can cause pain and stiffness in the joint.

osteoporosis—A crippling disease resulting from low bone mass and poor structural bone quality; increases the threat of bone fractures.

peak bone mass—The highest bone mass acquired prior to the age of 30.

peripheral vision—Vision outside of the center of gaze.

presbycusis—Age-related hearing loss.

primary aging—Age-related declines associated with healthy aging.

secondary aging—Changes that are the result of disease or environmental effects (e.g., emphysema or Alzheimer's disease).

senile plaques—Masses that form on the outside of neurons and have been related to memory loss.

slow-twitch fibers—Muscle fibers that have a slower contraction–relaxation cycle than fast-twitch fibers and are best suited for endurance activities such as long-distance running and swimming.

stroke volume—The volume of blood pumped through one ventricle during one contraction.

vertigo—A balance disorder with signs and symptoms that can vary from dizziness and vomiting to difficulty standing and walking.

visual search—The act of directing attention toward important cues in the environment.

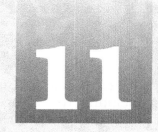

COGNITIVE DEVELOPMENT

After reading this chapter, you should be able to do the following:

- Explain Piaget's four stages of intellectual development.
- Discuss the ways declarative, procedural, and metacognitive knowledge and skill execution differ.
- Describe the developmental relationship between knowing and doing.
- Understand the development of attention and information processing.
- Describe the relationship between memory and knowledge and ways to improve memory for movements.
- Discuss the distinguishing features of an expert.

Even People of the Same Age Are Different

Michelle met her afternoon summer recreation group of 12-year-olds for the first time. She noticed a wide difference in body size and shape. These were among the structural constraints discussed in chapter 9. She directed a couple of basketball activities and observed the expected differences in skill level. Then she asked some questions about basketball rules and strategies and was overwhelmed with the range of basketball knowledge in her group. Two of the children could articulate subtle differences in offensive strategies, but a couple of others were unaware that five players from each team were on the court at the same time! Michelle wondered whether the highly skilled players also possessed this rich basketball knowledge and whether the knowledge had come simply as a result of playing. In high school she made the varsity team and remembered that her teammates differed widely in their knowledge of the game and other "smart" things such as attention and memory. One of the girls could recall a lengthy sequence of plays with remarkable accuracy and insight. Most of the players were not quite so sharp. How does cognition relate to basketball knowledge and basketball skills? More specifically for Michelle, what changes in skill and knowledge about the game might she expect over the summer in this group of 12-year-olds?

This chapter explores the developmental changes in functional constraints that affect the learning of physical skills, including the changes in intellectual development, knowledge acquisition, attention, and memory. We also briefly explain what it means to be an expert in sport. Awareness of these functional factors should clarify the skill and learning differences in the group of 12-year-olds mentioned in the opening scenario.

From birth, children move through phases of intellectual development, which is defined as the ability to understand, think, and conceptualize. This development is quicker in some children than in others, and it extends well into adolescence. It is not surprising that all 12-year-olds may not comprehend the subtle aspects of instruction or team play. Also, sport-specific knowledge is likely to assist performance, and some keen youngsters acquire an almost encyclopedic knowledge of their favorite sports. Moreover, children's developing ability to attend to detail and focus on two things at the same time interact in intriguing ways with physical skills. Finally, you may not have thought that we have a memory of movement, but the ability of older people to ride a bicycle after not doing so for many years suggests that we do. How can we assist learners with their memory of the physical skills we are instructing? In this chapter we explore the functional constraints related to thinking and learning.

Intellectual Development

Jean Piaget was a brilliant Swiss child psychologist who published his first paper at age 10 and received his doctorate at 21 (Crain, 1985). His passion was the origin of knowledge, which led to his developmental studies of children's thinking. Experimentally, he observed youngsters in spontaneous activities and discussed with them their logic in arriving at "wrong" answers. Younger children's thinking was not wrong, but it was quite different from older children. In addition, Piaget recorded in great detail, and interpreted, the activities of his three children. His theory of intellectual development emerged from this body of work.

Piaget's theory proposed four general stages of intellectual development (see table 11.1) to describe the qualitatively different ways children and adolescents think from birth to maturity (Crain, 1985; Ginsburg & Opper, 1969; Piaget, 1976; Shaffer, 1999). He proposed that children develop structures called **schemes** (or schema) for thoughts and action. The schemes are the result of children's actively constructing understandings of the world based on their experiences (Shaffer, 1999). Because cognitive experiences early in life are movement generated, movement development and cognitive development are interacting processes. Let's take a quick look at the four periods Piaget proposed: sensorimotor (0-2 years), preoperational (2-7 years), concrete operational (7-11 years), and formal operational (11 years and beyond).

In the first month of the **sensorimotor stage**, newborn schemes are based on reflexes, according to Piaget. By one month, children learn to self-initiate a movement that is similar to a reflex; for example, sucking in anticipation of a nipple. This is referred to as a sucking scheme. By four months, they repeat actions they enjoy, such as bringing a

Table 11.1 Piaget's Four Stages of Intellectual Development

Stage and age	Description
Sensorimotor (0-2 years)	Sensory experience and movement are coordinated to act on the world and generate knowledge.
Preoperational (2-7 years)	Thinking is symbolic but egocentric and often illogical from an adult perspective.
Concrete operational (7-11 years)	Thinking is logical but restricted to events experienced, seen, or heard.
Formal operational (11 years and beyond)	Logical thinking can now extend to ideas and hypotheses.

hand into view to watch it. These actions occur very close to the body. In this early developmental period, infants learn that their actions have an effect on their own bodies. From 4 to 10 months, this cause-and-effect link is extended outside the body; for example, the infant realizes that shaking a rattle results in a unique sound and that actions such as a crude throw of food produce a curious "splat" and interesting reactions from parents. By one year, children are experimenting with a host of actions that produce many fascinating outcomes. A rattle can be seen, reached for, grasped, and shaken. They also become aware that an object removed from vision still exists (object permanence). They find the object by thoughtfully searching around barriers and under coverings. By two years, children demonstrate a time lag before acting on a problem. Although the outcome remains a motor act, a thought process appears to precede the action. Of course, by age 2, children understand many words and requests and have been experimenting with expressive language for almost a year.

Piaget's **preoperational stage** is characterized by the use of symbols such as images and words. Language can reconstruct a previous event, explain the present, or predict the future. Children at this stage initiate pretend play and through action finally develop logical thinking. In most cases, however, children are not logical thinkers the way adults are. In Piaget's famous experiment on **conservation of liquids**, children were presented with two identical glasses that contained the same amount of water (Crain, 1985). When water from one glass was placed into a taller glass, the children were asked which glass now had the most water. They often responded that the taller glass had more water, suggesting that their logic was based on only one dimension—in this case, height.

It is not surprising that parents, therapists, and teachers who attempt to use adult logic with children are met with minimal understanding. In social situa-tions children are often egocentric in their thinking until quite late in the preoperational stage. *Egocentric* does not imply selfishness, but rather, that children are unable to view the world from a perspective other than their own. Thus, it makes little sense to the child to spread out on a playing field in the hope that someone will pass him the ball, or even to wait his turn on a playground. The child who tells the teacher on a Monday morning that her parents had a big fight during the weekend over the time she should go to bed cannot understand that sharing the story with the teacher is not desirable from the viewpoint of her parents. This period is also the time when children move from **parallel play** (playing alongside peers but not really interacting) to **cooperative play** (sharing a goal with other youngsters such as building a sandcastle).

Children in Piaget's **concrete operational stage** make much more logical use of thinking, albeit regarding real objects or events based on their experience. They can now master the conservation of liquid problem as well as other conservation problems; for example, they are aware that objects have more than one dimension. In sport, children in this stage can begin to think strategically about the intent of an opponent and the personal action required to counter their opponents' tactics (Payne & Isaacs, 2008). They also develop a less egocentric view of the world during this period, as they find that they must adopt the perspective of others if they want to be understood. Thus, they consider what they are saying and the needs of the listener. Rules of games that were unchangeable and determined by adults can now be viewed as plastic, modifiable to suit the needs of several people and the group.

The **formal operational stage** begins at about age 11 and continues until adulthood, according to Piaget. Thinking is no longer restricted to concrete objects; children can now deal with abstractions. In the conservation of liquid problem, children understand that water can be repoured into the original glass, and they know the outcome without performing the action. This affects a wide array of cognitions, in areas from science to sport to social values. Children can deal with science problems systematically by exploring many possibilities and hypotheses. A defensive player in a team sport can picture the oncoming players, predict outcomes, and decide on a defensive strategy.

Formal operations enable adolescents to ponder questions of the future and their own aspirations. In relation to this thinking, they can begin to set longer-term goals and realize that certain actions are needed now to achieve the ultimate goal. As we will see in the context of social development, prior to the formal operational stage, a child might brag about a parent as tall, athletic, and rich; during the formal operational stage, concepts of honesty, thoughtfulness, and integrity develop. Some aspects of egocentrism may reappear as adolescents ponder the vast array of life's possibilities. Eventually, experience and adultlike thinking enable self-realization as older adolescents learn their own limits and cognitive abilities.

Piaget's theory helps us appreciate the cognitive functioning of children and adolescents. Piaget advocated neither a strict maturational nor a strict environmental position. Rather than viewing knowledge as something to be provided by teachers or parents, he believed that true learning comes from active discovery. Materials of interest to children are critical but should be tailored to their stage of cognition so that they are drawn to them. The ages associated with Piaget's four stages vary

with each child. Some of the 12-year-old youngsters described at the beginning of the chapter may still be functioning in the concrete operational stage, whereas others may be well into formal operations. Thus, students in this group will vary a great deal in how they think and view the social and academic worlds. Piaget was primarily concerned with qualitative changes in children's thinking as they develop. But children also gain knowledge; they know things as they develop. We turn to this topic next.

Types of Knowledge

Influential papers by Chase and Simon (1973) and Chi (1978) prompted the exploration of knowledge and its relationship to memory and development. Chase and Simon asked people to look at a chess board and remember the positions of the chess pieces. The pieces were then removed, and the people were instructed to replace them in their original positions. Not surprisingly, perhaps, the chess experts remembered the positions of the pieces better than the nonexperts did. However, this excellent memory was apparent only when the chess pieces represented patterns seen in a game. When the chess pieces were randomly placed on the board, the chess experts could not recall their positions any better than the novice chess players could. The experts did not have any advantage in basic abilities or mental "hardware" (Ericsson, 2003), but their extensive knowledge of the game was responsible for their remarkable memory of actual chess patterns. This result has been replicated in studies in which expert athletes recalled patterns of game play in sports such as basketball, volleyball, and field hockey more effectively than sport novices did (Starkes & Allard, 1991).

Chi (1978) extended this thinking about the role of knowledge by challenging the long-held assumption that the memory of adults always exceeds that of children. She used the chess task and demonstrated that children who were chess experts could recall more chess positions than could adults who were novices in chess. Children can outperform adults when their knowledge is more extensive than that of the adults. This supported the impact of domain-specific knowledge on memory and led researchers to compare experts and novices in a wide range of areas such as chess, sport and refereeing, music, and science to gain insight into knowledge development and performance (Starkes & Ericsson, 2003). In this section we focus on knowledge in physical activity and sport (see table 11.2). The types of knowledge that have been identified include declarative, procedural, and metacognitive (e.g., Brown, 1975; Chi, 1981; Wall, McClements, Bouffard, Findlay, & Taylor, 1985).

Declarative knowledge about action is factual and conceptual information stored in memory that can influence the development and execution of skilled movement (Wall, Reid, & Harvey, 2007). Factual knowledge includes knowing the difference between a softball (which is not really soft) and a Nerf ball (which is actually soft) or between an underhand throw and an overhead throw. Factual knowledge begins to develop in preschool and is acquired through experience and facilitated by language. Conceptual knowledge developed by athletes and sport enthusiasts involves knowledge of the rules, equipment, and tactics of the game. This is affected by cultural norms: Canadians often have extensive knowledge of ice hockey; and the British, of cricket. Declarative knowledge is often assessed using written or verbal tests.

Procedural knowledge is about how to do something. It underlies an action and includes anticipation and prediction, decision-making, and response selection aspects of information processing (Wall et al., 2007). Catching a ball is influenced by perceptual knowledge of the trajectory, speed, and size of the ball; cues from the thrower; and the position of the catcher in relation to the environment. Experts pick up cues earlier than nonexperts do for perceptual processing (Abernethy, 1991; Wall et al., 2007), and children from 5 to 12 years old show improvement in the use of cues to predict the direction of a ball (Lefebvre & Reid, 1998). One researcher assessed the procedural knowledge of gymnastics judges by showing video clips of gymnasts performing with errors and requesting the judges to describe the error, as well as by monitoring their eye movements to determine where they were focused and for how long (Ste-Marie, 2003). French and Thomas (1987) studied decision making in basketball with

Table 11.2 Knowledge Influences in Movement Performance

Types of knowledge	Description
Declarative knowledge	Factual knowledge stored in memory: *The shortstop usually stands to the left of second base, so I should move to that location.*
Procedural knowledge	Knowledge underlying action such as decision making: *If the ball rolls slowly to me at third base and the runner on first is fast and has a good lead, I will throw to first base instead of second to get the sure out.*
Metacognitive knowledge	A higher level of declarative knowledge about how one learns: *I really want to make this team but my attention can wander, so I had better place myself in the front of the other players where I can see the coach.*
Metacognitive skills	A higher level of procedural knowledge about how one performs: *I am not doing very well in this race at the moment, but I will not stay with the leaders because I think they are going too fast and I know my strength is the final kick.*

an observation instrument that recorded whether the child shot, passed, or dribbled after receiving the ball; French, Spurgeon, and Nevett (1995) conducted a similar study in baseball.

The relationships between movement execution, declarative knowledge, and procedural knowledge are complicated. In chess, declarative knowledge is information about the game quite apart from actually playing. One would assess procedural knowledge by having people play the game to determine the extent of their knowledge of how to play. In chess, researchers are not typically concerned with the act of reaching and grasping the chess pieces and moving them to a new location. But movement scientists are very much interested in the act of reaching and grasping, not just declarative and procedural knowledge. Although some argue that procedural knowledge is synonymous with skill execution, it is probably wise to differentiate between movement execution, declarative knowledge, and procedural knowledge (e.g., French & Thomas, 1987; Kourtessis & Reid, 1997). If you have ever made a decision to execute a particular movement (procedural) but failed to accomplish it (execution)—that is, you didn't do what you meant to do—then you understand the distinction between procedural knowledge and movement execution.

Meta is a prefix that refers to a higher level. In the context of knowledge, it is a higher level of understanding knowledge.

It is not just more knowledge but personal reflection on one's knowledge, awareness of how one acquires knowledge, and awareness of one's strengths and weaknesses. University students demonstrate **metacognitive knowledge** when they realize that they must study in a quiet environment to do well on a test, or when they find it easier to learn subject A than subject B. Wall and colleagues (2007) distinguished between metacognitive knowledge (a higher level of declarative knowledge) and **metacognitive skill** (a higher level of procedural knowledge). A swimmer may know that her kick in the breaststroke is fine but that she needs more work on her arm action; this is an example of metacognitive knowledge about action. With development, metacognitive knowledge becomes more "organized, coherent, and accessible" (Wall et al., 2007, p. 267). Metacognitive knowledge is awareness of one's own strengths and weaknesses. Metacognitive skills are especially important in selecting and planning goal-directed learning. Much of what we describe later as self-regulation could be viewed as metacognitive skills. A budding athlete who intentionally continues to problem solve to push his personal performance limits is demonstrating metacognitive, or self-regulatory, skill.

Development of Knowledge

The development of declarative, procedural, and metacognitive knowledge likely

Exploring Types of Knowledge

Exercise 11.2

Establish a group with one or two of your classmates. In your group, pick an area of knowledge within movement (e.g., a sport, playing a musical instrument). It is best if you feel quite knowledgeable about this area. Your first task is to list examples of declarative knowledge, procedural knowledge, metacognitive knowledge, and metacognitive skill that are important in your sport or activity. For procedural knowledge, focus on decision making rather than skill execution. Second, can you think of professional players or other highly skilled athletes or musicians who are recognized as particularly strong in one of the types of knowledge?

follows that order (Brown, 1975, 1978; Wall et al., 1985). As children acquire language in the preschool years, they demonstrate factual (declarative) knowledge of early movements. Evidence of procedural knowledge then emerges. However, these knowledge types are related to quite specific actions (i.e., domain-specific knowledge), and therefore the extent of knowledge is based largely on experience rather than age. One of the children in the class mentioned at the beginning of this chapter might have extensive procedural and declarative knowledge of basketball as a result of playing the game so frequently. Therefore, just like the chess experts in the experiment of Chi (1978), who could remember the placement of pieces better than adults could, this basketball player may possess more declarative and procedural knowledge of basketball—not only beyond that of her age peers, but also beyond that of her teacher. Metacognitive knowledge is the last to develop and requires Piaget's formal operations, but much experience as well.

Knowing and Doing

Perhaps it does not surprise anyone that sport-specific declarative, procedural, and metacognitive knowledge are more elaborate in people who participate extensively in a given sport. Is it really unexpected that people who play baseball might know more about baseball than those who do not?

RESEARCH NOTES

Basketball Skills and Knowledge

French and Thomas (1987) published two studies that explored knowing and doing in basketball. In the first study, they examined declarative knowledge, skill development, and expertise. The participants were basketball players in age groups 8 to 10 and 11 to 12. The coaches completed a questionnaire to rate each player's basketball ability and designated the top third of each age group as experts and the bottom third as novices. All players completed a 50-item multiple-choice declarative knowledge test and a skills test of basketball. In addition, an observational instrument was used during games to assess control, decision making, and execution. Control referred to whether the player made a successful or unsuccessful catch. Decision making involved whether the player held the ball, passed, shot, or dribbled. Execution related to the success of the decision. The findings showed that the experts in both groups possessed more shooting skill and basketball knowledge and made more correct decisions than the novices did. The authors concluded that "development of sport-specific declarative knowledge is related to the development of cognitive decision-making skills or procedural knowledge, whereas development of shooting skill and dribbling skill are related to motor execution components of control and execution" (French & Thomas, 1987, p. 24).

The second study explored change in declarative knowledge, skills, and basketball performance (using an observational instrument) over a seven-week season. It also included a control group from middle school physical education classes. Basketball knowledge, cognitive decision making, and control components of performance improved; but performance on the skills test did not change significantly, nor did the execution component of performance. Because cognitive knowledge and decision making improved, the authors concluded that "children are learning what to do in certain basketball situations faster than they are acquiring the motor skills to carry out the action" (French & Thomas, 1987, p. 30).

But what about the armchair quarterback who might have much declarative knowledge about the game of American football but limited playing ability? Knowing and doing are obviously related, but precisely how they are related and how they change over time is not clear; the relationship is quite complex because knowledge and performance are dynamic, ever-changing factors.

That children might learn appropriate actions before attaining the ability to execute them was supported by Kourtessis and Reid (1997), who demonstrated that fundamental knowledge of catching preceded actual performance. In contrast, French and colleagues (1995) showed that in baseball players who were 7 to 10 years of age, skill contributed to expertise more than decision-making skills, possibly because baseball is a low-strategy sport compared to basketball. If sport experts have more declarative knowledge than novices, is it simply because the experts have more experience with the sport, or because they have more skill?

Williams and Davids (1995) tried to distinguish between **game experience** and **skills** by comparing high-skilled soccer players, low-skilled soccer players, and spectators who had a physical disability and therefore had never played the game but reported having watched hundreds of games. Arguably, the latter group had much experience with the game but minimal skill. Overall, the results showed that the high-skilled players had the most extensive declarative knowledge about soccer, suggesting that playing the sport was an important factor in developing declarative knowledge. It seems that declarative knowledge is part of skill rather than only a by-product of experience. Clearly, the relationship between knowing and doing is not simple, and at times knowing might be more advanced than doing. However, more research is needed to determine the best combination of cognitive and motor instruction.

Another aspect of the relationship between knowing and doing is the role of knowledge that accompanies skill acquisition. Experts have asserted for many years that well-learned skills become automatic, and we might assume that the impact of explicit knowledge would diminish or change with such automaticity. Stanley and Krakauer (2013) contended that even highly skilled performers continue to use knowledge as they seek new and improved actions to guide their performances. Knowledge is important for continued improvement and is used by elite athletes in practice sessions and preperformance routines in closed-skilled sports (Toner, 2014). Knowledge is also a critical dimension of sport education models (e.g., Hastie, Calderon, Rolim, & Guarino, 2013).

Attention

Attention has been investigated for over 100 years by scholars interested in motor performance and learning. Bicyclists navigating busy streets, students learning in noisy environments, typists working in open offices, and trauma patients trying to reacquire lost skills understand the need to pay attention. In chapter 2 attention was described from three viewpoints: capacity, selectivity, and focus. Here we focus on the development of attention.

Exercise 11.3

How do students' declarative knowledge, procedural knowledge, and metacognitive knowledge influence their ability to learn motor skills?

Development of Attention

The ability to manage information develops with age; there would seem to be little doubt that children are less able than adults to perform simultaneous tasks. In other words, attention (from a capacity viewpoint) is greater in adults than in children. The intriguing developmental question is, Why are adults more capable? The simple explanation is that overall capacity increases with age. A person is analogous to a container that changes over time from a pint to a gallon. This capacity-increase view has generally not received much support (Thomas, Thomas, & Gallagher, 1993). Rather, it is more likely, as Wickens and Benel (1982) concluded, that automation and deployment of attention skills explain developmental changes. Automaticity is the autonomous phase of learning described by Fitts and Posner (1967)—the point at which motor skills can be executed with almost no attention. Because this occurs after considerable practice, automation is not limited solely by age or maturation, but also by specific experience with the task. Think of the excellent downhill skier, young or older, who requires thoughtful attention only when he finds himself suddenly on dangerous terrain. Attention skills are strategies employed during the learning and performance of tasks that improve with age and experience. Later in this chapter we will see that children's memories improve when they intentionally engage in rehearsal strategies, such as rehearsing a telephone number presented to them verbally.

Newborns demonstrate some selective attention (Reynolds, Courage, & Richards, 2013). Frantz (1963, 1964) showed that newborns systematically stop looking at repeatedly presented stimuli (1963) and that they look longer (suggesting preference) at patterned than at unpatterned forms (1964). This suggests early perceptual processing of visual information. By three months there is rapid neurological development of the retina and visual pathways to the cortex, permitting expansion of the visual field, increased eye movements, and the ability to sustain attention for 5 to 10 seconds. By six months, infants can orient and focus on most environmental stimuli and are attracted to complex visual forms such as a caregiver (Reynolds et al., 2013). Infants differ in the amount of time they spend attending to stimuli. When "short lookers" were compared to "long lookers" at 24, 36, and 48 months of age, those who spent less time attending to events (short lookers) were superior to long lookers on tasks of inhibition, memory, and cognitive flexibility (Cuevas & Bell, 2014). The short lookers were likely more efficient information processors.

As the brain (particularly the prefrontal cortex) develops into the second decade of life, the ability to control selective attention and inhibit the processing of irrelevant stimuli continues to improve (Wetzel, 2014). Selective attention is important in information processing and required for learning, thinking, remembering, and gaining competence in the world. Atypical development of selective attention is linked to disorders such as ADHD (Atkinson & Braddick, 2012; Wetzel, 2014).

Thomas and colleagues (1993) presented a review of the development of selective attention for motor skills. Ross (1976, as cited by Thomas et al.) described overexclusive, overinclusive, and selective attention. Children five or six years of age are likely to be overexclusive; that is, they attend to a limited number of cues regardless of the importance of the task. Between 6 and around 11 years of age (approximately), children become overinclusive, directing attention to the complete display rather than focusing on task-relevant cues. Children older than 11 begin to selectively attend to the task-important cues and ignore the task-irrelevant cues. This is consistent with recent models of selective attention (Atkinson & Braddick, 2012; Wetzel, 2014).

Evidence also suggests that guiding learners' visual search can be an effective

Exercise 11.4

How does the development of attention make you rethink teaching students?

intervention (Ryu, Kim, Abernethy, & Mann, 2013). Teachers and coaches can help children and older learners focus on relevant cues, as explained in chapter 15.

Developmental Changes in Information-Processing Speed

Information-processing speed also shows clear developmental trends. In a **simple reaction time** experiment, participants remove a finger from a response key when a light comes on. Adults outperform children, or to put this more positively, children improve with age. In a more complex situation called choice reaction time, the finger is lifted from the key and moved to a second response key under two or more lights. Removing the finger from the initial response key is the same act in both simple and choice reaction time. Yet choice reaction time is longer than simple reaction time presumably because the decision to move to a specific response key is processed before the lifting of the finger. Hick (1952) demonstrated that reaction time increases as more choices are presented. Choice reaction time improves with age and is particularly slower in children than in adults at higher loads of information (Keogh & Sugden, 1985). Information-processing speed also improves with age on tasks involving feedback processing and decision making (Thomas et al., 1993). Children process information more slowly and less efficiently than adults do.

As in the case of attention, the intriguing question is, Why are children slower on information-processing tasks? It is unlikely that children have lower nerve impulse conduction speed or motor capacity than adults have (Thomas et al., 1993). Central information-processing mechanisms may account for the age difference

in processing speed. Keogh and Sugden (1985) suggested that this may occur in any part of the processing chain (e.g., perception, recognition, decision making). More research is necessary to determine whether the slower reactions of children are due to slower perception or slower decision making. It is also possible that children lack task-specific strategies and knowledge, which reduces their speed of processing (Thomas et al., 1993). Finally, several noncentral factors might be involved, such as attentiveness, incentive, and practice. That is, perhaps children do not perform as well on such speed tasks because they are not attentive enough during testing or have no great motivation to perform well.

Memory

Memory, defined as the ability to recall things, was introduced in chapter 2, where we discussed short-term, working, and long-term memories. For over 100 years there has been research and speculation about memory development (Schneider & Ornstein, 2015). The study of children's memory—specifically, strategies for encoding information such as rehearsal—received a boost from Flavell's research in the 1960s (e.g., Flavell, Beach, & Chinsky, 1966; Flavell, Friedrichs, & Hoyt, 1970). Strategies are defined as goal-directed and mentally effortful processes that enhance memory—that is, the acquiring and retrieving of information (Bjorklund & Douglas, 1997). Flavell and others demonstrated that strategies develop with age and that memory performance was closely aligned to the use of strategies. Older elementary school–aged children were shown to be more intentional than younger children in recalling information; they actively used strategies such as rehearsal, elaboration, and organization to remember. Strategies become more complex with age and contribute to age-related memory performance differences (Schneider & Ornstein, 2015). Researchers have also discovered that a significant contributor to memory development is the knowledge of how one's own memory works. In this section we describe more fully the relationship between memory and knowledge, as well as memory for movements.

Memory and Knowledge

Because long-term memory represents our personal knowledge, memory and knowledge have been categorized in a number of similar ways. Piaget believed that understanding, knowledge, and memory are inseparable. Tulving (1985, 2002) distinguished between **episodic memory** and **semantic memory**. The former refers to remembering personal events, going back in time, such as your first day at university. You might recall details of your feelings, your parents' reactions, the people you met, and your first class. Semantic memory refers to general knowledge built from life experiences and learning. Semantic memory includes everything from the concept of school to the name of the country north of the United States. Tulving (1985) also included procedural knowledge—that is, knowing how to do something. He viewed motor skills as a form of procedural knowledge that allows us to achieve goals in our environment, not just talk about what to do. We noted earlier that skilled movement should be differentiated from procedural knowledge of that skilled movement.

Developmental psychologist Brown (1975) described memory as three types of knowledge: knowing, knowing how to know, and knowing about knowing. **Knowing** is our knowledge base, which others have called semantic memory or declarative knowledge. From a developmental perspective, younger children are not expected to perform as well on memory recall tasks as older children, because the younger ones have less detailed knowledge that they can relate to the new information. When practitioners build links with previous knowledge, learners benefit. For example, a practitioner might say, "Remember how you learned to step forward when throwing a ball? With the football, you have to do the same thing."

Knowing how to know refers to control processes and strategies used for deliberate learning. These activities move information or action from working memory to long-term memory. Strategies include rehearsing information, naming (attaching a verbal label to stimuli), grouping information (e.g., tennis instructors may suggest you scratch your back with the racket rather than provide a lengthy list of actions), and searching long-term memory. Much learning, and hence knowledge, depends on strategic learning, according to Brown (1975). Her research demonstrated that young children and those with intellectual disabilities must learn to use strategies and become more active learners. Therefore, games that intentionally teach strategies such as getting into the open for a pass are important. Likewise, the common reminder in teaching the breaststroke (*Arms, legs, glide*) specifies the important coordination sequences and is a strategy learners can use on their own.

Finally, **knowing about knowing** is metamemory, or metacognition (Flavell, 1979); it is the knowledge of how our personal memory functions. If young children are asked if they can recall a list of 14 foods provided verbally, they are likely to say yes. Adolescents know that 14 items exceeds their memory capacity (seven plus or minus two). The teenagers know more about how memory works. They realize that they can recall a list of 14 only if they use a memory strategy, such as writing the list on paper or grouping food items (e.g., into fruits, vegetables, and grains). In a movement context, a person with excellent metamemory might know that she needs to read about a skill to learn the verbal labels

I Know That I Remember . . . but How?

Exercise 11.5

We don't often think about memory for movements we perform. But vision, the vestibular apparatus, and kinesthesis permit us to replicate movements we have experienced. Form pairs with classmates. One pair should volunteer to go to the front of the class and do a quick demonstration that proves we can replicate previously experienced movements. One student stands facing the class with eyes closed. His partner lifts one of his arms to form an angle (45 or 90 degrees) to the side of the body, then lowers the arm and asks him to return to the previous angle. The angle will not be perfect, but it will approximate the angle experienced.

After you have seen the demonstration, face your partner, with each of you at a desk. Place your elbow and forearm on the desk so that your forearm crosses your chest. Close your eyes. Your partner now slowly moves your hand around an arc with the elbow as a pivot point (really, a curvilinear path of the hand). After 20 seconds, your partner asks you to go back to the same spot. Your partner should select five distances to move your arm, such as 30, 60, 90, 120, and 150 degrees. Thus, there will be five trials consisting of (a) a movement, (b) 20 seconds, and (c) replicating the movement. After five trials, switch positions.

After each person has had five trials, discuss with your partner how you remembered the movements. Did you use any of these strategies: visual imagery, verbal labels, rehearsal, intention to remember, or subjective organization? Did you use techniques other than these?

and to gain some declarative knowledge, then practice alone to get the idea of the movements and rehearse the declarative knowledge, and then seek out a teacher to provide feedback after some trials. Others might know that they learn best by going to an instructor at the beginning. *Knowing how to know* develops after *knowing about knowing* and *knowing.*

Memory for Movements

Memory for movements may be assisted by **visual imagery**, **verbal labels**, rehearsal, intention to remember, and **subjective organization** (Magill, 2017). First, memory is influenced by the **meaningfulness** of the movement. We are not referring to meaningfulness in a motivational context, such as how important the movement is to the person. Rather, we are referring to the similarity of new movements to previous ones. Movements have space and time constraints. A meaningful movement is one that the learner can relate to because the new

movement is similar to something already known. Meaningfulness can be assisted by visual imagery and verbal labels. A swimming instructor could describe the biomechanics of the arm pull of the sidestroke or provide an image of picking an apple from a tree, bringing the apple down, and putting it into a basket. The visual image is preferable. If the new movement skill is similar to a previously learned skill, the instructor can provide that link for learners.

Verbal labels can also improve meaningfulness. Research indicates that learners can remember the end location of movements and the distance of movements. A verbal label for the end locations of movements, such as the position of the golf club driver at backswing, can be used to improve the memory of the swing. The moonwalk can help learners remember that the knee is straight when the leg begins to slide backward. Verbal labels for movements that match something well known are also effective, such as *Move your arm to the 2 o'clock position.*

Winther and Thomas (1981) and Weiss (1983) showed that children as young as five years old can benefit from labels. Magill (2017) offered four reasons images and verbal labels are effective: they reduce the complexity of verbal instructions needed to describe all movements, make an abstract movement more concrete, focus on the intended outcome of the movements rather than the movements themselves, and help in movement planning by using memories of previously learned movements.

Most children begin to use deliberate rehearsal strategies between five and seven years of age; over the childhood and early adolescent years, they become more efficient and intentional in their use (Ornstein & Naus, 1978). The conscious rehearsal of movements is also developmental (Reid, 1980a; Sugden, 1978).

RESEARCH NOTES

Rehearsal of Movements by Children

Gallagher and Thomas (1984) used four participant age groups (approximate ages were 5, 7, 11, and 19) in a study of movement rehearsal. The experimenters compared three rehearsal conditions: mature, childlike, and self-determined. The participants were required to grasp a handle that supported an arm and to move the handle in different angle and distance combinations. Specifically, the angles were parallel, 15 degrees, and 30 degrees, and the distances were 4 to 16 inches (10 to 45 cm). The distances and angles were determined by the experimenters. This is an example of a positioning task, which was typical of much of the research in that era. Essentially, participants made an initial movement that was constrained by the experimenter, remained at the end location, and then returned to the starting point and independently moved the handle to the end location once again. In other words, they tried to remember the first movement and then to reproduce it in the recall trial. The distance from the end location on the recall trial is considered the amount of error in such motor memory studies.

Gallagher and Thomas' participants were presented with a series of eight movements to recall, but in any order they chose. The childlike rehearsal condition, considered passive, involved remaining at each of the eight movements for eight seconds. The mature, or adultlike, condition was more active; participants remained at the first movement end location for eight seconds. At the end of the second movement, they remained for three seconds, but then moved to the first end location for three seconds followed by the second location for an additional two seconds. Subsequent new movements were rehearsed for two seconds and the previous two movements for two seconds each, followed by two seconds at the new movement. Thus, rehearsal was more active than in the passive childlike condition, but rehearsal time was a constant eight seconds. The self-determined condition had participants move to the end point of a movement for two seconds and allowed them to use the remaining six seconds any way they wished. The results showed that the youngest children remembered the eight movements as well as the 7- and 11-year-old children did when forced to rehearse like adults. In addition, participants using the mature strategy tended to recall movements from short to long, whereas those in the childlike rehearsal group were more likely to recall in random order. Thus, imposing an organizational strategy was effective. Overall, active rehearsal was shown to be important in the recall of movements.

Exercise 11.6

What role does memory play in learning movements? How can you help students remember movements?

Young children often do not spontaneously rehearse, but when they are instructed to use a memory strategy, performance usually improves. When presented with a sequence of movements to remember, five- and seven-year-olds who were taught to rehearse a subset of the movements (rather than perform instance-by-instance practicing) improved compared to those not receiving instruction (Gallagher & Thomas, 1984).

Lui and Jensen (2011) had 5- to 7-year-olds and 8- to 10-year-olds cycle on a stationery ergometer at three cadences (60, 80, 100 rpms). They were told they had to reach a particular cadence during practice trials. After practice they were told to reproduce each cadence and then asked how they remembered. The older children were superior to the younger children in terms of pedaling at the three cadences, and they used more strategies to remember. In a second experiment, the children with the most errors were assigned to either an experimental or control group. The experimental group was instructed to count with a metronome beat while pedaling. This strategy resulted in more accuracy recalling cadences than that exhibited in the control group. Memory strategy instruction is also effective for those with intellectual disabilities (Reid, 1980b) and learning problems (Hoover & Wade, 1985).

Another way to help memory for movements is to tell learners explicitly that they will be required to remember (e.g., *We will use this sliding action in the folk dance we will learn tomorrow*). Although incidental memory, or nonintentional recall, occurs, knowing that a test of memory will happen later often promotes the use of personal intentional memory strategies. Memory can also be enhanced by allowing participants to develop subjective organization. This is particularly useful in remembering a series of movements in sequence, such as dance steps or gymnastics moves. When faced with a sequence, novices are likely to view the sequence as a long list of individual movements (Magill, 2017). If there are 20 movements, the novice becomes overwhelmed. With practice, two or three separate movements might become organized into one, thus reducing the number of movements to remember from 20 to 7 or even fewer. Because experts might view the sequence of 20 in parts, it is no wonder they can remember the list more easily than novices can. Their knowledge of dance makes it easier because they really have less to remember. In a study by Starkes, Deakin, Lindley, and Crisp (1987), expert dancers recalled the eight steps of the sequence almost perfectly, whereas novices recalled about half correctly. And as in the chess study by Chase and Simon (1973), when the dance sequences did not conform to typical and expected dance sequences, the experts were no better able to recall the sequences than the novices were.

Sport Expertise

The study of sport expertise provides important insights into the nature of differences in sport participants but less information about how expertise is developed. **Expert performance** in sport has been defined as "consistent superior athletic performance over an extended period" (Starkes, 1993, as cited by Janelle & Hillman, 2003, p. 21). Janelle and Hillman suggested that experts are distinguished by excellence in four domains: physiological, technical, cognitive, and emotional and psychological (see table 11.3).

One of the factors that lead to expert performance is (quite unsurprisingly) practice. It is often noted that expertise requires 10-plus years and 10,000-plus hours of practice, although in sport this may be 3,000 to 4,000 hours (Côté, Lidor, & Hackfort, 2009). Moreover, there is greater variability across domains of expertise than captured by the simple 10,000 hours in 10 years (Ericsson, 2013). But, as we will see in chapter 14, this is not just a matter of practice itself, but of something called deliberate practice.

We mention sport expertise in this chapter on functional constraints because children and adolescents come to a learning or practice context with varying levels of skill, as well as declarative, procedural, and metacognitive knowledge. Simple observation of any physical education class attests to the existence of a wide

Table 11.3 Sport Expertise

Domain	Distinguishing features of the expert
Physiological	Exhibits appropriate anaerobic power and aerobic capacity, muscle fiber type, body morphology and body segment size, height, and flexibility; requirements are unique to each sport.
Technical	Exhibits sensorimotor coordination for refined, efficient, and effective patterns of movement, and has artistic and aesthetic values as required for the specific activity; movement becomes automatic after years of extended and deliberate practice.
Cognitive	Has an extensive base of knowledge to do such things as recognize structured game situations and match appropriate strategies and tactics to game situations; extracts the most relevant cues in the sport environment; avoids distracting cues; uses effective visual search strategies and signal detection; can make fast decisions.
Emotional and psychological	Is able to regulate emotions and anxiety as well as motivation regulation; sets realistic goals; maintains confidence and positive attitude; uses effective imagery and mental training; can self-regulate; uses metacognitive strategies.

Data from Janelle and Hillman 2003.

WHAT DO YOU THINK?

Exercise 11.7

As a physical education teacher, you may not have the time or resources to assist every student in becoming an expert. However, you can place your students on the path to expertise. Make a list of external factors that can contribute to expertise, and provide strategies you can implement.

External factor	Strategy
Deliberate practice	Provide social support and feedback. Provide many opportunities to practice skills of choice.

range of skill. Some of the youngsters, particularly adolescents, may be more skilled in a particular sport than the instructor because they have spent many hours practicing the sport skills. They might not be experts in the same way as professional athletes or Olympians, but they are highly skilled compared to their age peers and are sometimes referred to as experts in research studies.

Summary

This chapter outlined several functional constraints related to thinking and learning that help define a person at one point in time. Learners have different abilities in cognition, knowledge, personal skills, attention, and memory that affect them in motor learning and performance situations. Being familiar with these constraints can help anyone interested in understanding the individual differences in a class of children or adolescents. Age peers vary widely in both cognition and knowledge. Some young people have acquired a number of intentional memory strategies, and some have not. Experiences in a given domain or sport vary enormously, as the sport expertise literature demonstrates. Constraints in attention are also influential. To complicate matters even further, the functional constraints described in this chapter change over developmental time within an individual during the stages of development outlined.

Children are rather immature learners compared to adults. As children develop, their knowledge base increases; attention to relevant cues becomes more precise; skills become more automatized; decisions are made more quickly; and learning is more strategic and intentional. Thus, the wide individual differences noted by most instructors in a class of 30 students results from the structural constraints discussed in chapter 9 as well as from functional constraints that change over developmental time (e.g., cognition) or learning time (e.g., skill as a function of practice). The diversity of the recreation class of 12-year-olds described at the beginning of this chapter can now be understood in a new light. They may differ on many factors that influence their skill, enjoyment, and attention.

ONLINE LEARNING

Visit the web resource at www.HumanKinetics.com/MotorLearningAndDevelopment for an accompanying lab activity and exercises from the chapter.

LEARNING AIDS

Supplemental Activities

1. Arrange an interview with an accomplished occupational, physical, or athletic therapist. Ask this person to reflect on declarative knowledge, procedural knowledge, metacognitive skills, and metacognitive knowledge. Your interviewee might not use the terms per se, but can he or she see his or her daily work reflected in this conceptualization of knowledge? Do some areas of his or her work not fit into the knowledge perspective?

2. There are many popular books on memory and how to improve it. Find one and see what it suggests. Are some of the recommended strategies consistent with the contents of this chapter? Are some different?

Glossary

concrete operational stage—Piaget's third stage (ages 7-11) of intellectual development in which children develop logical thinking that is restricted to events or things experienced, seen, or heard.

conservation of liquids—Piaget's experiment demonstrating that, unlike that of adults, children's logic is based on one dimension.

cooperative play—Play in which children strive to achieve the same goal.

declarative knowledge—Factual and conceptual information about knowledge stored in memory.

episodic memory—Memories that are associated with personal experiences and are related to a specific period in time; the ability to remember personal events.

expert performance—Superior athletic performance over an extended period.

formal operational stage—Piaget's fourth stage (age 11+) of intellectual development, in which children develop logical thinking.

game experience—Knowing about a sport (i.e., declarative knowledge) without necessarily knowing how to perform the sport (i.e., procedural knowledge).

knowing—A person's base of knowledge.

knowing about knowing—Knowledge of how personal memory functions; also known as metamemory or metacognition.

knowing how to know—The use of control processes and strategies for deliberate learning.

meaningfulness—The degree to which a new movement relates to previous movements or knowledge.

memory—The ability to recall things from experience.

metacognitive knowledge—A higher level of declarative knowledge that includes an awareness of owns own strengths and weaknesses.

metacognitive skill—A higher level of procedural knowledge that is particularly important in selecting and planning goal-directed learning.

parallel play—Playing alongside peers but not really interacting.

preoperational stage—Piaget's second stage (ages 2-7) of intellectual development, which is characterized by symbolic but egocentric thinking.

procedural knowledge—Knowledge of how to do something; this type of knowledge underlies an action and includes anticipation and prediction, decision-making, and response selection aspects of information processing.

schemes—Structures developed by children for thoughts and action resulting from actively constructing understandings of the world based on their experience.

semantic memory—The ability to remember general knowledge built from life experiences and learning.

sensorimotor period—Piaget's first stage (ages 0-2) of intellectual development, in which children coordinate sensory experience and movement to act on the world and generate knowledge.

simple reaction time—The time to react on a task with only one stimulus.

skill—A learned ability to bring about predetermined results with maximal certainty, often with a minimal outlay of time, energy, or both.

subjective organization—The arrangement of information into memorable parts.

verbal labels—Words used to describe a part of a skill to improve memory.

visual imagery—Images stimulated by memory.

PSYCHOSOCIAL AND SOCIAL–AFFECTIVE DEVELOPMENT

Chapter Objectives

After reading this chapter, you should be able to do the following:

- Discuss the developmental changes in Erikson's stages of psychosocial development.
- Discuss Harter's view of development in the context of how people view themselves.
- Discuss the development of motor competence, perceived motor competence, health-related fitness, and physical activity, and how they interact.
- Explain how self-efficacy develops and how professionals can promote it.
- Describe self-determined motivation and explain how it develops.
- Discuss the relationship between emotional development and physical activity.
- Describe self-regulation and its relationship to physical activity.

It's Not All About Size

Rodney is a 270-pound (122 kg) defensive lineman who plays on a university American football team and possesses speed and agility. He is a starting player in every game and even makes an occasional tackle. His teammate Martin also plays on the line, but is 40 pounds (18 kg) lighter than Rodney and not as quick. Yet, Martin plays effectively against bigger men and makes more tackles than Rodney does, and with fewer penalties. Martin also seems to make more critical plays, leads the team with tackles, and is usually in the discussion for the defensive player of the game award. Quite simply, the smaller Martin outperforms the larger Rodney. What is happening? It is often said that Martin is always the first at practice and the last to leave. Martin is also driven, is confident of his abilities, and monitors his performances. Perhaps these attributes make up for his lack of size.

Participating in a sport is certainly influenced by structure (chapter 9) and functional constraints such as cognition, knowledge, attention, and memory (chapter 11). However, it is also influenced by how people view themselves, how competent they perceive themselves to be as athletes, the extent of their motivation to become better players, their awareness of emotional factors in this quest, and their ability to regulate much of their learning. These thoughts and feelings are largely shaped by psychological factors such as motivation, which have strong social and emotional influences and developmental roots that go back to very early ages. These powerful forces and experiences influenced Martin's approach and focus on football. This chapter is an extension of the discussion of cognitive development in chapter 11; it outlines psychosocial and social–affective functional constraints such as self-esteem, competence motivation, self-efficacy, self-determination, arousal, anxiety, and self-regulation.

Psychosocial Constraints

How we come to view ourselves is largely affected by our social experiences. We live in a social world from birth. Our initial interactions with our immediate caregivers are followed by interactions with extended family members, friends of our parents, and eventually our own friends and schoolmates. The increasingly extensive social networks influence our uniqueness, our sense of self, and how well we manage in the world. To explore these psychosocial factors more completely, we look at the development of psychosocial conflict as conceptualized by Erikson, self-perception and competence according to Harter, self-efficacy viewed by Bandura, and self-determination motivation as described by Deci, Ryan, and Vallerand.

Erikson's Psychosocial Development Theory: Childhood and Adolescent Stages

Erik Erikson was born in 1902 out of wedlock and was abandoned by his father at birth. He became an artist, teacher, and psychoanalyst, but eventually fled Europe for the United States when the Nazis gained power. He received an appointment at Harvard Medical School and went on to practice childhood psychoanalysis in Boston. Although he had studied Freudian psychoanalysis, he was also greatly influenced by work with Native American communities in South Dakota and California, civil rights groups, and combat soldiers (Crain, 1985; Shaffer, 1999). His views of psychosocial development became more social and more culturally influenced than Freud's. Erikson also stressed that children are active explorers of their world rather than simply passive reactors to biological urges; his research and experience culminated in 1950 with the first edition of his classic text *Childhood and Society*.

Erikson adopted a life span perspective in his work, which was unusual for the mid-20th century; his eight life stages extended into adulthood and old age. Each stage was viewed from the standpoint of a psychosocial crisis or conflict that had to be resolved to move to the next stage. This chapter addresses the first five stages; chapter 13, on psychosocial and cognitive constraints in adults, addresses the last three stages. Erikson (1963) described the stages very well and influenced thinking about social and emotional development as well as **self-esteem**. However, he has been criticized for not explaining the experiences that might resolve the conflicts and promote development (Shaffer, 1999). The first five stages of Erikson's psychosocial development theory are described as follows:

• *Basic trust versus mistrust (birth to 1 year)*. Basic trust in infants emerges from interactions with primary caregivers. Infants of parents who attend to feeding, cleaning, and comforting them learn to expect consistency and predictability in the world. The reliability and sameness of parent action produce a feeling of trust. Erikson (1963) claimed that "the infant's first social achievement . . . is his willingness to let the mother out of sight without undue anxiety or rage, because she has an inner certainty as well as outer predictability" (p. 247). An unreliable parent fosters a general sense of mistrust. However, some experience with mistrust actually strengthens the understanding of trust. This is because babies must also learn to trust themselves. Erikson suggested that babies may have an urge to bite while teething, but a grasp of the nipple rather than a bite is a sign of their trustworthiness. As they develop a sense of being trustworthy, infants form a sense of "being 'all right,' of being oneself" (p. 249). The social impact of self-concept begins very early in life.

- *Autonomy versus shame and doubt (1-3 years)*. The basic conflict in this stage is to become autonomous in action but within social regulations. Children from 1 to 3 years of age learn to stand on their own two feet (literally and figuratively), dress and feed themselves, and express their needs and wants with language. Their explorations of the world and growing independence are sources of cognitive development (see the discussion of Piaget in chapter 11) and also of awareness of social and cultural expectations. A 12-month-old will make a mess as she tries to feed herself, and parents are likely to accept messiness as part of the process of gaining autonomy. At age 3, however, parents are likely to insist on some degree of tidiness during eating; this is an early social regulation that is imposed on the child. Social expectations should not be acquired through shame and doubt. Shame is the conscious feeling that one is exposed and does not look good to others, and doubt refers to a sense of loss of personal control. Parents are primary social agents who attempt to carefully guide the learning of social behaviors without promoting lasting shame and doubt. They realize that "from a sense of self-control without loss of self-esteem comes a lasting sense of good will and pride" (Erikson, 1963, p. 254).

- *Initiative versus guilt (3-6 years)*. At age 3, enjoyment of new physical and mental powers propels the child to action. Behaviors can be goal directed and very imagina-

tive. As the child makes plans and tries to realize them, some plans come into conflict with others because the consequences of the actions are often unknown to the child and certainly not considered. There might be physically aggressive acts toward siblings or parents, as well as infantile jealousy and rivalry for parental attention. This may produce guilt. In other cases, the initial plan is beyond the child's capacities, and his autonomy is challenged by failure. As in the previous stage, the child must learn social regulations but now is ready, with the assistance of parents and siblings, to accept these as internal guides through self-observation, self-control, and self-punishment.

- *Industry versus inferiority (6-12 years)*. This stage occurs in the elementary school years when teachers and peers become important social agents. Children learn to win recognition by producing things in the wider culture of school. The need to produce mobilizes them beyond play to acquire cognitive skills such as reading and writing, as well as social skills appropriate to the culture. They learn to cooperate with others to achieve shared goals. Although Erikson did not mention physical skills, fundamental motor skills and game performance are valued in Western cultures and are sources of self-assuredness. In school, children are in a position to compare themselves to peers as never before. The danger is that a feeling of inferiority may result such that the child "considers himself doomed to mediocrity or inadequacy" (Erikson, 1963, p. 260). Teachers and coaches can contribute to resolving this conflict by truly valuing all students, encouraging a focus on personal improvement rather than comparison to others, and counseling those who are struggling to find niches of skilled performance.

- *Identity versus role confusion (12-20 years)*. This stage of adolescence is characterized largely by a new search for ego identity (Who am I?) in the social world (Erikson, 1963; Shaffer, 1999). The crisis that must be resolved is role identity versus role confusion. This conflict occurs in the context of a rapidly changing body and sexual awakening. Erikson contended that adolescents seek a new sense of continuity and sameness related primarily to social and occupational identities. Peer influence is significant, and teenagers worry about meeting others' expectations and the career roles they will assume as adults. Their ego identity is a social matter as they wonder about how others perceive them and about their social role in a larger social world. The conflict of Who am I? is resolved in part by identifying with others who appeal to them, celebrating personal accomplishments, and engaging in the sometimes challenging acceptance of their uniqueness in terms of strengths and weaknesses.

A number of themes are apparent in Erikson's (1963) model of psychosocial development: trust, competency, autonomy, self-concept, self-control, and social regulation. Although Erikson quite appropriately underscored the conflict in adolescence of self-identity, the development of a sense of self actually begins much earlier and is explained more completely by Harter's (1999) descriptions of change in self-representation during childhood and adolescence.

Harter's Self-Representation Stages

Harter (1999) viewed the development of self as a cognitive and social process that is thus influenced by the interaction of our own thinking about and evaluation of ourselves and feedback from caregivers, siblings, peers, teachers, and coaches. Harter acknowledged distinctions between self-descriptions (what I am) and self-evaluations (how good I am) but contended that most research deals with self-evaluations. The more common terms for self-evaluation are *self-esteem* and *self-worth* (Harter, 1999; Shaffer, 1999). Harter's six descriptive periods are very early childhood, early to middle childhood, middle to late childhood, early adolescence, middle adolescence, and late adolescence.

1. *Very young children* focus on the physical aspects of self, such as the color of their hair. They know their favorite foods and the color of their house. They are likely to view themselves, for example, as good jumpers or runners, but they do not generalize this to viewing themselves as good athletes or good at sports. They do not have a judgment of overall self-esteem and do not differentiate competence domains such as academic, social, and physical appearance. When they are aware of specific behaviors (e.g., jumping or speaking), they are usually unrealistically positive about themselves.

2. As they enter school in *early childhood*, children continue to overestimate their abilities and remain positive about themselves (LeGear et al., 2012), in part because they are not comparing themselves with others. They do not distinguish between ability and effort (e.g., *If I am working hard, I must be a good swimmer*). During this period they do become aware that others are evaluating them and that some can perform better than others can. Also, they can be good in several domains and are capable of personal comparisons over time; for example, they might think, *Last year I couldn't swim the length of the pool, but now I can.*

3. As children move toward *later childhood*, they are able to differentiate between additional competence domains such as academic, athletic, social, physical appearance, and behavior. With the aid of language and increased cognitive functioning, they are now aware of social comparisons as they interact with others in school and sport environments. They know others have an opinion of them, which influences their self-esteem (e.g., *I like myself because my parents and other kids like me*). They understand competence within domains;

Guess the Age Period

Exercise 12.1

Age is not always a perfect predictor of behavior or thinking. However, let's play a game about the self-representation age periods. Pair up with a classmate; both of you should have access to the descriptions of Harter's six stages of self-representation. One person makes a self-statement that represents one of the time periods. The other person has to determine which age period is represented by the statement. The two can debate the answer because a single statement might be argued to fall into two or more age periods. Try three statements each.

that is, they can be a good swimmer but a poor baseball player. At this point children have a more balanced and accurate view of themselves. A global evaluation of self-esteem begins to emerge (e.g., *Overall, I am a talented person*).

4. In *early adolescence*, domains of self continue to expand and include competence with romantic partners and close friends and in work. Children in this period become concerned about how others view them. They may have multiple selves; for example, "cheerful and rowdy with friends, depressed and sarcastic with parents" (Harter, 1999, p. 62). However, they do not give these seemingly inconsistent descriptions of the self much thought. In addition, they are very sensitive to the opinions and standards of people in different contexts.

5. *Middle adolescents* make even finer discriminations that now include self with close friends, self with a group of friends, and self with mother versus self with father. They continue to realize that their behavior and feelings can be quite different with each group (e.g., tolerant with friends but depressed with parents). A sport example is increased self-awareness of competence in basketball that suggests being outstanding in dribbling and shooting, but average in passing and decision making. Adolescents at this stage remain greatly occupied by what others, particularly peers, think of them. Some may believe that they will not be popular if they are too studious. As in Erikson's identity and role confusion stage, adolescents struggle with different levels of self-worth in different domains, potential conflict and confusion from perceptions of self versus others, and discrepancies between real and ideal self-concepts.

6. Finally, *late adolescence* is characterized by a clearer sense of direction as personal beliefs, values, and standards are internalized. Older adolescents better understand their strengths, weaknesses, and potential and are less influenced by the opinions of others. They may realize that they are ethical, desire independence, and are generally optimistic. Some conflict with parents may remain if parents' expectations and future hopes conflict with their own. Self-knowledge becomes internally rather than externally driven.

Competence Motivation

The development of self-representation deals with emerging self-esteem and related competence in various domains. The young toddler demonstrates an intrinsic interest in mastery of his world by spending hours playing with blocks, stacking them, lining them up, or placing them into and taking them out of a container. As success is achieved, feelings of competence and control develop. Harter (1978) formalized these observations into a model of competence motivation. Recent research has demonstrated that perceptions of motor competence are important in physical activity involvement (Babic, Morgan, Plotnikoff, Lonsdale, White, & Lubans, 2014; Bai, Chen, Vazou, Welk, & Schaben, 2015; Seabra et al., 2012), leisure participation in adolescence (Leversen, Danielsen, Wold, & Samdal, 2012), and enjoyment of physical education (Cairney, Kwan, Velduizen, Bray, & Faught, 2012); it is also one of the reasons children participate in sport (Bailey, Cope, & Pearce, 2013).

Competence motivation represents the fundamental desire of humans to be competent. This desire leads to participation in a domain (e.g., physical activities or a specific sport); such participation is referred to more formally as mastery attempts. Optimal challenges should exist; those that are difficult but realistic with respect to improvement with practice are preferred over those that are too hard or too easy. People very low in competence motivation may choose not to be involved (i.e., make no attempts at mastery), and they will remain inactive. Low perceived competence is related to reasons children drop out of sport programs (Balish, McLaren, Rainham, & Blanchard, 2014). If a person is successful in an attempt at mastery, an increase in perceptions of competence and control should result, as well as an increase in positive affect such as pride and happiness. When significant others such as parents and peers approve of and reinforce such mastery attempts, perceptions of competence and control are enhanced as well. One of the consequences of heightened self-perceptions is the seeking of further mastery attempts with effort and persistence (e.g., *If I believe I am improving in an activity valued by Mom,*

Dad, and myself, I will tend to practice more with considerable enjoyment and persist in achieving my goals in the face of a setback).

Weiss and Williams (2004) offered an overview of some of the critical developmental changes related to competence motivation. Competence domains are increasingly differentiated as children develop, which is consistent with the changes in self-representation discussed earlier. Toddlers have no sense of general self-esteem, but they can recognize skill in specific activities (e.g., *I am a good jumper).* School-aged children are aware of competence in social, academic, and athletic domains and begin to view themselves with a general sense of self-esteem. Older adolescents add domains such as romantic involvement and employment to those recognized at younger ages.

Developmental changes in perceived competence are also affected by the level and accuracy of perceived competence as well as information sources used to judge competence (Weiss & Williams, 2004). Level and accuracy of perceived competence relate to whether perceptions are high or low (level) and the relationship between perceived and actual competence (accuracy). Preschool-aged children are notoriously inaccurate in their perceptions of competence, but they become more realistic by 10 to 12 years of age. By ages 4 through 8, youngsters' perceived skill competence may reflect actual competence (Barnett, Ridgers, & Salmon, 2015).

Perceived competence in academic areas generally increases with age, but research is equivocal with respect to perceived motor competence; some studies show a positive increase with age and others a decline, and some demonstrate stability over childhood and adolescence. Among the reasons offered by Weiss and Williams (2004) for these contradictions are the public nature of physical performance and the unusual transition pattern through sport levels. Unlike most academic performances, physical skills can be viewed by anyone. As one practices in the gymnasium, performance is a public exercise.

Moving through academic levels is standardized for all ages (e.g., middle school to high school). Transition through sport levels, however, depends largely on skill as well as a willingness to devote more time to the activity. Three 11-year-old boys may be playing at three different levels of soccer (e.g., recreation, select, travel). Thus, their comparison groups are very different, and this may influence perceived competence.

Developmental changes in perceived competence may also be due to changes in information sources used to judge competence. Information sources include parent feedback, coach evaluation, peer comparison and evaluation, spectator feedback, performance statistics, and skill improvement (Weiss & Williams, 2004). Children under 10 years of age tend to rely on their parents, game outcomes, and spectator feedback. Even among 10- and 11-year-olds, parental encouragement and modeling have been shown to have a positive impact on physical activity and perceived competence (Maatta, Ray, & Roos, 2014). Ten- to 15-year-olds pay more attention to comparisons with peers and coach feedback than younger athletes do (Weiss & Williams, 2004). Older adolescents (aged 16-18) report greater use of self-referenced information such as skill improvement and attraction to the sport than younger adolescents do. This is consistent with the development of self-representation

---

RESEARCH NOTES

Information Sources for Perceived Competence Change With Age

McKiddie and Maynard (1997) conducted a study that showed an increase in the accuracy of perceived motor competence and changes in social information sources over age. They had 80 males and 80 females from two age groups (11-12 and 14-15) fill out two forms. The first, the Athletic and General Competence subscales from Harter's Self-Perception Profile for Children (Harter, 1985), measured motor competence in physical education classes. The second was the Sport Competence Information Scale (from Horn & Hasbrook, 1986), which determines sources of information young people use in arriving at a sense of motor competence. In addition, the actual motor competence of the 160 participants was measured with a rating scale completed by the physical education teachers. The first purpose of the study was to determine age differences in the accuracy of judgments of physical competence. The correlation between perceived and actual competence was .22 and .88 for the children and adolescents, respectively. This indicates that the perceived motor competence of the younger children was not closely related to actual competence, whereas the adolescents were quite accurate about their motor competence as rated by their teachers.

The second purpose of the study was to determine developmental changes in social sources of information about motor competence. The information scale measured sources such as peer comments, comparisons to classmates, teacher evaluations, parent judgment and feedback, attraction to physical education, and enjoyment of sport. The findings showed that the 11- and 12-year-olds used feedback from important adults and their attraction to sport to arrive at a level of perceived motor competence, whereas the adolescents relied more on peer comparisons and peer evaluations. Thus, developmental changes in information sources of perceived motor competence are evident.

discussed earlier, as well as Harter's (1978) assertion that self-regulation (self-judgment, self-goals, self-reinforcement) develops over time when parents and coaches encourage mastery performance and independence in learning.

Motor Competence

Perceived motor competence and actual motor competence became important parts of a developmental model to describe the relationship of motor skill competence to physical activity and health (Stodden et al., 2008). It has been known for many years that regular physical activity is positively linked to health-related benefits including reduced body weight and obesity. Stodden and colleagues proposed that being physically skilled should lead to more frequent physical activity, but the relationship between motor competence and physical activity may change over developmental time. They argued that the contribution of physical skill to physical activity and health had not received the emphasis warranted. Much has been learned about how to measure physical activity and its relationship to health, but with little focus on the impact of good or poor performance on physical activity. Recall that skillfulness was the top of the mountain of motor development described in chapter 4.

Stodden and colleagues (2008) proposed four interacting factors: motor competence, perceived motor competence, health-related fitness, and physical activity. They suggested that the relationship between motor competence and physical activity strengthens over developmental time. In early childhood (ages 2-5), physical activity influences motor competence. Parents, available environments, and socioeconomic status promote physical activity, which should lead to the acquisition of fundamental motor skills and other motor skills important in a culture (e.g., swimming). However, because physical activity is so strongly influenced by parents at this age, motor competence and physical activity are only weakly related. In middle childhood (ages 6-9) and later childhood

(ages 10-13), physical activity and motor competence should become more strongly related because those with moderate or greater skill are more able to participate in physical activities, games, dance, and sport. Those who are less able in motor competence engage in less physical activity. By late elementary or middle school ages (ages 12-15), motor skill competence drives physical activity levels.

Young children may perceive themselves to be quite competent if they are actively engaged and expending effort (Harter, 1999). They do not judge themselves accurately or in comparison to others. Thus, in early childhood the relationship between actual motor competence and perceived motor competence is quite low (Stodden et al., 2008). During middle childhood, opportunities for social comparison and cognitive growth have increased, resulting in more accurate comparisons to peers. At this point, perceived motor competence is more closely related to actual motor competence. Stodden and colleagues (2008) predicted that less skilled youngsters will become less active as they view activities as difficult. They begin to opt out of physical activity because it is not enjoyable. This is termed a negative spiral of disengagement, which even further reduces motor competence, perceived competence, and physical activity. In contrast, skilled youngsters become more active during middle childhood because they experience fun and rewards from participating; this is termed a positive spiral of engagement. More activity across the elementary school years should augment motor competence, perceived competence, and physical activity.

Physical fitness should be fostered in early childhood with the practice of fundamental motor skills (Stodden et al., 2008). The spirals of engagement or disengagement (positively or negatively) affect physical fitness from middle childhood through adolescence. Quite simply, those who are more physically skilled are more physically active and thus able to realize greater health-related fitness. Also, children who are more physically fit are able to engage in physical activity for longer periods of time and thus continue to progress in the development of movement skills. For those with lower levels of physical skills, lower levels of physical fitness are predicted. These children and youth have difficulty persisting in physical activities, which limits their gains in motor competence.

Obesity is both a product of Stodden and colleagues' (2008) four factors interacting and a mediating variable. Obesity is predicted as a result of the spiral of disengagement and associated low levels of physical and perceived motor competence that result in reduced physical activity levels and health-related fitness. But obesity is also a mediating variable because heavier children have difficulty performing motor skills, are less likely to be physically active, and experience less success when they attempt physical activities.

The postulates of Stodden and colleagues (2008) place new emphasis on the role of motor competence in perceived motor competence, physical activity, physical fitness, and obesity, which is a major health issue across the world. Learning motor skills during the developmental years is a good thing! Much research has been generated on issues related to the four factors, how they interact over developmental time, and their predictions regarding health (e.g., Barnett, Ridgers, & Salmon, 2015; Holfelder & Schott, 2014; Lloyd, Saunders, Bremer, & Tremblay, 2014; Lubans, Morgan, Cliff, Barnett, & Okely, 2010; Robinson, 2010; Stodden, Gao, Goodway, & Langendorfer, 2014). Although more research is needed, considerable support currently exists for the model and its predictions regarding the importance of skillfulness in promoting physically active lifestyles (Robinson et al., 2015).

Self-Efficacy

Bandura (1997) defined perceived **self-efficacy** as "beliefs in one's capabilities to organize and execute the courses of action required to produce given attainments" (p. 3). It is a belief that you can accomplish a specific task. Can you jump over that high jump pole at 6 feet (1.8 m)? Self-efficacy beliefs (*I can high jump 6 ft [1.8 m]*) are more specific than perceived competence beliefs (*In general, I am good at track and field compared to my peers*) and can be distinguished from each other by adults (Rodgers, Markland, Selzler, Murray, & Wilson, 2014). Bandura argued that there is little incentive to engage in an activity without the belief that you can achieve desired outcomes. Children with higher self-efficacy do seem to participate more in physical activity than those with lower self-efficacy (Chase, 2001). When self-efficacy is defined as confidence in the ability to be physically active in specific situations, it becomes the most consistently identified psychosocial determinate of physical activity in children, adolescents, and adults (Bauman, Reis, Sallis, Wells, Loos, & Martin, 2012). It is good to believe you can accomplish a task. One of the authors of this text admits that a 6-foot (1.8 m) jump is beyond his capabilities, and this lack of self-efficacy is motivation to remain on the couch rather than to jump.

Infants have little sense of who they are and must learn that their actions have consequences. Piaget's position (discussed in chapter 11) was that in the first four months of life infants begin to recognize that they are controlling the hands in front of their eyes. A few months later, these same hands can grasp and throw. The sense of self continues to improve as children understand language and realize that others refer to them by a specific name. From ages 8 to 14, there may be a decline in their perception of their capabilities in sport and physical education as they become more accurate in their perceptions (Chase, 2001). As children age, parents and family members, followed by peers and then school activities, have major impacts on their sense of personal capabilities. Bandura listed four sources of self-efficacy: past mastery experiences (successful actions, which increase self-efficacy), vicarious experiences (viewing others and comparing oneself to them, which may enhance or diminish self-efficacy), verbal persuasion (having others express faith in one's abilities), and physiological and affective states (personal judgments of arousal, fatigue, and mood states).

Much of the research on self-efficacy and movement behavior has occurred in the sport domain. Feltz, Short, and Sullivan (2008) provided practitioners with five techniques to increase self-efficacy in young novice athletes (see table 12.1). This reference also provides additional ideas for more advanced athletes and teams.

Self-Determined Motivation

Motivation to learn and participate in physical activity is obviously important. It influences whether people even begin an activity and how long they persist. As noted in the discussion of competence motivation, preschoolers and young children engage in play seemingly for no other reason than the sheer joy of participating. The two-year-old may play with pots and pans for hours, stacking, banging, and rearranging. Piaget's theory would argue that the children are learning important cause-and-effect relationships, linking language to actions, and creating and refining action schemes of exploring objects with the hands or the perceptual schemes of circles and rectangles. Harter (1978) suggested that they are motivated to have an effect on their environment and develop perceptions of competence. Actual competence was critical in Stodden and colleagues' (2008) model discussed previously. The notion of competence was also central to the thinking of Deci and colleagues (Deci & Flaste, 1995; Deci & Ryan, 1985; Ryan & Deci, 2000), who were fascinated with such behavior of young children and proposed self-determination theory as an explanation. The theory has been expanded as a hierarchical model of intrinsic and extrinsic motivation by Vallerand (1997, 2007).

Self-determination theory includes three types of motivation:

- **Intrinsically motivated behaviors** provide pleasure and satisfaction from participating, in the absence of

WHAT DO YOU THINK?

Exercise 12.2

How can you assist students in developing self-esteem, self-efficacy, and perceived competence?

Table 12.1 Promoting Self-Efficacy in Novice Athletes

Technique	Description
Instructional strategies and performance aids	Break down skills, modify equipment, use physical guidance and performance aids to ensure some initial success. Gradually remove aids so that learners take some ownership for success.
Feedback	Give feedback based on personal skill acquisition, not in comparison to others. Provide realistic verbal persuasion about ability.
Modeling	Use peer models to convey skill, attitudes, and behaviors (see chapter 15).
Imagery	Encourage imaging or rehearsing successful performance once learners have developed the concept of the movement.
Goal setting	Establish specific, measurable, and realistic goals. This provides objective evidence of increased competence on a specific task (see chapter 15).

Based on Feltz, Short, and Sullivan 2008.

material rewards or constraints. A long-distance runner who enjoys the peace and tranquility of the outdoors is intrinsically motivated.

- **Extrinsically motivated behaviors** provide a means to an end and are not engaged in for their own sake. Extrinsic motivation explains a host of behaviors, from completing additional fitness workouts to make a team, remaining on the job after 5 p.m. to impress a boss, or engaging in rehabilitation exercises to please a partner. If the behavior is extrinsic but valued by the person and outcomes are viewed as positive, it is referred to as **self-determined extrinsic motivation**. If the behavior is based on avoiding negative consequences, it is called **non-self-determined extrinsic motivation**.

- **Amotivation** is present when people do not see any relationship between outcomes and actions. In other words, people feel that whatever they do, nothing positive will result, so why should they bother? We certainly do not want children or adolescents to be amotivated toward physical activity.

Self-determination theory postulates that humans have basic needs to feel **competent**, **autonomous**, and **related** (that is, connected with other people). When these needs are met, psychological health is promoted, but when they are not met, psychological health is undermined (Vallerand, 2007). People engage in activities to satisfy needs. For example, children who spend hours in free play do it of their own accord (autonomy); they gradually become more skilled at tasks (competent) and particularly enjoy the time when parents join in (relatedness). To the extent that play satisfies these three needs, it is considered intrinsically motivated behavior. Maintaining a learning environment that emphasizes play and fun will likely keep children motivated to participate and to learn new skills. On the other hand, consider a child who begins snow skiing because he is told he must (i.e., no autonomy), whose initial attempts result in frequent falls and embarrassment (i.e., no competence), and who sees no one in the future with whom to ski (i.e., no relatedness). Without some intervention in the form of excellent instruction and support, this child is destined to become a dropout because his needs are not being met, and a state of amotivation may result. This is similar to the person who enters the negative spiral of disengagement described earlier in the chapter.

When children and adolescents are sampling activities and sports, a strong emphasis on intrinsic motivation is desirable. Coaches and teachers should offer a choice of activities, encourage achievable goal setting, emphasize personal improvement, and provide positive feedback. These ideas are explored further in chapters 14, 15, 16, and 17. Of course, people can participate for both intrinsic and extrinsic reasons. For example, someone can feel competent and also really want that team jacket. If extrinsic reasons dominate as children become older, the chances of their dropping out of sport increase. Côté, Baker, and Abernethy (2003) reported that highly skilled sport experts recall early practice activities connected with fun and experimenting with new ways of solving movement problems. Thus, practitioners and parents should be very careful not to turn fun practice into dreadful work for children.

Self-determination motivation theory is used in many areas related to kinesiology. The needs of autonomy and competence predict exercise behaviors, and intrinsic motivation is associated with long-term adherence to exercise (Teixeira, Carraca, Markland, Silva, & Ryan, 2012). In pedagogy, Sun and Chen (2010) promoted self-determination practices that lead to motor competence and relatedness/warmth with others, but acknowledged some conflict with satisfying the need of autonomy in an institutional environment.

They wondered whether students in physical education can be fully autonomous and how much autonomy is required to enhance learning. Van den Berghe, Vansteenkiste, Cardon, Kirk, and Hearns (2014) located 74 self-determination studies in physical education and recommended the usefulness of the theory to guide practice as well as the need for future research. Finally, 26 studies in motor learning and medical training were located in which at least one aspect of practice was controlled by the learner (Sanli, Patterson, Bray, & Lee, 2013). The advantages of self-controlled learning are well documented and discussed later in this chapter. Sanli and colleagues (2013) proposed that feelings of autonomy and competence are the likely reasons for the beneficial learning effects of self-control.

Social–Affective Constraints

A newborn is not likely to have a sense of self separate from the environment. But Piaget demonstrated that infants in the first two months of life begin to repeat pleasurable acts centered on their own bodies and to understand that they are responsible for some of the events that fascinate them (Shaffer, 1999). Their social world is primarily limited to immediate family members, and their crying as early as seven to nine months when held by strangers suggests that they distinguish between friendly folk and unknown people. They can recognize themselves in a mirror by 18 months, and by two or three years may issue self-concept statements such as, "I am a big boy, not a baby" (Shaffer, 1999). The impact of their social world is powerfully demonstrated by the emergence of language early in the second year of life. Yet they may remain egocentric thinkers until the end of the preoperational stage (ages 2-7), unable to imagine that their world view is different from others'. As a result, they have difficulty realizing that others in their world have different needs and desires from their own. As outlined in the sections on self-representation and competence motivation, children are affected by an increasing number of social agents over time that change in their relative impact, they develop a sense of self-esteem that can be strongly affected by motor competence, and they develop a repertoire of emotional reactions. We turn next to these functional constraints.

Emotional Development and Physical Activity

Participating in physical activities and sport competitions is often a significant emotional experience—pride, anger, satisfaction, and happiness can be experienced and expressed (Crocker, Hoar, McDonough, Kowalski, & Niefer, 2004). The model of competence motivation suggests that positive affect is an outcome of success at challenging activities and is related to competence motivation. Young athletes must also learn to control and express emotions that are socially appropriate and regulate them for optimal performance (Crocker et al., 2004). In the first six months of life, if not earlier, children demonstrate primary emotions such as interest, distress, anger, fear, joy, sadness, and surprise (Shaffer, 1999). Later, in the second year, they may display guilt, pride, envy, and embarrassment. Yet despite the honesty of a young infant's emotions, each society has "**emotional display rules**" (Shaffer, 1999, p. 394) that determine the circumstances under which emotions should or should not be expressed. Infants and toddlers begin to learn how to regulate their emotions, which is called **emotional self-regulation** (Garner & Waajid, 2012). A strategy adopted from age 2 to 6 is closing the eyes to control an unpleasant emotional arousal, such as when looking at a scary shark. Learning to control one's emotions may become context specific with development as all athletes realize that controlling their emotions is critical to performance (Crocker et al., 2004; Tamminen & Crocker, 2013).

Another important aspect of emotional development is recognizing the emotions of others, which facilitates social interaction. Preschool children learn to correctly interpret facial features, a skill that is called **emotional knowledge** (Garner & Waajid, 2012). Family conversations about emotions can help children deal with their feelings and to become aware of others. Children aged 3 and over begin to show awareness, and by age 5 can offer reasons a playmate is happy or sad. It may not be until age 6 or later that children understand that people can experience more than one emotion at a time.

Emotional knowledge and self-regulation are important skills to develop as children interact with others; these skills are related to educational and social outcomes in preschoolers (Garner & Waajid, 2012). It appears that all children, from 5 to 18 years of age, make affective judgments about engaging in physical activities (Nasuti & Rhodes, 2013). Perhaps not sur-

prisingly, among the emotions they seek from participation are pleasure and enjoyment. Physical activity programs are sometimes recommended as venues in which to learn positive emotional responses. Lubans, Plotnikoff, and Lubans (2012) found evidence for improved emotional and social functioning in at-risk youth as a result of participating in outdoor education, sport, or fitness programs. The authors added that a bias on the part of the respondents might have contributed to the positive findings.

Attributions

Attribution theory (Weiner, 1985) has implications for understanding emotion and motivation in achievement situations (Crocker et al., 2004). According to Weiner, emotion is a function of the outcome of achievement attempts (i.e., success or failure) as well as of people's attributions for outcomes. Positive emotions such as happiness are influenced by success, but also by attributions for the success. Attributions are explanations of why things turned out as they did. Common attributions are personal ability, effort, task difficulty, and luck; in sport, they include teamwork, injury, and referee decisions.

Weiner (1985) suggested that causal attributions have three dimensions: locus of control, stability, and control. Locus of control can be internal or external, the former referring to causes related to one's own behavior and the latter to causes that are beyond one's personal control (e.g., a lucky bounce or a teammate's play). Stability refers to attributions or factors influencing outcomes that are either stable from situation to situation (e.g., ability) or unstable (e.g., luck and effort). Effort is considered unstable because someone can try very hard and expend considerable energy one day but be much less involved on another day. The control factor refers to whether people perceive that they control the factors influencing outcomes (e.g., *If I work harder and obtain a personal trainer, I can make the team*) or consider the results uncontrollable (e.g., *Nothing I can do will influence my success*).

People who believe there is no relationship between effort and outcome (i.e., success or failure is unrelated to whatever they do) have developed **learned helplessness**, according to Seligman (1975). The person has minimal motivation to engage in the activity, but if forced to do so experiences anxiety and frustration. Learned helplessness may be domain specific; one of the authors of this text concedes that car problems are totally beyond his control and will not even open the hood if his car breaks down. Teachers and coaches can help learners by creating experiences that enhance success, even small successes, and encouraging them to take credit for the outcome (e.g., *You are working very hard, Charles, and you are getting faster on the track; you have improved by five seconds*). Horn (1987) also recommended helping learners understand that improvement comes with effort and practice, encouraging goal setting, and providing accurate feedback.

In general, positive emotions such as joy and pride occur as a result of success in a valued activity that is attributed to personal factors (Crocker et al., 2004). Consistent with the competence motivation model of Harter (1999), the positive affect resulting from success enhances competence motivation. Differentiating between ability, effort, luck, and task difficulty and hence making accurate attributions is developmental. Five-year-olds see no difference between effort and ability. By seven years of age, some children are capable of making causal explanations in some situations (Caprara, Pastorelli, & Weiner, 1997). Even at 11 years, children are limited in knowledge, the ability to process information, and reasoning (Crocker et al., 2004; see the discussion of information processing in chapter 11). Although clear developmental trends have not been identified (Crocker et al., 2004; Haywood & Getchell, 2014), attributions in achievement situations emerge more clearly and are more accurate during adolescence.

Arousal and Anxiety

One of the most important tasks of an athlete, or anyone learning a movement skill, is to control emotions in competition and during practice (e.g., Tamminen & Crocker, 2013). Optimal performance is unlikely for someone who is anxious, nervous, afraid of making a mistake, or worried about not succeeding. Heightened arousal (e.g., getting psyched up for a game) is usually beneficial to some extent. **Arousal** is different from **anxiety**. Anxiety refers to an emotional response to perceived threat and can involve cognitive concerns or physiological reactions (Crocker et al., 2004). On the other hand, arousal is a general state of activation or excitability (Magill, 2017; Schmidt & Lee, 2014).

The difference between arousal and anxiety was recognized over 100 years ago by Yerkes and Dodson (1908), who studied the relationship between performance and electric shock intensity in mice. Mild forms of shock produced an increase in performance, but at some point, increasing the intensity of the shock resulted in a decrease in performance. Optimal performance was assumed to be at a moderate level of arousal. This idea, which became known as the **inverted-U principle of arousal**, has been studied extensively in the field of motor learning (Schmidt & Lee, 2011). Coaches use pep talks to arouse players with the expectation that they will aid performance. However, if a player is too aroused or anxious, performance will likely be adversely affected, according to the inverted-U principle. The inverted-U principle has been criticized (Schmidt & Lee, 2011) for its simplicity, and some have proposed that some athletes require a very high level of arousal for optimal performance whereas others perform optimally with more modest arousal. Thus, individual differences are expected, and optimal arousal may be influenced by the nature of the task and environmental conditions. For the beginning learner of motor skills, modest arousal coupled with a desire to perform (motivation) would seem to be beneficial.

Self-Regulation

Guidance and feedback from therapists, teachers, and coaches are important for those in rehabilitation, recreation participants, and expert performers. However, learning and performing motor skills also occur through self-regulation—that is, practice and play without formal instruction. This begins at a young age when infants and preschoolers learn that their actions can affect the environment and that they can learn new skills by watching others. As a student, have you ever decided to read or study for 60 minutes before you take a break and call a friend? If so, you have engaged in two dimensions of self-regulation: goal setting (60 minutes) and self-reinforcement (calling a friend). As a fitness enthusiast, have you recorded your times on 5-mile (8 km) runs over a season, or listed the dates and durations of your workouts? These are examples of self-monitoring.

Zimmerman (2000) suggested that self-regulation is an inherently human endeavor because it helps us adapt to our environment. Although similar to metacognition, self-regulation also includes knowledge of one's motivation (self-motivation beliefs) and emotional reactions. More formally, self-regulation "refers to the self-generated thoughts, feelings, and actions that are planned and cyclically adapted to the attainment of personal goals" (Zimmerman, 2000, p. 14). People must set goals for self-regulation to function. They must then plan thoughts, feelings, and behaviors to attain those goals while also monitoring them along the way and changing them as necessary if they get off course. Self-regulation is thus an attractive concept in motor learning and

development. For example, a runner might set a specific time for a long race. However, during the race she realizes that she feels great and the humidity is low and thus decides to increase her goal and shoot for a personal best.

Zimmerman proposed a three-phase cyclical model of self-regulation: *forethought* leads to *performance or volitional control*, which leads to *self-reflection*. Being cyclical, self-reflection leads right back to forethought as greater self-regulation becomes possible. In a movement context, the participant plans an action (forethought), executes it (volitional control), and reflects on its success (self-reflection) (see figure 12.1). The self-reflection processes provide information for the forethought phase of the next trial for a discrete motor skill such as batting a ball, or later in the activity for a continuous motor skill such as swimming.

Forethought ("Plans an action" in figure 12.1) consists of task analysis and self-motivation beliefs. **Task analysis** includes setting personal goals for achievement and creating general strategies for achieving those goals. The **self-motivation beliefs** refer to the person's valuing of the activity, degree of intrinsic interest in the activity, degree of self-efficacy or belief in the ability

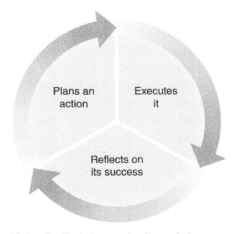

Figure 12.1 Cyclical phases of self-regulation.

Adapted from D.H. Schunk and B.J. Zimmerman (eds.), 1998, *Self-regulated learning: From teaching to self-reflective practice* (New York: Guilford Press).

to achieve the goal, and expectation of the outcome or awareness of the benefits that will occur if the goal is attained.

Performance control and **volitional control** ("Executes it" in figure 12.1) are the self-regulation strategies that can be applied during the learning trials or performance and include self-control and self-observation. **Self-control** includes self-instruction such as reminding yourself while swimming a length that the left arm must come farther out of the water, or focusing on your own motivation when you realize you might be attending to the noise of the crowd cheering for your opponents. Also included in self-control is the imagery of performance, or imagining yourself performing an action; this is a common technique used by divers and gymnasts just prior to performance. Also included in self-control are task strategies that can be altered during the game or event. **Self-observation** guides progress toward a goal, particularly self-recording of things such as the percentage of successful free throws during a basketball season, the types of food consumed during training, or independent steps accomplished in rehabilitation. Self-experimentation is a self-observation activity in which a new approach to performance or learning is attempted long enough to be able to perform a fair evaluation.

The final part of the cyclical self-regulation process is **self-reflection** ("Reflects on its success" in figure 12.1), which occurs at some point following a trial, a set of trials, a game, or a season. Self-reflection includes self-judgment and self-reaction. Self-judgment is self-evaluation in which the person assesses the degree to which the goals were achieved. Also included in self-judgment are causal attributions—that is, explanations for why goals were met or not met; these were discussed briefly under attributions. Questions might be: What did you think led most to goal success? Did you exert sufficient effort? and Did you try to accomplish the task without enough coaching? Finally,

self-reaction refers to being aware of one's degree of overall self-satisfaction. Even if the goal was not attained, a self-reflective person might ask herself: *Am I satisfied with my performance, with what I learned, and with the effort I expended?*

Is self-regulation important for learning and performance? Researchers have found that experts are more likely to engage in self-regulation than novices are (Cleary & Zimmerman, 2001; Kitsantas & Zimmerman, 1998). Singer (2002) suggested that self-regulation is just as important as skill in performance. Self-regulation is sometimes called self-control in motor learning studies. These studies reveal advantages in skill learning when learners control aspects of practice (Sanli et al., 2013) such as the following: when to receive knowledge of results (Chiviacowsky & Wulf, 2005; Janelle, Barba, Frehlich, Tennant, & Cauraugh, 1997), the delivery of augmented feedback (Aiken, Fairbrother, & Post, 2012), task difficulty (Andrieux, Boutin, & Thon, 2016), the relative timing of a movement sequence (Wu & Magill, 2011), physical guidance (Wulf & Toole, 1999), the amount of practice (Post, Fairbrother, & Barros, 2011), the amount of practice in a fixed time period (Post, Fairbrother, Barros, & Kulpa, 2014), and blocked versus random practice (Keetch & Lee, 2007). Even choices about the color of practice golf balls augmented skill learning (Lewthwaite, Chiviacowsky, Drews, & Wulf, 2015).

Self-controlled motor learning extends to children. Ten-year-olds were allowed to determine when they would receive knowledge of their results on a nondominant hand throwing task (Chiviacowsky, Wulf, de Medeiros, Kaefer, & Tani, 2008). They threw beanbags to a concentric-circle target. Benefits generally favored self-selected knowledge of results compared to an equal number of feedback trials that participants did not specifically request. The children tended to request feedback after good trials, and the authors suggested that feedback after poor trials may be ineffective and that self-selected feedback appears to have a motivational influence. As Sanli and colleagues (2013) suggested, the positive impact of self-controlled learning might be due to facilitating feelings of autonomy and competence.

There is also evidence that novices and those with learning difficulties show few signs of self-directed learning (Lloyd, Reid, & Bouffard, 2006; Zimmerman, 2000), so self-regulation is assumed to be very important in the learning process. Also encouraging is the fact that self-regulation appears to improve as a result of instruction, including of those with a disability (Jokic, Polatajko, & Whitebread, 2013; Kitsantas & Zimmerman, 1998; Zimmerman & Kitsantas, 1997).

How does self-regulation develop? There is not much research available on this question, but a developmental model from Zimmerman (2000) has proved helpful. He proposed a social–cognitive model in which new skills are initially acquired via social means and then progress through steps that represent increasing metacognitive, motivational, and behavioral regulation. The four developmental levels are observation (observing and listening to proficient models for major features of the skill), emulation (mimicking the model's style and skill with social assistance), self-control (mastering the skill of a model in structured settings), and self-regulation (adapting the use of the skill across changing environments and interpersonal states).

Observation, the first level in the development of self-regulation, includes witnessing skills of peers or older children or hearing about them from teachers. These are largely vicarious experiences that provide an image of the skills and

---

RESEARCH NOTES

Self-Regulation and Developmental Coordination Disorder

Lloyd and colleagues (2006) explored self-regulation in children with and without developmental coordination disorder (DCD). DCD is a formal diagnostic term for those who have considerable difficulty performing movement skills at age-expected levels that is not due to factors such as cerebral palsy or intellectual disability. Some authors have described these people as awkward or clumsy. DCD is associated with low self-concept and withdrawal from physical activity. The authors postulated that DCD might be related to poor self-regulation. Therefore, they compared a group of 10 boys without DCD to 10 boys with DCD. The mean age of the boys was 11.5. The investigators used two tasks: a sport-specific problem-solving task of shooting indoors at a hockey net with a rubber puck and an educational problem-solving task of peg solitaire in which the goal was to remove all wooden pegs from the holes on the board by jumping over a peg and then picking it up. Participants were taught to use a think-aloud verbal report in which they articulated their thought processes during the activity. Their thoughts were transcribed and then categorized into self-regulation categories such as goals, knowledge, monitoring, emotion, and evaluation. Among the salient results was the finding that the boys with DCD expressed less knowledge about the shooting task, had fewer error correction plans, and had more total emotion and negative emotion; additionally, 25 percent had fewer action plans. On the peg solitaire task, the only difference was less planning ahead by the boys with DCD. The authors concluded that the results were consistent with a self-regulation deficit in children with DCD and that, with the exception of planning, the difficulties did not appear on nonmotor tasks.

Another Peek at Those Self-Regulation Strategies
Exercise 12.4

In groups of two or three, review the strategies in each of the three phases of self-regulation that might improve studying behaviors. The identified strategies might be ones you currently use or might use.

awareness of rewards received by models. Thus, children may be motivated to engage in the activity (e.g., jumping down from a height, skiing, or roller skating) and will maintain some persistence during initial learning trials. Observational learning is described more fully in chapter 15. **Emulation**, the second level, refers to adopting a model's style of skill rather than mimicking exact response components. Thus, the learner performs a skill but in his own unique way and using self-regulatory skills. The motivated four-year-old will ice skate at the rink with a fairly upright posture and minimal glide on the skates. This style maintains stability, but with practice, the body lean and glide increase. As we will see in chapter 15, research has demonstrated that children who fear water can benefit from exposure to models by emulating the coping strategies of models (Weiss, McCullagh, Smith, & Berlant, 1998). According to Zimmerman (2000), this produces sensorimotor feedback and internal standards of correct performance that are necessary for the next two steps. This process is similar to the creation of a generalized motor program, which has a recall dimension for initiating movements but also a recognition dimension for evaluating the movement based on expected sensory consequences.

Self-control refers to the use of one's own strategy as a planned and self-monitored process. At this level, people practice by themselves without a model present. Their personal representation or image of the skill is their guide, and their motivation is largely self-rewards and personal reactions to attaining standards. Hence, they may go to the gym and shoot at the basketball net while focusing on how they are performing (e.g., placement of feet, arms, and hands or how many baskets they get). The highest level is **self-regulation**, in which skills can be adapted to changing environmental demands (e.g., a hostile crowd, rain during a track meet) and interpersonal states. At this level, people need not focus on how they are performing but on their performance outcomes, such as how many of their shots are successful. With experience at this level, self-efficacy and self-motivation toward mastery should increase.

Research with motor and other skills has demonstrated that students can be taught more effective self-regulation and that they do progress through the four levels of self-regulation (Kitsantas & Zimmerman, 1998; Zimmerman & Kitsantas, 1997, 1999). Kolovelonis, Goudas, Hassandra, and Demitzaki (2012) used emulation and self-control instruction with fifth- and sixth-graders who were learning basketball dribbling. The success of the self-regulation groups in comparison to control groups provided support for the developmental model and evidence that self-regulation is amenable to instruction. Self-regulation must become a more prominent research topic in motor development for a clearer development picture to emerge.

The use of self-regulation processes, much like the development of expertise and knowledge, is primarily task dependent. The following recommendations

Exercise 12.5

1. Imagine that you are teaching an elementary school physical education class. Provide specific examples of how you could help your students develop self-regulation. Now imagine that you are teaching a high school physical education class. How would you facilitate self-regulation among these students? Do your ideas differ for these two groups? Explain. If you are an occupational or physical therapist, how might you include self-regulation in your interventions?

2. Define the term *self-regulation* in your own words. Provide at least three examples of times when you used self-regulation to succeed in a sport or physical activity.

may enhance self-regulation by children and adolescents (in part from Petlichkoff, 2004):

- Promote self-observation, which includes self-monitoring progress toward a goal and monitoring behavioral outcomes and processes such as cognitive strategies generated internally and available from models.

- Set process goals before outcome goals. This means focusing on skill improvement rather than a specific outcome such as 10 points in a game.

- When skills become automatic, shift to outcome goals that are within reach.

- To assist in self-judgment processes, expose learners to peer coping models rather than expert models (see chapter 15), and encourage them to focus on personal improvement (self-comparison) rather than comparing themselves to peers. This should help them view themselves favorably.

- Teachers, coaches, and parents should model self-regulatory strategies such as self-instruction and goal setting.

- Demonstrate and promote problem solving for tasks that have more than one movement solution, such as guarding an opponent one-on-one or executing an offensive two-on-one situation.

- Encourage self-reinforcement.

- Discuss attributions of success and failure. What influenced the outcome? What can be done immediately to counteract a failure? What factors should be considered in the longer term?

Summary

This chapter outlined several functional individual constraints that people bring with them to motor learning and performance situations. The constraints included psychosocial and affective constraints as well as those having to do with self-regulation. The psychosocial model of Erikson (1963) outlined the development of autonomy, initiation, and identity while simultaneously coming to terms with social expectations and regulations. Identity, or self-representation, was also the focus of Harter's description of self-esteem. There are many individual differences in the timing and ultimate level of achievement of Erikson's and Harter's phases, and thus children and adolescents demonstrate considerable heterogeneity with regard to perceptions of self.

Perceptions of competence affect physical activity, but researchers have argued that actual competence in motor skills is the most important factor leading to physical activity (Robinson et al., 2015; Stodden et al., 2008). Based on experiences with a host of social agents and environmental factors, self-efficacy and intrinsic motivation vary in children and adolescents, and both affect performance. In a physical activity context, some learners show behaviors consistent with seeking competence motivation experiences and intrinsic motivation, while others have little interest in learning or participating in physical activity because their previous experiences and social influences have been negative. Finally, self-regulation represents a host of strategies that learners can adopt to self-direct learning. When learners are allowed to control aspects of practice, learning is frequently enhanced.

Rodney is the 270-pound (122 kg) talented American football player who does not play as well as Martin, his smaller peer, does (see the chapter-opening scenario). Can you see some reasons for this difference? Despite his smaller stature, Martin likely possesses a stronger sense of self, higher perceived competence and self-efficacy, and greater intrinsic motivation for the game than Rodney does. Moreover, Martin is almost assuredly engaged in self-regulation of his practices and games. Overall, Rodney possesses the structural constraints to play, but not the functional ones to excel.

ONLINE LEARNING

Visit the web resource at www.HumanKinetics.com/MotorLearningAndDevelopment for an accompanying lab activity and exercises from the chapter.

LEARNING AIDS

Supplemental Activities

1. Spend some time talking to an elementary school-aged child (5-12 years of age)—a younger sibling, a cousin, or the child across the street. Ask the child to describe him- or herself. See which age period of self-representation most closely matches your interviewee's comments. Even better, then talk with an older person, perhaps an adolescent, to confirm development in self-representation.

2. Self-determination is a major motivational theory as described in this chapter. But it has other meanings. Search the Internet for pre-20th-century philosophical interpretations of self-determination; then find political meanings of self-determination that were important in the early 20th century.

Glossary

amotivation—Lack of any motivation; present when a person does not see any relationship between outcomes and actions.

anxiety—An emotional response to perceived threat; can involve cognitive concerns or physiological reactions.

arousal—A general state of activation or excitability.

autonomous—Referring to engaging in a task by free will, without external influence from others; autonomy is one of three basic needs according to self-determination theory.

competent—Having the ability to realize success in a given domain; competence is one of three basic needs according to self-determination theory.

emotional display rules—Socially defined circumstances in which emotions should or should not be expressed.

emotional knowledge—Recognizing the emotions of others.

emotional self-regulation—Modifying ones emotions.

emulation—The adoption of a model's style of skill rather than imitating an exact response; Zimmerman's second level in the development of self-regulation.

extrinsically motivated behaviors—Behaviors engaged in as a means to an end and not for their own sake.

forethought—The phase of Zimmerman's cyclical model of self-regulation that involves planning an action and consists of task analysis and self-motivation beliefs.

intrinsically motivated behaviors—Behaviors that provide pleasure and satisfaction from participation in the absence of material rewards or constraints.

inverted-U principle of arousal—The idea that optimal performance occurs at a moderate level of arousal.

learned helplessness—A belief that there is no relationship between effort and outcome.

non-self-determined extrinsic motivation—Motivation toward a behavior based on avoiding immediate negative consequences.

observation—Witnessing the skills of peers or older children or hearing about them from others; Zimmerman's first level in the development of self-regulation.

performance control—The phase in Zimmerman's cyclical model of self-regulation that involves self-control and self-observation.

related—Being connected with other people; one of three basic needs in self-determination theory.

self-control—The use of personal strategies as a planned and self-monitored process; Zimmerman's third level in the development of self-regulation.

self-determination—A theory of motivation proposing that the basic needs of competence, autonomy, and relatedness drive people to action.

self-determined extrinsic motivation—Motivation based on extrinsic reasons.

self-efficacy—(1) The belief in personal capabilities to successfully execute the action required to achieve identified goals. (2) The belief that one can successfully perform a desired behavior given various instrumental barriers.

self-esteem—A self-evaluation of competency, successfulness, and worthiness.

self-motivation beliefs—The perceived value of an activity, the degree of intrinsic interest in the activity, the degree of self-efficacy or the belief in the ability to achieve the goal, and the expectation of the outcome or the awareness of the benefits that will occur if the goal is attained.

self-observation—The process that guides personal progress toward a goal, particularly self-recording.

self-reflection—The phase of Zimmerman's cyclical model of self-regulation that involves reflecting on the success of an action and consists of self-judgment and self-reaction.

self-regulation—(1) "Self-generated thoughts, feelings, and actions that are planned and cyclically adapted to the attainment of personal goals" (Zimmerman, 2000, p. 14), or informally, the ability to practice and play without formal instruction. (2) A complex process whereby athletes or exercisers engage in voluntary goal-directed behaviors over time and context by initiating, monitoring, sustaining, and achieving certain thoughts, feelings, and behaviors (Weiss, 2004, p. 385).

task analysis—The process of setting personal goals for achievement and creating general strategies for achieving those goals.

volitional control—A phase of Zimmerman's cyclical model of self-regulation; self-regulation strategies such as self-control and self-observation that can be applied during learning or performance.

PSYCHOSOCIAL AND COGNITIVE FACTORS IN ADULTHOOD

Chapter Objectives

After reading this chapter, you should be able to do the following:

- Identify psychosocial factors in adulthood.
- Explain the adulthood stages in Erikson's psychosocial development theory.
- Demonstrate an understanding of self-regulation, including Kirschenbaum's self-regulation model and self-regulation strategies.
- Identify sociocultural factors of development in adulthood.
- Describe age-related changes in cognitive function.

Winning Is a State of Mind

Ja'rell was an athlete in her youth, and she played at the Division 1 level in college (university). After college, she missed the competitive environment and sought a similar experience. She started running at age 35 and registered for her first race, a 10K, shortly after she began running. During the race, she found herself thinking: *I can't do this. I'm so slow. Maybe I should just quit now.* Ja'rell wasn't expecting the race to be so difficult and likely wasn't physically (or perhaps mentally) prepared for the race. Although she never considered herself a runner, she was used to being one of the top athletes in her younger years and was not expecting to be passed by so many other runners, some much older than she was. However, she continued to run. On the last mile, her mentality changed and she began to enjoy the experience, changing her negative thought pattern to a positive one. Her pace quickened, and she made it across the finish line with a smile. This experience was humbling, but her change in attitude pushed her to the finish and was the impetus for beginning a long and impressive career as a distance runner and triathlete.

The mind can have a very powerful influence on performance. Mental toughness (tuning out distractions while keeping anxiety low and attentional focus high) can take many years to master. Maintaining a positive attitude and using positive self-talk can provide huge advantages, because negative thoughts can not only prevent improvement but also be the downfall of even the most skilled athletes. Although only the elite may experience performance at such high levels, all of us, whether we are competitive or not, are affected by psychosocial and cognitive constraints. In this chapter, we discuss how performance in adulthood is affected by many functional constraints, how those constraints change with age, and how older adults compensate for these changes. We extend the functional constraints discussed in chapters 11 and 12 to adulthood and include discussions of self-efficacy, self-regulation, motivation, Erik Erikson's psychosocial development theory (adulthood stages), sociocultural factors and social support, and age-related changes in cognitive function including attention and memory.

Psychosocial Factors

Changing self-perceptions and declining physical abilities related to aging can affect social interaction and social approval, which can, in turn, significantly affect mental health and well-being. Much evidence supports the benefits of physical exercise for adults, physically, psychologically, and socially (Spirduso, Francis, & MacRae, 2005). Participation in group physical activities can be particularly beneficial because they have been found to improve fitness level, a sense of well-being, and mood (Biddle, Fox, & Boutcher, 2000). Many of these health benefits result from the psychosocial benefits of participating in recreational physical activity and sport.

Psychological Factors

Numerous psychological factors interact with the physical domain. Most of the research has focused on exercise adherence, including intention to exercise, self-efficacy, and locus of control. Older adults experience different barriers to exercise than children and adolescents do. Motivational factors also change throughout adulthood from a focus on weight management and appearance to a focus on maintaining health and physical function.

Intention to Exercise

One of the greatest factors affecting exercise adherence is the person's intention to exercise. According to the **theory of planned behavior**, attitudes toward a behavior depend on two factors: (1) the belief that the behavior will produce a specified outcome and (2) the person's desire to attain the specified outcome (Ajzen, 1985). Adults who do not place much value and importance on exercise are much less likely to adhere to a regular exercise program (Motalebi, Iranagh, Abdollahi, & Lim, 2014). Intention is the main determinant of behavior because it reflects both motivation and willingness (Ajken, 1991; Kosma, 2012). Intention comprises three concepts: (1) the attitude toward the behavior, (2) perceived social pressures about the behavior, and (3) perceived behavioral control (White et al., 2012). Someone who has a positive attitude toward exercise and perceived social pressures as well as behavioral control will have a much higher intention to exercise than someone who does not. Researchers have discovered a negative relationship between age and exercise intention in older adults (Yardley, Donovan-Hall, Francis, & Todd, 2007). This is likely the result of decreasing positive attitudes toward exercise with age and a reduced belief in the ability to perform exercises in this population. Because older adults tend not to meet physical activity related guidelines (see chapter 10), improving their attitudes toward physical activity, and therefore their intention to exercise, is critical for improving exercise behavior (Hausenblas, Carron, & Mack, 1997).

Self-Efficacy

Self-efficacy is also an important factor when people adopt an exercise program (McAuley, 1992). Self-efficacy, which is very similar to a "situation-specific form of self-confidence" (Weinberg & Gould, 2003, p. 316), is the belief that the person can perform a desired behavior leading to anticipated outcomes (Bandura, 1997). According to **Bandura's social cognitive theory**, self-efficacy determines (a) whether the person is even going to attempt a task, (b) how persistent the person will be amid challenges, and (c) the final outcome (e.g., either successful maintenance of an exercise program or failure to adhere to the program). Adults with higher self-efficacy typically engage in physical activity longer than those with lower self-efficacy (Litt, Kleppinger, & Judge, 2002). Older adults have significantly lower self-efficacy than young adults have, perhaps because they perceive that they have reduced control in exercise situations (Dishman, 1994) and are afraid of injury (Stephens & Craig, 1990).

Self-efficacy is such a positive mediator for physical activity that it can reverse common barriers to exercise. In a study of older Filipino adults living in Hawaii, lack of health became a motivator to exercise (Ceria-Ulep, Serafica, & Tse, 2011).

Locus of Control

Locus of control is "the extent to which people believe that they have control over their own fate" (Thomas, Sorensen, & Abby, 2006, p. 1057). People who believe they have some personal control over their health are more likely to adhere to an exercise program. Specifically, those with an **internal locus of control** (i.e., who believe that their actions affect the environment) are more likely to eat well and exercise regularly than those with an **external locus of control** (i.e., who believe that their actions do not affect the environment and that events happen by chance) (Cobb-Clark, Kassenboehmer, & Schurer, 2014). It is not surprising, then, that people with

an external locus of control are less likely to adhere to an exercise program. If they do not believe that exercise can change the way they look and feel, why would they do it?

Barriers to Exercise

The barriers to exercise most commonly reported by adults are the same for both exercisers and nonexercisers (e.g., lack of time, laziness, and work responsibilities). Barriers to exercise in older adults, not surprisingly, are different because older adults no longer have the time constraints of work and raising children; however, many have physical limitations. In the over-65 age group, the most common barriers reported by nonexercisers were fear of falling, laziness, and lack of motivation, whereas the barriers reported by exercisers were time constraints, physical ailments, and laziness (Lees, Clark, Nigg, & Newman, 2005). A study of older adults who were afraid of falling found that in addition to a lack of motivation, they reported reduced health status, bad experiences with exercise, and other environmental factors (Lindgren De Groot & Fagerström, 2011). Barriers reported by older adults also differ based on socioeconomic status. Those of higher socioeconomic status reported time, facilities, and transport as the three biggest barriers to physical activity; those of lower socioeconomic status reported health conditions, neighborhood safety (including fear of crime), and facilities (Gray, Murphy, Gallagher, & Simpson, 2016).

Given that those who exercise and those who do not reported the same most common exercise barriers, it is likely that these are perceived barriers (i.e., personal priorities) rather than actual barriers. Adults who place a higher priority on exercise or do not perceive the barriers to be insurmountable are much more likely to continue exercising in spite of them. Adults who do not make exercise a priority may be using these external barriers to avoid a physically active lifestyle (Valois, Shephard, & Godin, 1986). Women participate

Exercise 13.1

For each of the following examples, list several possible barriers to exercise and strategies for removing these barriers.

1. A 25-year-old woman with little previous movement experience who does not exercise
   a. Barriers:
   b. Strategies:
2. A 44-year-old man who played a lot of sports in high school and university but has not exercised or participated in sports since then
   a. Barriers:
   b. Strategies:
3. A 70-year-old woman who exhibits interest in going to the gym but is intimidated by all of the equipment
   a. Barriers:
   b. Strategies:

in less physical activity and report more barriers to participating in physical activity than men do (Stephens & Craig, 1990). When walking, women reported more environmental concerns such as heavy traffic, unattended dogs, and lack of safety in comparison to men. They also reported less enjoyable scenery and fewer people exercising in their neighborhoods.

Creating a successful exercise program requires an understanding of the greatest barriers to exercise. If practitioners focus older adults' attention on the benefits of exercise and reduce their perceptions of exercise barriers, older adults are more likely to maintain a physically active lifestyle (Rhodes, Martin, Taunton, Rhodes, Donnelly, & Elliot, 1999).

Motivation

Motivation (a set of reasons that determines behavior) is not something that is simply present or not; it isn't just turned on or off like a light switch. Rather, motivation exists along a continuum (see figure 13.1 and chapter 12 for further information and definitions) that includes amotivation, non-self-determined extrinsic motivation,

self-determined extrinsic motivation, and intrinsic motivation (Dacey, Baltzell, & Zalchkowsky, 2008). The most extreme example would be someone who has no desire to engage in any type of exercise or physical activity (this person would be considered amotivated). The main difference between non-self-determined extrinsic motivation and self-determined extrinsic motivation is that, in the latter, the extrinsic reasons are personally valued and the outcomes are generally viewed as favorable (e.g., practicing yoga to reduce stress). Intrinsic motivation is optimal and occurs when behaviors are performed because of a personal interest in and an enjoyment of engaging in the activity.

Dacey and colleagues (2008) found that the amount of physical activity older adults engage in is affected by their type of motivation for exercise. Intrinsic and self-determined extrinsic motivation are positively correlated with increased physical activity. Self-determined extrinsic motivators included health and fitness, stress management, and social–emotional benefits. Weight management and appearance were considered non-self-determined

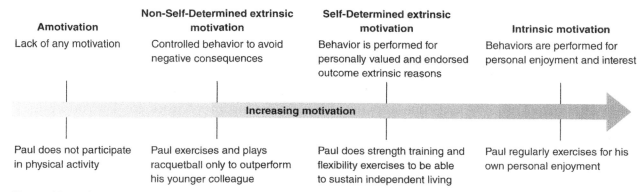

Figure 13.1   Motivation continuum showing an example of an older adult's motivation for participating in physical activity.

WHAT DO YOU THINK?

Exercise 13.2

1. Classify the following adults according to their type of motivation toward physical activity (amotivation, non-self-determined extrinsic motivation, self-determined extrinsic motivation, intrinsic motivation).

    a. Sandeep is a 53-year-old man who regularly plays racquetball at the local recreation center. Even though the games are noncompetitive, Sandeep is very competitive when he plays. Outside of racquetball games, Sandeep does not participate in any form of regular physical activity or exercise.

    b. Jessica is a highly active 32-year-old who exercises six or seven times per week and regularly competes in local and regional running races. She thoroughly enjoys the highs she feels from both her workouts and the competitions.

    c. Jose is a 68-year-old man who has recently started an exercise program that includes resistance training, cardio workouts, and stretching. Jose began the exercise program to maintain his functionality and reduce age-related physical declines.

2. Devise an example of a person who demonstrates amotivation toward physical activity.

extrinsic motivators because they reflect a desire to attain social approval or enhance the ego. The results of this study revealed that, regardless of the participants' level of motivation, appearance and weight management were motivators. However, appearance became less important with advancing age. This suggests that weight management and appearance are least likely to induce long-term behavior change. Better motivators for older adults to increase physical activity levels could include the social benefits of a game of

tennis with a friend or a group exercise class or the fitness benefits of increasing flexibility through stretching exercises.

Self-Regulation

The importance of self-regulatory skills is not limited to athletic adults trying to improve or maintain their skills. All adults, regardless of age, health, or fitness level, need self-regulatory skills. For example, these skills are also important for the inactive adult who is trying to initiate and adhere to an exercise program or for the

Watch More Television to Improve Healthy Behaviors?!

We've all heard that too much television can cause people to become couch potatoes by encouraging poor health behaviors such as eating more junk food, exercising less, and sometimes even getting less sleep. Considering that the average American watches 151 hours of television per month (Thomas, 2009), television alone could play a major role in the obesity epidemic. Many studies back the notion of the negative effects of television, but is it possible for television to fight a sedentary lifestyle and even foster healthy behaviors? To examine this possibility, Nabi and Thomas (2013) randomly assigned 253 female undergraduate university students to watch either a health-oriented reality program, a non-health-oriented reality program, or a health-themed sitcom with embedded healthy or unhealthy food commercials. The results revealed that the type of program affected the participants' motivations to choose either healthy or unhealthy foods as well as their motivation to exercise. The women who viewed the health-oriented reality program were the most likely to choose a healthy snack following the program. These results indicate the power of advertisements and programming. This research reveals that watching television may actually decrease sedentary behavior and even increase motivation and self-efficacy for healthy behaviors such as healthier eating and exercise when health-oriented programs are watched.

injured adult who is going through rehabilitation. Self-regulation is a complex process in which athletes, patients, or exercisers engage in voluntary goal-directed behaviors by initiating, monitoring, sustaining, and achieving certain thoughts, feelings, and behaviors (Weiss & Gould, 2015).

Through management of short- and long-term goals, adults self-regulate their behavior in both exercise and sport. Adults who decide to start an exercise program, improve their skills, or recover from an injury through a rehabilitation program go through a series of steps, as depicted in Kirschenbaum's self-regulation process (1984), to achieve the necessary self-regulation skills. To facilitate self-regulation skills in their students, patients, or athletes, practitioners need to understand these steps.

Kirschenbaum (1984) developed a five-stage model of self-regulation (see figure 13.2). The first stage is the **problem identification stage**. During this stage, adults must not only identify the problem, such as a need to improve their softball skills or to start an exercise program, but also decide

Stage 1: Problem identification
Sierra needs to improve her golf drive.

Stage 2: Commitment
Sierra is willing to make the sacrifices necessary to relearn how to perform a drive in golf.

Stage 3: Execution
Sierra sets goals and monitors her progress.

Stage 4: Environmental management
Alternative practice locations are found for possible inclement weather.

Stage 5: Generalization
Goals are reevaluated. Sierra may now focus on other aspects of her game.

Figure 13.2 Kirschenbaum's five-stage model of self-regulation.

whether the change is possible and worth the effort. During stage 1 the person must be willing to take responsibility for solving the problem. Stage 2 is the **commitment**

RESEARCH NOTES

What Separates the Experts From the Rest?

Kitsantas and Zimmerman (2002) conducted a study to compare the self-regulatory processes of novice, nonexpert, and expert volleyball players. Thirty female university students participated in the study. The experts were university varsity team players; the nonexperts played in a volleyball club; and the novices had played volleyball only informally. The experts used more self-control strategies (e.g., self-instruction, imagery, attention focusing, and task-specific strategies) than the nonexperts and novices did. The experts also prepared their serves with more forethought and set more specific process goals than those in the other two groups did. The novices did not even report any goals. Focusing on technique, as the expert volleyball players did, can help learners decrease the amount of time they need to learn a motor skill (Locke & Latham, 1990).

The expert volleyball players spent more time on self-reflection than the nonexperts and novices did. Self-reflection is essential to improve performance of a motor skill. The experts were much more likely to attribute their errors to improper form or technique (e.g., *It was a bad toss*), which enabled them to appropriately self-correct for the subsequent serve. Only half of the nonexperts and none of the novices attributed their errors to form or technique; rather, most attributed their poor serves to insufficient power.

The expert players also spent more time preparing for their serves with warmups, pepper drills, and specific skill training. The nonexperts used only one of these components, and the novices did not use any. The experts spent significantly more time reflecting on their performances and were more likely to adapt their serves than were those in the other two groups. Furthermore, the experts were more likely to seek assistance from coaches or teammates. It is perhaps not surprising that the novices were unlikely to seek assistance. Even the nonexperts, who played on a team through a club, were only moderately likely to seek help. Seeking help is not a sign of weakness on the part of athletes; rather, it is an essential element of self-regulation. Athletes must focus on their errors and ask for help.

Understanding how experts, nonexperts, and novices differ in their self-regulatory behavior can help instructors prepare self-directed practice. At minimum, instructors should encourage their learners to set specific goals and reflect on their performances. They should also encourage them to seek assistance when they notice errors they cannot correct.

stage. To commit, the person must be willing to make the sacrifices necessary to persevere through the process.

Once a commitment has been made, the person moves to the **execution stage**, which is the active stage of behavioral change. During this stage, the person must develop self-expectancies for success through goal setting and continually self-evaluate and self-monitor his performance with respect to these goals. In addition to goal setting, he should plan ways to reinforce continued improvement and potentially even punishment for deviating from goal attainment. An athlete trying to improve his swim for triathlons might set a goal to swim 40 minutes, four times per week, or to decrease his swim time by 10 percent by the next competition. He could log when he swims and the duration and distance of each swim. If he meets his goals, he could reward himself by buying new gear or an athletic watch. In therapy settings, physical and occupational therapists work closely with patients during the execution phase, developing goals with them and continually evaluating their progress.

The fourth stage is the **environmental management stage**. In this stage, adults prepare strategies to deal with potential environmental or social barriers to attaining their goals. The triathlete may schedule some practices in open water but have an indoor pool option as a backup during inclement weather. Social barriers could also affect performances or practices. For instance, someone who relies on a friend for moral support to exercise could lose motivation when her friend decides to cancel a workout session. Having backup plans, such as other people to walk with or group exercise classes to participate in, could keep unforeseen changes from affecting an exercise routine. Therapists must also help patients set up their home environments, providing them with the knowledge and equipment they need to continue their treatments at home.

Stage 5 is the **generalization stage**, during which people focus on sustaining their efforts for long periods of time. They may change some of their goals. For instance, the triathlete may notice that his swim times have improved but may need to focus on his run. Or he may want to increase his strength and thus begin a weightlifting program. A woman who has successfully adhered to her exercise program may want to shift her focus to improving her diet while continuing her exercise program. Therapists may help patients develop at-home plans to continue

their treatments after completing their rehabilitation programs.

The five stages in Kirschenbaum's (1984) model emphasize the importance of self-monitoring in self-regulation. People must continually evaluate their performances and progress toward their goals. Self-regulation is also strongly influenced by personality styles and dispositions. Optimistic people with high self-esteem are much more stable and likely to continue self-regulatory behavior, whereas pessimistic people with low self-esteem are more likely to see changing social and environmental conditions as barriers to continuing with the program (Waschall & Kernis, 1996).

Self-Regulation Strategies

Although there are many self-regulation strategies, the most commonly used are self-monitoring, goal setting, self-talk, and imagery (Weiss & Gould, 2015). Self-monitoring and goal setting are critical skills in self-regulation because they keep people focused on attaining their performance goals (Massey, Meyer, & Naylor, 2015). We are almost constantly engaging in some form of self-talk. Therefore, regulating self-talk has a strong influence on all of our behaviors, from sport performance to social situations. Imagery can also be a powerful form of self-regulation that can help us improve performance and control emotion.

Self-monitoring Self-monitoring is the systematic observation of oneself (Kirschenbaum, 1987). Methods of self-monitoring

WHAT DO YOU THINK?

Exercise 13.3

1. How would a recreational hockey goalie likely differ in self-regulatory strategies from a Division I (university) hockey goalie?
2. What self-regulatory skills would you encourage a recreational hockey goalie to focus on?

include recording behaviors or performances and making self-observations. Performances can also be self-monitored through the use of tangible items, such as putting a nickel in a jar for every mistake. The purpose of self-monitoring is to become more aware of one's behaviors, which can not only improve performance, but also decrease anxiety and boost confidence (Crews, Lochbaum, & Karoly, 2000). Self-monitoring can be either positive (e.g., recording successful performances) or negative (e.g., recording poor performances). Research has shown that positive self-monitoring is beneficial for difficult tasks because it enhances the performer's expectancies and improves performance. On the other hand, well-learned and simple tasks benefit more from negative self-monitoring, such as focusing on failures and mistakes (Kirschenbaum, 1987).

Goal setting   Perhaps the most critical self-regulation skill is goal setting. Setting goals focuses the learner's attention on attaining a set level of proficiency. It is especially important to set specific and measurable goals that must be achieved by a predetermined time (e.g., throwing 10 percent farther by the first meet of the track and field season). Goals that either are not specific or cannot be measured are ineffective. Goals are further discussed in chapter 15.

Self-talk   Another useful self-regulation skill is the management of self-talk. Considering that people engage in a lot of self-talk every day, it is not surprising that managing self-talk can assist in regulating behavior. Athletes may say to themselves, *I can't do this, I am the worst player* or *I'm going to mess this up.* On the flip side, positive self-talk can improve confidence, increase motivation, correct bad habits, and focus attention (Williams & Leffingwell, 1996). Most skilled athletes have learned how to manage their self-talk, even to the point of changing negative thoughts to positive thoughts, as Bjorn Borg did in the following example at the Wimbledon final against

John McEnroe in 1980, a match that has often been referred to as legendary:

> As [Bjorn] Borg took his position for the fifth set, he said to himself, 'This is terrible. I'm going to lose.' But then thought, 'If you lose a match like this, the Wimbledon final, after all those chances, you will not forget it for a long, long time. That could be very hard.' It was his serve to start the last set. He lost the first two points. 'But then,' Borg recalls, 'I say to myself, "I have to forget. I have to keep trying, try to win."' He served the next point and won. And again and again. (Deford, 1980)

The mind can have a very powerful influence on performance. Negative thoughts can not only prevent improvement but also be the downfall of even the most skilled athletes. Maintaining positive thinking and clearing the mind can provide an athletic advantage. Managing self-talk can divert people from negative, unproductive thoughts and guide them toward positive thoughts. Self-talk management strategies include stopping self-talk that is negative or irrational; changing negative self-talk to positive self-talk; internally reasoning to counter negative self-talk; and reframing, which is changing one's perspective on the situation (Zinsser, Bunker, & Williams, 2001).

Imagery   **Imagery**, the visualization or cognitive rehearsal of a movement, has been found to be a very effective self-regulatory skill and performance enhancer. It provides additional rehearsal of the movement pattern and can be implemented as part of a regular practice schedule. Imagery can be either internal (i.e., viewing through your own eyes) or external (i.e., imagining you are an external observer watching yourself). Imagery training directs attention to the movement, promotes self-monitoring, and assists with positive self-reinforcement (Kirschenbaum, 1987). Refer to exercise 13.4 for some guidelines for effective imagery training.

Imagery Training

Exercise 13.4

Imagery Process

1. *Visualizing simple objects.* The ability to visualize images and scenes takes time and practice. When you first attempt imagery, it is best to simply practice visualizing stationary objects. For instance, look closely at an object in the room, at its size, shape, color, and texture. Now close your eyes and try to visualize the object. Try to remember all of the details you noticed with your eyes open. Then open your eyes and compare your image with the object. Were you able to easily visualize this object? Were there details that you missed? Next, try visualizing an object in another room without looking at it first. After visualizing the object, go into that room and compare your image with the object. Did your visualization closely resemble the object?

2. *Visualizing yourself completing daily activities.* The next step in imagery training is to practice controlling images of your movements in the environment. It is best to start with simple activities such as your morning routine. Close your eyes and imagine yourself lying in your bed. If you use an alarm, hear your alarm sound. What does it sound like? How does your body react to the alarm? Then follow your normal morning routine in your mind. What do you do next? Be sure to include all of your senses. What does your shampoo smell like? How does the water feel on your skin? Can you hear the sound of the shower?

3. *Visualizing yourself in a competitive event.* Once you can control images in a simple environment, you can practice imagery for a more complex environment such as a competitive event. During this practice, begin by imagining the entire scene before the competition even begins. What are the sights, sounds, and smells? Now move into imagining the entire event. Try to control the outcome. It is important that you visualize yourself performing well, because this will increase your confidence and motivation. If you find yourself having trouble controlling the images, or if you are visualize poor performances, go back and practice visualizing simple objects and movements. Imagery is a learned skill, and developing it may take some practice.

Questions

1. How vivid were your images? Which details seemed the most vivid? Did you visualize any unintentional images?
2. Did you incorporate all of your senses (sight, sound, smell, touch)?
3. Were you able to control your movements and the outcome in the competitive event?
4. Did you use internal imagery or external imagery?

Sociocultural Factors

Social and cultural influences on physical activity behaviors continue across the life span. Prior to adulthood, the primary socializing occurs in home and school settings. The dominant socializing influences during adulthood include the media; significant others; friends; and community members, including instructors and health professionals (Gabbard, 2012). Physical activity and sport participation are also largely affected by life cycle changes, including marriage, the birth of children, career, retirement, and other transitions (Mihalik, O'Leary, Mcguire, & Dottavio, 1989).

Most people attain peak physical performance during young adulthood. Many continually test their physical abilities during this stage. On the other hand, many adults do not engage in adequate physical activity because they believe they are already healthy and are not concerned with the lifelong benefits of physical activity. Once this attitude is established, it can be difficult to overcome, especially as people begin to decline physically (Gabbard, 2012). As they approach middle adulthood, around the age of 35 to 40, many people become increasingly concerned about their physical abilities and appearance. One of the main causes of these heightened concerns is the media, which often emphasize youth, beauty, and vitality. On a positive note, the media have also flooded society with educational information on healthy behaviors through advertisements, websites, and community medical organizations. The increased promotion of healthy behaviors and the focus on youthful appearance have had a very positive impact on young and middle-aged adults' attitudes toward physical activity. See the sidebar Watch More Television to Improve Healthy Behaviors?! for a research study on the positive effects of television and healthy behaviors. Now more than ever, people are realizing the benefits of a physically active lifestyle, including decreased risks for cardiovascular disease, high cholesterol, high blood pressure, and type 2 diabetes.

Unfortunately, ageism (i.e., the stereotyping of older adults based on their age) still exists in today's society. One sign of it is decreased expectations of older adults professionally, physically, and cognitively. These negative perceptions devalue older adults, often affecting their opportunities, choices, and lifestyles. Someone who is expected to become increasingly sedentary with age is likely to fulfill that prophecy.

Social Theories of Aging

There are two main theories of aging: activity theory and disengagement theory. **Activity theory** suggests that adults who maintain social interactions and active lifestyles can not only maintain their life satisfaction but may even increase it (Rook, 2000; Schaie & Willis, 1991). **Disengagement theory** asserts that older adults must gradually withdraw from society by participating in fewer activities and decreasing their personal relationships. Disengagement theory suggests that older adults need to separate themselves from society to maintain their integrity by accepting their changing status and physical decline. Because participation in physical activity often involves social interaction, increased physical activity would be considered counterproductive according to the disengagement theory because it asserts that older adults need to *decrease* personal relationships. Activity theory, however, suggests that active and productive lifestyles are necessary to sustain happy and satisfying lives. Physical activity often involves social interaction, helping older adults to remain attached rather than detaching from society (Gallahue, Ozmun, & Goodway, 2012). Activity theory also asserts that adults should continue their roles throughout life. If they discontinue a particular activity—for example, when they retire—they should find other activities to replace it.

Social Support

Perceived social support of family, friends, and community members is a significant factor in young adults' (Darlow & Xu, 2011) and older adults' exercise adherence (Chogahara, O'Brien Cousins, & Wankel, 1998). Perceived social support is the anticipation of help from one's social network. This may be different from the actual social support received. Most research in the area of social support focuses on the benefits of perceived social support rather than actual received social support (Rackow, Scholz, & Hornung, 2014).

Those who provide social support and affect a person's adherence to a healthy lifestyle, including physical activity, are termed **socializing agents**. Socializing agents change across the life span: parents are the primary socializing agents for infants and children, and peers become the primary socializing agents for adults.

When compared to younger adults, older adults generally have poorer social networks (Stephens & Craig, 1990). Ageism may contribute to reduced social support from family members, and peers are often less active themselves. Given the decreased support of older adults, physical activities that involve social interaction may be most

---

RESEARCH NOTES

My Friend Laura

Social networks are unquestionably important for helping older adults adhere to exercise programs. However, as previously mentioned, many older adults do not receive much, if any, social support. Many live alone and are fairly isolated from society. Given the ubiquitous presence of technology today, it is not surprising that computer-animated images have been designed to motivate adults to increase their daily physical activity. These computer-animated images, termed relational agents, are also designed to build long-term social–emotional relationships with them.

Bickmore Caruso, Clough-Gorr, and Heeren (2005) conducted a two-month study with 21 adults between the ages of 62 and 84 to see whether a relational agent would increase the daily number of steps walked. The relational agent maintained conversations with the participants, encouraged them to be physically active, and discussed their progress. The results revealed that the relational agent, Laura, increased the older adults' physical activity levels. According to some of the participants, not only did Laura motivate them to increase their physical activity, but they also formed a social bond with her. The relational agent "may be an ideal platform to provide an effective automated health educator with unbounded patience and empathy for . . . patients" (Bickmore et al., 2005, p. 733).

The following is part of a sample conversation between a user (U) and the relational agent (A):

A: Hello, Bertha. Great to see you.

U: Hi, Laura.

A: How are you feeling today?

U: I'm not feeling so great.

A: I am sorry to hear that. Tell me more about how you are feeling.

U: I'm tired.

A: How tired are you feeling?

U: I'm pretty beat.

A: Good grief, I hope you're not getting sick. Can you get some rest soon?

U: I think so.

A: That is great. I hope you come back feeling refreshed.

U: Me too!

A: So, are you from the East Coast originally?

helpful. Older adults with mutual interests in particular activities may be able to encourage each other to continue participating. Adults who live in active neighborhoods in which people are outside walking and gardening may be more inclined to be active themselves. Day-to-day interactions with neighbors can complement other social networks such as family and friends (Gardner, 2011).

Erikson's Psychosocial Development Theory: Adulthood Stages

As discussed in chapter 12, Erik Erikson's psychosocial theory (1963, 1980) on human development consists of eight stages. Each stage is represented by a conflict that must be resolved before the person can advance to the next stage. Although no one perfects a stage, resolving each stage increases the likelihood of further progress in advanced stages. Table 13.1 provides a summary of Erikson's last three stages of psychosocial development (Erikson, 1963). The first five stages, which have to do with psychosocial development from infancy to early adolescence, were discussed in chapter 12. This section describes the final three stages of psychosocial development during adulthood, beginning in late adolescence. We also consider implications for motor development.

Intimacy Versus Isolation

Erikson believed that during young adulthood (ages 19-40), people focus on exploring personal relationships. At this stage of life, it is vital for people to form personal and committed relationships. Young adulthood is a transitional period in which people acquire more responsibilities and liberties than they had during childhood and early adolescence; they move out of their parents' homes and start making their own decisions. This experience is often quite liberating and allows young adults to better understand who they are as individuals and how they fit with and influence other people.

Table 13.1 Erikson's Psychosocial Stages of Development

Approximate age	Psychosocial conflict
20 to 40 years	Intimacy versus isolation
40 to 65 years	Generativity versus stagnation
65 and over	Integrity versus despair

Adapted from E.H. Erikson, 1963, *Childhood and society*, 2nd ed. (New York: W.W. Norton), 263-269.

Young adults also form relationships through group recreational and sporting experiences. Those who cannot work cooperatively on a team may feel a sense of isolation, whereas those who can develop relationships with a team or group members will likely feel a greater sense of intimacy. Keep in mind that Erikson's psychosocial stages are like building blocks. One must be in place before the next one is formed. People must form their own identities during adolescence (stage 5) before they can develop intimate relationships. Young adults who have not developed a strong sense of self often have less committed relationships and are likely to feel lonely and isolated.

Generativity Versus Stagnation

Erikson believed that during adulthood (ages 40-65), people's focus shifts to career and family. Adults during this stage are less interested in their own problems and more interested in how they can affect future generations by nurturing their own children, helping other children through education or other support systems, or having a positive influence on society. Adults interested in movement and physical activity may focus on improving society by increasing physical fitness, or by passing on to their peers or even future generations the self-fulfillment of involvement in recreation and sport. Adults who shift their concentration from self-interests to the interests of others during this stage feel fulfilled because they have contributed to future generations in their local communities or globally. Successful adults experience feelings of usefulness and accomplishment, whereas adults who fail during this stage often have a shallow sense of self. Self-absorbed adults experience increased difficulties dealing with their changing capabilities through middle and old adulthood.

Integrity Versus Despair

The final Erikson psychosocial stage occurs during late adulthood (beyond 65 years). This stage is marked by reflecting on one's life. Successful adults in this stage can reflect with a sense of fulfillment, whereas adults who fail at this stage experience much regret, which leaves them feeling bitterness and despair. Adults who reflect on their life with a feeling of accomplishment and sense of satisfaction attain a sense of integrity. Successful adults at this stage also gain a sense of wisdom that reaches beyond their own lives. In the movement domain, those who are successful can adapt their movements to their changing capabilities, enabling them to sustain an independent lifestyle. Rather than feeling despair about their declining function, they maintain an active lifestyle, continuing to walk, swim, play tennis, or stay involved in other recreational or sport activities. This allows them a much greater sense freedom and enjoyment of life. Adults who sustain active lifestyles have accepted their changing physical capabilities and maintain their competence rather than feeling despair about their declining physical bodies. Those who feel despair often limit their physical activities, which results in further physical decline.

Cognitive Function

The many age-related structural changes in the brain include a daily loss of thousands of brain cells, which progressively decreases the size and weight of the brain. Also, many detrimental changes occur within the neurons, including plaques and tangles (see chapter 10), which affect cognitive function. Given the many large structural changes that occur in adulthood, cognition is surprisingly only minimally affected.

The two cognitive functions most affected by aging are attention and memory. Age-related changes in attention and memory are not uniform; some areas are well maintained in older adulthood, whereas others exhibit substantial declines. Deficits in these areas can have significant effects on sport performance. Older adults may be able to maintain their performance levels during training sessions but have more difficulty performing with increased arousal, such as during a competition. This is because their attentional capacities are already decreased due to age-related declines.

Attention

Humans are limited in the amount of information they can process at one time. This is referred to as attentional capacity (see chapter 2 for more information on attention). We can attend to or concentrate on only one thing at a time. If people try to process more information than their capacity can hold, interference occurs. When someone attempts to perform two activities at the same time, whether it is juggling while unicycling or simply holding a conversation while walking, interference will occur if attentional capacity is exceeded.

Interference can be either cognitive or structural. When physical structure limits a person's actions, **structural interference** has occurred. Humans have two hands, which limits the number of activities they can do at any given time with their hands. For instance, typing while catching a ball would cause structural interference. The performance of one activity would be impaired, most likely the typing in this case. The person would

have to briefly stop typing to catch and toss the ball before resuming typing. We are also structurally limited by our eyes. We can visually focus on only one thing at a time. A person cannot see a pass happening behind her if she is focusing on the defender in front of her. These limitations are not the result of attentional capacity; rather, they are imposed by our physical bodies.

Given these structural limitations, when multiple activities are performed, the decrement that occurs is to the result of limited central capacity, or **cognitive interference**. Attentional capacity, although limited, is flexible. With practice and increasing skill, the attentional capacity necessary to perform a particular skill can increase. You may have observed that older adults often slow down when they are engaged in conversation. Most young adults can hold conversations while walking without interference, but if one task becomes increasingly difficult (e.g., answering a difficult question), even young adults' attentional capacities may be exceeded. This can cause them to either slow down or take longer to answer the question.

Attention is also selective. Selective attention is the ability to focus on selected sensory information while ignoring irrelevant information (Määttä, Pääkkönnen, Saavalainen, & Partanen, 2005). Selective attention can be either intentional or incidental (Eimer, Nattkemper, Schröger, & Prinz, 1996). We can choose to attend to something (intentional attention), such as reading a paper, holding a conversation, or learning to juggle, but our attention can then unexpectedly be directed to something else (incidental attention) such as a phone ringing, our name being called, or the sound of a referee's whistle.

Age-Related Changes in Selective Attention

Intentional attention declines with increasing age as a result of age-related reductions in attentional capacity (Van Gerven

& Guerreiro, 2016). Envision an older woman browsing the Internet, which is not a familiar task. While searching for some information, she is continuously bombarded with pop-ups and advertisements. Dealing with all of the distractions is likely challenging. Perhaps in addition to the many distractions on her computer, she is also in a noisy coffee shop with people coming and going, coffee grinding, conversations happening, and possibly even some background music. For this woman, a simple Internet search may become an overwhelming challenge.

Because of their reduced attentional capacity, older adults have been referred to as cognitive misers because they tend to focus specifically on one component of a task while ignoring others (Hess, Follett, & McGee, 1998). You may have noticed this in an older adult such as your grandfather to whom you had to repeat a message multiple times when he was focused on another task such as reading a newspaper or watching television. Older adults are even more impaired in their auditory selective attention (i.e., focusing on voices or music) when there is a visual distraction (Van Gerven & Guerreiro, 2016).

Focusing on one task while ignoring others is a compensation mechanism. Older adults realize that they have fewer cognitive resources than they had when they were younger and must focus only on the most relevant information. Their ability to attend is also affected by other factors such as the time of day; it is significantly worse in the morning than in the afternoon (Lustig & Meck, 2001). For instance, older adults may perform worse in a morning game of tennis than in an afternoon game because they are more

WHAT DO YOU THINK?

Exercise 13.6

Looking at the illustration, list all of the activities that the multitasker is completing. Give two examples of structural and cognitive interference that are affecting his performance on one or more of these tasks at any given time.

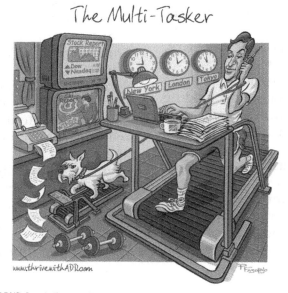

easily distracted; they attend to irrelevant cues rather than focus on relevant cues such as the ball speed, the position of the opponent, and the angles of the hits.

Arousal and Attention

A strong relationship exists between arousal and attention. This is explained by the cue-utilization hypothesis (Easterbrook, 1959). (See chapter 2 for further information on arousal and attention.) This hypothesis states that attentional focus progressively decreases with increasing levels of arousal. With low arousal levels, attentional focus is very broad. This is detrimental because it causes people to be easily distracted. For example, in American football, a cornerback with a very broad attentional focus could be easily distracted by players on the sidelines, the crowd, or other environmental noise (irrelevant stimuli) rather than focusing on the movements and positions of the quarterback and receiver (relevant stimuli). As arousal levels increase, attentional focus becomes progressively narrower. At a moderate arousal level, irrelevant cues are ignored, and the person can solely focus on task-relevant stimuli. Some refer to this as being in the zone. If arousal levels continue to increase, attentional focus will become too narrow, and relevant cues will be lost. The cornerback whose arousal levels are too high may miss a cue from the quarterback, preventing him from blocking a pass. This progressive reduction in attentional focus is termed **perceptual narrowing**.

The cue-utilization hypothesis can explain the inverted-U principle of arousal with regard to performance and arousal levels. When the arousal level is too low, the person is distracted by irrelevant stimuli. Attention becomes progressively narrower with increased arousal. Performance initially improves with increasing arousal because irrelevant cues are being eliminated, helping the performer to focus on the relevant cues and not be distracted by irrelevant cues. Performance peaks at a moderate level of arousal. (The optimal level of arousal is task dependent.) If the arousal level continues to increase, the performer will begin to miss relevant cues. When the arousal level becomes too high, performance is degraded because the person's perception is too narrow to include all of the necessary task-relevant cues. Once task-relevant cues begin to be eliminated, performance worsens.

Age-Related Changes in Arousal and Attentional Capacity

Age-related differences are found with increases in arousal. Studies have shown that young, middle-aged, and older adults exhibit parallel increases in arousal levels when performing in competitive events in comparison to relaxed settings as measured by heart rates and subjective anxiety ratings (Molander & Bäckman, 1989, 1994). Although the young adults performed similarly or even better with increased arousal levels, middle-aged and older adults performed significantly worse during competitive events than during training (Molander & Bächman, 1994). These effects may be task or skill dependent, however, because less competitive anxiety has been reported in more skilled amateur golfers competing at a World Amateur Golf championship in comparison to less skilled golfers. The more skilled golfers also reported greater use of psychological skills such as imagery, positive self-talk, and goal setting, as well as less worry and negative thinking than the less skilled golfers did (Bert, Petrie, MacIntire, & Jones, 2010).

Molander and Bäckman (1994) examined the effect of age and increased arousal in miniature golf. Young adults performed well in competitive environments, whereas middle-aged and older adults performed significantly worse. Even though all age groups showed a similar increase in arousal levels from training sessions to competition, the middle-aged and older adults may have experienced declines in their performance because they had higher arousal levels during training than the younger adults had. It is possible that they were already in the zone during training, and so further increases in arousal led to performance declines (Molander & Bächman, 1994).When their arousal levels increased even further during the competitive events, they were losing task-relevant stimuli. Because the young adults had lower arousal levels during training, the increase in arousal levels may have either kept them in the zone or brought them up to the zone.

The results of this study also indicate that age-related changes in performance as a result of stress (arousal levels) occur during middle age and that no further declines are found in older age. The authors explained that this change may be due to a shift from an external attentional focus in young adulthood to an internal (self-reflective) attentional focus. Middle-aged and older adults reported being distracted more than the younger adults and spent significantly less time

concentrating prior to swinging. This is especially surprising given that miniature golf is a self-paced motor skill, and there is no pressure to initiate the swing early. Furthermore, although the young adults increased their concentration time in increasingly stressful situations, middle-aged and older adults decreased their concentration time. This may also be explained by a reduction in attentional capacity under stressful conditions with increasing age.

Memory

Memory is often divided into short-term memory and long-term memory. Short-term memory stores information for only approximately 20 seconds, whereas long-term memory is seemingly limitless. Information in short-term memory can become stored in long-term memory by rehearsing the information and associating it with meaning. For instance, associating some-

RESEARCH NOTES

Can Older Adults Improve Their Attentional Capacities With Training?

Older adults perform significantly worse in dual tasks (performing two tasks concurrently) than young adults do. This is not surprising given that older adults have significantly reduced attentional capacities, including selective attention and divided attention (i.e., the ability to attend to more than one sensory input at a time; Verhaeghen, Steitz, Sliwinski, & Cerella, 2003). Bherer, Kramer, and Peterson (2008) investigated whether training would improve older adults' performances in dual tasks. A total of 88 adults (44 younger and 44 older) performed a task involving two visual tasks (color discrimination [yellow or green] and letter discrimination [B or C]) and two motor responses. Participants were given one of three instructions on how to prioritize their responses: (1) Respond to the color first; (2) respond as fast as you can on both tasks; (3) respond to the letter first. Each instruction was given twice per session. The results revealed that both younger and older adults significantly improved their performances on the dual tasks. Both groups also performed well on a slightly different task, indicating that this training program was generalizable. The authors suggested that cognitive plasticity (changes in the organization of the brain as a result of experience) in attentional capacity is possible at any age through training.

one's name with a name from your favorite movie may help you move this information into long-term memory. See chapter 2 for more on memory.

Short-Term Memory

Short-term memory can be subdivided into primary memory and working memory. Both are responsible for holding small amounts of memory for short durations, but information that is also manipulated is in working memory. Recalling a list of words is an example of using **primary memory**. Very little decline is seen in primary memory with age. Reorganizing the list of words alphabetically is an example of using working memory, because you must not only recall the list but also manipulate the order of the words. Working memory does decline with advancing age (Luo & Craik, 2008). This is likely due to the increased effort required to remember and manipulate information.

Long-Term Memory

Long-term memory can be subdivided into declarative and procedural memory. **Declarative memory** refers to memories that are consciously available through recollection or recall. Declarative memory includes episodic and semantic memory. **Episodic memory** refers to memories that are associated with a time, such as the tragic events of 9/11 or memorable events such as your high school graduation day. It is likely that many people not only remember what 9/11 refers to, but even specifically remember where they were and what they were doing when they heard that the Twin Towers had been hit by airplanes. **Semantic memory** refers to general knowledge and memories that are not associated with time, such as knowing your school colors, the function of scissors, or personal experiences. **Procedural memory** refers to memories about how to perform tasks such as tying shoes, starting a car, or shooting a layup.

Older adults often complain of memory changes with advancing age (Vestergren & Nilsson, 2011). However, objective measures of memory indicate that only some types of memory decline with age (Nyberg, Lövdén, Riklund, Lindenberger, & Bäckman, 2012). Some of the changes associated with age-related memory declines were actually more strongly due to mood than age (Mowla et al., 2007). In addition, not all areas of memory decline at the same rate. Procedural memory, the type of memory that enables the acquisition and performance of motor skills, shows little change with age. This is likely because procedural memory is largely automatic and cannot be verbalized (Luo & Craik, 2008). In general, semantic memory also holds up well with age; however, certain things, such as names, can become hard to recall. The greatest age-related decline in memory is found in episodic memory, such as remembering personal experiences.

Recall and recognition are both long-term memory processes, but only one is affected by aging. **Recall** refers to retrieving long-term memories with very few cues, which requires much conscious effort. **Recognition** requires both conscious and unconscious processes and is considered easier than recall because it provides environmental support (Craik, 1986). An example of recognition is choosing a word from a list rather than remembering it without any cues. An intense memory search is not required for recognition, but it can be for recall. Memory tasks that are strategic or effortful are more difficult for older adults, such as recalling a particular word, a person's name, or items on a grocery list (Zelinski & Kennison, 2001). However, older adults are very good at recognizing items or names.

Adults can use many strategies to improve long-term memory.

- *Group it.* People can memorize up to about seven items fairly well. The key to memorizing larger amounts of information is to group, or chunk, items. For instance, if you have a grocery list, group the vegetables, the meats, and the dairy. It is much easier to remember 15 items if you know you have five in each of the three categories. It's also much easier to remember a phone number if you are already familiar with the area code.

• *Repeat, repeat, repeat.* For information to move from short-term memory to long-term memory, it must be rehearsed. This is why it is so easy to forget the name of a person you just met. If someone says her name but you do not repeat it in your head or back to her, it will likely be lost. By simply repeating the name in your head once or twice or associating it with a sentence or something or someone familiar, you will be much more likely to remember it.

• *Make a jingle.* If you can make a tune out of the information or associate it with a familiar tune, you are much more likely to retain the information. For instance, if you have just met someone and know a song with the person's name in the title, you will probably not forget the name if you sing the song in your head. Think about it. You probably still sing the alphabet song when you need to alphabetize something!

• *Concentrate.* If nothing else, simply concentrate when you are receiving the information. It's a no-brainer that if you are not focused, you are simply not going to remember.

Summary

This chapter discussed functional constraints in adulthood including psychological, sociocultural, and cognitive factors. It is important to distinguish psychological and sociocultural factors in adulthood from those in childhood, because they can change quite considerably. Adults have different intentions and barriers with respect to exercise. Older adults generally place less value on exercise and perceive more barriers. Socializing agents change throughout adulthood as well. Young adults are more likely to have a strong social structure that can have a very positive influence on their attitudes toward physical activities and their motivation to engage in them. These are important factors to consider when developing a program for adults.

It is important to remember that adults vary widely, and that this variability increases with age. With increasing age, adults are affected by more and more experiences and at the same time dealing with age-related structural and functional changes. These factors combine to make adults increasingly unique with age. To further complicate matters, cognitive function declines at different rates. The greatest basic cognitive changes occur in attention and memory; however, the two are not uniformly affected. Some types of attention and memory are largely unaffected, whereas others decline significantly. And again, the amount of decline depends on the person. Some people maintain most of these abilities through late adulthood; others show decline decades earlier. It is perhaps even more important to assess adults on an individual basis than it is to assess children and adolescents on an individual basis.

ONLINE LEARNING

Visit the web resource at www.HumanKinetics.com/MotorLearningAndDevelopment for an accompanying lab activity and exercises from the chapter.

LEARNING AIDS

Supplemental Activities

1. Memory Tests
    a. Conduct an Internet search on both long- and short-term memory tests. Complete at least two of them. Describe the tests and report how well you performed on them. Do you believe these tests are valid? Explain your answer.
    b. Search the Internet for strategies to improve memory. Describe at least two of them. Do you believe these strategies would improve memory? Explain your answer.
2. There are many infomercials for products that advertisers claim can slow age-related declines (e.g., enhance memory or attentional focus, perhaps even motivate older adults to be more active). Refer to the research note My Friend Laura in this chapter, which is about a socializing agent designed to motivate adults to be more physically active. Discuss some products that are designed specifically to assist with age-related psychosocial or cognitive changes (or both). Do you think these would be effective? Is there anything you would change about the product? Is the marketing targeted specifically to older adults or to any adults?

Glossary

activity theory—A social theory on aging that suggests that adults who maintain social interactions and active lives can not only maintain life satisfaction, but also perhaps even increase it.

Bandura's social cognitive theory—A theory asserting that self-efficacy determines (a) whether someone is even going to attempt a task, (b) how persistent the person will be amid challenges, and (c) the final outcome (e.g., either successful maintenance of an exercise program or failure to adhere to the program).

cognitive interference—A decrease in performance as a result of exceeding one's attentional capacity due to a limitation in central capacity.

commitment stage—Stage 2 of Kirschenbaum's self-regulation process, in which the person commits to making the sacrifices necessary to persevere through the process of making a change.

declarative memory—Memories that are consciously available through recollection or recall, including both episodic and semantic memory.

disengagement theory—A social theory on aging that asserts that older adults must separate themselves from society to maintain their integrity by accepting their changing status and physical decline.

environmental management stage—Stage 4 of Kirschenbaum's self-regulation process, in which adults prepare strategies to deal with environmental or social barriers that may prevent them from attaining their goals.

episodic memory—Memories that are associated with personal experiences and are related to a specific period in time; the ability to remember personal events.

execution stage—Stage 3 of Kirschenbaum's self-regulation process, the active stage of behavioral change. During this stage the person develops self-expectancies for success through goal setting.

external locus of control—The belief that actions do not affect the environment and that events happen by chance.

generalization stage—Stage 5 of Kirschenbaum's self-regulation process, in which people focus on sustaining their efforts for long periods of time.

imagery—A form of mental practice that involves a visual or kinesthetic representation of performance; the visualization or cognitive rehearsal of a movement.

internal locus of control—The belief that actions affect the environment.

locus of control—People's perceptions of their influence on the environment.

motivation—A set of reasons or a personal drive that determines behavior.

perceptual narrowing—A progressive reduction in attentional focus with an increased level of arousal.

primary memory—Information that is actively available in short-term memory.

problem identification stage—Stage 1 of Kirschenbaum's self-regulation process, in which adults identify the problem and must decide whether the change is possible and worth the effort.

procedural memory—Memories about how to perform tasks.

recall—The ability to retrieve long-term memories with very few cues, requiring much conscious effort.

recognition—The retrieval of long-term memories, requiring both conscious and unconscious processes, with the help of environmental support.

semantic memory—The ability to remember general knowledge built from life experiences and learning.

socializing agents—(1) People who affect someone's adherence to a healthy lifestyle, including physical activity. (2) People who influence the development of someone's social role, such as parents, teachers, and coaches. One of the major elements of the socialization process.

structural interference—Interference that occurs as a result of a physical structure.

theory of planned behavior—A theory that asserts that attitudes toward a behavior depend on two factors: (1) the belief that the behavior will produce a specified outcome and (2) the person's desire to attain the specified outcome.

PART IV

Designing Developmentally Appropriate Programs

Now that you understand the foundational concepts in motor learning and motor development and have explored life span changes including structural and functional constraints from infancy to older adulthood, you are ready to learn how to design developmentally appropriate programs. In part IV, we strongly encourage you to use the knowledge you have gained to individualize programs for each learner.

It is quite clear that practice is essential for acquiring a motor skill, but the amount of practice that is necessary and how it should be organized are probably much less obvious. Part IV explores key factors in arranging both physical and mental practice. Scheduling practice is a complex topic. Variables such as age, experience, and the type of skill affect whether a particular form of practice will actually accelerate learning. We consider when and how to use variable, part, and whole practice and also discuss the distribution of practice. Next, we consider feedback. Feedback helps performers execute the proper movement patterns, motivates them, and reinforces successful performances. It is perhaps obvious that feedback is critical when people are learning a new motor skill, especially a complex one, but as with practice, many considerations come into play. Each of these issues is examined, including the type, frequency, and timing of feedback.

As a practitioner, you must learn how to manipulate constraints to encourage the appropriate movement patterns in your learners. Before implementing a program, you will have to make many instructional decisions, including what teaching style to use, how to optimize motivation, and how to develop tactical skills and decision making. Part IV begins by describing how to structure the environment, which includes physical, affective, and instructional factors (chapter 14). Then we explore these prepractice variables that affect performance and learning: goal setting, demonstrations, verbal instruction, directing attention, and physical guidance (chapter 15). Of course, this is only the beginning of your role as a practitioner. You must also arrange physical practice (chapter 16) and provide appropriate feedback (chapter 17).

Part IV concludes with case studies (chapter 18) to show you how what you learned in this book can be applied in practice. These case studies present real-life situations on a variety of topics ranging from physical education and adapted physical education to the instruction of older adults and rehabilitation.

PHYSICAL, AFFECTIVE, AND INSTRUCTIONAL FACTORS

Chapter Objectives

After reading this chapter, you should be able to do the following:

- Explain why instructors should incorporate problem solving in their instruction.
- Describe physical factors that instructors can manipulate.
- List affective factors that might improve instruction.
- Identify ways to enhance learner motivation.
- Explain how play, learning, and competitive environments differ.
- Describe ways instructors can promote decision making.

How Do We Remain Contemporary?

The Pinegrove Soccer Association has existed in Springfield for 40 years and has overseen player, coach, and referee development in a program for youngsters 5 through 18 years of age. Longtime president Bill is stepping step down after 15 years at the helm. Bill is respected for his leadership and commitment, but he is definitely "old school"; he believes that all players should perform skills just like the pros and therefore that practices should emphasize repetition. He also believes that drills should be done in straight lines because the volunteer coaches have an easier time managing when they are organized that way. A parent representative on the association board, Tony, played university soccer with a coach who did not insist that everyone dribble and kick exactly the same way. His coach also used lots of fun drills such as keep-away and one-on-one challenges rather than repetitive line drills. Tony wonders if some of that thinking might be appropriate for younger players in the Pinegrove association. He volunteers to find out more.

This chapter explores the notion that all players should demonstrate an identical motor pattern, such as with kicking. Should practices focus on repetition and hold players to a gold standard for kicking? Or should coaches (such as in soccer) expect that each player will develop a unique kick and plan practices that involve a lot of self-discovery and self-direction, as long as the players are getting the ball to their teammates? How can coaches prepare the learning environment in terms of equipment, and what impact does this have on learning motor skills? Also, how do coaches address the emotional side of learning? Teachers and coaches have many instructional decisions to make, some of which they can make prior to instruction, including optimizing motivation and considering how to develop tactical skills and decision making. We explore these issues in this chapter.

Gold Standards Versus Variability

Instructors of physical skills sometimes teach with a template in mind (e.g., the movement pattern of a highly skilled athlete). After all, doesn't it make sense to imitate the best? A skiing instructor might encourage her students to emulate the style of the last Olympic champion, and the track coach might highlight the running pattern of Usain Bolt. Because the assumption is that everyone should strive for the gold standard, instructors' feedback is often directed at making everyone similar. However, motor learning theories challenge this gold standard thinking.

As discussed in chapter 3, most motor learning theorists agree that if every movement were stored in memory as a simple motor program, humans would have a storage problem. In addition, the single motor program idea does not provide a logical or theoretical explanation for how novel movements are produced. These questions about storage and novel movements led to the notion of a generalized motor program (see chapter 3) (Schmidt, 1975).

The generalized motor program is argued to contain the skeleton, or abstraction, of a movement pattern rather than a specific movement. For example, an overhead throwing action, as described in chapter 7, might be a motor program that contains feet placement, arm flexion, sequential trunk rotation, weight transfer, arm follow-through, and visual contact with a target. As previously described, the generalized motor program likely includes information about the sequence and relative timing and force of actions. Performers use that program when the task calls for an overhead throw, but it can be modified to meet specific environmental demands. Thus, in baseball, the second baseman throws the ball to first base with less arm flexion than the third baseman uses because the distance of the throw is shorter, and both know to "hurry the throw" when the runner is particularly quick. These situations require variations of the generalized motor program and produce different movement skills that can accomplish the task of getting the ball to the first baseman before the runner. Teachers and coaches need to include throwing variation in their practices to help learners develop generalized motor programs so that they can respond to a variety of movement situations.

Supporters of ecological and dynamic systems thinking also promote variation in movement patterns in practice but for different theoretical reasons than those of supporters of information processing. Variability is viewed very positively in dynamic systems thinking because each person is considered to have a unique signature, or style, in most motor patterns. As a result of varying intrinsic dynamics, such as body size, strength, and experience (chapters 9 and 11) and the self-organizing nature of systems, people are expected to solve movement challenges in different ways. For example, basketball players have been shown to have quite distinct shooting patterns (Button, MacLeod, Sanders, & Coleman, 2003). People with cerebral palsy will certainly walk or reach differently than others do, even those who also have cerebral palsy. Observation of ice hockey players skating quickly reveals unique patterns even to the naked eye. Practice experiences must recognize these differences by presenting opportunities for learners to build on their personal and current capabilities. An instructor may demonstrate one way to shoot a basketball or ice skate, but should anticipate that other patterns will naturally emerge. At other times, an instructor may watch a class and determine that a very direct comment about performance is necessary, perhaps because some learners are struggling. At other times a more direct approach may be necessary to ensure safety in activities such as gymnastics, skiing, and diving. Although **guided discovery** has many benefits, the skilled instructor knows when to be more direct.

Variability in practice is also viewed positively by ecological and dynamic systems thinkers because it mirrors the actual situations in games and sport. Particularly in open sports, participants must frequently adapt their movements to their opponents' actions. Constant practice of the bounce pass in basketball without movement and opponents will not prepare players to lean left and pass around a moving opponent. More formally, if the attractor state for a bounce pass in basketball is too stable, the player will have difficulty with the phase shift necessary to solve the dynamics of the game. Similarly, physical and occupational therapists who may be concerned with improving walking must design practices on surfaces that vary in size and slope.

Davids, Button, and Bennett (2008) summarized these thoughts about variability when they wrote: "Practitioners' traditional emphasis on reducing errors during skill practice by encouraging consistency in motor patterns should be revised to acknowledge the valuable goal of variability in moment-to-moment control as well as long-term learning" (p. 151). According to Davids and colleagues, less time should be devoted to teacher-directed promotion of identical motor patterns, and more time should be devoted to problem solving, discovery learning, and self-regulation. As noted previously, this does not mean that a more direct instructional approach is never appropriate. These authors proposed the term **nonlinear pedagogy** as the foundation of instruction based on dynamic systems—"nonlinear" because of findings that learning is often characterized by rather sudden changes in performance (e.g., to new and more mature motor patterns) rather than by linear increments, as traditionally proposed by most other learning theorists.

Consistent with the principles of the dynamic systems approach, nonlinear practitioners recognize that a learner's solution to a movement challenge is a unique coordination pattern resulting from the self-organization of numerous body systems. Variability among people is natural, and therapists, teachers, and coaches should design practices with this in mind. Also, by changing task, environment, and personal constraints, practitioners can nudge people to new levels of performance and can better replicate in practice the dynamics that exist in real games or life contexts. Of course, in some circumstances, a therapist or instructor will intervene with a particular person and suggest a change in movement pattern, but this is quite different from expecting everyone to perform skills in identical ways.

Davids and colleagues (2008) also proposed that teachers and coaches be called **hands-off practitioners** to reflect a new role consistent with the dynamic systems approach. The hands-off practitioner is just as involved as the traditional practitioner, only in different ways. Davids and colleagues suggested that practitioners using traditional methods present drills to perfect a gold standard of performance for all, use practice skills outside the real context of performance, provide too much instruction and feedback, and overly manage the practice environment. The hands-off practitioner creates "a learning environment for the discovery of optimal solutions by manipulating constraints, interpreting movement variability, and nurturing learners in their search activities" (p. 100). Because there is no one movement solution for all learners, the hands-off teacher or therapist allows greater opportunity for learners to find appropriate personal motor patterns within practice. This prepares them to deal with changing dynamics in real performance situations, particularly in open sports and games. However, even in more closed activities such as bowling and golf, movement patterns must change subtly to accommodate changes in the physical environment or in psychological functioning.

Problem solving, discovery learning, and self-regulation are embraced in dynamic systems thinking as well as in generalized motor programs theory and knowledge-based perspectives, although the

WHAT DO YOU THINK?

Exercise 14.1

1. You just read about generalized motor programs. Choose two skills and complete the following table. (The overhand throw is provided as an example.)

Skill	Sequence of actions	Task goal	Parameters
Overhand throw	Foot placement, arm flexion, sequential trunk rotation, weight transfer, arm follow-through, and visual contact with a target	Getting the ball to first base before the runner	Increased arm flexion to throw far; decreased arm flexion to throw a short distance

2. Describe the role of the practitioner according to the dynamic systems approach.
3. Considering your own beliefs about teaching and coaching is important. This chapter presents a role of teachers and coaches that you were likely not exposed to as a child. Will you adopt this role easily, or will you be tempted to take on a more traditional role? For example, will you provide opportunities for students to make choices based on their interests, or do you prefer to be in control? Explain and justify.

theoretical explanations differ (Wall, Reid, & Harvey, 2007). Even thoughtful educational philosophers (e.g., Dewey, 1916) have acknowledged for many years that the most effective learning occurs through discovery and problem-based activities. So, how can the physical, affective, and instruction dimensions of the learning environment be manipulated to encourage problem solving, discovery learning, and self-regulation?

It might not need stating, but just in case—the learning environment for motor skills should be structured to promote fun. Children, adolescents, and adults list other reasons for participating in sport and physical activity (Gould, Feltz, & Weiss, 1985; Weiss & Williams, 2004), but fun is often at the top of the list. Recall that intrinsic motivation is based on the pure joy of participating, and fun activities would seem to promote this. If you have seen a toddler making noise and repeating actions while playing with toys, or an elementary school gymnasium during a class, you may realize the value of fun and the notion of intrinsic motivation.

Physical Factors

Many physical factors of the environment constrain movement patterns; some can be easily manipulated to create variability in practice and promote discovery learning and problem solving, and others are more difficult to modify. Physical factors can be described as control parameters that may cause a change in an attractor state. Wind, temperature, and humidity cannot be easily changed but surely influence performance. A runner racing with a strong wind in her face will likely alter her motor pattern by leaning a bit more forward than usual, and she will not expect a personal best time. Such environmental constraints are difficult for a teacher or coach to manipulate (moving indoors, if possible, is one option). However, if weather conditions might be a factor on game day, it is best to practice under such conditions.

Factors such as humidity, altitude, and pollutants necessitate that athletes train under similar conditions or acclimatize for some time at the event site, or both, before the competition.

Therapists and teachers can rather easily manipulate physical factors such as the hardness, shape, or size of the surface. Placing a mat on the floor immediately changes the dynamics of jumping, landing, or walking. A teacher who wants the children to look up while dribbling a basketball or stick handling in ice hockey may move everyone into a half or a quarter of the playing space. To avoid bumping into others in the small space, the players have to lift their heads. Of course, they might lose the ball or puck, but that is part of the fun. The game manipulates a control parameter (lifting the head), which should force the player to focus on haptic sensations for dribbling. With time, a new attractor state of dribbling without visual contact with the ball is acquired.

One of the most important task constraints, and one that is quite easily manipulated, is the size and mass of equipment relative to the person. This is often referred to as body-scaled equipment (see chapter 3; Davids et al., 2008; Haywood & Getchell, 2014). Think of a young T-ball player swinging a bat the size and weight of a bat used by a professional baseball player. *Swinging* is probably the wrong word, because the child would likely hold the bat with the hands some distance apart and push the bat forward to hit the ball. The bat is simply too heavy and too long to grasp and swing with a movement pattern approximating that of a baseball player. By changing to a smaller and lighter bat, the T-ball player can swing at the ball with a very different movement pattern (i.e., holding the bat at one end with both hands). Simply by changing equipment size relative to learners (control parameters), practitioners can modify movement patterns and attractor states. Yet limb length, arm strength, experience, and the size of bat relative to the child are factors that may make one child's swing pattern look different from another's. If balls and bats are far too large and heavy, skill acquisition may be adversely affected. Research has demonstrated that hitting performance improves when six- to eight-year-old boys and girls play with body-scaled rackets and low-compression balls (Buszard, Farrow, Reid, & Masters, 2014).

The ideal learning environment has sufficient equipment and targets of different sizes, shapes, and textures, and participants are encouraged to explore. One of your authors challenged a group of fourth-graders to choose a ball, find a space, and throw the ball as high as they could as long as they could catch it. They chose from among small balls, soft Nerf balls, and larger playground balls. Some students threw with one hand and others with two, and throwing technique varied widely. Skilled youngsters tossed the ball almost to the gymnasium ceiling, and others achieved more modest heights. Children were encouraged to change balls as they saw fit, and occasionally, the activity was stopped and some of the children were asked to demonstrate to their peers. With new ideas and another ball, they then began the task anew. This is a simple example of a task with a specific goal (throw the ball up and catch it) that can be accomplished in many different ways by children of diverse skill levels. Also, children were encouraged to challenge themselves at their own level of

RESEARCH NOTES

Children Selecting Equipment for Children

Beak, Davids, and Bennett (2000) described an interesting study in which 10-year-olds showed remarkable ability to select equipment that was best for them. The researchers compared three groups, 10-year-olds inexperienced in tennis, young adults who were also inexperienced, and adults who were experienced in tennis. By placing a 1.8- ounce (50 g) weight at various points along the longitudinal axis, the researchers manipulated the moment of inertia of six rackets (i.e., the resistance of the racket to being rotated). The task was to select the racket that would allow the participants to swing and hit a sponge tennis ball a maximal distance with a forehand drive. Each of the three groups wielded the rackets with and without vision for as long as they wished. Vision of the rackets was occluded by having the participants place the arm through a screen to grasp the racket. Thus, the participants swung the six rackets before choosing a racket to hit the sponge tennis ball. Generally, the children selected rackets with the weight nearer the lower end of the handle, which reduced the moment of inertia. In other words, they were sensitive to their own intrinsic dynamics and could reliably pick the best racket for their own bodies. In fact, the children showed less variability in their choices without vision—that is, when they handled the racket and relied only on haptic cues. It seems they had difficulty integrating visual and haptic cues. The authors suggested that for novice children to become skilled at picking up haptic cues, to which they appear quite sensitive, they need to explore a variety of tennis rackets.

The research of Beak and colleagues (2000), Buszard and colleagues (2014), and the instructor in the story who allowed children to select their own balls with a task in mind provide support for structuring the learning environment with equipment of many sizes and shapes. Instructors who do so will be better able to accommodate a wide variety of skill levels and promote self-discovery and the exploration of movement patterns.

Exercise 14.2

Think of your favorite activity or sport. Using the following example (dribbling a basketball) as a guide, name the environmental, task, and individual constraints involved.

Sport or activity	Environmental constraints	Task constraints	Individual constraints
Dribbling a basketball	Temperature, amount of light, floor surface	Size of the ball, shooting at a large versus small target	Height, limb length, strength, motivation

skill and explore new throws and equipment. This produced variability in throws, and they had multiple practice trials. An information-processing advocate would say that the students were learning a generalized motor program, whereas a dynamic systems thinker would argue that the changes in task constraints were control parameters that pushed the participants into a new attractor state as they explored the perceptual–motor landscape, which better prepared them for a game context that would require them to solve a movement problem.

Almost any equipment can be modified to introduce new physical task constraints to the learning equation. Targets can change in size, amount of movement, and color. Lower the basketball net and see the difference; 5-year-olds can now use a two-handed underarm throw and reach the net, whereas 12-year-olds will try to dunk. Balance beams can be wide or narrow or inclined, with or without obstacles. Racket handles can be long or short, narrow or thick. Gymnastics equipment can be lowered. In rehabilitation settings, the incline of a slope can be changed for infants and toddlers learning to crawl or walk, or the height of the steps can be scaled to the person's size.

This section has stressed how manipulating control parameters in the physical environment may produce a phase shift in the attractor state or movement pattern. The environment can also affect attention and memory. Wide-open, busy, and noisy environments make it difficult for children to attend to the key elements of a lesson if they have not learned selective attention skills and memory strategies. In addition, instructors can manipulate the environment to reduce the difficulty of open skills (e.g., T-ball removes the need to predict the flight of a pitch) or to add challenge and difficulty to a skill practiced in a closed manner (e.g., soccer dribbling around a person who offers token resistance and forces the performer to react after dribbling the width of the field without obstructions).

Affective Factors

A learning environment also has emotional factors. Think of a situation in which you felt at least somewhat confident of success if you persisted, aware that if you made an error it would not be embarrassing. It would be a situation in which you were encouraged to solve movement problems, and the focus was on your personal improvement and performance rather than comparisons with other folks. Now think of another situation in which you had little confidence of success, failure would be public and perhaps embarrassing, and the instructor clearly dictated all class activities and expected your movements to conform to everyone else's. Can you feel the difference? Learners of all ages approach movement tasks with a variety of emotional reactions, and it seems highly likely that the stress of the second scenario would adversely affect learning.

Schmidt and Lee (2014) promoted familiarization and open communication early in the learning experience. Familiarization with the physical environment and the instructor's expectations and style should help to alleviate concerns and facilitate communication between the instructor and learners. Collier (2005) also reminded us that a learning environment is more than a space with equipment; it also possesses emotional dimensions. A positive emotional environment is one in which everyone belongs, is valued, and is treated with dignity. Activities occur in positive, affirming ways to embrace individual differences. This is not restricted to respectful treatment of all learners by the instructor in a top-down manner. A positive emotional environment is also characterized by behaviors among the learners themselves and the behaviors of learners toward the instructor. Mutual respect should be acknowledged and practiced.

Hellison's (2003) model of teaching personal and social responsibility (see table 14.1) may provide guidance for promoting a respectful learning environment. It was originally designed for youth at risk who demonstrated little interest in school, physical activity, or respect for others (Hellison, 1995), and it has been recommended for those with attention-deficit/hyperactivity disorder (ADHD) (Harvey, Fagan, & Kassis, 2003). The five-level model places greater emphasis on the values of self-respect, personal control, self-direction, and respect and caring for others than on traditional curricula of skill and fitness.

Five general strategies help move learners through these levels. **Awareness talks** remind learners about the levels of responsibility, which have been explicitly discussed and posted on the walls. During the lesson itself, responsibility is taught; for example, a cooperative game may be appropriate for a level 1 learner, whereas a level 4 learner is encouraged to help others. **Individual decision making** is the second strategy and is used at each level. A learner at level 1 who senses that she is frustrated and might hit someone in a game decides instead to sit on a bench. A level 5 learner might decide to volunteer at a local Saturday morning community activity program. A **group meeting** involves a discussion of what constitutes self-control and responsibility and is used to establish self-control rules. The students are central to this discussion and arrive at fundamental rules

Table 14.1 Social Responsibility Model

Level	Focus
1. Respecting the rights and feelings of others	Students are taught self-control and personal responsibility to prevent physical and psychological harm to others and to respect the feelings of classmates. Conflict resolution and the right to be included are also components.
2. Participation and effort	Emphasis is on physical activity participation rather than nonparticipation and assuming responsibility for self-motivation. Students are encouraged to determine whether effort is related to improvement and not to give up. Success as a personal accomplishment or degree of effort is explored.
3. Self-direction	Students take more responsibility for their choices and work independently when not supervised. They establish their own goals and plans to achieve those goals, and they evaluate their plans. With stronger self-identity, peer pressure will be resisted.
4. Helping others and leadership	Students are encouraged to support and assist others with compassion and sensitivity, helping those who want help, including conflict resolution. They take leadership roles such as reciprocal teaching and develop the inner strength to make decisions that might not be popular.
5. Outside the gym	Students are encouraged to transfer responsibility for learning in their physical education classes to other areas such as teaching younger students, participating in service projects, and being role models for others.

Adapted from Hellison 2003.

Exercise 14.3

Review Hellison's model. Provide specific examples of how you could move learners through each level.

Level	Example
1. Respect rights and feelings of others	
2. Participation and effort	
3. Self-direction	
4. Helping others and leadership	
5. Outside the gym	

in the gymnasium that all are prepared to accept. **Reflection time** occurs at the end of each lesson, at which point learners contemplate what went well or not so well in the session. They are encouraged to write in their personal journals, complete checklists, and engage in discussions with others. The final strategy is called **counseling time**, which is time devoted to a discussion of problems identified by the teacher and learners (or the therapist and the client). For example, a teacher might observe that some learners are expending little effort during the physical education class, which is part of level 2. He wants to reinforce the goals the students have established for themselves and communicate that their expenditure of time and effort is not sufficient to reach these goals.

Structuring a positive affective environment of mutual respect among learners and teacher, or between the patient and clinician, is necessary for productive motor learning. People who are highly anxious about the session, fear for their physical or psychological safety, and have little hope of success are not likely to enjoy the lesson or to learn very much. A positive emotional atmosphere conducive to learning involves acceptance of individual differences in skill and an opportunity for students to make decisions, set goals, and self-direct some aspects of learning, all while knowing that effort and personal improvement will be rewarded.

Instructional Factors

There are a number of instructional factors to consider when structuring the learning environment. This section addresses motivation; play, learning, and competitive environments; and decision making and tactical learning.

Motivation

The learning environment must be structured with motivation in mind. Motivation influences initiation and persistence. Self-motivation is also an important dimension in the forethought phase of self-regulation (Zimmerman, 2000). Motivational ideas for practitioners emerge from competence motivation theory (Harter 1978, 1981), self-determination theory (Deci & Ryan, 1985, 2000; Vallerand, 1997, 2007), self-efficacy theory (Bandura, 1997), and achievement goal theory (Nicholls, 1989). Teachers, therapists, and exercise leaders can enhance and maintain participation in physical activity by following the steps explained next (Kilpatrick, Hebert, & Jacobsen, 2002; Ntoumanis, 2001; Vallerand, 2007). Developmental differences are noted as appropriate. Many of the recommendations are cast in self-determination theory because teachers and therapists can influence factors such as achievement and choice. An extensive body of research supports the notion that these factors affect perceived competence, autonomy, and relatedness, the three needs posited in self-determination theory. Also, when the learner is permitted to control aspects of practice, feelings of autonomy and competence are likely to increase (Sanli, Patterson, Bray, & Lee, 2013). The following list is theoretically sound and manageable by instructors.

- *Promote achievement.* The learning environment should provide much opportunity for successful experiences. Not surprisingly, positive achievements enhance personal self-efficacy and competence and are important mediators of intrinsic motivation. Professionals can increase success by creating the positive affective environment discussed earlier, manipulating environmental and task constraints, and encouraging learners to be actively involved in the discovery learning process. This does not mean manipulating the environment to avoid failure on all attempts or trials, because learning can result from analyzing why something went wrong and trying a new way. However, repeated failure in a physical activity is destined to decrease motivation and result in little interest in that activity. Learners seek opportunities in which to demonstrate their competence and are usually intrinsically motivated to learn physical skills. Even observing someone succeed who is similar to oneself can have a positive impact on self-efficacy and performance (Bandura, 1997).

- *Promote a mastery climate.* A **mastery climate** is one in which participants are encouraged to improve their skills, and success is judged by a positive change in performance, not in comparison to others. This contrasts with an **ego-involved climate**, in which participants are encouraged to improve their skills to outperform others. In the ego-involved climate, success is defined in comparison to other people in the group or some idealized model. Generally speaking, before children begin school, they are largely unaware of how they compare to others in terms of movement skills. Most are intrinsically motivated to move

and are eager to explore and learn. From ages 5 to 12 years there are many opportunities for comparison in physical education classes or community sport and physical activity programs. If the star athlete is always held up as the idealized example of performance, the underlying message is that others should aspire to such skill levels. Children who adopt this perspective as truth may conclude that they are incompetent and experience reduced intrinsic motivation. The mastery climate champions personal improvement as the important measure of success. Teachers, fitness professionals, and clinicians who point out improvement, regardless of how their charges perform, create a mastery climate that is conducive to self-determined forms of motivation.

- *Provide positive feedback.* Positive feedback promotes learning, intrinsic motivation, and self-confidence with the given task, particularly with more accurate versus less accurate trials (Badami, VaezMousavi, Wulf, & Namazizadeh, 2011, 2012). As we will see in chapter 17, positive feedback is not needed on every trial, but in general, most people of all ages appreciate a therapist or parent saying, "Good effort, I see you are working hard" or "Yes, you have it; that step with the throw really added distance." Verbal feedback or encouragement that is not realistic will teach learners that their capabilities do not match the words of others. Negative feedback is usually associated with a decrease in intrinsic motivation. Henderlong and Lepper (2002) cogently pointed out that other dimensions of praise can have unexpected consequences. For example, praise that is not considered sincere can have the effect of negative feedback. Also, the way feedback is presented is important. If the words convey autonomy (e.g., *You should do this to improve performance*), the participant will feel in control. On the other hand, if the message is controlling (e.g., *You have no choice but to do this*), intrinsic motivation will likely decrease.

- *Provide choice.* Choice facilitates intrinsic motivation. Teachers can allow participants to select their own music to accompany exercise; the size, color, or texture of a ball; or in some cases the task (e.g., *When the music stops, move to the locomotor skill station of your choice and practice the activities on the task card*) (Kilpatrick et al., 2002). Choice promotes autonomy and intrinsic motivation (Lewthwaite, Chiviacowsky, Drews, & Wulf, 2015; Wulf & Adams, 2014; Wulf, Chiviacowsky, & Cardozo, 2014). Physical education teachers and therapists may be constrained to some extent by required curricula or traditional practice, but choice can still be afforded the students or patients within the required activities. With adults, every effort should be made to include them in a broader decision-making process of selecting the activities, as well as the amount of time for instruction, self-directed practice, or play.

- *Promote goal setting.* Preschool children do not require goal setting because they generally play and practice for intrinsic reasons. If an instructor senses that younger school-aged children might benefit from setting goals to promote activity and provide a barometer of success, the children will need assistance in selecting realistic and specific goals (e.g., *You swim the length of the pool with the backstroke in 40 seconds; do you want to aim for 35 seconds?*). Goal setting is consistent with a mastery climate in which personal improvement is emphasized (Kyllo & Landers, 1995). Participants should be encouraged to set moderately difficult personal goals, and adults may benefit from both short-term and long-term goals. The instructor may say, "Yes, I agree that you should try to bump the volleyball 6 times to yourself today, but 10 times with Fred can probably wait for a few sessions." Setting one's own goals is consistent with autonomy. The achieved goals provide a sense of satisfaction, competence, and hence, intrinsic motivation. We discuss goal setting further in chapter 15.

- *Use competition wisely.* Competition with others will arise at some point in many physical activity programs. However, competition should not be a huge part of all programs; rather, practice should emphasize personal skill improvement (e.g., in swimming, skiing, or gymnastics) outside the context of competition. A run can be conceived as a personal method of having a good workout or as a race against others. Realistically, however, competition will be part of units of track or basketball, because even one-on-one drills are inherently competitive. The early literature on motivation with physical tasks showed that competition had a detrimental effect on intrinsic motivation. The sport literature confirmed this finding in those who lost. For winners, and those who did well, intrinsic motivation was enhanced (Vallerand, 2007). Practitioners are cautioned against using too much competition or placing too much emphasis on the outcome when only a few can "win."

A series of basketball studies by Tauer and Harackiewicz (2004) is informative. The researchers assessed the impact of competition, cooperation, and intergroup competition on children's enjoyment of a basketball free throw task. In the competitive situation, enjoyment increased for the winners but decreased for the losers. This was consistent with the intrinsic motivation literature. It was expected from earlier research that cooperation would lead to more enjoyment than competition, but competition and cooperation did not differ in this respect. In fact, intergroup competition resulted in the highest levels of enjoyment. Even though intrinsic motivation and enjoyment are different constructs (although related), Vallerand (2007) tried to explain these surprising findings by postulating that "trying to do well" was emphasized by the researchers. Perhaps the children did not perceive the competitive environment as one of "win at all costs" and thus did not perceive a controlling dimension, so enjoyment was not reduced. In summary, too much competition in a program and excessive importance placed on winning may be viewed as controlling and therefore reduce intrinsic motivation in many participants. Rather, learners should view competition as one way to extend their skills, recognizing that competitors who try their best against them will make them better players.

- *Provide a rationale for activities.* Providing reasons for some activities (e.g., *Many of our activities today are designed to help improve range of motion in your knee and will speed up your recovery*) should provide knowledge about the activities and facilitate a sense of competence and autonomy (Kilpatrick et al., 2002). Therapists and instructors should encourage questions and discussions about the rationale of activities.

- *Promote social interactions.* The desire to be with friends and make new friends is a motive many children mentioned for participating in sport (Weiss & Williams, 2004). Social interaction, or relatedness, is also a need postulated by Deci and Ryan (1985) in self-determination theory. It is expected that creating social relationships in physical activity environments will enhance enjoyment of the activity. Ways to accomplish this include partner and small-group activities that promote new interactions.

- *Use rewards wisely.* The use of rewards has been extensively researched in laboratory tasks (e.g., Deci, Koestner, & Ryan, 1999, 2000). Rewards (e.g., trophies or other tangible items rather than positive verbal feedback) decrease intrinsic motivation if they are presented for participating or completing an activity or for reaching a certain level of performance. They undermine autonomy. If the rewards are unexpected and not related to achievement, they do not decrease intrinsic motivation. Thus, a participant trophy or certificate of practice given to all team members at the end of the year is unlikely to undermine intrinsic motivation if it is unexpected. However, if people participate in sport or exercise to receive a trophy or money from parents, intrinsic motivation toward that activity will likely decrease. This effect is even greater in children than in university-age students (Vallerand, 2007). Likely reasons are that children begin at a higher level of intrinsic motivation or that because of inexperience they do not expect any reward for something they enjoy. Rewards may be useful for people who are reluctant to participate, and the hope is that once they attempt the activity, it will become appealing in itself. More research is needed on this issue, but the thoughtful therapist, teacher, or coach should use rewards sparingly and with awareness that they may detrimentally affect intrinsic motivation, which in turn will lead to a decrease in participation.

Play, Learning, and Competitive Environments

Play has been described as an essential component of optimal human development for many years (e.g., Piaget, 1976; Vygotsky, 1978), and it is a right of every child, according to the United Nations (Milteer & Ginsburg, 2012). Most scholars believe that play contributes to social, cognitive, physical, and emotional well-being (e.g. Ginsburg, 2007). More specifically, play may enhance cooperation, persistence, problem solving, creativity, language development, imagination, negotiation skills, and persistence and the development of strong and healthy bodies. Play is often described as an experience free of an immediate purpose that is inherently enjoyable. Young infants may gaze at their moving hands; by 12 months they may reach and grasp objects (e.g., take pots from accessible cupboards). The 18-month-old may throw a ball and a year later may place favorite cars in a careful line. By age 4, children climb on playground apparatuses, hide in tunnels, and learn self-propulsion on swings. These play activities are repeated time and time again but never in exactly the same way; the children must be having fun! Also, as noted in chapter 11, Piaget argued that cause-and-effect relationships are learned, and in chapter 12 we spoke of autonomy and competence as among the outcomes of early play. Thus, although play seems inherently enjoyable and rather spontaneous, a great deal of social, cognitive, physical, and emotional learning is likely going on. To put it more simply, play is serious stuff.

Get Motivated

Exercise 14.4

Recommendations for enhancing intrinsic motivation are listed in the bulleted paragraphs in the preceding Motivation section. In groups of three, select a sport or physical activity and generate specific examples of how you could use each of these recommendations in teaching and coaching settings. The first example is provided.

Enhancing intrinsic motivation	Example
Promoting achievement	Consider task, individual, and environmental constraints.
Promoting a mastery climate	
Providing positive feedback	
Providing choice	
Promoting goal setting	
Using competition wisely	
Providing a rationale for activities	
Promoting social interactions	
Using rewards wisely	

Developmental stages of play have been proposed since the 1930s (Parten, 1932) to reflect social, cognitive, and emotional changes, but there is no universal agreement about the specific stages. The banging of a rattle at one year is play, but how is it different from two seven-year-olds who amuse themselves with a train set? Table 14.2 outlines some suggested developmental tendencies and types of play.

Table 14.2 emphasizes the social dimensions of play. Some research supports a change from predominately solitary to **parallel** to **cooperative** play as development occurs (e.g., Bakerman & Brownlee, 1980; Dyer & Moneta, 2006; Parten, 1932; Smith, 1978). Of course, adults can engage in solitary play even though cooperative play is well developed. Parents and other social agents affect when such types of play might begin. More recent research into play has begun to include emotional and cognitive growth, in addition to social change, from the perspective of pretend play (e.g., Lillard et al., 2013). In pretend play, a person creates a fantasy role such as that of a superhero.

A **game** is usually defined as having an element of competition and some semblance of rules or guidelines, but players can change the rules to suit the conditions. One-on-one competitions or spontaneous 3v3 basketball games are examples of physical games. A rule requiring all three players to touch the ball prior to a shot can be implemented and repeated the next time the group assembles (or not). Games are more structured than play but less formal than sport. Of course, there are board games and computer games as well.

Sport emerges when coaches, referees, schedules, and standardized rules enter the fray. Organized sport for children and youth has been present for decades in the United States and Canada in forms such as Little League baseball, minor hockey, and age-group swimming and gymnastics. Not unlike play, sport has been argued to have positive outcomes related to physical health, social and psychological well-being, and intellectual involvement (Eime, Young, Harvey, & Payne, 2013; Fraser-Thomas, Côté, & Deakin, 2005; Weiss, 2008). More precisely, increased motor development, reduced obesity, increased perceived competence, a sense of autonomy, initiative, fun, positive social interactions, cooperation, good sporting behavior, and moral reasoning may be associated with sport participation.

How do children become involved in play, games, sport, and physical activity in general? Haywood and Getchell (2014) list three elements: **socializing agents** such as family members, peers, coaches, and teachers; **social situations** such as play environments and toys; and **personal attributes** such as perceived sport ability. The child's immediate social network of parents and siblings and the availability of social environments such as playgrounds influence physical activity play in preschoolers (Haywood, & Getchell, 2014) and children (Fredricks & Eccles, 2004). Parents who value swimming are likely to take their children to the pool, enroll them in swim lessons, and play in the water as a family. Likewise, a backyard or basement with balls, swings, and tricycles provides opportunities for movement competence to grow. Young children may watch parents and older siblings participate in physical activities, listen to them talk about such activities, or both. Ultimately, this will

Table 14.2 Development of Play

Type of play	Development begins at...	Description
Solitary	1 month	The child plays by himself (e.g., filling up a container with sand).
Parallel	2 years	The child plays in near proximity to others on a personal task, seldom interacting with the other children (e.g., playing in the same sandbox as another but focused on her own task).
Cooperative	4 years	Two or more children work together to achieve the same goal (e.g., building a sandcastle together or playing throw and catch).

influence their initial selection of activities and contribute to what they come to value. Personal attributes were discussed in chapter 12 and refer to the child's sense of perceived competence, self-efficacy, and self-regulation. Those who are effective and confident are drawn to activity.

When children begin school, peers are added to the list of socializing agents and will continue to influence physical activity participation into the adult years (Weiss & Stuntz, 2004). Like parents, peers can encourage or discourage participation in specific activities. Coaches and teachers, although not as influential as parents, siblings, and peers, also have a significant socializing influence in childhood. Adults other than parents can have a detrimental impact on participation if they place too much emphasis on winning, embarrass and criticize children, or create tasks and challenges that are too difficult. Fredricks and Eccles (2004) wisely suggested that parents have the most positive impact on the sport participation of their children when they maintain a moderate level of involvement and are neither disinterested nor overinvolved. In adolescence, the role of parents as socializing agents decreases as the impact of peers and coaches increases (Fredricks & Eccles, 2004). Likewise, peers and coaches become a source of information about motor competency after age 10, whereas younger children rely more on their parents (Weiss & Williams, 2004).

The roles played by parents may also change as a function of the dedication to sport. Côté, Baker, and Abernethy (2003) showed that athletes who became highly talented recalled their parents as supportive in allowing them the freedom to practice, formally or not. These experts recalled participating as children in several sports and physical activities, and their parents were often coaches, chauffeurs, and sometimes coparticipants. As dedication to a particular sport began, the parents were seldom coaches but remained supportive by helping the athletes structure practice routines, join fitness clubs, or set up weight rooms at home. As the athletes committed to one sport, the parents' direct role diminished; they may have continued to assist in practice, but most often their roles became relegated to financial support.

Great strides have been made in recent decades to encourage young girls to participate in sport, with considerable success (Hardin & Greer, 2009). Many parents equally support the participation of their children of both sexes. Yet research conducted in the United States and France still suggests that university students (Clement-Guillotin, Chalabaev, Fontayne, 2011; Hardin & Greer, 2009) and parents (Fredricks & Eccles, 2004; Heinze, Heinze, Davis, Butchart, Singer, & Clark, 2014) continue to endorse the belief that sports are more suited to and more important for males than females. Also, the sex stereotyping of sports (e.g., gymnastics or figure skating rather than ice hockey or rugby for girls) continues to influence parents regarding their daughters' participation in sport (Heinze et al., 2014). Practitioners should recognize that these beliefs still exist and attempt to counteract them by providing equal opportunity and encouragement to girls and boys.

Weiss and Williams (2004) proposed a number of reasons children and adolescents participate in sport. These personal attributes in the socialization process (noted earlier) include motor competence (e.g., learn skills, achieve goals), social acceptance (e.g., be with friends, achieve social status), and enjoyment (e.g., have fun, feel excitement). Competence and relatedness dimensions of self-determination are evident in these reasons for participation. Teachers, coaches, and parents should always remember fun because it is mentioned in almost all research as a reason children participate in sport. Saying that fun is a reason is another way of saying that intrinsically motivated behaviors provide enjoyment and pleasure. Although more research is required, it appears that reasons to participate may differ based on age (Haywood & Getchell, 2014). For example, older teens and young adults may place more emphasis on social status and fitness as reasons to participate in sport than younger children or older adults do.

Fitness is a major reason for middle-aged adults to participate in sport, but not for children and older adults.

The positive outcomes of sport for children and youth do not occur magically; rather, they depend on the input of parents and coaches, participant resources, and the structure of the programs (Côté, Lidor & Hackfort, 2009; Petitpas, Cornelius, Van Roalte, & Jones, 2005). If the sport experience is too focused on winning, creates stress in the participants, reduces feelings of competence, produces conflict with peers and coaches, and does not provide fun and playing time, youngsters may become depressed, burn out, and drop out (Bergeron, et al., 2015; Coakley, 1980; Eime et al., 2013; Fraser-Thomas et al., 2005; Orlick & Botterill, 1975). Concern has been expressed that youth sports might be becoming too expensive, competitive, and elitist (Fraser-Thomas et al., 2005) and can be associated with overuse and overtraining injuries (Bergeron et al., 2015; Caine, DiFiori, & Maffulli, 2006).

This chapter discussed many factors to consider to create an optimal learning environment. Although we have downplayed the role of competition as a motivational technique during the acquisition of movement skills, there are certainly times when competition is at the heart of the activity. As such, participants need to be prepared for all aspects of the competitive event or game. The learning and practice environments of athletes are quite different from those of novice participants struggling with learning new movement patterns.

Côté (1999) and colleagues (Côté, Baker, & Abernethy, 2003, 2007; Côté, Lidor, & Hackfort, 2009) proposed the developmental model of sport participation. The model was inspired by Bloom (1985), whose pioneering research in science, art, and athletics determined the antecedents of experts' high level of skill. It appears that sport experts progress toward excellence in much the same way that musicians, chess players, and scholars do (Janelle & Hillman, 2003), but they require 3,000 to 4,000 hours of practice rather than the 10,000 hours often cited as necessary for expertise in other domains. Like Bloom, Côté and colleagues (2003) identified three phases of development: the **sampling years** (ages 6-12), the **specializing years** (ages 13-15), and the **investment years** (16 plus).

The sampling years are characterized by exposure to many fundamental motor skills (see chapter 7) and a wide range of sports with an emphasis on fun and excitement. In the specializing years, the young adolescent begins to spend more time on one or two sporting activities. Skill development takes on a higher priority than during the sampling years, but fun remains a critical component. Côté and colleagues (2003) suggested that the activities pursued at this point are a function of "positive experiences with a coach, encouragement from an older sibling, success, and simple enjoyment of the activity" (p. 93). Adolescents who move into the investment years want to achieve elite levels of performance. The main focus is strategy, competition, and skill development within a context of deliberate practice directed and assisted by a coach.

Côté and colleagues (2003) proposed that the sampling, specializing, and investment years in sport are anchored in the concepts of **free play**, **deliberate play**, **structured practice**, and **deliberate practice**. Table 14.3 provides a comparison of these four types of physical activity participation across six dimensions. Briefly, children move from the free play of infancy and early childhood to deliberate play in which some rules are established and monitored by children or adults. The concept of free play was intentionally included to incorporate play as conceived by Piaget and other developmentalists, and deliberate play has much in common with games, as described previously. From deliberate play, children may elect to participate in the structured practice of a sport in which skill improvement assumes a higher priority than in deliberate play and games. Finally, some highly motivated adolescents move to deliberate practice. Deliberate practice usually includes much hard work,

Table 14.3 Comparison of Free Play, Deliberate Play, Structured Practice, and Deliberate Practice Activities

	Dimensions			
	Free play	**Deliberate play**	**Structured practice**	**Deliberate practice**
Goal	Fun	Fun	Improve performance	Improve performance
Perspective	Process (means)	Process (experimentation)	Outcome (ends)	Outcome (ends)
Monitored	Not monitored	Loosely monitored	Monitored	Carefully monitored
Correction	No correction	No focus on immediate correction	Focus on correction (often through discovery learning)	Focus on immediate correction
Gratification	Immediate	Immediate	Immediate and delayed	Delayed
Sources of enjoyment	Inherent	Predominantly inherent	Predominantly extrinsic	Extrinsic

Reprinted, by permission, from J. Côté, J. Baker, and B. Abernethy, 2003, From play to practice: A developmental framework for the acquisition of expertise in team sports. In *Expert performance in sports: Advances in research on sport expertise*, edited by J.L. Starkes and K.A. Ericsson (Champaign, IL: Human Kinetics), 95.

RESEARCH NOTES

Memories of Elite Athletes

Investigating the time devoted to organized sport, deliberate play, and deliberate practice is difficult because it requires excellent athletes to look back in time. Such a retrospective study was conducted by Soberlak and Côté (2003), who interviewed four 20-year-old athletes who had signed contracts to play in the National Hockey League. Arguably, these were elite athletes. The in-depth interviews of the four players were corroborated by three of the parents to ensure validity of the athletes' recollection of other sports played and time devoted to them. The researchers explored the type of sporting activity, age and level of initial involvement, hours per week and months of the year participating in the activity, and age when participation ended. Among the findings were high engagement in deliberate play (hours per week) during the sampling period, a reduction during the specializing period, and a decline to little or no deliberate play during specialization. As expected, deliberate practice increased in time over the sampling, investment, and specializing periods. During the sampling period of 6 to 12 years of age, the athletes actually increased the number of sports played (from three to six), but they decreased to about three sports in the investment period. The athletes remained at two or three sports in the specializing period, but in addition to ice hockey, participation in recreational activities such as golf and water skiing was typical. Overall, the results supported the three periods of sport development proposed by Côté and colleagues (2003) and suggested that early sport specialization is not necessary to reach elite levels of achievement.

often monitored by a coach; performance outcome is the prime goal.

Figure 14.1 displays the results from a study of the number of hours of participation in various forms of physical activity by young professional ice hockey players. Consistent with predictions, many hours were devoted to deliberate play during the sampling years, which began to decline in the specializing years. Hours devoted to deliberate practice increased during the investment years, at which point there was less involvement in other games. Other research with athletes who perform at outstanding levels supports the value of sampling and specialization prior to significant investment. Overemphasis on one sport at a young age is not usually desirable unless

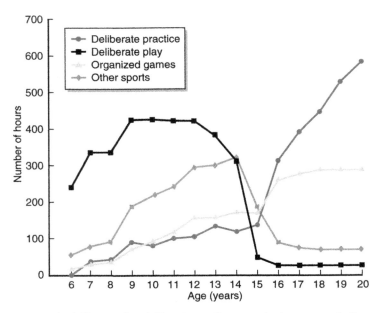

Figure 14.1 Hours spent per year in deliberate play, deliberate practice, organized games, and other sports.

peak performance is usually achieved prior to maturation, as in female gymnastics.

The developmental model of sport participation (Côté et al., 2009) proposes early diversification of sport participation (deliberate play and structured play) until the teenage years, when specialization and deliberate practice may be desirable for some participants. A consensus statement on youth athletic development from the International Olympic Committee (Bergeron et al., 2015) concurs that a variety of age-appropriate physical activities (diversification) in early development is associated with continued involvement in more intense activities later in life, elite performance itself, and continued participation in sport. In other words, diversification does not detract from elite performance in later years if that becomes a personal goal and is less likely to be linked to sport drop out and other negative aspects of youth sport noted previously. Diversification is also associated with intrinsic motivation, self-regulation, positive well-being, and long-term sport involvement. Using the developmental model of sport participation as a framework of youth sport organization and philosophy, coupled with parent and coach education, may go a long way to support the children and youth who entered sport in the first place to improve motor competence, enjoy social acceptance, and have fun (Weiss & Williams, 2004). In addition, it may reduce the negative aspects of youth sport (e.g., stress and drop out) while advancing the positive.

Ericsson (2003) proposed an extension to Fitts and Posner's (1967) three-stage motor learning model (described in chapter 4) to explain one of the mechanisms of expert performance. He asserted that most people arrive at the autonomous level of performance more easily than Fitts and Posner thought. For example, 50 or so hours of training and experience is likely to enable one to ski or drive a car with little effort—that is, relatively autonomously. Most people are satisfied with this level of performance because they have no need to continue working hard—their performance is quite stable, and they can thoroughly enjoy recreational skiing and daily driving. Those aspiring to expert levels of performance, however, are not satisfied with this autonomous stage, and they begin to use cognition once again to move toward sport expertise. In other words, they deliberately try to find better ways to perform the tasks required in their sport. Usually, with the help of a teacher or coach, the person practices with the primary goal of improving performance; this is deliberate practice (Ericsson, 2003). Such practice requires effort without an immediate reward and may not be enjoyable (Côté et al., 2003). The idea of lack of enjoyment during practice may seem disturbing to potential teachers, coaches, parents, and psychologists. The authors of this text are not suggesting that practitioners adopt such deliberate practice as a regular methodology and go out of their way to make practice and training unpleasant. In fact, it seems that in the sport context, as opposed to the musical world, practice for most participants seeking expertise remains rather fun (Deakin & Cobley, 2003).

Free play, deliberate play, structured practice, and deliberate practice share features with three types of environments proposed by Wall and colleagues (2007) to promote a greater depth of knowledge and performance in physical activity. These three environments (instructional, practice, and competitive) capture the additional challenges and social pressure experienced when moving from an environment for novices to one for athletes. "The instructional, practice, and competitive environments can be viewed as a continuum; seeing them this way underscores the need to recognize and assess the performance capabilities of learners in different performance environments" (Wall et al., 2007, p. 270).

Instructional environments are relatively closed and supportive environments that provide instruction, feedback, and encouragement to explore movement options. Such instructional learning environments are typically present in physical education, where ample practice opportunities (and the manipulation of the physical factors noted earlier) are provided. Students are encouraged to move to progressively more difficult tasks and environmental conditions. **Practice environments** are more demanding because more emphasis is on the proper execution of specific skills under increasingly demanding space and time constraints. An instructor or leader controls the practice session by determining the number of players involved, the player roles, the equipment, and the space. In **competitive environments**, the performance expectations and social pressure increase as individuals or teams compete against each other. The performance expectations are lower in younger recreational settings than in older and more elite settings, where expectations can be very high. Aspects of deliberate practice may be present in elite contexts with older participants. Recall that deliberate practice includes more control by the coach, the goal of improving performance, and more effort in practice. Competitive environments can include the stress of evaluative fans, and outcomes may be linked to social prestige and future opportunities in the sport.

Decision Making and Tactical Learning Environments

Physical activities require decision making, which can vary from a simplistic yes or no decision to the complexity of choices inherent in competitive situations. At a minimum, Grehaigne, Godbout, and Bouthier (2001) argued that any voluntary action involves the decision of whether to initiate the action (e.g., *Do I go for a walk or do I remain in front of the TV?*). Exercise

WHAT DO YOU THINK?

Exercise 14.5

Does the developmental model of sport participation reflect your experiences? Do you think it would be a helpful model to adopt to reduce the criticisms of youth sport regarding too much emphasis on winning, too much stress, and athlete burnout?

psychologists are very concerned with factors that compel us to move. Grehaigne and colleagues (2001) offered an interesting example in a more complex life situation. You make a decision to move a heavy object, but you then have to decide how to move it (e.g., pull, push, carry it in your arms, or carry it in a wheelbarrow). This decision will be based on such factors as your perception of your strength, the form of the object, the availability of helpers, and the characteristics of the surroundings. Children's play includes many decisions such as which climbing apparatus to use and how to move along those with wall bars.

In the competitive sport context, important decisions are made even when not simultaneously competing against opponents. Divers must decide which dives to execute given the degrees of difficulty, their confidence in performing a dive well, their perceived ability of the competitors, the current scores of competitors, and so on. The golfer must select the club and decide on the subtle mechanics of the shot with factors such as the wind and the shape of the fairway in mind. Team sports may involve the most complex decisions, because many have open environments in which players can go almost everywhere on the playing surface and intercept or block balls and pucks. Broader team tactical decisions, such as zone or one-on-one coverage in basketball, can be made prior to a game, but countless times during actual play, players (individually or with a teammate or two) must decide how to execute a play based on the placement of opponents, the perception of the opponent's strength or weakness, the time, or the score.

Tactics are organized actions by individuals, pairs, or groups engaged in to acquire an advantage over an opponent. In the context of soccer, these might include actions to defend a goal or open space, moving to a passing lane to receive the ball, maintaining possession of the ball, or supporting the dribbler, as well as offensive and defensive strategies. **Decision making** is the selection from a variety of choices knowing the consequences of the choice. Examples of decisions in physical activity and sport contexts underscore the fact that choosing the correct course of action at the correct time is as much a determiner of success as executing the action well. Awareness is growing that decision making and tactics should be directly taught (Davids et al., 2008; Grehaigne et al., 2001; McPherson & Kernodle, 2003; Vickers, 2007). Skilled movement execution and physiological readiness are important, but so is decision making. Practices should be constructed with decision making in mind.

How to include decision making and tactics as part of instruction is a matter of some debate. Traditionally, coaches and teachers have focused on ensuring that participants possess the correct motor patterns before introducing tactical skills. For example, the bounce pass in basketball is often taught with much repetition, feedback from the instructor, and minimal promotion of thought on the part of the learner about when to use the pass. In addition, the drills are often rather static; the game-like context is intentionally removed on the assumption that one cannot be tactical without appropriate technique. Only after the technique is well developed are tactics and decision making introduced in the actual game. Teachers and coaches who express great disappointment during a game (*They could do it in practice!*) may have used this traditional approach. Critics claim that children taught with this emphasis on technique achieve little success, know little about game strategy, are too inflexible, make poor decisions, and rely too much on the coach or teacher (Holt, Strean, & Bengoechea, 2002; Werner, Thorpe, & Bunker, 1996). An alternative to this approach is called Teaching Games for Understanding, or TGfU (Bunker & Thorpe, 1986; Butler, Griffin, Lombardo, & Nastasi, 2003; Griffin, Brooker, & Patton, 2005; Werner et al., 1996).

Advocates of TGfU argue that game tactics and decisions are best taught in modified games prior to teaching movement techniques, which will emerge to some extent through the games designed to teach the tactics. The modified games enhance game tactics and skill as learners are prepared for real game play. Teaching Games for Understanding conceptualizes four types of games: target (e.g., bowling, golf), striking or running (e.g., baseball, cricket), net and wall (badminton, squash), and invasion (e.g., basketball, American football, water polo). In each category, the tactics may be quite similar across the sports. The techniques can be explicitly taught after the tactics, and learners may be more receptive to learning techniques when they understand the context in which a technique might be required. In contrast to traditional methods, TGfU encourages students to solve problems and make decisions inherent in the actual game.

Summary

Tony, in the chapter-opening scenario, agreed to find out more about contemporary soccer practices for his local soccer association. This chapter would have assisted him in understanding the pros and cons of aspiring for gold standards for soccer skills and in understanding how to structure the physical, affective, instructional, and sport environments to enhance players' enjoyment and learning. We discussed the need of learners to be exposed to variability in practice so that they can respond in novel ways if the performance situation dictates. We then discussed a number of ways the physical environment, including equipment, can be manipulated to modify performance. We also highlighted the affective factors that contribute to a positive learning environment and provided an overview of motivation as well as of play, competitive, and instructional environments. We finished by arguing that decision making and tactical learning should receive greater emphasis within the motor learning context.

ONLINE LEARNING

Visit the web resource at www.HumanKinetics.com/MotorLearningAndDevelopment for an accompanying lab activity and exercises from the chapter.

LEARNING AIDS

Supplemental Activities

1. Arrange an interview with an accomplished athlete. Ask your interviewee about her (or his) early years in the sport. Did she participate in many activities before she began to specialize in her current sport? What role did Mom and Dad play? Does her current practice reflect deliberate practice? Estimate the number of hours she has devoted to her sport. Is it close to 3,000 to 4,000 hours?

2. Motivation is such an important topic in human performance that the Internet is full of images, quotes, and tips about it. Search for these and try to find a quote or image to match our list of motivation topics. Also, see if you can add to the list of motivations.

Glossary

awareness talks—Talks in which learners are reminded about the levels of responsibility explicitly discussed and posted in the learning environment; one of the strategies in Hellison's personal and social responsibility model.

competitive environment—An environment in which individuals or teams compete against each other. Performance expectations and social pressures are high.

cooperative play—Play in which children strive to achieve the same goal.

counseling time—Time devoted to a discussion of problems identified by the teacher or students; one of the strategies in Hellison's personal and social responsibility model.

decision making—Making a selection from a variety of choices knowing the consequences of the choice.

deliberate play—Activities in which some rules are established and monitored by children or adults.

deliberate practice—Activities designed to improve current levels of performance; they require much effort and are not necessarily enjoyable.

ego-involved climate—A climate that encourages participants to improve their skills in order to outperform others. Success is defined in comparison to other people in the group or some idealized model.

free play—Activities engaged in exclusively for intrinsic reasons, often during infancy and early childhood.

game—Any form of playful competition, undertaken singly or in combination, whose outcome is determined by physical skill, strategy, or chance.

group meeting—A meeting that includes a discussion of what constitutes self-control and responsibility and is used to establish self-control rules; one of the strategies in Hellison's personal and social responsibility model.

guided discovery—An approach to learning in which the teacher creates an environment and tasks to help learners find their own solutions.

hands-off practitioner—Based on the dynamic systems approach, a practitioner who incorporates problem solving, self-discovery, and self-regulation into the learning environment to encourage learners to discover appropriate personal motor patterns.

individual decision making—The practice of learners of being in control of their own actions and decisions; one of the strategies in Hellison's personal and social responsibility model.

instructional environment—A closed and supportive environments that includes ample instruction, feedback, and encouragement to help learners explore movement options.

investment years—The years characterized by achieving elite levels of performance. The main focus is strategy, competition, and skill development within a context of deliberate practice directed and assisted by a coach.

mastery climate—A climate that encourages participants to improve their skills and judge success by positive changes in their individual performances.

nonlinear pedagogy—The foundation of instruction based on the dynamic systems approach, in which practitioners promote problem solving, discovery learning, and self-regulation.

parallel play—Playing alongside peers but not really interacting.

personal attributes—Individual qualities that influence the development of a social role.

play—Deliberate and repetitive activity motivated by the need for an experience of competence and autonomy.

practice environment—An instructor-controlled learning environment that emphasizes the proper execution of specific skills under increasingly more demanding space and time constraints.

reflection time—Time at the end of each lesson in which students contemplate what went well or not so well, which may involve writing in personal journals, completing checklists, or engaging in discussions with others. This is one of the strategies in Hellison's personal and social responsibility model.

sampling years—The years characterized by exposure to many fundamental motor skills and a wide range of sports with an emphasis on fun and excitement.

socializing agents—(1) People who affect a person's adherence to a healthy lifestyle including physical activity. (2) People who influence the development of someone's social role, such as parents, teachers, and coaches.

social situations—Contexts in which socialization takes place, such as school and home.

specializing years—The years during which people spend significant time on one or two sporting activities. Skill development takes on a higher priority than during the sampling years, but fun remains a critical component.

sport—A competitive event guided by standard rules; usually with coaches, referees, and schedules of play.

structured practice—Activities in which skill performance assumes a higher priority than in deliberate play.

tactics—Organized actions by individuals, pairs, or groups engaged in to acquire an advantage over an opponent.

PREPRACTICE CONSIDERATIONS

15

Chapter Objectives

After reading this chapter, you should be able to do the following:

- Describe three types of goals and principles of goal setting.
- Explain when demonstrations are effective and when they are not, and why.
- List the pros and cons of expert and learning models.
- Discuss the relationships between verbal instruction and both implicit and explicit learning.
- Describe guidelines for using verbal cues.
- Discuss attention in terms of being broad or narrow and external or internal.

Challenging Traditional Thinking

Donaya is a thoughtful coach of a young ski team of 11- and 12-year-olds. She realizes that much practice will be necessary to improve their times as they descend the mountain, but she worries that if she talks too much, they will not have enough time to practice—and on cold days their attention will wander for sure. On the other hand, she knows a great deal about skiing and wants to share her knowledge. She also wonders about demonstrations. As a former national-level skier, she is confident of her ability to demonstrate, and part of her wants the boys to realize that girls *can* ski. But Donaya remembers from her coach education program that demonstrations by other children can be as helpful as expert demonstrations. She also remembers learning that demonstrations are overrated in some situations. Is that really possible? She knows that practices should include verbal instructions and physical demonstrations, but she decides to research more so she doesn't talk too much and waste time on ineffective demonstrations. Her hope is that this will result in optimal use of their precious practice time on the mountain and lead to faster skiing.

This chapter explores several prepractice variables that affect performance and learning. Prepractice refers to actions of instructors, therapists, and coaches immediately prior to physical practice rather than more general issues of structuring the environment (as discussed in chapter 14). Prepractice actions include goal setting, demonstrations, verbal instruction, directing attention, and physical guidance. Of course, the role of the instructor does not end here. It also includes arranging physical practice (addressed in chapter 16) and deciding how to provide feedback during or after physical practice (discussed in chapter 17). Somewhat surprisingly, there is little scientific consensus about the role of prepractice information such as demonstrations and verbal instruction in motor learning (Hodges & Franks, 2002).

Goal Setting

Theories of motor learning and self-regulation assume that learners are goal directed. They want to achieve something. As we saw in chapter 14, the purpose of free play and structured play is fun, and as adults we do not want to turn child's play into anything else by inserting goals of achievement. We can modify the environment to present activity challenges and encourage exploration by supporting and interacting with children, but we should allow their natural sense of fun and intrinsic motivation to flourish while they play. In structured practice or deliberate practice, the situation changes and performance improvement becomes more important. In these situations, goal setting is likely to enhance performance and learning. Goal setting has also become an important treatment component in those who have had a stroke (Langhorne, Bernhardt, & Kwakkel, 2011) and those with cerebral palsy (Sorsdahl, Moe-Nilssen, Kaale, Rieber, & Strand, 2010).

In practice situations, instructors often have a tendency to encourage students to do their best. At first glance, this seems sensible, because the instructor knows that a goal for the whole class or team (e.g., perform 15 push-ups or 10 throws that hit a target) will result in some students failing and others barely being challenged. **Goal setting** is a self-regulatory skill that allows people to monitor progress toward a self-determined goal (Zimmerman, 2000). Instructors and therapists should encourage goal setting because people tend to commit to goals they set for themselves (Schmidt & Lee, 2014). In general, research demonstrates that goals are most effective when they are specific, attainable, challenging, and realistic (Gould, 2006). Goals direct attention to important elements of the skill, produce greater effort and persistence, promote new learning strategies, and influence psychological characteristics such as confidence and anxiety (Gould & Chung, 2004). As adults age, goals remain motivational and affected by self-efficacy, but become attenuated when ability declines (West, Edner, & Hastings, 2013).

The types of goals are outcome goals, performance goals, and process goals (Schmidt & Lee, 2014). **Outcome goals** emphasize the results of performance, often in comparison to others (e.g., *I want to be first*). Such goals may provide direction, but outcomes are often beyond the person's control; someone else might win because of outstanding but unexpected performance. **Performance goals** focus on improvement relative to one's own performance, whereas **process goals** specifically emphasize particular aspects of skill execution or selected strategies. (See table 15.1 for examples.) Weinberg and Gould (2011) recommended setting specific, moderately difficult goals to which the person is committed. Goals should be realistic and used for practice and competition and for the short and long term. Moreover, goals should be recorded and periodically evaluated.

Most early research in goal setting compared the instruction *Do your best* or *Give*

Table 15.1 Examples of Outcome Goals, Performance Goals, and Process Goals

Activity	Outcome goals	Performance goals	Process goals
Basketball	Win the district championship.	Increase foul shoot percentage from 50 to 70%.	Don't look at teammate to whom you are passing the ball.
Cross country running	Finish in the top 3 of the state championship.	Improve time on state championship course by 10%.	Lean forward on the downhill to take advantage of the momentum of the hill.
Golf	Qualify for regional championship.	Score under 85 in practice rounds.	Concentrate on a smooth putt and ignore the crowd.
Folk dance	Make no errors with the 10-step sequence and win the community dance-off.	Improve from 3 to 7 correctly sequenced moves.	Maintain a straight back and keep the head up during the do-si-do move.
Therapy	Walk independently 20 yards without crutches and with a gait pattern.	Improve from 3 steps with crutches to 10 yards without crutches.	Concentrate on a heel landing and improve toe takeoff with the injured foot.

it 100 percent to more specific and challenging but achievable goals in industrial settings (e.g., Locke & Latham, 1985). The results showed clearly that the latter type was superior to the former. Similar comparisons between *Do your best* and more specific personal goals have been made in sport and exercise psychology research (see the review by Kyllo & Landers, 1995). The findings are similar to those in industrial settings but not quite as dramatic in sport. Schmidt and Lee (2011) speculated that in *Do your best* sport situations, people may secretively set their own goals, thus overshadowing the experimenter's manipulations. They also pointed out that most of the goal-setting research has ignored the difference between performance and learning, with the exception of Boyce (1992). The task was rifle shooting, and Boyce used three groups. Those in the first group were encouraged to do their best; those in the second were encouraged to set specific but individual goals; and those in the third were given individual goals set by the experimenter and based on previous performance. Those in the *Do your best* group performed better than those in the other groups only during the first practice session, whereas the specific goal-setting procedures in the latter two groups were equally effective during performance and

retention. It would seem that goal setting has a positive impact on both performance and learning.

A study of self-regulated dart throwing by adolescent girls showed some evidence that process goals lead to more improvement than performance goals do (Kitsantas & Zimmerman, 1998; Zimmerman & Kitsantas, 1996); however, setting process goals and then shifting to performance goals resulted in the highest performance (Zimmerman & Kitsantas, 1997). In younger children, the results of goal setting have been equivocal. A study by Kolovelonis, Goudas, and Dermitzaki (2011) showed no difference between performance and process goals with 11-year-olds, but youngsters who self-recorded had superior performances. In a subsequent study (Kolovelonis, Goudas, & Dermitzaki, 2012) with children of the same age, those who used self-talk with either performance or process goals outperformed those in a goals-only group and those in a control group. Goal-setting research has not frequently compared groups of different ages, and hence few developmental trends have been noted. Practitioners might wish to encourage individual goal setting but to check goals periodically to ensure that they are realistic. More research into development and goal setting is clearly needed.

Demonstrations

Demonstrations, modeling, and *observational learning* are terms often used interchangeably. These activities are so common in physical activity instruction and therapy that we do not give them much thought. The term *demonstration* is more closely aligned to motor learning and instruction, whereas *modeling* and *observational learning* are terms more frequently used in the context of social learning and sport psychology. In any case, practitioners often demonstrate a skill such as a forward roll, provide some verbal cues, and then send the class or team off to practice it. The notion that a picture is worth a thousand words seems true for learning motor skills.

In addition to demonstrations by the instructor, video clips of good performers and even photos of correct actions may be used (Schmidt & Lee, 2014). Under certain circumstances, demonstrations are effective in teaching motor skills (Hodges & Franks, 2002; McCullagh & Weiss, 2001; Schmidt & Lee, 2011; Scully & Newell, 1985). However, we seldom ask how different task goals or task types might make demonstrations effective or ineffective, who should perform demonstrations, what learners are supposed to see in demonstrations, or how demonstrations affect learning. We turn to these topics now.

Demonstrations and models may serve three functions (Weiss, Ebbeck, & Wiese-Bjornstal, 1993). The first is to *help learners acquire new skills,* such as a forward roll, or new behaviors, such as returning equipment to its proper storage spot. This is the main focus of this section. The second function is to *elicit already learned behaviors,* such as going out for a walk or cheering for your team. The third function is to *reduce avoidance behavior* such as fear by using models that manipulate psychological factors such as self-confidence, motivation, and anxiety.

Effectiveness of Demonstrations

A demonstration provides a visual template, or model, of a desired movement pattern (Hodges & Franks, 2002) and can inform the learner about the nature of the task and its requirements. If a task is very simple and the learner has previous knowledge of the criteria for performance, a demonstration may have no impact (Newell, 1981). How simple the task is depends on both the task itself and the skills of the learner. Tasks such as dance steps or gymnastics actions might not require a demonstration as individual skills; but if they need to be sequenced in a particular order, a demonstration may convey such cognitive information (Hodges & Franks, 2002).

Whether a demonstration of more complex tasks is effective likely depends on the task goal and the measurements of effectiveness used. In closed skills, the movement form is often the primary learning goal. In gymnastics, synchronized swimming, diving, and figure skating, how one performs is critical to success. Demonstrations may help learners acquire new patterns of coordination because they must practice the pattern or technique repeatedly until performance is automatic (see table 15.2).

A meta-analysis compared results from observational studies using movement form measures and movement outcome measures (Ashford, Bennett, & Davids, 2006). Meta-analysis is a mathematical technique that standardizes findings from many studies. As you might imagine, one researcher may use a basketball shooting task and another may use a badminton task; it is difficult to combine such studies quantitatively. Meta-analysis transforms the results from different tasks into a standard result called an effect size (ES). The ESs from each study can then be combined to determine an overall effect of the treatment—in this case, the difference between using demonstrations and not using demonstrations during practice. Combined with statistical significance,

the ES provides a quantitative snapshot of treatment effects. Many researchers use Cohen's recommended interpretation of ES: an ES of .80 or higher is a large difference, an ES of .50 or higher is a moderate difference, and an ES of .20 is a small difference.

Ashford and colleagues (2006) measured form, or how the model performed the task. Outcome measures included accuracy (or error) scores. A moderately large effect size (.77) was reported for form; that is, practices with demonstrations were more effective than practices without demonstrations when form was measured. A significant but smaller effect size (.17) resulted with outcome measures. That is, practices with demonstrations were still superior to practices without demonstrations, but not to the same degree when assessed with movement technique.

Table 15.2   Effectiveness and Noneffectiveness of Demonstrations

Demonstration may be effective when . . .	Demonstration may not be more effective than other types of information when . . .
• The person is acquiring a new pattern of coordination. • The person requires a template of the movement pattern. • The person is learning a movement sequence. • The person is learning strategies and decision making. • The person is learning to cope with difficult emotional situations.	• The task is simple. • The person already knows the task and its requirements. • The new task involves a change in parameters. • The outcome is more important than how the movement is performed. • The outcome is clear and performance feedback is available.

TRY THIS

Focus, Focus

Exercise 15.2

Demonstrations are usually helpful when learners are acquiring new coordination patterns. Pair up with another student and crumple up a piece of paper to throw. One person demonstrates a throw, and the other person observes and then tries to copy the demonstrator. As you learned in chapter 7, a mature throw for distance involves a step with the contralateral leg, a backward swing of the throwing arm, trunk rotation, a lag of the throwing arm, and follow-through. The demonstrator should perform one aspect of the throw in a unique way (e.g., step with the ipsilateral leg) to demonstrate a new pattern of coordination. After a couple of demonstrations, the other person tries to replicate the new throw. Discuss whether the observer was successful and how the demonstration could be enhanced. Did you find it easy, moderately difficult, or very difficult to replicate the throwing pattern of your partner? Why?

It appears that in the early phase of learning, movement technique is more sensitive to the influence of demonstrations than is the outcome of the movement. To state this simply, initial learning is associated with learning how to assemble the movement pattern, but its effect on outcome is not as obvious. People have to learn how to perform before their movement pattern has an effect on the outcome. Movement dynamics were more sensitive to the impact of demonstrations than movement outcomes for serial, continuous, and discrete tasks as well (Ashford et al., 2006). Attention to the end of the movement form (e.g., the hand and forearm in a basketball set shot) may be particularly helpful (Breslin, Hodges, & Williams, 2009). Early in the learning of a new movement, several demonstrations are likely necessary to begin building the template, followed by practice with additional demonstrations thoughtfully interspersed (see Weeks & Anderson, 2000). If the task is an old pattern of coordination and learners are required to perform new parameter characteristics (e.g., the same pattern faster), demonstrations may be no more effective than other forms of instruction (Magill, 2017).

With open skills, the primary goal is the movement outcome (not how it is accomplished). The successful basketball pass to a teammate is the desired outcome, but the movement form of the pass (i.e., how it was executed) is much less important. With many open skills, as discussed in chapter 14, variability in practice is desirable. There is less need for demonstrations that replicate the solutions of others and a greater need to emphasize discovering novel tactical solutions. Williams and Hodges (2005) contended that demonstrations may be no more effective than verbal descriptions when the goal is problem solving, because the outcome does not depend on replicating a specific movement pattern or technique. When instructors believe that a demonstration is needed in open skills, they should combine it with the outcome effect. This provides information for learners to use as they solve problems and determine how their actions relate to results. Williams and Hodges also recommended that instructors use verbal instruction expressing the intended outcome of the skill before offering a demonstration (e.g., *Can you pass the basketball from out of bounds to the high post area?*). A demonstration can then be used to guide the learning process.

Hodges and Franks (2002) described several of their motor learning studies involving novel bimanual movements, as might be found in juggling or playing musical instruments. In these situations, they concluded that "movement demonstrations and instructions relating to the movement of the limbs convey little useful information in the early stage of acquisition, if information about goal attainment is available through feedback" (p. 805). Thus, if the desired outcome is clear and performance feedback is available, demonstrations may not be necessary. Of course, bimanual movements are only one class of movements.

Demonstrations and video presentations may help learners develop strategies and decision making based on perceptual information. Martens, Burwitz, and Zuckerman (1976) used the task of trying to move a ball placed on top of two rods up an incline by manipulating the distance between the rods. The ball could fall into any of eight holes beneath the rods, and the hole at the end of the incline earned the highest score possible. Two approaches were modeled. A creep strategy involved slowly adjusting the rods, which produced consistent but moderate success. A ballistic strategy involved moving the rods very rapidly, which resulted in variable levels of achievement but very high scores when successful. Observers tended to replicate the strategy they had observed.

Weeks (1992) argued that most observational research had studied internally paced skills such as locomotor skill sequences or serial arm movements, and suggested that more open, externally paced tasks should shed light on the impact of observation on perceptual processing and decision making in more complex tasks. In a coincident timing task, participants had to displace a barrier at the same time the final light was illuminated on a runway of lights. Three modeling groups were created. One group received modeling that focused on the perceptual demands of the task, and a second group received modeling that focused on the motor demands of the task. The perceptual modeling participants used 10 observations of the runway lights to assist in timing the arm action to the lights, although their hands had to remain on their knees during the prepractice observations. Motor modeling participants received 10 demonstrations of a person hitting the barrier. A third group received both motor and perceptual models, and a fourth group received no prepractice modeling. Groups in perceptual modeling conditions performed better than those in only motor task modeling

conditions, which suggests that perceptual demands can be modeled and that they are very important in externally paced activities. Weeks recommended that instructors of externally paced tasks such as batting and groundstrokes in racket sports include training on the perceptual characteristics of ball flight. Thus, demonstrations may help learners focus on relevant perceptual cues and strategies of action.

Another line of research used video-recorded models of children coping with difficult situations (McCullagh & Weiss, 2001; Weiss, McCullagh, Smith, & Berlant, 1998). This represents the third function of modeling noted earlier, reducing avoidance behaviors. One approach is to show models exhibiting negative cognition, affect, and behavior as they perform in difficult or fear-evoking situations such as learning to swim. Over repeated trials, the models verbalize more positive thoughts and also improve their performance. For example, statements that change from *I can't do this* to *I can do this* convey a shift from

RESEARCH NOTES

Observational Learning and Anxiety

Weiss and colleagues (1998) investigated the impact of observational learning on swimming performance and the psychological responses of children who were fearful of swimming. Twenty-four children (average age of 6.2 years) participated. They were matched on age and swim lesson experience and then randomly assigned to one of three model types: control, peer mastery, and peer coping. The control group watched cartoons on days of the swimming lessons, but the cartoons provided no information on swimming. The peer mastery group observed a video of a similar-age peer who verbalized positively and was technically correct in swimming. The peer coping group video showed a peer who expressed increasingly positive comments and showed gradual improvement in swimming. Three days of swimming lessons were used, and the researchers evaluated the children's swimming skills, fear of swimming, and swimming self-efficacy, in addition to producing field notes. The coping and mastery groups were superior in swimming performance, were higher in self-efficacy, and showed more change in fear compared to the control group. Coping models had a stronger effect on self-efficacy than mastery models did. Thus, the use of modeling may help young learners deal with movements involving some inherent degree of fear and produce change in associated psychological variables.

lower to higher self-confidence (Weiss et al., 1998). The models demonstrate how they are learning to cope through problem solving and the impact on their motivation. This has the potential to influence self-confidence and motivation.

Wrisberg and Pein (2002) explored the self-regulation of how often to view a demonstration of a badminton long serve by novice university students. One group watched a video of a model prior to each practice attempt, one group chose when to see the video, and one group never saw the video. The first two groups acquired the correct form of the serve and retained that form better than the group that did not see the video did. The group with the option of requesting when to see the video requested it only 9.8 percent of the time, primarily during the first half of the trials on the first day. This suggests that demonstrations may be most effective for novices early in learning. The motor learning benefits of learners controlling when and how often they view a demonstration (Wulf, Raupach, & Pfeiffer, 2005) has also been supported. Self-regulation of demonstrations may be an effective practice for promoting learning. Whether these findings would be the same for children must await further research.

Performance of Demonstrations

Professionally created videos of top athletes performing the perfect throw or swing create the impression that an expert, or at least a very skilled person, should be performing the demonstration. This makes sense if the goal is to present the ideal movement pattern that all learners should mimic. These expert models often enjoy high status, and their demonstrations are often accompanied by verbal cues and explicit highlights of the correct technique (Darden, 1997). Consistent with the formation of a perceptual trace, or template, to which performance will be compared to detect errors, it is often assumed that more frequent expert demonstrations will create

stronger blueprints. However, chapter 14 highlighted the value of using variability in practice and promoting problem solving, and questioned whether a gold standard of movement patterns actually exists. These ideas are at odds with the logic of having all learners mimic one movement pattern and raise the question of the necessity of an expert model. In fact, there is some consensus that demonstrations by unskilled people may be more effective than those by experts (Darden, 1997; Hodges & Franks, 2002; McCullagh & Weiss, 2001; Ste-Marie, Law, Rymal, Jenny, Hall, & McCullagh, 2012). Of course, learners should have some idea about the correct movement pattern and understand that what they are observing contains errors.

Learning models have been shown to be as effective as expert models and in some cases more effective for learning (e.g., Lee & White, 1990). A learning model is a novice who practices the skill and receives feedback from an instructor or coach. The demonstration is of the model trying to acquire the task, receiving feedback, and then using the feedback to construct the next performance effort. By definition, a learning model demonstrates variability in performance. Learners might identify with the learning model because of similarity in status (both are learning) and realize that the demonstrated skill level is within their reach. It seems that learning can occur from watching others make errors (Domurachi, Wong, Olivieri, & Grierson, 2015). In addition 10-year-olds learning a five-skill trampoline routine benefited more from a video of themselves than from verbal instructions alone (Ste-Marie, Verles, Rymal, & Martini, 2011).

It is also possible that what is being modeled is not the movement pattern per se, but a process of problem solving. This latter idea was originally put forth by Adams (1986), who argued that the learning model was actively, rather than passively, involved in his own learning and that this would produce performance benefits. Andrieux and Proteau (2013,

Exercise 15.3

The section has probably made you realize that using demonstrations effectively is much more complex than you previously thought. Describe how you could use demonstrations to teach the following:

- Students who are being introduced to the skill of overhand throwing for the first time
- Students who are learning to dive
- A student with a hearing impairment

2014) showed that both novice and expert models together are more effective than either alone, likely because more cognitive effort is expended in acquiring the skill through identifying a standard (expert model), witnessing the errors of a novice (learning model), and learning how to avoid those errors. In summary, there are motivational, attention, and learning explanations for the beneficial impact of learning models or mixed models.

Learning models could be incorporated into a class through the use of reciprocal teaching or learning groups in which all students are both observers and models in a problem-solving activity. Magill (2017) also recommended presenting a checklist of key aspects of the skill to the pairs or groups to guide observation and feedback.

Theoretical Explanations of Demonstrations

Thus far we have discussed several demonstration issues: when demonstrations are effective, who should perform demonstrations, and what the learner is viewing. Under some circumstances, demonstrations are very important. But questions of when, who, and what do not deal with how or why demonstrations are effective. How and why are theoretical questions. We now look at motor learning, social learning, and ecological theories to see how each explains why demonstrations are helpful to learners.

Motor Learning Theories

Demonstrations are a part of classic theories of skill acquisition, including the closed-loop theory of motor control (Adams, 1971) and schema theory (Schmidt, 1975). In Adams' closed-loop theory, a perceptual trace, or template, of the movement develops with practice. Sensory feedback during subsequent movements can be compared to the perceptual trace to ensure correct execution. A second memory trace was also posited that initiates the movement because the same perceptual trace could not initiate and evaluate the correctness of a response. Schema theory is an open-loop account of motor control. Not unlike Adams, Schmidt postulated two types of schemas: a recall schema for response production and a recognition schema for response evaluation. If a template of movement already exists (that is, the perceptual trace of Adams and the recall schema of Schmidt), then a demonstration will likely refine the template to which feedback during movement execution will be compared (Hodges & Franks, 2002). For example, if a throwing schema exists, the demonstration will provide information about the specific type of throw, its force, and its direction. If the movement template is not established and the task is novel, the demonstrations may help learners engage in cognitive processes similar to those that occur in physical practice (Blandin & Proteau, 2000).

The stages of motor learning, according to Gentile (1972) and Fitts and Posner (1967), are discussed in chapter 4. Each provides some insight into how movement templates might be established in the early stages. Gentile (1972) referred to early learning as "getting the idea of the movement"; and Fitts and Posner's first stage was termed cognitive because the learner attends to cues and feedback to develop an executive program. In both of these theories, a demonstration may present the idea of the movement and the cues that are necessary for initial learning of the movement skill.

Social Learning Theory

Social learning (Bandura 1986, 1997) theory is perhaps the most detailed account of demonstrations, although *modeling* and *observational learning* are preferred terms. Bandura's original focus was the social learning of behaviors rather than motor skills. He contended that people learn most about their social world through observation and that practice is not essential for developing social or cognitive behaviors. This makes sense for simple responses that are already in people's repertoires, such as a sequence of movements. If the movements can already be accomplished, the activity becomes more cognitive than motoric (Hodges & Franks, 2002). A demonstration of the sequence might help at the beginning of the learning process.

Bandura (1986, 1997) asserted that modeling is information processing with four subprocesses that transfer, or code, information from the model into a template of correctness to which future movements are compared. The first subprocess is attention to the modeling. This is affected by the observer's cognitive capabilities and arousal level. Attention is also influenced by characteristics of the modeled event (e.g., its complexity). For complex movement patterns, the observer should focus on relevant cues via verbal directives or alternating good and poor performances. Retention, the second subprocess, involves reformulating the event into a memory representation. It is assumed to be an abstraction of the event and likely verbal or visual, depending on the task. The third subprocess is production. As McCullagh and Weiss (2001) pointed out, this was not well developed in Bandura's original writings because he was concerned with explaining social behaviors that might be dichotomous (i.e., either performed or not). Motor learning specialists are concerned with movement quality, and demonstrations may convey spatial and timing aspects of importance. The final information-processing subprocess is motivation, given that the person must be motivated to exhibit the behavior. Reinforcement of observed models or actions by the observer enhances the motivation of the observer to reproduce the action demonstrated. These four processes are developmental; the first three are cognitively oriented, and the fourth is motivation oriented (Weiss et al., 1993). Observation learning is therefore expected to improve with age because of critical developmental changes in attention, retention, production, and motivation.

Ecological Perspectives

As we have discussed in several chapters, practice from the ecological theoretical viewpoint is designed to enable the learner to explore the perceptual–motor landscape and to assemble functional coordination patterns that offer solutions to movement problems. Movement variability is highly valued, and demonstrations that highlight variability rather than one ideal movement pattern should be effective. This theory views perception as direct, and ecological researchers try to determine what information is available and useful for the learner in demonstrations without cognitive interpretations and transformation of information as put forth by Bandura (1986, 1997). They place more emphasis on the information learners glean from a demonstration than on how the information should be presented (Hodges & Franks, 2002). It has been proposed that observers are sensitive to the relative motions of movements and that this information can be used to assemble coordination patterns (Scully & Newell, 1985).

Support for the ecological perspective and the information gleaned from demonstrations comes from research using point-light displays (e.g., Williams, 1989). A point-light display is a video from a motion analysis system showing dots of light placed at a person's joints. Williams provided a point-light display of a throwing motion with dots placed on the wrist, elbow, and shoulder. The observer saw the movement of only the dots, not the arm or ball. Almost 90 percent of children and adults reported seeing a throwing action after four trials. This research suggests that observers attend to information about the relationships of limb components in the movement pattern. In ecological terms, these relationships are invariant relative motions (Scully & Newell, 1985). Recall from chapter 3 that invariant features include the sequence of action, relative timing, and relative force. The sequence of movements such as the rotation of the trunk, the backswing of the arm, and the step with the contralateral foot, followed by forward rotation, was apparently conveyed to the adults and children by the moving dots.

Magill (2017) reviewed similar studies of walking patterns in which people distinguished individual gaits on the basis of unique relative motions rather than a single factor such as walking velocity. It seems that learners do perceive and use invariant relative motions in observational learning (Magill, 2017). However, the movements used in most of this research were rather common and well practiced, such as throwing, walking, and running. It is not yet clear how instructors might help learners focus on the relative motions of skills that are not yet mastered or are very novel, because the perception of the invariant relative motions is likely learned without consciousness.

Learning From Demonstrations

What learners see in a demonstration is likely influenced by the nature of the task. In addition, the interpretation is influenced by the theory behind the research. Schmidt and Lee (2011) suggested that demonstrations can lead to learners' acquiring movement strategies, spatial information, and temporal information. Strategies might include task-specific approaches such as the creeping and ballistic movements described by Martens and colleagues (1976) or throwing a basketball from the foul line with one or two hands. More general problem-solving skills suggested by learning model research would be exemplified by a student receiving teacher feedback about the front crawl and then saying to herself, *I have to raise my elbow higher during recovery*. Modeling of coping strategies led to performance improvement but also to enhanced psychological function such as self-efficacy. These coping strategies helped learners acquire a more positive psychological approach.

Spatial information can also be picked up, as shown in a series of studies on learning sign language through modeling (Carroll & Bandura, 1990). Relative motion also involves spatial and temporal information about body parts moving in relation to each other or to the environment, and strong evidence suggests that learners are aware of this information (Ashford et al., 2006). Temporal information (i.e., information about the timing of movements) has been demonstrated in a number of studies (Magill, 2017). Think of the instructor who claps his hands in the rhythm of a skipping motion that young students happily try to imitate. This research presents auditory information about movement timing or rhythm and has led to gains in rhythmic timing of movement sequences as might occur in dance.

Mirror neurons in the premotor cortex were discovered in the 1990s (Lago-Rodriguez, Cheeran, Koch, Hortobagyi, & Fernandez-del-Olmo, 2014). As part of the motor system, these unique neurons fire both when an action is observed and when it is performed. An infant may grasp a cup and view Mom grasping the same or a very similar cup. The mirror neurons fire in both situations; hence, observing a movement may strengthen the neuronal path of action. Mirror neurons have been proposed as the neurological link between the observation of movement and the creation of motor commands (Lago-Rodriguez et al., 2014; Ste-Marie et al., 2012).

Developmental Considerations in Demonstrations

Chapters 11 and 12 dealt with functional constraints such as cognitive functioning, attention, knowledge, self-regulation, and memory. These constraints are developmental, in that they improve with age, experience, and knowledge of the task. Adults, adolescents, and those with sport-specific knowledge are more likely to use self-regulated learning strategies and have access to other capacities that have resulted from years of experience dealing with educational and movement challenges. These functional constraints, coupled with structural constraints, give adults and adolescents an advantage over children when faced with unfamiliar tasks. Experienced observers are more likely to produce closer approximations of a model early in learning. As Ashford, Davids, and Bennett (2007) stated, "Adults can adapt existing coordination tendencies but in a way that results in the acquisition of a new coordination pattern suited to the goals of a task" (p. 548). McCullagh and Weiss (2001) provided the corollary that motor skill instruction for children under 12 years of age should facilitate task-relevant attention (*Try not to look at the ball when you're dribbling*), strategies (*Watch me. . . . After I kick the ball to a teammate, I run quickly to a spot where I can receive a pass*), and knowledge (*Let me show you an offside*), and that these factors must be considered in observational learning.

McCullagh and Weiss (2001), in a detailed review of studies that shed light on children's ability to benefit from models, underscored the point that the effectiveness of models is multifaceted: it depends on the age of the observer; how performance is measured; and whether acquisition, retention, or transfer is assessed. We have also discussed that the impact of demonstrations is affected by the type of task and task goals. Therefore, developmental generalizations to guide practice are difficult to generate. With children four or five years of age, a show-and-tell model can be effective for teaching a sequence of movements (Weiss, 1983). Show and tell is a demonstration and explanation of what should be done and is helpful for children who do not spontaneously attend to task-relevant cues, such as stepping forward with the foot opposite the throwing arm. It may also use verbal rehearsal strategies for remembering the order of events (e.g., *Arms, legs, glide* for the breaststroke). In an obstacle course task, children were encouraged to use verbal self-instruction by "thinking aloud"— that is, saying phrases such as *Jump and clap* and *Jump-jump* that matched the activity (Weiss, 1983). Older children may benefit from show and tell but not more than from a visual demonstration without suggested rehearsal strategies. With novel tasks requiring new patterns of coordination, such as juggling, Meaney (1994) showed that both children and adults benefited from verbal rehearsal and cues combined with a demonstration, whereas adults improved following only the visual demonstration. The adults' physical performances were better than those of the children, and the adults used more strategies. These studies support the premise that the cognitive developmental level of children should be considered with demonstrations, and that children benefit from instruction focused on relevant cues and from engaging in intentional memory strategies.

Wiese-Bjornstal and Weiss (1992) showed that girls as young as seven to nine years old could watch a demonstration of a softball fast pitch and recognize a correct model from one of four video alternatives, could engage in verbal cues similar to the model, and could show some of the model's form (e.g., stride length, release body angle). Having learners restate the main points about a demonstration and verbal cues following show and tell would be good teaching practice. Watching the model more frequently and engaging in more practice resulted in better recognition of the correct form and in performances that resembled the model's. Self-regulation and observational learning research also supports the cognitive–developmental changes that occur during childhood and the influence on demonstrations. Younger children

from 5 to 7 years of age may benefit more than older children from verbal cueing and rehearsal strategies used along with a demonstration, because the older children already possess the language skills to use strategies spontaneously (Ste-Marie et al., 2012). The older children (11 years old) appeared to have greater awareness of their own learning, as evidenced by the fact that they requested more observations of a model than younger children did (8 years old) when rehearsing a dance sequence (Cadopi, Chatillon, & Baldy, 1995). The older children also used more verbal self-instruction, which is a self-regulated strategy.

A final developmental factor regarding modeling is the tendency for children to focus on task goals rather than movement form during demonstrations. Earlier, we stated that movement dynamics (approximation of the movement form) are more sensitive to the impact of demonstrations than movement outcomes (outcome performance such as accuracy or time) earlier

---

RESEARCH NOTES

Developmental Self-Regulation

Bouffard and Dunn (1993) explored whether developmental differences existed in children's use of self-regulation while learning the movement sequences of American Sign Language (ASL). They compared children 6 and 7 years old to children 9 and 10 years old; both groups had unlimited time and unlimited trials of watching a tape with the ASL sequence. The length of the sequence was 1.5 times longer than an estimated memory span for each child. When each child thought he had learned the sequence, he rang a bell, which signaled the researchers to enter the testing room to watch the child perform the sequence. Thus, this study explored what children do spontaneously in response to a demonstration without any guidance from the teacher. The older children displayed better recall of the sequences than the younger children did. In addition, the older children watched the demonstration videos more frequently than the younger ones did, and they used more strategies for learning the sequences (e.g., miming the gestures and rehearsing movements). Further, the 9- and 10-year-olds used more instances of language, indicating that they monitored their own learning more frequently. It appears that models can assist in self-regulation development and that older children spontaneously use self-regulation more often than younger children do.

WHAT DO YOU THINK?

Exercise 15.4

Review what you learned in chapters 11 and 12 about cognitive functioning, attention, knowledge, self-regulation, and memory. How do these act as constraints for children who are engaging in observation learning? What structural constraints should be considered?

in skill acquisition for serial, continuous, and discrete tasks (Ashford et al., 2006). It seems that developmental factors affect this generalization. Ashford and colleagues (2007) conducted a meta-analysis of 55 studies that compared children and adults with regard to their awareness of movement dynamics, movement outcome, or both, in demonstrations. The ES of movement dynamics for adults (.80) was larger than that for children (.24) when demonstrations were compared to practice-only conditions. This indicates that adults benefited more than children from demonstration and practice, compared to practice without demonstration, when measures of movement form were employed in the research. In fact, although the ES for the children was positive (.24), it was not significant. The opposite was found for measures of movement outcome: the ES for adults was negligible (–.02), and that for children was more substantial (.48). In other words, children seem to benefit more from demonstrations when assessed on movement outcome, thus adding a developmental caveat to the earlier generalization that initial learning is associated with learning how to assemble the movement patterns. Children seem to be more aware than adults of movement outcomes than of movement form in demonstrations. Thus, therapists and instructors should feel comfortable using demonstrations with an emphasis on movement outcomes with children.

Although modeling can facilitate the acquisition of closed skills, the magnitude of the effect depends on age and the measure used to quantify learning. Children can discern and benefit from movement form, but they have a tendency to focus on movement outcome. The extent to which instruction can focus children from movement outcome to movement form remains unknown. Hence, teachers and coaches should be sensitive to their students' and athletes' natural tendencies and help them focus on movement form if they believe that the youngsters possess the necessary cognitive functioning, attention, knowledge, self-regulation, and memory.

Verbal Instruction

Verbal instruction is a frequent and expected prepractice element that is often used in conjunction with demonstrations. Verbalization and demonstrations may provide redundant cues, but they may also provide different information to learners (Huff & Schwan, 2012; McCullagh & Weiss, 2001). Instructions could be in written form such as a task card, but more often they are spoken. Verbal instructions and cues are assumed to facilitate learning and to establish safe practice settings; however, they must be brief (e.g., *Bend your knees*). Magill (2017) recommended presenting only one or two instructions about what to do because learners have to remember the instructions and then perform the skill. Instructors should not exceed their charges' attention capacity. This is particularly important for novice learners and children.

Verbal information conveys the nature of task requirements, just as demonstrations do (Lee, Chamberlin, & Hodges, 2001). Examples include the correct and consistent movement form of a closed skill such as a dive, the creation of a smooth sequence of movements in the correct order in learning to stand independently while recovering from an accident, or the movement outcome goal of a successful pass to a teammate in an open sport. More specifically, Schmidt and Lee (2005, 2014) indicated that verbal information provides an initial orientation to a new skill, an overall idea or image of a movement, a means of recognizing one's own errors (e.g., checking the wrist on a follow-through), details of how to hold an apparatus or implement, information on where and how to move in a game, cues that are most important (e.g., the seams of a baseball), and the results performers should try to achieve (see the section Goal Setting earlier in this chapter). A verbal phrase may simplify a rather complex movement in the tennis serve (e.g., *Scratch your back with the racket*) or reinforce the order of movements in the breaststroke (e.g., *Arms, legs, glide*). Instructors may also promote the transfer of related, previously learned movements and strategies through verbal means. Feelings that should be expected from a movement can also be conveyed (e.g., *If you are stretching properly you should feel a slight pull in the calf muscle*).

Implicit and Explicit Learning

The examples in the previous paragraph underscore the many instances in which clear instructions would appear to be important in skill acquisition. Yet, there is not a great deal of research supporting these common purposes and outcomes of verbal instruction with respect to motor learning beyond specifying the task requirements, such as speed, accuracy, or both; movement form; or movement outcome (Hodges & Franks, 2002; Lee et al., 2001). In fact, research suggests that in some situations verbal instruction may not be helpful beyond personal practice and may be detrimental to learning. Some of this research deals with **explicit learning** and **implicit learning**.

Gentile (1998) extended the cognitive learning distinction between explicit and implicit learning to motor learning. The term *explicit* refers to conscious awareness of such factors as goal attainment and developing the relationship between the learner and the task. The aim of verbal instructions is to help learners become explicitly aware of some aspects of the skill (e.g., *The goal of this skill is to . . .* or *Hold the ball with your fingers along the stitching*). This is similar to declarative knowledge. Implicit learning is not conscious and likely deals with issues such as force production. For example, consider a young toddler who is offered a tricycle and initially cannot contract and relax the appropriate muscle groups at the correct time and order, and with the appropriate force, to move the vehicle. She does learn to cycle, but is not aware of how she does it. Even adults are unaware of the physical principles that govern bicycle riding, and they can have a hard time explaining how to tie shoelaces. Much motor learning is implicit, and knowing mechanical principles is not likely to assist such learning.

Hodges and Franks (2002) proposed that tasks with high perceptual–motor demands or complex response requirements would benefit less from explicit instructions. Some experimental support exists for this proposal (e.g., Farrow & Abernethy, 2002; Sanchez & Reber, 2013). Farrow and Abernethy (2002) manipulated the amount of time participants viewed a tennis ball after a serve. The participants were asked to predict whether the ball would fall to their forehand or backhand. The implicit instruction group received no information about the server's action and the direction of the ball. The explicit instruction group received specific information through videos, verbal and written information, and feedback during practice trials. Not surprisingly, those in the explicit group were able to write more rules and strategies that were important for returning serves than those in the implicit group were. The two groups performed equally well in predicting the direction of the ball, but the implicit group had an advantage at ball contact (i.e., when no ball flight was evident). It seems that those in the implicit group used the anticipatory information to predict the direction without conscious awareness and without advanced cues.

The potential detrimental effect of verbal information was shown by Green and Flowers (1991) in a study in which participants had to manipulate a joystick to catch a ball that moved across a monitor. An explicit instruction group received information about expected pathways and their probability. The implicit group received no information other than the goal of the game. During 800 trials, those in the group that received explicit instruction actually performed more poorly than those in the implicit group, presumably because those in the explicit group devoted more attention to remembering the rule and looking for its occurrence, which disrupted their performance. It seems that instructors should use verbal instructions cautiously when a task has a high degree of perceptual input (e.g., video games) and involves complex responses (e.g., catching a ball that is thrown fast).

A number of studies have used a ski simulator task to explore explicit and implicit motor learning, as well as discovery learning. The participants' goal is usually to move the platform as far to the left and right as possible for a specified time and with a constant cycle time (e.g., for 60 seconds; each cycle takes 3 seconds).

In a study by Wulf and Weigelt (1997), one group—on the basis of previous research on participants who demonstrated high performance—was given explicit instructions to exert force once they moved beyond the center of the simulator platform. The second group was told only the goal of the activity—in this case, to move the platform as far to the left and right as possible for 90 seconds, with each cycle taking 2 seconds. This group was considered a discovery or implicit learning group. On performance and transfer tasks, the discovery group performed better. These participants apparently learned the technique (exert force once beyond the center) in an implicit manner.

A number of studies have used the ski simulating apparatus as well as other complex motor tasks to explore the impact of both demonstrations and verbal instruction compared to discovery learning (see Hodges & Franks, 2002; Lee et al., 2001). In general, the results support the effectiveness of allowing learners to discover how best to achieve task goals. It seems that instructions may interfere with learning if attention is misdirected by either demonstrations or verbal instruction. Of course, this assumes that the task goal is understood and that performance feedback of

TRY THIS

Can you Make Tying Shoe Laces Explicit?

Exercise 15.5

Create groups of two or three. We assume that all members of the group can tie their own shoelaces. It is a common activity that we do regularly, and university students have had many years of practice. Create two columns on a sheet of paper, one labeled Explicit and one Implicit. For the first phase of this activity, the group lists explicit information about how to tie shoelaces. This will be a bit of a challenge because you have had so many years of practice with this task. After you generate some explicit knowledge, actually tie your shoelaces a couple of times and see if you can add to the explicit list and begin to identify implicit factors. Select a sport skill and repeat the exercise.

some form is present in the learning situation. This research usually included novice adult learners, but even with fourth- and fifth-grade children learning a soccer loft kick, discovery learning has been shown to be more effective than explicit instructions (Gredin & Williams, 2016).

Ringenbach and Lantero (2005) extended this line of thinking regarding self-discovery. They asked typically developing children and adults, as well as adults with Down syndrome, to draw circles with both hands. First, in an exploratory phase, participants performed the task any way they wished. Then the three groups were instructed to draw the circles either symmetrically (in-phase) or asymmetrically (anti-phase). Adults without a disability responded without problems. However, the children and the adults with Down syndrome, who had performed symmetrically in the exploratory, or self-selected phase, performed less symmetrically when they were requested to perform symmetrically. This demonstrates that even with children and people with an intellectual disability, self-selected or exploratory instructions may be best.

Verbal Cues

Verbal cues are commonly used by coaches, instructors, and therapists. They are brief and concise phrases that direct attention to regulatory conditions in the environment, prompt key skill components, or initiate activity (Magill, 2017; Ste-Marie et al., 2012). The classic phrase, *Look at the ball* directs attention; *Bend your knees* focuses on a skill component; and *Ready, set, go* prompts activity. Magill (2017) offered the following suggestions for using verbal cues to enhance their effectiveness. Cues should be one to three words in length, be easily related to aspects of the skill, be used only for the most critical elements, not interfere with performance, be rehearsed by the learner, and direct shifts of attention and the rhythm of movement sequences.

Directing Attention and Providing Guidance

One of the uses of verbal cues is to direct attention. Previously presented research warned that explicitly directing attention to optimal or correct coordination of the limbs may not facilitate learning and may even be detrimental. How can we help learners focus on their bodies or the environment to promote skill acquisition, and what are the developmental implications? As mentioned in chapter 11, one of the concepts of attention is **visually searching** for environmental cues necessary for performance (Magill, 2017; Schmidt & Lee, 2011). Attention may be broad or narrow and external or internal, as discussed in chapter 2.

An external focus produces greater accuracy, consistency, and efficiency in learning compared to an internal focus. This is consistent with the positive view of discovery learning and the potential detrimental effects of incorrect attentional focus via demonstrations and verbal

WHAT DO YOU THINK?

Exercise 15.6

1. Choose two skills. Describe how you could implement verbal instruction to facilitate student learning. Provide examples of verbal cues.

2. Can you recall instances when an instructor, perhaps even your professor in this course, seemed to go on and on verbally and finally you said, "So that's what you mean?" What made this difficult? Was it simply too much detail, or was the goal of the activity unclear?

instructions regarding coordination patterns. Unlike some variables in motor learning, the superiority of an external focus exists for both performance and learning (Wulf, 2013).

The external focus viewpoint is a rather robust finding for novice as well as experienced learners (Wulf, 2013). Research with children has provided unambiguous support for external focus on a soccer throwing task (Wulf, Chiviacowsky, Schiller, & Avila, 2010) and with target throwing (Avila, Chiviacowsky, & Wulf, 2012). External focus superiority also extends to children with ADHD (Saemi, Porter, Wulf, Ghotbi-Varzaneh, & Bakhtari, 2013) and intellectual disabilities (Chiviacowsky, Wulf, & Avila, 2012). It seems reasonable for instructors to consider using some internal focus with children.

Visual selective attention (often called a visual cue) refers to directing visual attention to environmental information to help people prepare for and perform an action (Magill, 2017). Important visual cues to guide movements are available in central vision (where the eyes focus) and peripherally. Much evidence suggests that experienced or expert performers in competitive sports are better able to attend to cues than less experienced or novice performers are, and that they pick up the cues earlier, thus enabling them to anticipate their opponents' movements and prepare their own responses. The cues depend on the situation. Waiting for the serve in tennis, experts actually watched for cues in the few seconds prior to initiating the serve, particularly in the head and shoulder and trunk regions (Goulet, Bard, & Fleury, 1989). Experienced players in

soccer attended more to the hip region of an opponent in one-on-one situations than less experienced players did (Williams & Davids, 1998).

Lefebvre and Reid (1998) asked boys and girls aged 6 to 12, with and without coordination difficulties, to watch a video and predict whether the ball thrown by a child would land to the left, to the right, or at the catcher. The older children were more effective predictors with less visual information available; boys were generally more effective than girls; and those without coordination problems were more effective than those with coordination problems. The authors concluded that experience is a significant factor in the development of attention to early cues. Because the cues are quite specific to the activity context, instructors can assist by directing learners' attention to relevant cues as well as providing sufficient practice to use such cues (Magill, 2017). Video-based visual search programs have also shown some promise as a teaching tool (e.g., Williams, Ward, Smeeton, & Allen, 2004).

Summary

This chapter would provide Donaya, the ski coach featured in the chapter-opening scenario, with some guidance about factors to consider prior to hitting the slopes with her students. Goal setting, demonstrations, verbalizations, and attention directing and physical guidance have been used effectively to promote performance and learning. Demonstrations and verbalizations are advantageous when there is need to explain a task goal, outline a movement sequence, promote the use of strategies, deal with a fearful learning situation, or point out an important cue. If the task goal is outcome oriented in a team sport, too many demonstrations and words might detract from the processing of team tactics. Demonstrations and verbalizations as means to acquire patterns of coordination with closed skills may best be described as overrated, assuming that the task goal is known and performance feedback is available. Implicit learning characterizes much motor learning. Our female ski coach can feel comfortable using carefully placed demonstrations, sometimes in concert with player demonstrations, and verbal cues to guide action and attention. She was correct in her questions about the potential detrimental impact of too many words and too many expert demonstrations.

ONLINE LEARNING

Visit the web resource at www.HumanKinetics.com/MotorLearningAndDevelopment for an accompanying lab activity and exercises from the chapter.

LEARNING AIDS

Supplemental Activities

1. Some of the suggestions in this chapter might appear contradictory to common practice. For example, research on the impact of demonstrations suggests that they are not as beneficial in as many situations as we might have thought. Interview an experienced and excellent teacher or coach. Determine where your interviewee agrees and disagrees with some of the generalizations in this chapter. Can you resolve the areas of disagreement?

2. Goal setting is so important in many walks of life that the Internet has extensive quotes and images related to it. Locate some and see if you can match them to outcome goals, performance goals, and process goals. You will also find steps and guides to goal setting. Do these match some of the goal-setting principles discussed in the chapter? Do some of them go beyond the goal-setting principles?

Glossary

explicit learning—The conscious awareness of learning a task.

goal setting—A self-regulatory skill that allows people to monitor progress toward a self-determined goal. Goals should be specific, attainable, challenging, and realistic.

implicit learning—Learning without consciousness.

learning model—A model who demonstrates variability in performance. In physical education, this usually refers to a novice who practices the skill and receives feedback from an instructor. Learners likely identify with the learning model because of similarity in status or as a result of watching the model engage in the problem-solving process.

outcome goals—Goals that focus on the results of performance in comparison to others.

performance goals—Goals that focus on improvement relative to one's own performance.

process goals—Goals that focus on particular aspects of skill acquisition.

verbal cues—Brief and concise phrases used by teachers, coaches, and therapists to direct attention to regulatory conditions in the environment, prompt key skill components, or initiate activity.

visually searching—An aspect of attention that involves detecting the environmental cues necessary for performance.

PRACTICE

After reading this chapter, you should be able to do the following:

- Discuss what research has revealed about the amount and timing of practice that results in the most learning.
- Explain variable and constant practice and the contextual interference effect.
- Describe block and random practice by explaining how they are used in instruction.
- Explain part and whole practice and their respective challenges for transferring to real-life learning situations.
- Discuss mental practice and imagery and how they may enhance learning and performance, and explain how instructors can mass or distribute practice.

Optimal Practice for Maximal Results

As a new physical therapist, Javier knows that he is ready to diagnose and treat many skeletal and muscular problems. But his boss has asked him to teach Lailani, a young woman, how to walk with new prostheses. She lost both legs just above the knees, and thankfully her legs have healed after the operation. She is eager to get out of the wheelchair she has been using since her operation because prostheses will allow greater mobility. As a snowboarder in high school, she wonders whether she will be able to enjoy the sport once again. The insurance company has informed Javier's clinic of the total number of billing hours, and Javier is concerned that unless Lailani makes some immediate progress, she might slip into a depression. Thus, he wants to maximize his time with her within the total hours available and within the specific sessions that his boss has already established. Javier realizes that he has to plan the practice time efficiently. He wonders what practice options are available.

This chapter focuses on many types of practice, or how practice can be organized, including variable, constant, random, blocked, part, whole, mental, massed, and distributed practice. That is a lot of practice types! The learner, instructor, or therapist can manipulate these types to augment learning. We provide the scientific support behind each type of practice and address issues regarding practice organization that might be relevant to Javier. Variables such as age, experience, and type of skill affect whether a particular form of practice actually accelerates learning compared to another.

The one practice variable of penultimate importance is, not surprisingly, practice itself (Schmidt & Lee, 2011). "If anything is certain in motor learning it is that there is no better, faster, or more efficient way of achieving it than with practice" (Lee, Chamberlin, & Hodges, 2001, p. 136). So, to learn racquetball, downhill skiing, or how to use new prostheses, you need to practice. That is not telling you anything you did not already know. But how much practice is necessary and how practice should be organized are more complicated questions. There is also increasing support for self-controlled practice, which may enhance learners' sense of autonomy and competence of the learner (Sanli, Patterson, Bray, & Lee, 2013).

Is it just a matter of repeating movements many times to become skilled, such as practicing walking with prostheses over and over again? If the basketball skills of dribbling, shooting, and passing need to be improved, should you focus on one skill for a considerable time before practicing the next skill? What advice can we give the coach who has her soccer team practice fun drills over and over again, only to see the players incapable of executing the skills in a real game?

Research findings relevant to practitioners sometimes depend on the type of task involved. When motor learning was in its infancy, simple tasks with which people had little experience were often used. This made sense because simple tasks could be investigated in controlled laboratories in which only the experimenter and participant interacted. Novel tasks were preferred because researchers did not want their findings affected by previous learning and experience. In fact, early motor learning specialists helped create tasks such as linear positioning, pursuit rotor, coincidence anticipation, and stabilometer tasks. The required responses sometimes included only one degree of freedom or were as simple as pressing a button. Occasionally, an inquisitive young researcher questioned whether the results from controlled laboratory environments could be applied to real environments—for example, a physical education class in which one teacher works with 30 students who influence each other and have different experiences with skills to be learned, which are often complex. The practice organization literature therefore has included discussions of findings from laboratories using controlled conditions versus real-life tasks and situations.

Amount of Practice

Practical reasons have restricted the number of motor learning studies that use extensive practice, but those conducted have been very insightful. Bryan and Harter (1897, 1899) investigated telegraphic skills over months of practice; Snoddy (1926) required participants to practice a mirror drawing task for 100 days; and Crossman (1959) reported performance changes in cigar rolling over seven years of practice. Self-controlled practice was not investigated in these early motor learning studies. However, when permitted to choose the amount of practice (Post, Fairbrother, & Barros, 2011) or the amount of practice in a fixed time period (Post, Fairbrother, Barros, & Kulpa, 2014), learners demonstrated superior learning to those who practiced under experimenter-controlled conditions.

These studies, among others, have led to a number of general conclusions, including the following:

- Early improvement in skill acquisition is generally very large and becomes smaller with additional practice.
- All things being equal, more learning will occur with more practice (power law of practice; Schmidt & Lee, 2011).
- Plateaus in performance may occur during skill acquisition.
- Improved performance, however minute, may be apparent after many years of practice.
- Motor learning is enhanced when learners control aspects of the practice (see chapter 12; Sanli et al., 2013).

As we mentioned in chapter 11, experts often have had countless hours of practice, and a significant portion of those hours have occurred under deliberate practice conditions (Ericsson, 2003). Deliberate practice involves activities designed to improve performance that require much effort and are not necessarily enjoyable. Because research has not compared deliberate practice with other forms of extensive practice, it is difficult to claim that expertise can be achieved only by deliberate practice. Also, athletes have often reported enjoyment while making deliberate attempts to improve performance (Deakin & Cobley, 2003). In any case, the amount of practice is a significant contributor to expert performance.

Although questions of deliberate practice remain, Lee and colleagues (2001) astutely observed, "The deliberate practice hypothesis does serve to refocus the practitioner's attention onto the importance of practice, rather than 'natural talent' when identifying individuals as potentially future experts" (p. 117). Of course, expert levels of performance may not be a motivating factor for many people, either children or adults. They may be motivated to downhill ski so that they can participate with friends and manage a single-diamond hill

safely; a desire to compete and to be faster than everyone else is not a factor.

One of the authors of this text would be pleased to break 100 in golf, but has no aspirations to challenge Jordan Spieth. Although the amount of practice required to achieve some personal criterion of success will be influenced by individual goals and motivation, the author should not underestimate the amount of practice that would be required to break 100.

Variable Practice

Variable practice is practice that includes variations of the skill itself or the context of the skill. Three variations of a forehand shot in tennis are a return at full force because the ball comes directly to your forehand where you are standing, a high lob because you had to scamper to the back line, and a volley before the ball hits the ground near the net. When these forms of the forehand are practiced in mixed order during a practice period, the practice is called **variable practice** (Schmidt & Lee, 2014). The order of practice (pattern) of the three variations might be BCACBAACBC. The learner may never use the same shot twice in a row, but certainly the instructor will project the ball to intermingle the three shots during a practice session. When the same skill is practiced repeatedly, the practice is referred to as **constant practice** (Schmidt & Lee, 2014).

In constant practice, the tennis instructor has the learner repeat many trials of the forceful forehand return with minimal lateral body movement before changing to the lob. The constant practice schedule is more intuitive and the one many of us have experienced as learners: a fixed amount of time or number of trials on one skill before moving to the next. This may seem reasonable because the learner can concentrate on one skill and benefit from feedback and time to refine the movement.

Somewhat surprisingly, perhaps, variable practice has actually been shown to be superior to constant practice for learning a wide range of motor skills when a novel variation of the skill is required (James & Conatser, 2014; Lee et al., 2001; Magill, 2017; Schmidt & Lee, 2014; Yao & DeSola, 2009). Variable practice is advocated by each of the major models of skill acquisition described in chapter 4, albeit for different reasons (Magill, 2017). Variable practice develops schema and generalized motor programs so that people can respond to novel movement situations, according to the cognitive schema perspective of Schmidt (1975). Such practice provides the necessary variation of regulatory and nonregulatory contexts in Gentile's stages model (1972, 2000). Finally, it gives learners the opportunity to explore and discover the perceptual motor landscape so that they can assemble functional motor patterns, according to the dynamic systems and ecological approaches (Davids, Button, & Bennett, 2008).

Constant practice may be beneficial if the ultimate movement goal remains consistent across trials. For example, free throws in basketball always occur from the same distance with noninterfering opponents; hence, a novel response is not required. A free throw is a unique action within the general category of throwing. Breslin, Hodges, Steenson, and Williams (2012) demonstrated the benefit of constant practice over variable practice following 300 trials of a basketball free throw. Baseball pitching, 3-meter diving, and much of competitive gymnastics involve consistency across time and context rather than novel responses to changing environments. Such skills are referred to as **especial skills** (Keetch, Schmidt, Lee, & Young, 2005). Also, emerging evidence suggests that constant practice may be superior to variable practice in acquiring force output patterns (King & Newell, 2013). See Ranganathan and Newell (2012) for a more complete discussion.

The variability of practice hypothesis was first postulated by Schmidt (1975) in the context of generalized motor programs and schema development. When faced with a goal-oriented movement, the person retrieves a generalized motor program from long-term memory and then selects parameters that will dictate how the action will be executed (e.g., how forceful, how long). A generalized motor program is largely defined by invariant features—that is, characteristics of the movement that remain constant despite changes in parameters (see chapter 3). For example, a throw usually has a stepping action, trunk rotation, arm action, wrist movement, and follow-through (Schmidt & Lee, 2014). Those are the invariant features of the throw and constitute the generalized motor program.

A throw has many variations depending on factors such as the object (e.g., ball or disc) and the intended distance of the throw. Variable practice involves variability in the parameters of the movement, not different movements. Different versions or variations of the basketball dribble might include parameters such as different dribbling speeds, ball heights, and player movements during a dribble. The movement **schema** is an abstract or general memory representation of a set of rules that connect a person's actions to the parameters needed to produce the outcome (Schmidt & Lee, 2014; see Schmidt, 1975, or Schmidt & Lee, 2011, for a more detailed account of schema). Consider a basketball player's decision, or desired outcome, to dribble around an opponent rather than shoot or pass during a game. This is achieved by using a generalized motor program of dribbling, with the addition of *quickly changing hands so that the ball is on the outside, driving quickly to the left of the opponent, and keeping the ball low.* The variations of the dribble (in italics) are the parameters that can change if the goal and context of the next dribble are different (e.g., the player decides to drive to the right because she knows this opponent does not move quickly to that side). Thus, a solution to a movement problem involves selecting the correct parameters from a generalized motor program (Schmidt & Lee, 2014).

With practice, the rules, or schema, are developed and used to determine the parameters required for different versions of a generalized motor program. Practice is variable because different parameters of the movement are included. Over time, the person learns relationships—for example, that different intensities and directions of forces generated by the hand produce successful dribbles for different running speeds and heights. Variable practice requires the learner to select new parameters for each movement trial; much less effort is required in constant practice because the same parameters are selected for many trials in a row. Strong schemas enable the person to select the appropriate parameters in novel contexts.

Much research supports the increased benefit of variable over constant practice when learning is assessed on tests of transfer and retention (Lee et al., 2001). Using an example from Schmidt and Wrisberg (2008, p. 274), suppose that a movement class is throwing a ball to different distances. Constant practice groups are created, and each one throws 60 balls at one of the distances (e.g., throws of 20, 30, or 40 yards). A variable practice group throws 20 balls at 20 yards, 20 balls at 30 yards, and 20 balls at 40 yards. Thus, each group has the same amount of practice, 60 throws. During the initial practice, the constant practice groups usually perform better than the variable group. The reason is likely that the constant practice groups are concerned with only one distance and hence one movement, whereas the variable practice group is attempting to produce three versions of a movement in an intermingled way. When the groups later switch to a new version of the movement such as a throw of 25 yards, the variable group usually performs better, or at least as well as the constant variable groups.

Thus, the benefits of variable practice may not appear in immediate performance but rather on later tests of transfer and retention. In other words, variable practice may appear to be adversely affecting performance during learning trials, but will ultimately enhance learning (for a reminder of the differences between learning and performance, see chapter 1; to compare retention and transfer, see chapter 5). Variable practice may seem very sensible with open skills because they inherently include variability. After all, tennis players try to make it difficult for you to return the ball by hitting it with unexpected direction and force, and those nasty folks called opponents are always trying to prevent you from receiving a pass from your basketball teammate. But even in closed skills, there are benefits from variable practice that might not seem so obvious at the outset. Golfers must perform under various wind conditions, on different fairway layouts, and also under anxiety in competition, and they must make appropriate decisions, from the selection of clubs to how to putt given the layout of the green. Golfers may have a great deal of time to decide on a course of action, but shots must be "parameterized" to the physical and psychological playing conditions.

Moxley (1979) provided an early example of the positive impact of variable practice on children. She asked six- to eight-year-olds to throw badminton shuttlecocks to a target on the floor. Half the children threw from a constant location (constant practice), and half threw from four different locations (variable practice). As predicted by schema theory, the variable practice group was more accurate than the constant practice group on a novel variation of the task. Consistent with schema theory, Green, Whitehead, and Sugden (1995) demonstrated that 11-year-old girls in a variable practice group who used four different rackets (tennis, squash, badminton, and short tennis) performed better on an accuracy transfer test than did girls in a group that practiced only with a tennis racket and those in a group that changed rackets on each block of trials.

Neither Moxley nor Green and colleagues investigated children of different ages or experiences.

Additional studies with children support the advantage of variable practice in motor skill learning (e.g., Gerson & Thomas, 1977; Kerr & Booth, 1978; Wulf, 1991; Zetou, Papadakis, Vernadakis, Derri, Bebetsos, & Filippou, 2014). However, other studies provided mixed or minimal support (e.g., Jarus & Goverover, 1999; Pease & Pupnow, 1983; Pigott & Shapiro, 1984; Wrisberg & Mead, 1981). The equivocal nature of these findings led Yan, Thomas, and Thomas (1998) to conduct a meta-analysis on the variable versus constant practice issue with children. The researchers located 39 effect sizes (ESs) in nine studies that included 272 boys and 336 girls ranging in age from 3 to 11. The overall ES between variable and constant practice with regard to transfer to a new task was .28, a relatively small effect. That is, although variable practice was generally superior, the difference from constant practice was not great. The authors were also interested in the impact of age, type of task (rapid timing versus slow positioning), and type of movement (simple linear positioning versus complex or real sport movements such as throwing a beanbag). Age had a strong mediating influence on the advantage of variable practice over constant practice; there was a large ES (.80) for young children aged 3 to 5 but a relatively small ES for those between 6 and 11 years of age. The transfer benefits of variable practice over constant practice were greater for more ballistic tasks than for slow movements as well as for more complex real-world movements than for simple movements. One can see that research findings can be quite complex and that generalizations and suggestions for practitioners might depend on age and the type of task or movement.

Yan and colleagues (1998) concluded that younger children might benefit more from variable practice than older children. Consistent with the intrinsic dynamics of self-regulation and expertise outlined in chapters 11 and 12, the authors suggested that across childhood, youngsters improve in cognitive performance, gather movement-related knowledge, and use strategies effectively. Thus, because older children have already developed a number of movement schemas, variable practice therefore has less benefit for them. In contrast, younger children likely have fewer and less well-developed schemas and thus benefit more from variable practice. Overall, the authors concluded that variable practice is better than constant practice for

TRY THIS

Throwing for Dollars

Exercise 16.1

In this activity you compare variable and constant practice on a variation of Moxley's (1979) shuttlecock throwing task. Tape a dollar bill to the wall. Measure distances of 4, 8, and 12 feet (1.2, 2.4, and 3.7 m). Create groups of six. Three people form the constant practice group and throw 30 shuttlecocks from 8 feet. The other three form the variable practice group and throw 10 shuttlecocks from 4 feet (1.2 m), 10 from 8 feet (2.4 m), and 10 from 12 feet (3.7 m). Count the number of times each person hits the dollar bill in 30 throws. This number is the performance score. Was there a difference between the constant and variable groups? Now have everyone throw 20 times from 6 feet (1.8 m; transfer task) and again count the number of hits. This number is the learning score. Was there a difference between the constant and variable groups? If not, what is your explanation?

RESEARCH NOTES

Variable Practice Across Age

Douvis (2005) investigated variable practice on a forehand drive in tennis with 9- and 10-year-olds and 18- and 19-year-old university students. There were 40 males in each group, and no one had experience with tennis prior to the study. Practice sessions were one hour, three times per week, for a total of 18 practice sessions over six weeks. Trained instructors led the practice sessions; they provided a warm-up, taught the technique of the forehand drive, and served the ball to the participants for 100 return drives per session. There were four practice targets on the far side of the net, differing in distance from the participants, as well as a fifth transfer target. Each age category consisted of four experimental groups. Group 1 performed the 100 trials at the transfer target. Group 2 practiced at four targets (25 trials at each), group 3 practiced 20 trials at each of the five targets, and group 4 executed 100 trials but without a specific target and thus constituted the control group. The transfer test occurred 72 hours following the final practice session at the end of the six weeks and consisted of 60 trials. The older students performed better than the younger students, but variable practice conditions proved superior to constant practice for both groups on a transfer test. That is, groups who practiced with four or five targets outperformed groups who practiced with one or no specific target. These findings support the value of variability of practice.

children's motor skill learning; although the magnitude of the effect may be small, they advised practitioners to consider variable practice conditions for children and young athletes.

Yan and colleagues' (1998) results do not mean that variable practice will have no benefit for older elementary school–aged children. The tasks included in Yan and colleagues' study were relatively simple. Although they distinguished between simple linear positioning tasks and more complex real-world tasks such as throwing a beanbag, the latter were likely rather easy for the older children (ages 6-8 and 9-11) despite being classified as complex. When learning new movements skills in real games and sport, older children may well develop new movement schemas more efficiently with variable practice. In addition, research with children (e.g., Pigott & Shapiro, 1984; Wrisberg & Mead, 1983) has occasionally demonstrated that some combination of variable and constant practice might be most effective. Wrisberg and

Mead (1983) showed that 6- to 8-year-olds who received six repetitions of a movement speed on a coincident timing task during practice, before moving to additional movement speeds, were more capable on a transfer task than children who performed completely random or variable practice. There is some agreement that variable practice is likely to be more productive after the learner has some notion of the skill and has moved beyond the cognitive stage of the Fitts and Posner (1967) learning model, or the getting the idea of the movement stage of Gentile's model (2000). One does not want to overwhelm the learner with too much variability too early (Boyce, Coker, & Bunker, 2006; Schmidt & Lee, 2014). Of course, consistent with knowledge and expertise perspectives, deciding when to introduce variability should be based not so much on age as on experience with the task. Boyce and colleagues (2006) recommended several pedagogical practices that lend themselves to using variable practice; they are outlined in table 16.1.

Table 16.1 Variability of Practice and Pedagogy

Pedagogical method	Explanation and examples
Movement concepts	Students practicing bouncing a ball are encouraged to bounce it slow or fast.
Challenges	Challenges are extensions of the current skill with criteria for success (e.g., dribbling a basketball for 30 seconds without looking down at it).
Additional skill	Dribbling with the feet is extended to dribbling and passing.
Variety of settings or contexts	Following Gentile's (2000) regulatory conditions, learners practice skills in a gamelike context such as one on one or in small groups after practicing in isolation. Learners practice nonregulatory conditions as well, such as performing a dance in front of a class after practicing alone.
Natural variability in open skills	For example, grade 3 students practice catching in pairs, trying to throw directly to a partner. Natural variability of speed and accuracy of throws will be present.

The original variability of practice hypothesis proposed that variability existed in movement parameters in a single generalized motor program. But what is known about organizing practices when variability appears as different movements related to a sport or activity, such as passing, shooting, and dribbling in soccer? Should a given practice include a mixture of the three skills, much like variable practice, or is it more effective to focus on only one of the skills for a considerable period of time before moving to the next skill? The area dealing with these nuances, known as contextual interference, addresses blocked, random, and serial practice.

Contextual Interference Effect

Battig (1979) introduced the term **contextual interference** to refer to an unexpected research finding on the cognitive task of learning word lists. Contextual interference refers to the interference in performance resulting from repeating multiple skills within the context of practice (Lee, 2012; Magill, 2017). In other words, during practice a negative impact is likely when attempting to learn several tasks at the same time, such as a soccer kick, pass, and dribble. Battig also demonstrated a **contextual interference effect**—in this case, a benefit in learning resulting from practicing multiple skills (Magill, 2017). Despite creating problems with performance during practice, contextual inter-

ference positively influenced learning as measured by retention and transfer (Lee, 2012; Magill, 2017).

Contextual interference research often uses blocked, random, and serial practice (Lee et al., 2001; Magill, 2017; Schmidt & Lee, 2014). **Blocked practice** is rehearsal of one skill repeated over a fixed block of time before moving to the next skill. It is similar to constant practice as described in the previous section because one skill is practiced over and over again, as often seen in repeated drills. **Random practice** is a practice sequence in which several skills are mixed in a random order. An attempt is made to avoid rehearsal of the same skill twice in a row. In some ways this is like variable practice, but random practice uses different skills rather than variations of the same skill as in variable practice. The organization of **serial practice** is similar to that of random practice in that various skills are intermingled during practice, but in a fixed format. Table 16.2 shows how these forms of practice might appear across three 30-minute sessions of soccer.

The contextual interference effect is a paradox, because a random practice schedule can be detrimental during acquisition but have a positive effect on learning. Two main theories have been proposed to explain this paradox: the **elaboration and distinctive hypothesis** and the **forgetting and reconstruction hypothesis** (Lee, 2012; Lee & Magill, 1985; Schmidt & Lee, 2014; Shea & Morgan, 1979).

Exercise 16.2

1. Pick two activities. Describe how you would teach them using each type of practice. The overhand throw is provided as an example.

Activity	Type of practice	Practice session
Overhand throw	Constant	Throw 60 balls 20 yards.
	Variable	Throw 20 balls 20 yards. Throw 20 balls 40 yards. Throw 20 balls 60 yards.
	Constant	
	Variable	
	Constant	
	Variable	

2. Choose one skill. Using table 16.1 as a guide, provide examples of how you would use each of these methods to facilitate variable practice.

Skill:	
Method	**Example**
Movement concepts	
Challenges	
Additional skills	
Variety of settings or contexts	
Natural variability in open skills	

Table 16.2 Three Soccer Classes With Three Skills and Three Practice Formats

Type of practice	Amount of contextual interference	Duration for each skill (in minutes)	Class 1	Class 2	Class 3
Constant	Zero	30	All passing	All shooting	All dribbling
Blocked practice	Low	10	Passing	Passing	Passing
		10	Dribbling	Dribbling	Dribbling
		10	Shooting	Shooting	Shooting
Serial practice	Moderate	5	Passing	Passing	Passing
		5	Dribbling	Dribbling	Dribbling
		5	Shooting	Shooting	Shooting
		5	Passing	Passing	Passing
		5	Dribbling	Dribbling	Dribbling
		5	Shooting	Shooting	Shooting
Random practice	High	Total of 30 for all skills	Dribbling Dribbling Passing Shooting Passing	Passing Shooting Dribbling Shooting Dribbling	Shooting Shooting Passing Dribbling Passing

The elaboration and distinctive hypothesis was proposed by Shea and Morgan (1979). They suggested that random practice results in more cognitive strategies such as comparing and contrasting movements in working memory. As the person shifts from one skill to the next, the distinct nature of each becomes clearer and more meaningful in long-term memory. This cognitive effort has a deleterious effect during acquisition, but is advantageous later when learning is assessed. Of course, during blocked practice, people are not challenged to compare and contrast skills because they perform many repetitions of the same skill.

The second theoretical account, the forgetting and reconstruction hypothesis, was proposed by Lee and Magill (1985). They argued that the key explanation for the contextual interference effect is the action planning required for each skill. In random practice, the person must abandon the action plan used on the previous skill because a new one must be constructed. Thus, the action plan is forgotten initially but is renewed each time that skill is repeated later during practice. Random practice forces the learner to practice action planning, which is absent in blocked practice.

Both the elaboration and distinctive hypothesis and the forgetting and reconstruction hypothesis enjoy research support (Brady, 1998; Lee, 2012; Magill, 2017). Time will tell as to which one emerges as the more effective explanation, or whether some combination of the two is proposed.

The contextual interference effect is a relatively robust finding based on a great deal of empirical research (Lee, 2012) that included children (discussed later in this section), adults (e.g., Feghhi, Abdoli, & Valizadeh, 2011), and older adults (e.g., Lin, Wu, Udompholkul, & Knowlton, 2010). Practitioners should feel comfortable using random practice in most learning situations. Despite this general statement, though, some research findings have provided no, or limited, support for the contextual interference effect (e.g., Cheong, Lay, Grove, Medic, & Razman, 2012).

Unfortunately, clear and unequivocal guidelines that might tell us that skill A under condition X will not yield the interference effect do not exist. More research is needed on this issue. But neither does the research suggest that blocked practice

Contextual Interference

Shea and Morgan (1979) conducted the first motor learning study that provided evidence of the contextual interference effect. The basic task was to move an arm and grasp a tennis ball and then knock over three of six small wooden barriers as quickly as possible and return the tennis ball to a final resting position. Participants had to learn three movement patterns (skills A, B, and C); patterns were illuminated by different-colored lights.

Two groups of university-aged students practiced the three arm and hand movements under blocked or random conditions. The blocked group had 54 practice trials: 18 consecutive trials for skill A, then 18 trials for skill B, and then 18 trials for skill C. The random group also had 54 trials to acquire the three skills, but practiced them in random order, never performing a skill twice in a row over the 54 trials. As shown in figure 16.1, the blocked group produced quicker movements during the practice phase.

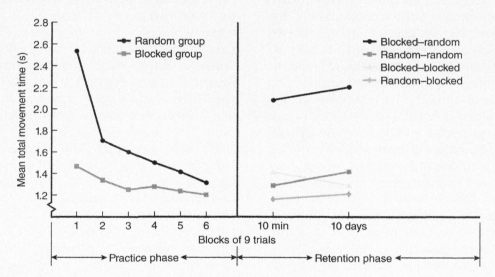

Figure 16.1   Performance on movement–speed tasks under random and blocked practice conditions. The relative amount that the groups learned is indicated by their retention performance at the right.

From J.B. Shea and R.L. Morgan, 1979, "Contextual interference effects on the acquisition, retention, and transfer of a motor skill," *Journal of Experimental Psychology: Human Learning & Memory* 5(2): 179-187. Reprinted by permission of the American Psychological Association.

To assess learning, the researchers required the participants to perform a retention test, one immediately after practice (10 minutes) and one 10 days later. The retention tests were performed under both blocked and random formats. Figure 16.1 clearly demonstrates that the participants who had practiced under random conditions became much quicker than those who had practiced under block conditions. In fact, the random group maintained the speeds accomplished during acquisition, whereas the blocked group showed very poor performance during randomly ordered retention trials. In line with contextual interference predictions, blocked practice produced faster immediate performance, but random practice resulted in more learning.

is generally more effective in motor skill acquisition than random practice. When the contextual interference effect fails to enhance learning, the research usually shows a nonsignificant difference between blocked and random practice, not the superiority of blocked practice. A number of mediators have been proposed that cast doubt on the general benefit of contextual interference. These include age, skill level, type of skill, personality, motivation, and amount of interference.

The contextual interference effect has been investigated with children. The superiority of random practice was shown on a handwriting task with 5- to 7-year-olds (Ste-Marie, Clark, Findlay, & Latimer, 2004). However, mixed results were found for the contextual interference effect for the forehand tennis groundstroke in two groups of 26 children aged 8 to 9 and 10 to 12 (Farrow & Maschette, 1997). The contextual inference effect was evident for the 10- to 12-year-olds in the retention phase on the preferred hand, and the random group was superior to the blocked group. However, the expected superiority of the blocked group during acquisition was not observed, and interference effects were not evident for the 8- and 9-year-olds. This mixed pattern of results with children is evident in other studies as well (Bortoli, Spagolla & Robazza, 2001; Del Rey, Whitehurst, & Wood, 1983; Edwards, Elliott, & Lee, 1986; Pollock & Lee, 1997; Vera, Alvarez, & Medina, 2008).

Brady (2004) conducted a meta-analysis on the contextual inference effect that provides insight into age as a moderator. He located 139 effect sizes (ESs) from 61 studies. The overall ES (i.e., across all ages and skills) was .38. Three age groups were compared: adults, adolescents, and children. The ESs were .50, .10, and .09, respectively. It appears that despite some research demonstrating the advantage of random practice to motor skill learning in children and youth, the overall effect is quite small. The explanation for the low ES for the children might be similar to

that given in the previous discussion of variable and constant practice in children. Young children may be overwhelmed with random practice because of their limited information-processing capabilities and the complexity of sport skills (Brady, 2004).

Newell and McDonald (1992) asserted that random practice would have more impact later in the process of learning, and Wulf and Schmidt (1994) suggested that random practice for novices may produce too much variability. In concert with these views, Herbert, Landin, and Solmon (1996) found that low-skilled university students performed forehand and backhand tennis strokes better on a retention test following blocked practice. From a practical viewpoint, it might be wise to use some blocked practice during early stages of learning, regardless of age, before inserting some random practice. On the other hand, even young children might benefit from random practice when practicing skills with which they have some experience and knowledge (e.g., a talented soccer team of eight-year-olds).

Beyond age and skill, the amount of interference might be an important variable when we seek to understand the sometimes equivocal nature of the contextual interference research. Perhaps contextual interference is more like a continuum between the two polar opposites of random practice (high interference) and blocked practice (low interference). Magill (2017) asserted that between the extremes falls moderate contextual interference, such as the serial order of trials of all task variations, the random repetition of short blocks of trials, and the serial repetition of short blocks of trials. Proteau, Blandin, Alain, and Dorion (1994) demonstrated the superiority of moderate contextual interference over high (random practice) or low (blocked) interference with a barrier knockdown task, and Landin and Hebert (1997) produced similar results with a basketball shooting skill. Pigott and Shapiro (1984) used an underhand toss with children and also found that a moderate contextual interference condition was superior to high or low interference. It seems that some repetition of a skill allows learners to make adjustments over a limited number of trials but that moving to another skill may invoke elaboration or action plan reconstruction to optimally benefit from some interference.

Another variable that is entering the random and block discourse is self-regulation. Four groups of participants learned a task of moving a cursor through a sequence of squares on a monitor as quickly as possible, but they had to stop at each square long enough to click the mouse button (Keetch & Lee, 2007). One group received blocked practice and a second received random trials. A third group used a self-regulated strategy—a mixture of random or blocked trials determined by the individual. The final group was yoked to the self-determined group, thus receiving the same order as in self-regulation but not deciding individually on the mixture of random or blocked

trials. Self-regulation did not provide any special benefits during acquisition, but the self-regulation group was superior to the other groups during retention.

Brady's (2004) meta-analysis also compared contextual interference effects on laboratory tasks and applied, or real-world, tasks. The ES for laboratory tasks for all ages was a moderate .57, whereas it was a small .19 for applied research. As shown in another review study, 60 percent of the studies in applied settings failed to demonstrate contextual interference (Barreiros, Figueiredo, & Godinho, 2007). Reasons for these findings in applied settings may be the complexity of skills in applied compared to laboratory settings, or the fact that students in physical education classes have a wide range of skill level (certainly some were novices in the task studied), or both (Landin & Hebert, 1997). It is also possible that the number of hits or baskets made with applied tasks is too gross a measure to detect differences from findings for laboratory tasks, which can be measured

WHAT DO YOU THINK?

Exercise 16.3

1. Describe in your own words the two theories that attempt to explain the contextual interference effect.

2. Choose two sports and indicate how you would teach the skills associated with each using blocked, serial, and random practice.

Sport 1: Associated skills:				
Practice type	**Time**	**Class 1**	**Class 2**	**Class 3**
Blocked				
Random				
Serial				

Sport 2: Associated skills:				
Practice type	**Time**	**Class 1**	**Class 2**	**Class 3**
Blocked				
Random				
Serial				

to a millisecond (Goode & Magill, 1986). Although the ES for real-world tasks is small across studies, randomized practice schedules are favored when differences do emerge from research (Brady, 2008). Practitioners must judge whether randomized practice can be efficiently implemented in their context, and they might wish to consider moderate contextual interference rather than the extremes of the practice schedules (Brady, 2008).

Other mediating variables might be motivation and attention (Lee & White, 1990). Because random practice necessitates more effort than blocked practice, tasks that are tedious or lacking in intrinsic interest might profit from contextual interference. A final potential mediator proposed by Brady (1998) is personality. He reviewed several studies whose results were consistent with the assertion that impulsive people might particularly benefit from random practice because such practice suppresses impulsivity, causing them to adopt a more reflective style.

Practice Specificity

Promoting the advantages of variable and random practice might seem at odds with the concept of specificity of learning described in the Types of Transfer section in chapter 5. Specificity of learning is the idea that practice experiences should reflect the movement components and environmental conditions of the target skill and target context. To state this differently, if we practice to develop skills for game play or individual competition, our practice should resemble the game or competition as much as possible. Specificity of practice is one of the longest-standing principles of human learning (Magill, 2017; Thorndike, 1914; Thorndike & Woodworth, 1901).

Specificity of practice may have two forms, sensory and motor specificity and context specificity (Schmidt & Lee, 2011). The idea of sensory and motor specificity has emerged largely from the research of Proteau and colleagues (Proteau, 1992; Pro-

teau, Marteniuk, Girourd, & Dugas, 1987; Soucy & Proteau, 2001). Primarily using aiming tasks such as placing a stylus on a target, they have manipulated the type and amount of feedback using techniques such as occluding vision of either the arm or the target. It is often assumed that over many practice trials, the need for sensory feedback diminishes or changes; for example, the learner depends less on visual feedback as kinesthetic feedback assumes more importance (Schmidt, 1975b). However, Proteau's research challenges this assumption, because the findings show that performance deteriorates on a transfer task even following extensive practice if the transfer task includes more or less sensory feedback than in the practice conditions. Proteau (1992) stated, "Withdrawing or adding a significant source of information after a period of practice where it was respectively present or absent results in a deterioration of performance" (p. 96). Thus, if practice included restricted vision, providing more visual information on the transfer task will actually result in poorer, rather than better, performance. It is proposed that this effect of specificity of practice occurs because the learner develops a sensorimotor representation during practice that is disrupted if the "real" game (transfer task) adds or reduces sensory information. Performance is optimal when the practice conditions match the transfer conditions.

This line of thinking was supported in several studies that used a balance beam walking task (Robertson, Tremblay, Anson, and Elliott, 2002). The authors challenged some common practice rituals of teachers and coaches that do not match performance conditions. For example, it is fine to direct participants to visual cues on the beam, which should not differ in competition, but probably not to cues on the home gymnasium ceiling or floor, which are most certainly going to be different in competition. They also challenge the coaching practice of talking an athlete through a routine. This added auditory stimulation cannot occur during competition and therefore should be used cautiously during practice. The authors also recommended that therapists in rehabilitation settings emphasize function- and goal-directed activities rather than isolated muscle actions. Therapists should determine the sources of information required in the functional task and manipulate those in therapy. Studies of gross motor skills that have supported the specificity of practice hypothesis have used powerlifting (Tremblay & Proteau, 1998), ball interception (Tremblay & Proteau, 2001), and basketball free throws (Moradi, Movahedi, & Salehi, 2014).

Proteau's sensorimotor representation logic can be extended to a broader sense of context specificity. We often hear about the need to practice a task over and over again as if to stamp it into the brain (Schmidt & Lee, 2014). This type of thinking appears to coincide with the thousands of hours of practice that experts report (see chapter 11). Without question, slap shots in hockey, golfing tee shots, and new ways of getting out of bed after an accident are often practiced hundreds of times over only a few weeks. But more than one coach has noted that some players perform wonderfully in practice but cannot perform in the game or competition. One of the difficulties with constant and blocked practice is that the target skill may not be practiced in the target context (Schmidt & Lee, 2014). Dribbling a basketball while walking is simply not the same skill as the dribbling required in a game. In a similar vein, practicing skating in hockey with control of the puck and passing to a teammate might be useful as a quick reminder of some passing or puck control techniques, but ignores the reality that the timing of the pass is often dictated by the positioning of moving opponents and teammates. Athletes must be prepared to produce particular movements in various situations. The target context also refers to such things as elevated anxiety on the first hole of golf compared to the driving range because this is now competition and the person wants to impress the other players in the foursome. Table 16.3 includes other features of a skill that might be different in the target context and blocked practice.

The idea of specificity of learning is to practice in a manner that brings learners as close as possible to the target skill and target context. Practitioners must consider the developmental level of the learners (i.e., age and skill level) and their degree of motivation (i.e., a team of elite 10-year-olds will be different from a grade 5 class). There will certainly be times when teachers or therapists believe it is appropriate to use constant and blocked practice, but over time they should remember that such practice is unlikely to mimic the target skill and context. As Schmidt and Wrisberg (2008, p. 264) stated, "The main point is that many *repetitions* in practice are essential for highly skilled performance—but *repetitiveness* in practice is not effective."

Table 16.3 Skill Differences Between the Target Context and Blocked Practice

Target context	Blocked practice
Preceded by regular variable conditions	Not preceded by regular variable conditions
Requires the generation of a solution on each attempt	Requires the generation of a solution only on the first attempt
Allows only one chance for success	Allows many chances for success
Same movement not repeated on successive attempts	Same movement repeated on successive attempts
Corrections not allowed on next attempt	Corrections allowed on the next attempt

Reprinted, by permission, from R.A. Schmidt and C.A. Wrisberg, 2008, *Motor learning and performance: A situation-based learning approach*, 4th ed. (Champaign, IL: Human Kinetics), 264.

Part and Whole Practice

Motor skills are often complex and difficult to learn, particularly for children, novices, and others who lack motivation or the structural constraints that match the skill. Instructors are faced with the decision of whether to teach a skill as a whole or break it into parts and teach the parts before combining them into the whole. Skills that overwhelm a learner, elicit some degree of fear, or even pose a real danger should certainly be broken into parts. The key assumption is that practicing one part of a skill will transfer to performing the whole skill (Lee et al., 2001). In fact, whether part practice transfers to performance of the whole skill is the ultimate test of its effectiveness (Schmidt & Lee, 2005). Concepts in this area of motor learning research very much depend on the nature of the task.

The literature on part and whole practice was advanced by Naylor and Briggs (1963), when they distinguished between task complexity and task organization (Magill & Anderson, 2013). **Task complexity** refers to the number of parts or components and the amount of attention required (information-processing demands). Serving a tennis ball, batting a baseball, and performing a dance routine are complex skills because they demand much attention and have many components. Low-complexity skills have few components and require little processing, such as picking up a ball or walking. Of course, whether a task is complex also depends on the person's experience with that task.

Task organization deals with the relationships of the skill components. The layup in basketball is a skill with a high level of organization because the parts are interdependent in terms of time and space. Other examples are juggling, ski racing, and the golf drive. The time and space performance characteristics of one part depend on those of the part performed just prior to it. If part A is not performed well, part B cannot be performed well, and so on. Tasks with a low level of task organization are those in which the performance of each component is relatively independent. For example, a folk dance has many components, but each task is more or less independent of the one preceding

---

WHAT DO YOU THINK?

Exercise 16.4

Think of one task in each of the four quadrants shown. Tasks could be high in both complexity and organization, high in neither, high in complexity but low in organization, or low in complexity but high in organization.

	High organization	Low organization
High complexity		
Low complexity		

it; someone who is a bit shaky with the gallop at one point in the dance can still perform the dance.

For skills that are low in complexity and high in organization, experts often recommend teaching the whole task because the high interdependency of the parts makes it difficult to practice parts outside the whole skill context. On the other hand, for skills that are high in complexity and low in organization, part practice can be effective because the interdependence of the parts is not critical and part practice can reduce the information-processing demands (Magill & Anderson, 2013; Naylor & Briggs, 1963). Teachers and coaches must therefore analyze tasks to judge their complexity and organization.

As noted, the person's experience with the task affects the complexity of the task and its level of organization for that person. In the case of children, task complexity and organization is likely to be influenced by their physical and cognitive functioning. The benefits of part or whole practice might be influenced by age, but few studies of whole and part practice have included participants who differed in development. An exception is Chan, Luo, Yan, Cai, and Peng (2015), who had first-, third-, and fifth-graders practice a three-beanbag juggling task. Whole practice involved 40 trials per day for six days, and part practice involved juggling with one ball for the first two days, two balls for the next two days, and three balls for the last two days. Based on the results from a retention test, the first-and third-graders benefited the most from part practice, and the fifth-graders retained more with whole practice. Juggling is a task of high complexity and organization, and authors reasoned that the fifth-graders (almost 11 years of age) could benefit from whole practice because of advanced neuromaturation, information processing, and motor coordination. More developmental studies of this nature are warranted.

As you completed exercise 16.4, you might have realized that some skills are not easily categorized as high or low. There may be some intermediate level of both organization and complexity, and thus the general guidelines for high organization–low complexity and low organization–high complexity may be difficult to follow. Did you identify any skills that were both low or both high on each factor? The skill classification of continuous, discrete, and serial may help here.

Continuous skills are usually high in complexity but may be either high or low in organization; however, more often they are also high in organization because of the interdependence of the parts (Magill & Anderson, 2013). Discrete skills may be low in complexity from the viewpoint of the number of parts, but some will still demand a great deal of attention. Schmidt and Lee (2014) made the point that rapid discrete skills such as a bat swing and bimanual skills such as the toss and swing in a tennis serve might be the least likely candidates for part practice. They argued that such skills can be broken down into parts, but that the parts are quite arbitrary, and practicing them in isolation contributes little to whole-task performance (the ultimate goal). For example, practicing the backswing of a golf shot by itself produces different dynamics than are produced in the whole swing because of the stop at the end of the backswing. Serial skills may be high or low in organization based upon the discrete skills that are part of the sequence but often are high in complexity because of the sheer number of skills in the sequence.

Lee and colleagues (2001) also argued that despite the challenge of learning highly interdependent parts (high organization), the research literature does not generally demonstrate instances of negative transfer from part practice; rather, some benefits of part learning are usually described. In other words, if a task has high organization but would overwhelm and discourage a learner, some form of part practice might be necessary. The issue becomes which part practice technique to use. Four part practice techniques have been proposed: fractionation, segmentation, simplification, and attention cueing (Lee et al., 2001; Magill & Anderson, 2013).

Fractionation

Fractionation is part practice that separates parts of an action that normally are executed simultaneously; for example, swimming instructors often have part practice drills for either the arms or legs for a given stroke. This seems to work because the arms and legs perform different movements, and instructors frequently move back and forth between the part and the whole. However, breaking a symmetrical movement like that of the arms of the breaststroke down into drills for each arm is likely counterproductive because the arms perform the same movement and the task is high in organization.

Lee and colleagues (2001) reviewed studies with video games, tapping, tracking, and bimanual aiming tasks. The overall results indicated that part practice was shown to be ineffective in promoting positive transfer to the whole task. This is likely because of the high degree of coordination and interdependence of the parts. With bimanual sport skills such as the sidestroke in swimming and the tennis serve, the evidence is mixed, with some support for both part and whole practice (Magill & Anderson, 2013). If asymmetrical bimanual tasks must be broken down, practicing with the limb that has the more difficult and complex task should probably come first. Bimanual rhythmical tapping tasks, as used in music, are likely best learned with whole practice, but part practice has shown some effectiveness for pianists when rhythm and melody are separated (Lee et al., 2001).

Segmentation

Segmentation is part practice that is possible when a task can be segmented, or broken into parts along the dimension of time. Usually the segments can be practiced by themselves but are reconnected into the whole by methods referred to as part whole, repetitive part, or progressive part (see table 16.4). For example, a folk dance may be segmented into five segments or steps. In part whole practice, the five steps would be practiced separately, and then all the parts would be gathered into the whole task of the folk dance. Progressive part practice involves practicing the first segment alone and then the second segment alone, followed by the first and second segments together. The whole task is achieved by progressively practicing larger versions of the whole task. Finally, in repetitive part practice, the first part is practiced alone and then the first and second parts are practiced together before the third part is added to the first and second. The three types of part practices are outlined in table 16.4, using the layup shot in basketball as the skill.

Part practice can be achieved by either forward or backward chaining. Forward chaining is the practice of the parts in their timed order: part 1, parts 1 and 2, and so on. Learning the folk dance with forward chaining gradually assembles the whole dance. Backward chaining is practice in the reverse order, starting with the final part. This might create motivation because the learner accomplishes the goal at the beginning of practice. For example, backward chaining of the basketball layup begins with the shot, then proceeds to the step–shot combination, the dribble–two-step–shot combination, and so on for several dribbles (Lee et al., 2001). Backward chaining has been demonstrated to be most effective when the end point of the chain requires accuracy, as in the layup

Table 16.4 Steps in the Types of Segmented Practice

Part whole	Repetitive part	Progressive part
1. Dribbling 2. Two-step combination 3. Shot 4. Dribbling, two-step combination, shot	1. Dribbling 2. Dribbling, two-step combination 3. Dribbling, two-step combination, shot	1. Dribbling 2. Two-step combination 3. Dribbling, two-step combination 4. Shot 5. Dribbling, two-step combination, shot

(Lee et al., 2001). Forward chaining is more effective in tasks such as folk dances, in which each segment contributes equally to the task goal.

Magill and Anderson (2013) pointed out that progressive part practice takes advantage of both part and whole practice methods. Part practice reduces attention demands of the whole task so that the learner can concentrate on one aspect. Building toward the whole has the advantage of coordinating parts that may have some degree of interdependence.

Simplification

Simplification, a pedagogical principle that teachers have been using for decades, involves practicing an easier version of the task. Six ways in which skills can be simplified (Magill & Anderson, 2013) are as follows:

1. Reduce object difficulty (e.g., juggle with scarves, catch a larger ball, bat with a large plastic bat).
2. Reduce attention demands (e.g., provide physical assistance such as support in gymnastics).
3. Reduce speed.
4. Add auditory cues (e.g., clap to the rhythm of a skipping action).
5. Sequence skill progressions (e.g., hit baseballs from a tee, then a pitching machine, and later a pitcher).
6. Use simulators (e.g., rebounders in basketball) and virtual reality.

WHAT DO YOU THINK?

Exercise 16.5

Choose your favorite sport or frequent therapeutic activity. Try to provide specific examples of how you could implement each part practice technique.

Sport or activity:	
Practice techniques	**Example**
Fractionation	
Segmentation	
Simplification	
Attention cueing	

Although simplification is a common practice, research support of it is rather limited (Lee et al., 2001). If simplification creates a new task or changes the dynamics of the task dramatically, then part practice may not be effective. Mane, Adams, and Donchin (1989; as cited by Lee et al., 2001) manipulated the speed of a video game. A slower speed transferred positively to the performance of the game at regular speed, but there was a limit. At some point, the reduced speed was ineffective, presumably because the game became quite a different one.

Attention Cueing

Attention cueing is not strictly a part practice method because the whole skill is performed. However, the performer directs attention to a specific part of the whole—for example, the backswing of the slap shot in hockey or the elbow on the recovery of the crawl stroke. Attention research supports the fact that selective focus is possible (Lee et al., 2001).

Mental Practice and Imagery

It may surprise you to learn that just thinking about certain aspects of a skill can have performance and learning benefits (Lee et al., 2001; Schmidt & Lee, 2014). **Mental practice** is cognitive rehearsal of a physical skill without overt physical movements (Magill & Anderson, 2013). **Imagery** is a form of mental practice that involves a visual or kinesthetic representation of one's own performance. These forms of practice should be considered when physical practice is inconvenient or impractical. In general, mental practice is used to aid skill acquisition, whereas imagery usually serves a performance preparation role.

Mental practice has a rather long history and usually involves rehearsing procedural or symbolic aspects of the skill. Rehearsing procedures could follow the series of movements in therapy or in a gymnastics or dance routine. Rehearsal

might also be related to response selection procedures such as the technique for the arm action of a swimming stroke, or a decision-making strategy (e.g., *If my opponent backs away, I will keep the puck and drive to the net*). Recall the discussion of procedural knowledge in chapter 11.

Symbolic aspects of skills refers to such things as remembering to follow through when throwing a ball. Mental practice research usually compares mental practice conditions to a physical practice condition and a no-practice condition. Some studies have incorporated experimental conditions combining physical and mental practice. With regard to learning the physical skill, the results typically demonstrate that mental practice is better than no practice but certainly not as effective as physical practice. The latter is hardly surprising given all that we have said about physical practice in this chapter. Yet, mental practice is recommended in combination with actual practice in recovery from stroke (Nilsen, Gillen, & Gordon, 2010) and to improve surgical performance (Cocks, Moulton, Luu, & Cil, 2014) and music performance (Bernardi, De Buglio, Trimarchi, Chielli, & Bricolo, 2013).

Some studies have shown that a combination of physical and mental practice is almost as effective as physical practice alone (e.g., Hird, Landers, Thomas, & Horan, 1991; Kolh, Ellis, & Roenker, 1992). Combined groups may have almost half the physical practice that physical practice groups do. Magill and Anderson (2013) explained these findings from a cognitive problem-solving perspective. During mental practice, learners engage in cognitive practice strategies that normally are used during physical practice, but can be developed during mental practice as well. From a developmental perspective, the review of mental practice studies conducted many years ago by Feltz and Landers (1983) showed that mental practice was effective regardless of the skill level. In a finger opposition task, mental practice was as effective as physical practice for imme-

Exercise 16.6

You just learned that mental practice has performance and learning benefits. How could you incorporate mental practice into instructional or therapeutic settings? When would be the most appropriate times to encourage the use of mental practice in each of these settings? Explain.

diate and long-term learning with 9- and 10-year-olds (Asa, Melo, & Piemonte, 2014).

Mental imagery is frequently used by athletes and dancers as they prepare for performance. Divers mentally view themselves rotating, twisting, and opening prior to the actual dive. Martin, Moritz, and Hall (1999) concluded that there is "tentative support" in the research literature for imagery as a preparation for competition strategy. Moreover, imagery is effective for both high-performance athletes and beginners. They distinguished between cognitive and motivational imagery. Cognitive images can be specific, such as performing a golf shot, or more general, such as a strategy to overcome a full-court press in basketball. Motivational images can also be specific (e.g., winning a medal for first place) or more general (e.g., to foster confidence or focus). Finally, motivational images also deal with arousal, relaxation, and anxiety (Martin et al., 1999).

Magill and Anderson (2013) described three generally accepted hypotheses for why mental practice and imagery are effective. A neuromuscular hypothesis links the mental practice of an action such as bending the elbow to electromyographic (EMG) activity in the muscles responsible for the bending. This may activate the neuromotor pathways involved in learning. The brain activity hypothesis comes from brain scan results indicating that motor pathways activated during imagining an action are similar to those activated during actual performance (Jeannerod, 1999). The third explanation is the cognitive hypothesis, which asserts that the first stage of motor learning involves a high degree of cognitive activity as people struggle with

performance-related questions. Recent evidence suggests that mental practice is tied to planning rather than execution, which provides some support for the cognitive hypothesis (Bach, Allami, Tucker, & Ellis, 2014).

Distribution of Practice

Is it better for learning to have fewer but longer practice sessions, or more but shorter practice sessions? Distribution of practice refers to the amount of practice during each period and the amount of rest between practice sessions to ensure optimal learning of motor skills (Magill & Anderson, 2013). This body of knowledge usually compares schedules of practice called massed and distributed. **Massed practice** involves longer practice sessions that involve many practice trials. This is contrasted to **distributed practice**, which has fewer practice trials in shorter practice sessions. Massed practice schedules have fewer practice sessions than distributed practice schedules have. To compare distributed with massed practice, the total number of practice trials must be equal; therefore, there will be more frequent distributed practice sessions in research. When the time between trials is a focus, massed practice has minimal or short rest periods, whereas distributed practice has longer rest intervals.

Many educational, recreational, and rehabilitation situations have specified practice times, and practitioners have little flexibility in allotting practice time. For example, teachers know the number of days during the week on which a given class will have physical education, and youth soccer teams are often allotted the practice fields in a predetermined fashion. As Magill and Anderson (2013) pointed out, little research addresses the optimal number and length of practice sessions, but in general, researchers recommend more frequent and shorter sessions, as would occur in distributed practice (e.g., Kwon, Kwon & Lee, 2015). This recommendation is supported by three hypotheses: Massed practice may result in more physical fatigue compared with distributed practice, may reduce cognitive effort compared to distributed practice, and provides less time for the memory representation of the motor skill to be consolidated. In medicine there is a tradition of full-day training of surgical skills. Three 75-minute sessions massed in a single day were compared to three 75-minute session distributed over three weeks (Spruit, Band, & Hamming, 2015). The distributed practice was superior to massed practice in terms of skill acquisition as well as short- and long-term retention.

A study by Dail and Christina (2004) also supports distributed practice for novice golfers. The task was a golf putt, and each participant had 240 trials. A

Throwing With the Nondominant Arm

Exercise 16.7

Let's compare massed and distributed practice for a throwing task using the nondominant arm and hand. The throw is an underhand toss of a badminton shuttlecock to an archery target of concentric circles 10 feet (3 m) away. A direct hit in the center scores 5 points, one in the next circle scores 4 points, and so on. Split the class in half, with half throwing with a massed condition and the other half with a distributed condition. The massed practice participants throw 40 times in succession. Record the scores from the 40 trials. The distributed group throws in four sessions of 10 blocks with two minutes between blocks. Again, record the scores from the 40 trials. Compare the massed and distributed groups. Did you find differences that are consistent with the content in the Distribution of Practice section?

Exercise 16.8

You just learned about distributed and massed practice. Fill in the following table by indicating whether the skills can likely be taught more effectively under distributed or massed practice conditions.

Skill	Massed practice	Distributed practice
Dancing		
Long jump		
Chest pass		
Riding a bicycle		
Skipping rope		

massed practice schedule group performed all the trials on one day, with a short break after each block of 10 trials; the distributed group had 60 trials on each of four consecutive days. At the end of the 240 trials, 24 hours later, and seven days later, the distributed group putted better than the massed group.

Most of the research on distributed practice has investigated the length of the inter-trial interval (i.e., the rest time between trials) (Magill & Anderson, 2013). Reviews of this literature point to the importance of the type of task. Continuous skills are learned better with distributed schedules of practice than with massed, whereas the reverse is true of discrete skills. Thus, swimming, dancing, and skiing would benefit from distributed practice, and hitting a golf ball or baseball would benefit from massed practice. Continuous tasks likely benefit from distributed practice because they can be physiologically fatiguing, whereas discrete tasks have naturally occurring breaks between trials.

Summary

Physical practice is by far the most important factor in learning motor skills. And Javier now realizes that the ultimate goal of practice is to perform the skill outside the therapeutic practice venue, in the context of activities of daily living, recreation, or competition. To some extent, the amount of practice depends on the learner's goals and aspirations. The research evidence suggests that more practice is necessary as higher levels of performance are sought. Will Javier's client be satisfied when she can walk to the store, or might she aspire to becoming a Paralympian?

How to organize and schedule practice sessions so that people can reach their goals was the focus of this chapter. We explored variable, constant, random, blocked, part, whole, mental, mass, and distributed practice and attempted to describe the best practice conditions. However, sometimes the research is incomplete, and the results are controversial or equivocal. Although we would like to have offered simple summary statements on exactly how therapists, teachers, and coaches should organize their practices, learning motor skills is simply too complex and is influenced by a host of factors beyond practice schedules. So we highlighted the moderating factors available from the research, including age, level of skill, type of task (laboratory or real world), type of skill, motivation, attention, and personality.

ONLINE LEARNING

Visit the web resource at www.HumanKinetics.com/MotorLearningAndDevelopment for an accompanying lab activity and exercises from the chapter.

LEARNING AIDS

Supplemental Activities

1. Biographies of highly skilled athletes and musicians often speak to the issue of practice. Select an athlete, dancer, musician, or other skilled mover you admire or would like to know more about, and read his or her biography. What are the person's reflections about practice?

2. Locate an experienced therapist you know and ask for an interview about practice. Does this person distinguish between the many types of practice discussed in this chapter? Does he or she see instances of the contextual interference effect? Does he or she use mental imagery?

Glossary

blocked practice—A practice sequence in which one skill is repeated over a fixed block of time before moving to the next skill. This is usually contrasted to random practice, which involves different skills intermingled during a designated time period.

constant practice—Very similar to blocked practice because one skill is repeated for a fixed amount of time or number of trials before moving to the next skill. This is usually contrasted to variable practice, which includes variations of a skill intermingled during a designated time period.

contextual interference—The memory and performance disruption that results from performing multiple skills or variations of a skill within the context of practice. This disruption has a negative effect when people are attempting to learn several tasks at the same time.

contextual interference effect—The learning benefit resulting from performing multiple skills using a high contextual interference practice schedule.

distributed practice—Practice that typically involves a short session with few practice trials and long rest intervals.

elaboration and distinctive hypothesis—The idea that random practice results in the use of cognitive strategies. When learners shift from one skill to another, the nature of each strategy becomes clearer and more meaningful in long-term memory. This cognitive effort has a deleterious effect during skill acquisition but is beneficial to skill learning.

especial skill—A skill with a single action sequence that is consistent across time and environments.

forgetting and reconstruction hypothesis—The hypothesis that the key to understanding the contextual interference effect is to consider the action planning required for each skill. Random practice forces learners to practice action planning, because they must reconstruct a new action plan each time they learn a new skill.

imagery—A form of mental practice that involves a visual or kinesthetic representation of performance; the visualization or cognitive rehearsal of a movement.

massed practice—Long practice sessions with many practice trials.

mental practice—The cognitive rehearsal of a physical skill without overt physical movements.

random practice—A practice sequence in which several skills are mixed in a random order. Rehearsal of the same skill twice in a row is avoided.

schema—An abstract or general memory representation of a set of rules that connect a person's actions to the parameters needed to produce an outcome.

serial practice—A practice sequence in which skills are performed in a mixed order but in a fixed format.

task complexity—The number of parts or components of a skill and the amount of attention required to complete the skill.

task organization—The relationships of the skill components.

variable practice—A practice sequence in which several variations of the same skill occur in a mixed order.

FEEDBACK

Chapter Objectives

After reading this chapter, you should be able to do the following:

- Explain why extrinsic feedback is an essential component of motor skill acquisition.
- Provide examples of types of extrinsic feedback.
- Identify the main functions of extrinsic feedback.
- Understand feedback schedules including when and how to use them.
- Describe factors that should be considered to provide feedback effectively.
- Explain how the timing of feedback following a performance attempt affects motor learning.

Are You Ready for Feedback?

Vera Jones' love of basketball began with her first basketball at age five. Throughout her childhood, she found herself playing not only basketball but virtually any sport she could, including some in which she was the only girl on the team. In high school she excelled as an athlete and was highly sought after as a top basketball recruit to play for Syracuse University in New York State on a full scholarship. Feeling on top of the world, Jones expected to begin her college career on the starting lineup. Instead, she found herself on the bench. Her coach told her that although she was good at making baskets, she played defense very poorly. While on the bench, she started analyzing the game, noticing that when the ball is passed to one side, the defense shifted and the corner was wide open. She thought, *When I get my opportunity, I'm going to go to that open spot.* She deeply yearned to play and started listening to her coach's feedback to focus on her defense. She did just that, and the rest is history (Jones, 2011).

Although feedback is an important part of the learning process, accepting it and making the necessary changes is not always easy. You've likely experienced a situation, perhaps like Jones', in which you didn't agree with the feedback you received or felt frustrated even hearing it. If so, you are probably not surprised to learn that when a learner is not open to receiving feedback, it is not going to help. So, how can instructors, coaches, and therapists provide critical feedback in these situations? What are the most effective methods of providing feedback? Siedentop and Tannehill (2000) reported that the feedback delivered in athletic and clinical settings is often not optimal in terms of type, accuracy, and frequency. This chapter discusses the many variables that determine the appropriateness and effectiveness of feedback to people of varying ages and skill levels, and based on skill difficulty. It also presents some common myths about feedback delivery.

Feedback is critical when learning new motor skills, especially complex ones. It is also necessary for highly skilled athletes such as Vera, as well as injured people trying to reacquire motor skills, whether they are sport-specific skills (e.g., making sharp cuts on the basketball court following an anterior cruciate ligament tear) or relevant life skills (e.g., relearning to walk, write, or even brush one's teeth). Injured people often have to either relearn a motor skill, modify a motor skill, or learn a new motor skill. Occupational and physical therapists must understand how to provide feedback in a way that maximizes patients' learning. When practitioners are providing feedback to facilitate motor learning, regardless of the situation (e.g., an unskilled person learning a new motor skill, or someone recovering from injury or illness), they must consider the type, frequency, and timing of their feedback.

Functions of Feedback

The three main functions of extrinsic feedback are information, motivation, and reinforcement (see figure 17.1). Feedback that provides information helps learners understand how they are moving, what they are doing correctly or incorrectly, and how they can correct errors. This information can guide them to better perfor-

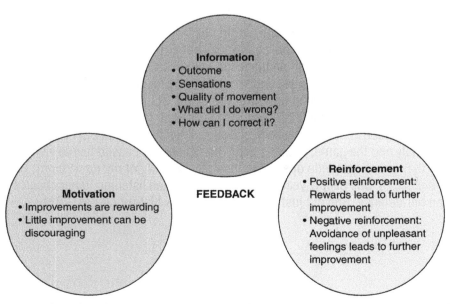

Figure 17.1 Extrinsic feedback has three main functions: guiding the learner to better performances, providing an incentive to motivate the learner, and reinforcing the movement.

mances. Feedback to correct performance errors addresses the performance outcome (knowledge of results), sensations produced by the movement (intrinsic feedback), the nature of the errors (descriptive feedback), and suggestions on how to correct errors (prescriptive feedback). For example, a pole vaulter will receive information about his movement from multiple sources. He will see the outcome of the vault, hear the pole make contact with the vaulting box and hear it fall if it hits too hard, feel whether he pulled his body up and around the bar or he hit the bar, and likely know the outcome before he is even near the bar. These are all types of intrinsic feedback. The pole vaulter may also receive extrinsic feedback from a coach or a teammate who describes his form or provides corrective information.

Feedback also functions to motivate learners. When learners receive feedback on their movement performances, they can compare it with their performance goals. Those who are progressively improving should receive feedback that they are moving closer and closer to their goals. Improved performance is very rewarding and provides an incentive to continue practicing to achieve further success. Conversely, learners who see little improvement or actually get worse often become frustrated with the task. Frustrated learners are likely to decrease their effort or even quit. To increase motivation, instructors can provide more feedback on correct aspects of the performance attempts than on errors to reduce some of the frustration learners may be experiencing.

The third function of feedback is reinforcement. Reinforcement occurs when the feedback following a performance attempt increases the probability of similar performance attempts in the future. Feedback can provide positive and negative reinforcement. **Positive reinforcement** following a performance attempt can be rewarding. This reward is intended to increase the likelihood that successful attempts will occur more consistently; however, it must be provided immediately following the attempt to be beneficial. Positive reinforcement can be given verbally through compliments or praise (e.g., *Great job on the backswing* or *You're getting there! You can do it!*), which can motivate learners to continue their efforts. These phrases should be used sparingly and only when deserved. If a learner is having very little success, the instructor should find at least some aspect of the movement pattern, however small, to praise. Nonverbal gestures can also provide positive reinforcement, such as a smile, a thumbs-up, or a pat on the back.

For extrinsic feedback to be positively reinforcing, the learner must perceive it as a reward (Rose & Christina, 2006). Consider a coach who increases the intensity or duration of practice because she believes the athlete is capable of improving to the next level. If the coach does not explain the reason behind the change, the athlete may perceive the added workload as a punishment. Similarly, a coach may switch a player's position because of the player's well-rounded athleticism. However, the athlete may interpret the change as suggesting an inability to play the position well rather than an enhanced capability to play multiple positions.

Feedback that evokes unpleasant feelings that the learner will want to avoid at all costs is **negative reinforcement**. Negative reinforcement can be derived simply from embarrassment over a poor performance, such as a missed shot, a poor throw, or a missed catch. A hurdler with a knee injury may avoid hitting the hurdle with his trail leg at all costs to avoid the pain. An inexperienced driver learning how to drive a car with manual transmission may initially cause the car to jump or stall. The embarrassment this causes can serve as negative reinforcement, strengthening the desire to learn. A golf teaching aid can provide negative reinforcement to eliminate lunging. The aid is placed just ahead of the lead leg; during the swing, the learner must stay behind the pad through ball impact. Hitting the pad tells the learner that she has moved ahead of the ball (negative reinforcement).

Another common negative reinforcer is the beeping or dinging sound in a car indicating that the seat belt is not fastened. Fastening the seat belt (correct movement) is reinforced to avoid hearing the annoying sound. To decrease the length of a batter's step, a coach can place a wooden barrier on the ground; contacting the barrier with the foot indicates that the step is too long. Shorter steps (correct movement) are because the batter wants to avoid making contact with the barrier (negative reinforcer).

Types and Modalities of Feedback

The two most general types of feedback are intrinsic feedback (i.e., derived from sensory systems) and extrinsic feedback (i.e., provided by external sources). Effective extrinsic feedback is an essential component of clinical, educational, and athletic programs. The only variable more important than extrinsic feedback in learning a motor skill is practice (Bilodeau, 1966). We will take a closer look at these two types of feedback but focus mostly on extrinsic feedback.

Intrinsic Feedback

The production of the task itself generates intrinsic feedback. **Intrinsic feedback** includes any feedback received through the sensory systems, including vision, proprioception, and audition. A basketball player receives information from each of these sensory systems when he takes a 3-point shot. He feels the release of the shot and the force with which he made it (proprioceptive intrinsic feedback). He sees the trajectory of the ball and whether it hits the rim, hits the backboard, or is "nothing but net" (visual intrinsic feedback), and he hears it hit the rim or (ideally) hears the swoosh of the ball through the net (auditory intrinsic feedback). A skilled basketball player often knows whether he is going to make the shot long before the shot even approaches the net. Intrinsic feedback can be supplemented by coaches, instructors, peers, and equipment.

Extrinsic Feedback

Feedback that is supplemental to the intrinsic sources of feedback is termed **extrinsic feedback**. Any feedback provided by an instructor, trainer, therapist, coach, or even a friend is extrinsic feedback. A fitness trainer who tells her client that her reps are too fast, or a fencing coach instructing his student to lunge more when striking, is giving extrinsic feedback. Equipment (e.g., stopwatch, heart rate monitor, video replay system) also provides a type of extrinsic feedback.

Providing appropriate feedback is one of the most important responsibilities of an instructor. Important considerations for extrinsic feedback are determining the most appropriate type, precision, and frequency of feedback, as well as when to schedule the presentation of feedback. Extrinsic feedback can result in quick learning and enhance retention while also increasing learner motivation. Learners who cannot detect their own errors may spend countless hours trying different techniques, which would not be necessary if they received a simple tip from an instructor who had observed their attempts.

Extrinsic feedback is pivotal in rehabilitation settings as well. Patients with perceptual or cognitive deficits may only be able to use limited intrinsic feedback (Flinn & Radomski, 2002). They may rely on extrinsic feedback to even understand how they are performing because they cannot accurately feel the movement or see the outcome.

Extrinsic feedback occurs in many forms. Most simply, it can be provided verbally or nonverbally. Nonverbal forms of extrinsic feedback include a buzzer that sounds following poor performances or a stopwatch that displays a race time. Extrinsic feedback can be provided either during the movement (**concurrent feedback**) or following the movement (**terminal feedback**). A 1-mile (1.6 km) race time is terminal feedback. However, running splits (i.e., race times during set intervals such as a quarter mile or half mile) are examples of concurrent feedback because the runner receives pace information during the run. To optimize and accelerate motor learning in learners, athletes, or patients, practitioners should manipulate factors such as task complexity, feedback designs, and feedback modalities—such as visual (videos, head-mounted displays), auditory (speakers, headphones, timers, practitioners), and haptic (robots, vibrotactile actuators), or a combination of them (Sigrist, Rauter, Riener, & Wolf, 2013).

Verbal Feedback

Perhaps the most common type of feedback is verbal. We often think of a coach providing feedback in terms of what athletes did incorrectly (e.g., *You didn't throw the shot put with a whipping motion*), how they can perform better the next time (e.g., *You need to hit down on the golf ball, not up*), or the outcome of the performance (*You jumped 19 feet 2 inches in your last long jump attempt*). Verbal feedback provides

knowledge of results (KR) or **knowledge of performance (KP)**. These give learners feedback regarding the outcome (KR) and the quality of their performances (KP).

Knowledge of results is terminal feedback that describes the outcome of the movement (e.g., a gymnastics score, the distance of a punt, the score on a sit and reach test, the speed of a pitch). Knowledge of performance provides specific feedback about the quality of the movement. It informs the learner about the components of the movement pattern that led to the outcome (e.g., the need to shift the weight more, use more force with the follow-through, or use more torso rotation when throwing). Most instructors and clinicians emphasize the outcome of the performance (KR) and fail to provide appropriate feedback regarding the movement itself (KP) (Fishman & Tobey, 1978). Outcome-based feedback is often inadequate in guiding the learner to perform the skill correctly (Newell & Walter, 1981; Sharma, Chevidikuunan, Khan, & Gaowgzeh, 2016).

There are two types of knowledge of performance: descriptive feedback and prescriptive feedback. **Descriptive feedback**, as the name implies, describes the movement pattern. This type of feedback is useful for explaining what learners are doing incorrectly. One of the most common errors in golf is an exaggerated twist of the backswing. Novice golfers often incorrectly assume that a greater twist of the backswing will help them generate more force. Instructors can provide descriptive feedback by describing this exaggerated twist.

Prescriptive feedback provides suggestions to correct the error. An instructor could tell a novice golfer, "By exaggerating your twist, you will not be able to stay in the same swing plane, which will be very difficult to compensate for. You need to maintain perfect posture and swing fluidly. This will help you to maintain contact with the ball and avoid twisting too far on the backswing." The appropriate type of feedback depends on the skill level of the

Providing Verbal KR

Exercise 17.2

1. Form pairs. Each pair has three different-colored pens (or markers or pencils), a piece of paper, and a blindfold. One student is the participant, and the other is the experimenter, providing feedback.

2. On the piece of paper, the experimenter draws a basketball hoop and a stick figure of a person about to shoot the basketball.

3. The participant then puts on the blindfold and draws a line from the hands of the stick figure to the hoop using a typical basketball shot trajectory. The participant does this 10 times with no feedback and without looking at the picture, although the experimenter does place the pen at the starting point after each attempt. The participant remains blindfolded throughout the experiment.

4. For a second group of trials, the participant uses a different-colored pen and completes the same task 10 times, but during these trials, the experimenter provides KR (outcome feedback, such as *You missed the hoop*) after each attempt. The participant remains blindfolded throughout the experiment.

5. For a third group of trials, the participant uses a different-colored pen and completes the same task 10 times, but during these trials, the experimenter provides KP (feedback on the quality of the movement, such as *You need more arc and need to continue the line farther*) after each attempt. The participant remains blindfolded throughout the experiment.

6. When you are finished, switch roles with your partner and complete the activity again.

7. Compare your results after receiving no feedback, KR, and KP.

Questions

1. How detailed was the feedback you and your partner provided for KR or KP?

2. Do you think the detail of feedback from your partner may have affected your results during the KR and KP trials?

3. What other factors do you think may have affected your results for each condition?

Exercise 17.3

Label each of the following examples as either KR or KP.

1. You are releasing the ball too early.
2. You just missed the archery target by 2 inches (5 cm).
3. Your plant foot landed 3 inches (7.6 cm) over the takeoff board for the long jump.
4. You just cut two seconds off your mile.
5. You are not bending at the knees enough.
6. You need to straighten your back when you bring the weight down.

learner. Novice learners need more prescriptive feedback than skilled performers do, because they have not yet learned how to correct errors. Regardless of skill level, a combination of both descriptive and prescriptive feedback is most effective. When given both types of KP, learners begin to associate the causes of errors with the appropriate corrections.

Nonverbal Feedback

Although we often think of feedback as verbal, most people use many forms of nonverbal feedback. Nonverbal feedback includes visual feedback (e.g., pictures or videos) and auditory feedback (e.g., a buzzer, a metronome, or a sound consequent to a movement). An example of a consequent sound is the sound of a racquetball hitting the wall. This sound can provide the player with information regarding the ball's speed and even trajectory. Consequent sounds can also provide information about the rhythm of a movement, such as double dutch jump roping, a skill in which the rhythm is crucial. The following sections will discuss nonverbal feedback in the forms of equipment, biofeedback, and visual feedback.

Equipment Feedback can be provided from a wide variety of equipment. An example is equipment for monitoring performance, such as radar guns to monitor the speed of a pitch. Nowadays, many people have activity-tracking apps or watches that monitor their physical activity levels, including number of steps, distance run, pace, splits, and even heart rate. Many devices have been developed to improve the golf swing, perhaps even more so than for any other motor skill, such as helping to eliminate swaying and lunging and facilitating proper impact. Equipment is also critical for therapists to assist clients with walking, regaining balance, and increasing strength.

Biofeedback **Biofeedback** is extrinsic feedback that provides concurrent information related to physiological processes (Magill, 2017). Biofeedback has been well known since the 1950s (Schwarz, Olson, & Andrasik, 2003) and is used to shape behavior during performance. One of the most commonly used forms of biofeedback is the heart rate monitor. Heart rate monitors, readily available at department or sporting goods stores and integrated into popular activity trackers, continuously display the person's current heart rate. They help people adjust their intensity levels throughout a workout based on their heart rates. Blood pressure monitors and chronometers are other sources of biofeedback. Blood pressure may be continuously monitored for people with cardiovascular problems. Chronometers provide swimmers with real-time, nonverbal biofeedback without interfering with their performances (Pèrez, Liana, Brizuela, & Encarnación, 2009). Providing feedback during water sports has been particularly difficult because of the pool environment. Chronometers have been found to be beneficial for improving swim times while also allowing the instructor to focus on other aspects of the performance or on other swimmers.

Biofeedback is also commonly used in rehabilitation settings. Feedback can be provided for muscular activation and joint angle excursions. By viewing electromyographic (EMG) biofeedback, patients have increased voluntary activation in particular muscle groups (Brucker & Bulaeva, 1996) and relearned how to walk following a stroke by changing their walking patterns (Intiso, Santilli, Grasso, Rossi, & Caruso, 1994). Biofeedback devices can improve postural control and gait using audio-biofeedback, which reports the amount and direction of postural sway (Dozza, Chiari, Peterka, Wall, & Horak, 2011). Unfortunately, these benefits are generally lost once the biofeedback is removed; thus the use of these devices should be limited so that learners do not become overreliant on them.

Visual Feedback   Visual feedback, which can be very beneficial during the learning process, can take the form of visual displays of kinetic and kinematic feedback. Kinetic and kinematic feedback, types of knowledge of performance that provide information in addition to intrinsic feedback, have been shown to be more effective than knowledge of results (Newell & Carlton, 1987; Young & Schmidt, 1992).

Kinematic feedback provides information on the observable aspects of the movement (e.g., the space–time properties of a performance) and can be very beneficial during the learning process. The most commonly used forms of kinematic feedback are pictures, illustrations, and video replays of limb position, velocity, or acceleration (see figure 17.2). For example, illustrating the aiming trajectory of the rifle barrel, an essential aspect of shooting performance (Konttinen, Lyytinen, & Viitasalo, 1998), provides information on the movement of the barrel and supplements intrinsic feedback (Mononen, Viitasalo, Konttinen, & Era, 2003). **Kinetic feedback** provides information on the underlying processes of the movement, such as force. Graphs illustrating force–time curves for a motor skill have been found to be useful for such actions as the jump out of starting blocks for sprinters and the trigger squeeze and release for rifle shooters. Learners can see whether they need more or less force and learn the appropriate timing in relation to the amount of force required.

For kinematic feedback to benefit the acquisition and retention of motor skills, it must supplement the feedback regarding goal achievement (KR) (Rucci & Tomporowski, 2010). The goal for most motor skills is to induce a change in the environment through a particular movement or set of movements, such as batting in baseball. Because separating the movement patterns in batting (the kinematics of the swing) from the outcome (where the ball was directed and landed, or KR) is easy, learners are likely to benefit from kinematic feedback. For other tasks, such as gymnastics, dance, and figure skating, the information on movement production and goal achievement would be the same (Newell, Quinn, Sparrow, & Walter, 1983). In this case, rather than *affecting* goal achievement, the movement pattern *is* the goal achievement. For these tasks, then, the kinematics of the movement and goal achievement cannot be separated.

The most effective kinematic patterns are generally known for most sporting activities, and kinematic feedback is very commonly provided to optimize learners' movement patterns. Feedback on some kinematic variables is more beneficial to learning than is feedback on others. Although the most appropriate feedback is on kinematic variables that are motor skill specific, feedback on spatial characteristics (positional information) tends to be more effective for learning than feedback on temporal aspects (Young & Schmidt,

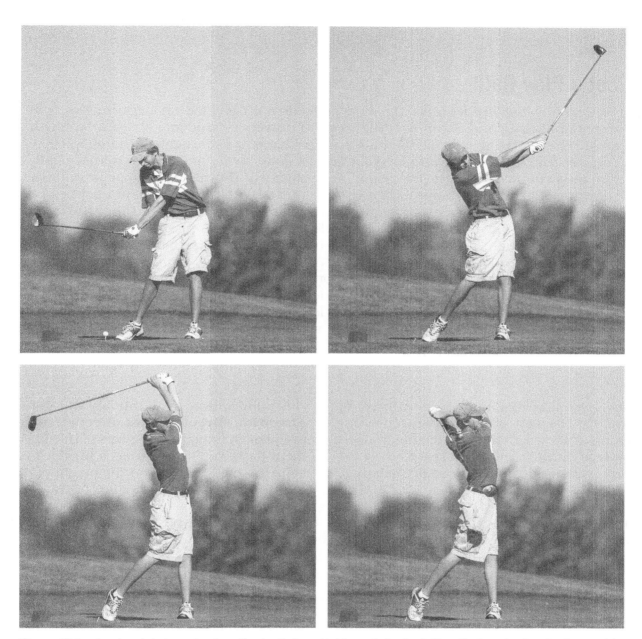

Figure 17.2   A series of photographs of a golf swing that provide kinematic feedback. They illustrate the changing form and the correct alignment of the body relative to the club throughout the swing.

1992). It is probably easier for learners to visualize where to place and move body parts and equipment, such as a racket, than to understand the timing of the movement, because this is more abstract and harder to conceptualize.

Video Feedback   Learners may believe that they are performing a task correctly until they see for themselves via pictures or a video that they are not. Although video feedback can be quite useful, practitioners must consider several factors when using it, such as the time period during which the video is presented, the skill level of the learner, and whether the video is supplemented with feedback from the instructor.

Video feedback is more useful when it is provided over an extended period of time. Because this type of feedback provides so much information, learners need time to fully benefit from it. The longer time period

Let's Play Ball!

To examine the influence of the type of feedback provided on performance and retention, Young and Schmidt (1992) had 60 university students strike a ball with a bat. The goal was to strike the ball to propel it as far as possible. Although people can use any of a number of movement patterns to strike a ball, they achieve optimal performance when the bat has a high velocity at the coincidence point and the trajectory of the bat is appropriate in relation to the ball. Participants performed the task 100 times over two days and completed a retention test on the third day. Feedback was provided on four kinematic variables, and each variable improved during acquisition. However, feedback on only one of these variables (mean reversal position information) improved learning. Although feedback on the other variables influenced performance during acquisition (short-term effects), it did not have long-term learning effects. Feedback that provided spatial information conferred a more permanent benefit than feedback that provided temporal information did. The authors concluded that feedback on a kinematic variable may influence performance and still not necessarily benefit learning.

also gives learners more opportunities to practice the motor skill. Research studies have shown that video feedback used for less than five weeks resulted in no improved performance (Rose & Christina, 2006).

Providing video feedback without cueing the learner to specific aspects of the movement is also ineffective, especially for novice learners, and it may actually be detrimental (Kernodle & Carlton, 1992; Rucci & Tomporowski, 2010). This is likely because video feedback provides too much information. Video feedback is not effective for learners who do not understand what they should be looking for in the video or how to interpret the information. Skilled performers, on the other hand, know the aspects of the movement pattern they need to focus on and can benefit from viewing videos of their performances with little to no supplementation.

Minimally, novices should be given attention-directed cues (Newell & Walter, 1981) when they view videos. Because they have little experience with performing the movement pattern correctly, they may become overwhelmed with all of

the information available on the video. **Attention-directed cues** direct attention to the most important aspects of the movement pattern. For instance, a juggler may be instructed to focus on the height of the toss; a golfer, on the position of the club during the backswing; and a soccer player, on the plant foot position. The benefits of attention-directing cues are not limited to novice performers. Highly skilled athletes have also benefited from these cues when viewing videos (Menickelli, Landin, Grisham, & Hebert, 2000).

Although attention-directed cues have been found to improve performance following video feedback, attention-focusing cues provide the greatest benefit (Kernodle & Carlton, 1992). **Attention-focusing cues** not only direct the learner's attention to specific aspects of the movement pattern, but also include error correction suggestions. For instance, rather than simply directing the juggler's attention to the toss, the instructor could inform the learner that she needs to make tosses that peak between the shoulder and the head. The golf instructor could inform novice golfers that they need to avoid overswinging the club because they will lose control of it, preventing them from staying in the same plane of motion. A soccer coach could inform novice players that the position of the plant foot is critical to dribbling. Cor-rectly positioning the plant foot allows the player to control the speed and direction of the dribble. See table 17.1 for examples of attention-focusing and attention-directed cues.

Table 17.1 Attention-Focusing and Attention-Directed Cues (Suggested Corrections) for a Back Handspring

Attention-focusing cues	Attention-directed cues
1. Focus on the position of your arms.	1a. Tighten your arms. 1b. With your arms straight and behind your body, drive them toward your feet, then up past your head. 1c. Your arms should be near your ears.
2. Focus on planting your hands on the floor.	2. When you plant your hands, put your weight into your hands, fingers, arms, and shoulders for support; don't put it all into your hands.
3. Focus on swinging your legs over your hands.	3. Swing your legs over your hands while keeping your feet together with your toes pointed. Your knees should have a slight bend.

RESEARCH NOTES

Who Needs Verbal Cues Anyway?

Kernodle and Carlton (1992) illustrated the benefits of supplementing video feedback in a study of participants who threw sponge balls at a target with their eyes closed. Participants were separated into four groups. One group was provided only KR (the distance the ball was thrown, no video); one group was provided only KP (a video); one group viewed the video and received attention-directing cues (e.g., *Focus on the hips during the throwing phase*); and the final group viewed the video and received attention-focused cues (e.g., *Rotate the hips from left to right during the throwing phase*). Although all groups started at approximately the same level, the greatest gains in performances were seen in the group that received the attention-focusing cues (video + correcting cues). Significant benefits were also found for the attention-directed cues (video + attention cues) over the KR-only and KP-only groups. No significant differences were found between the KR-only and KP-only groups, which indicated that providing video feedback without attention-focusing or attention-directing cues provides no more benefit than simply providing KR (e.g., *You threw the ball 35 feet*).

A more recent study (Rucci & Tomporowski, 2010) revealed similar results for learning the hang power clean over six training sessions. Participants were separated into three groups: visual feedback only, verbal feedback only, and verbal and video feedback. Dartfish video analyses revealed that the video-only group did not significantly improve, whereas the other two groups did.

These studies indicated that video feedback that is not supplemented with verbal cues is not effective for novices. Most learners need some form of verbal cues to improve their skills. Videos should be supplemented by an instructor who can direct learners' attention to the most important cues and describe how they can correct their errors to maximize learning.

Table 17.2 Video Feedback Learning Stages

Stage	Learner characteristics	Instructor's role
Shock	Learners are preoccupied with appearance.	Allow learners to become familiar with viewing videos. Hold off on further instruction until learners are ready.
Error detection	Learners critically observe their performances. They identify some performance errors.	Distinguish relevant and irrelevant cues. Provide attention-focusing cues.
Error correction	Learners can now identify their errors. They know the causes of their errors. They focus on learning how to correct the identified errors.	Encourage problem solving.
Independence	Learners detect and correct their errors. They have little to no dependence on the instructor.	Recognize a minimal or nonexistent supplemental role. Provide encouragement.

Four stages have been described for learners who are introduced to video feedback: (1) shock, (2) error detection, (3) error correction, and (4) independence (see table 17.2; Darden, 1999). When learners are introduced to video feedback, they are often more focused on their visual appearance than on their movement patterns or performances. Because of this preoccupation with irrelevant factors (overall appearance rather than movement patterns), this stage has been termed the **shock stage**. Darden stated that until learners have adjusted to viewing themselves on video, further instruction is ineffective. During stage 2, the **error detection stage**, instructors should supplement the video feedback with attention-focusing cues. This is especially important for novice learners who may not know the task-relevant cues for the motor skill and may be focusing on irrelevant cues. These cues enable them to begin to critically analyze their performances and prepare them to detect and correct their errors. Learners who can identify their errors and understand the causes of their errors have advanced to stage 3, the **error correction stage**. During this stage, learners are developing error correction strategies. With learners in this stage, the instructor's role is to focus on problem-solving skills. The **independence stage** is the final video feedback learning stage. Learners who reach this stage require minimal to no video supplementation by an instructor. Skilled performers know exactly what to look for when viewing the videos and can identify and correct their errors.

Providing Effective Feedback

Instructors and clinicians often spend much time preparing the learning situation by properly setting up the environment, setting goals, and designing the practice sessions, but many do not provide effective feedback. Important factors include the frequency, timing, and scheduling of feedback.

RESEARCH NOTES

Using Video Feedback in Practical Settings

Roberts and Brown (2008) described how to best use video feedback to assist in aquatic instruction. An intermediate swim class met twice a week for 50-minute sessions. The first day of class was an orientation session in which students were informed of all of the skills and expectations but did not enter the pool. The students' current skill levels were assessed during the second session. Instructors demonstrated the skills and then recorded the students using digital cameras and underwater cam sticks. Following the completion of each skill, the students viewed their performances at poolside while the instructor provided attention-directed cues. Students then practiced the skill again and often showed immediate improvement. One student said, "The video *really* did help. I'm doing things in my underwater swim that I am totally not aware of! I had no idea that I flutter-kicked some and my kick is kinda tilted toward the side."

Student performances were also contrasted with videos of skilled demonstrations. Using video-editing software, the researchers were able to show the two videos together, allowing the students to compare their performances with those of the model. They were encouraged to watch these videos as much as they liked.

It is key for instructors to remember the importance of including attention or correcting cues (or both) with videos. Instructors could also provide this additional feedback through written questions, giving students another opportunity to reflect on their performances (Herbert & Landin, 1997). Reflection is an important component in improving error correction. In the Roberts and Brown (2008) study, five to eight online questions were combined with the videos for each skill using an online questioning tool (Webassign). This allowed students to critique their own skills as guided by the questions. This video feedback model saved instructor time while also enhancing student learning and decreasing learning time. Students of all levels have benefitted from this type of video technology (Roberts & Brown, 2008).

Corrective or Error-Based Feedback

Instructors must determine whether to provide feedback on the correct aspects of the movement pattern or instructional cues on the learner's errors. The effectiveness of error versus corrective feedback largely depends on the learner's skill level, motivation, and interest. For novices, feedback focused on errors can be very effective. This guides them to the correct movement patterns. Learners who are not very motivated toward or interested in the activity benefit more from feedback on the correct aspects of the movement pattern. This feedback encourages them

to continue their efforts by confirming their progress.

Tzetzis, Votsis, and Kourtessis (2008) examined the effect of different corrective feedback methods on badminton performance for a low-difficulty and high-difficulty skill. Participants were separated into four groups: a control group and three practice groups. Group 1 received positive feedback and instructional cues on how to correct technique, group 2 received only instructional cues on how to correct technique, and group 3 received positive feedback, instructional cues on how to correct technique, and instructional cues on errors. The group with all three (group

3) improved the most in the high-difficulty skill, but groups 1 and 2 performed better in the low-difficulty skill. The authors concluded that the feedback that is most appropriate might depend on the level of difficulty of the motor skill.

In general, it is optimal to provide feedback on *both* the errors and the correct components of the movement. The sandwich approach (see figure 17.3) is a recommended strategy for providing feedback on both errors and correct components (Fischman & Oxendine, 2001). In the sandwich, the bread is praise and constructive criticism is the meat. Initially, instructors praise the learner's strengths to reinforce correct performance (e.g., *Good! You kept your eye on the ball, and you had good timing*). Improvements are then suggested based on the learner's errors (e.g., *Next time, spread your feet a little wider*). The instructor concludes with motivational information, encouraging the learner by discussing the benefits of correcting the error (e.g., *Spreading your feet wider will help your balance*).

Feedback Frequency

Traditionally, researchers believed that the more frequently feedback was provided following performance attempts, the greater the gains in learning would be (Thorndike, 1931). This line of thinking developed because performance tends to increase more and at a faster rate when extrinsic feedback is given most or all of the time. However, current research has indicated that too much feedback is detrimental to learning (Anderson, Magill, Sekiya, & Ryan, 2005). The **guidance hypothesis** asserts that novices benefit from high-frequency KR initially, even as much as feedback on every attempt; then, as they improve, the frequency of feedback should be gradually reduced. If extrinsic feedback is given frequently for too long, learners can become overly dependent on it, often relying more on the extrinsic feedback than on their own sensory sources of feedback. This promotes passive learning; that is, learners do not develop the critical problem-solving skills necessary for performing the motor skill without extrinsic feedback. On the other hand, learners who receive extrinsic feedback at a lower frequency become much more active in the process. They reflect and evaluate their movements. This active process helps them perform the motor skill without feedback. It should be noted that feedback frequency is task and skill dependent. How much to reduce the feedback is not a one-size-fits-all variable. More complex tasks require additional feedback, and reducing the frequency of feedback can degrade learning under certain practice conditions (Wu et al., 2011).

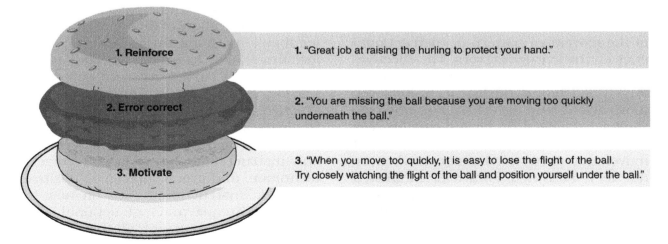

Figure 17.3 The sandwich approach to providing error feedback.

Exercise 17.6

1. Using the sandwich approach, change the following statement: *You messed it up again! How many times do I have to tell you to follow through? You never listen!* You can choose any motor skill for which following through is a key component. Be sure to add something that the learner did correctly and discuss the benefits of following through.

2. Devise a feedback example using a motor skill of your choice using the sandwich approach.

3. Describe how each step in your example of the sandwich approach benefits the learner.

Feedback Precision

Adjusting feedback precision based on the skill level of the learner is also important. Feedback should be less precise for beginners. When learners are introduced to a task, they are simply trying to obtain a broad understanding of the movement pattern. More general instructions can be effective during this stage. As they progress from the cognitive stage to the associative stage, their focus shifts to refining the task. At this time, more precise feedback is more meaningful.

Feedback given only when performance is outside a particular range is referred to as **bandwidth feedback**. For example, in American football, a long snapper may receive feedback only when the snap exceeds a range of correctness, such as above the chin or below the knees of the kicker; a volleyball player may receive feedback only when the ball is tossed beyond a foot in front of the shoulder; and a long jumper may receive feedback on his take-off only when his foot lands more than 3 inches (7.6 cm) behind the line. These players know that if they do not receive feedback, they have performed satisfactorily. With this method, the absence of feedback provides positive reinforcement and can be motivational.

Bandwidth feedback eliminates the provision of too much feedback because learners receive feedback only when they are outside a predefined range of correctness. Bandwidth feedback has been found

to promote significantly more retention than both high- and low-frequency KR (Lai & Shea, 1999; Lee & Carnahan, 1990; Sherwood, 1988) as well as the learning of complex motor skills such as a gymnastics sequence (Sadowski, Mastalerz, & Niznikowski, 2013). These benefits may result from the fact that the strategy inherently involves a fading schedule. Novice performers require more feedback than skilled performers do because they are performing outside of the satisfactory range much more often. With practice and increased consistency of movement, learners perform more and more in the satisfactory range, so they receive progressively less and less feedback. The benefit of bandwidth feedback can be further increased by providing positive feedback when the learner is within the bandwidth. In this case learners are receiving less quantitative, or error-based, feedback as they progress, while also receiving the motivational benefit of positive feedback with better performances (Agethan & Krause, 2016).

Choosing an appropriate bandwidth is an important consideration for instructors. Depending on the task, it may be better to have a larger bandwidth for beginners. As learners progress, the bandwidth can be slowly decreased. The goal is to provide the most feedback initially, but the task should not be so challenging that the learner does not achieve any success or see much progress. Tasks that are perceived as too challenging can cause learners to quickly lose motivation or interest in the activity.

Feedback Schedules

Although providing too much KR continuously can be detrimental, so can providing not enough KR during the initial stages of learning (see figure 17.4). Novices who receive very little KR do not receive the guidance they need to improve movement patterns. Beginners do not yet know what they are doing correctly or incorrectly and may spend significant amounts of time trying new strategies. Those who do not receive enough KR during these initial stages require significantly more time to improve and may lose motivation or interest during the process.

Although research has determined that the traditional concept of the more, the better is not valid for providing KR, no optimal reduced-frequency feedback schedule has been found to be most effective. This section describes several reduced-frequency feedback schedules. The appropriateness of each depends on the complexity and duration of the task and the intrinsic factors of the learner.

Faded Feedback

Winstein and Schmidt (1990) developed a feedback schedule in which the amount of feedback is based on the skill level of the learner; it is appropriately termed **faded feedback**. Beginners receive high-frequency feedback to guide their movements and reinforce the correct aspects of their movements. An effective amount of feedback for a beginner may be as high as 80 to 100 percent relative frequency of KR

depending on the complexity and duration of the motor skill. The **relative frequency of KR** is the percentage of performance attempts in which KR is provided. To calculate the relative frequency of KR, the number of trials with KR (i.e., the **absolute frequency of KR**) is divided by the total number of trials. This number is then multiplied by 100 percent. For example, if a gymnast receives feedback following four out of eight vaults, then the absolute frequency is four attempts and the relative frequency is 50 percent, because she received feedback 50 percent of the time. As learners improve, the relative frequency of KR should be progressively reduced. This feedback schedule should be tailored to the learner and should not be reduced until the learner has reached a certain level of proficiency. Children may require longer periods of practice than adults do, and their feedback should be reduced more gradually than that of adults (Sullivan, Kantak, & Burtner, 2008).

Summary Feedback

Summary feedback is feedback following a set number of performance attempts in which the instructor summarizes each attempt. For example, a gymnast could complete an entire floor routine, after which the coach would provide feedback on each of the moves. Similarly, a learner could perform a set number of attempts for a discrete skill, such as shooting a foul shot or throwing a shot put, before receiving summary feedback. Videos are also a source of summary feedback. Learners

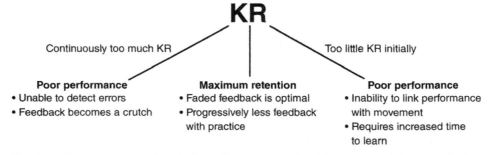

Figure 17.4 Negative outcomes can result from both continuously providing KR and not providing enough KR.

can watch a video following the completion of a series of moves and preferably receive attention-directed feedback regarding their performance attempts. The number of performance attempts appropriate for a motor skill would depend on the complexity and duration of the task. Fewer trials should be summarized with longer or more complex motor skills.

Average Feedback

Average feedback is very similar to summary feedback in that both occur following a set number of performance attempts. However, rather than providing feedback on every attempt or movement, the practitioner discusses only the average performance error(s) or the essence of the performances with the learner. Summary and average feedback also differ with respect to the amount provided. Average feedback provides less, more focused feedback than summary feedback does. Summary feedback and average feedback have been found to be equally effective (Weeks & Sherwood, 1994), but average feedback may be more appealing to practitioners. Given the demands and time constraints imposed on most instructors, clinicians, and coaches, it is unlikely that they can devote attention to many performance attempts for one learner and provide specific feedback on each attempt. Providing a description of the quality of the performances overall (average feedback) is more practical. Average feedback is also advantageous to learners because they are less likely to become overwhelmed with too much information.

Learner-Regulated Feedback

All of the feedback schedules we have considered so far are designed and implemented by the practitioner. One feedback schedule, which has been the focus of many research studies, puts learners in control of feedback by allowing them to decide how often to receive extrinsic feedback, and after which trials. This is called **learner-regulated feedback**. Shifting the control of the provision of feedback from the instructor to the learner resulted in more learning than in matched participants who received feedback at the instructor's discretion (Chiviacowsky, Wulf, Laroque de Medeiros, Kaefer, & Wally, 2008). The only difference between the groups in this study was that one group decided *when* they would receive feedback. The possible benefits to learner-regulated feedback are (a) a more active role, providing learners with more opportunity to process the movement and the feedback cognitively (Wulf, Clauss, Shea, & Whitacre, 2001), and (b) increased motivation (Chiviacowsky & Wulf, 2007). The frequency with which learners request feedback largely depends on their characteristics, including skill level and age, as well as characteristics of the task such as complexity and duration. As previously discussed, beginners require more feedback until they obtain a certain level of proficiency. More feedback is also required for more complex and longer tasks.

Do Children Require More or Less Feedback?

Chiviacowsky and colleagues (2008) investigated the effectiveness of learner-regulated feedback in 10-year-olds, comparing the frequency of their requests for feedback with their learning. The investigators also sought to determine whether children would choose the "optimal" frequency of feedback. Previously, it had been found that children who requested feedback (learner-regulated group) learned the task more effectively than did children who received feedback on the same schedule but did not control when they received it (Chiviacowsky & Wulf, 2006). On the basis of the results, participants were separated into two groups—a more KR group (requested 39.3 percent KR on average) and a less KR group (requested 8.4 percent KR on average). The more KR group showed enhanced learning in comparison to the less KR group. The authors suggested several reasons children require more feedback than adults do. First, because they have less movement experience, learning new motor skills is more challenging than it is for adults. Children also have shorter attention spans and are less able to process information than adults are (Lambert & Bard, 2005). Processing speed increases from age 3 to adolescence, so children require more time to process information than adults do.

These results indicate that, although children significantly benefit from learner-regulated feedback (Chiviacowsky & Wulf, 2006), they may not always choose an optimal frequency. Because of their limited movement experiences, reduced attentional capacity, and slower processing speeds, children require more frequent feedback than adults do. Learner-regulated feedback may be the most optimal feedback schedule for children if the instructions encourage them to request more feedback for more difficult tasks, because children have a tendency to request feedback at a lower-than-optimal rate (Chiviacowsky et al., 2008).

It is also important to consider the type of feedback that is appropriate for children. Typically, positive feedback is very effective; however, this may not be the case for all positive feedback. In a study of 10-year-olds performing kicking and throwing tasks, those who received generic feedback such as feedback reflecting inherent ability (e.g., *You have natural talent*) improved less than did those who were given specific feedback on the movement pattern (Chiviacowsky & Drews, 2014). These effects provided both short- and long-term benefits. Feedback that teaches children that they are in control of their performances was more likely to change their performances, which led to improvements.

Extrinsic Feedback Timing

Another critical issue is the timing of extrinsic feedback (see figure 17.5). In other words, when is it most appropriate to provide extrinsic feedback? Many instructors and clinicians assume that feedback is most effective immediately following a performance attempt. Although one might expect immediate feedback to be most beneficial because it allows learners to link the performance with the outcome or quality of the movement before their memory of the movement production fades, immediate feedback actually prevents learners from reflecting on the movement. Just as the provision of high-frequency KR (i.e., 80-100 percent relative KR) eliminates active processing, feedback provided too soon after a performance attempt promotes passive learning. The learner will become reliant on the feedback and will not develop the

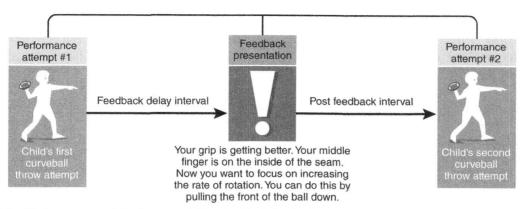

Figure 17.5 Timing components for the presentation of extrinsic feedback.
Based on Coker 2009.

critical problem-solving skills necessary for performing the motor skill without the guidance of the extrinsic feedback.

The time period between one performance attempt and the next is termed the **interresponse interval**. This time period is broken down into two other temporal intervals, the feedback delay interval (the time between the first attempt and the provision of feedback) and the postfeedback delay interval (the time between the provision of feedback and the second attempt). The following sections describe these intervals further, because their duration has important implications for learning.

Feedback Delay Interval

Researchers have examined the timing of feedback to determine the most effective time lapse between the completion of a performance and the provision of KR. The time between the completion of an attempt and the presentation of feedback is termed the **feedback delay interval**. The length of the feedback delay interval is a critical component in the presentation of extrinsic feedback. The learner needs adequate time to focus on proprioceptive, auditory, and visual feedback from the attempt (Magill, 2001). If the feedback delay interval is too long, then the learner will have forgotten much about the movement production. On the other hand, if the feedback delay interval is too short, the learner will not have time to engage in the cognitive operations needed to detect errors and create

correction strategies (Salmoni, Schmidt, & Walter, 1984; Swinnen, Schmidt, Nicholson, & Shapiro, 1990).

The key question is How long should instructors and clinicians wait before providing extrinsic feedback? The feedback delay interval does not need to be lengthy. It simply needs to be long enough to allow learners to process and evaluate their own intrinsic feedback. Learners need to think about how the movement felt, how they performed, what errors they may have made, and how to correct them. Even just a few seconds can be long enough to do this. However, research has indicated that longer delays do not adversely affect learning (Bilodeau & Bilodeau, 1958). Although a longer feedback delay interval is less likely to negatively affect learning than immediate extrinsic feedback (a very small feedback delay interval), motor forgetting can occur during this time, which makes it more difficult for learners to link their performances to extrinsic feedback.

Consider an instructor who has chosen a feedback delay interval of five seconds. How does he know that the learners are reflecting during this time and not simply waiting for his feedback? The truth is that he doesn't know, unless he asks. Prompting learners to self-reflect and evaluate their performances during this break leads to increased retention (Swinnen et al., 1990). To promote self-evaluation following a performance attempt, the instructor should ask learners directed questions.

The questions could be general, such as *How do you think you did?* or *What do you think you did wrong [or right] during that attempt?* The instructor could then follow up by asking, *How did you come to the conclusion that [a particular aspect of the movement] was correct [or incorrect]?* or *What about that movement was incorrect?* or *How could you correct that mistake?*

Self-evaluation is a learned strategy that takes time to develop. It may be more effective to ask specific questions, especially with beginners, because they will likely not know the causes of their errors or how to correct them. For example, an instructor could ask leading questions, such as, *Do you think you followed through the release of the ball?* or *Where did you make contact with the ball? Was it the correct location?* As learners develop better self-evaluation strategies and improve their performances, the questions can become more general. Eventually, they will be able to self-evaluate with little to no help from the instructor.

Postfeedback Delay Interval

The time between the presentation of extrinsic feedback and the subsequent performance attempt is called the **postfeedback delay interval**. In contrast to the feedback delay interval, learners are likely focusing more on evaluating the feedback just received than on their own intrinsic feedback (Magill, 2001). However, if this interval is too short, learning can be negatively affected (Gallagher & Thomas, 1980). Learners need sufficient time to process the information provided through extrinsic feedback and to plan the next attempt (Rose & Christina, 2006).

The appropriate length of the postfeedback delay interval depends on the age of the learner; children require longer intervals (Barclay & Newell, 1980). As previously mentioned, children have greater processing limitations than adults have. Increased postfeedback delay intervals give young learners more time to develop the error detection and correction mechanism necessary for learning motor skills.

Conversely, older adults are negatively affected by longer postfeedback delay intervals (Liu, Cao, & Yan, 2013). Older adults are not only affected by longer feedback delay intervals, but delays of even three or six seconds longer in duration in the postfeedback delay interval degraded their performance. This is likely due to their reduced attention and working memory capabilities. Older adults may switch their attention from their intrinsic feedback to the KR in short intervals and overrely on KR feedback (Yan & Dick, 2006).

To facilitate cognitive processing during the postfeedback delay interval, the instructor can ask learners how they are going to execute the next attempt, or more specifically, what they are going to do differently from the previous attempt. By encouraging learners to further process this information, the instructor can check how well they understand their performance errors and the effectiveness of the feedback.

Misconceptions About Feedback

Now that you've looked at various types and schedules of feedback, it's important that you also understand some misconceptions about feedback. Table 17.3 outlines three common misconceptions about feedback and provides best practices to address each.

Summary

Feedback is one of the most important factors in skill acquisition, second only to practice. Feedback helps guide performers toward executing proper movement patterns, motivates learners, and reinforces successful performances. Feedback received via the sensory systems is intrinsic feedback, whereas feedback that has been given in addition to sensory sources is extrinsic feedback. The two main forms of extrinsic feedback are knowledge of results (performance outcome) and knowledge of performance (quality of the movement pattern). Knowledge of performance

Table 17.3   Misconceptions About and Best Practices for Extrinsic Feedback

Misconception	Best practice
More is better: The more feedback provided, the better the learning.	Fade the amount of feedback provided.
The faster, the better: Providing feedback immediately following the performance attempt is most effective.	Allow processing time after the performance attempt and after providing feedback.
Increased precision is better: Decreased size of the bandwidth is more effective.	Fade the bandwidth (expect progressively better performances as skill level increases).

Note that for each best practice of feedback, considerations should be made in regard to the skill level of the learner, the difficulty of the motor skill, and the age of the learner.

can be descriptive or prescriptive, but providing both is most effective.

Novice learners require more extrinsic feedback than skilled learners do. Feedback during the initial stages of learning can decrease learning time by helping learners link successful performances with the movement patterns produced. As learners progress, the amount of feedback provided should decrease, which is known as faded feedback. Practitioners can accomplish this by progressively providing less relative KR or by providing bandwidth KR, because more skilled learners will perform within the bandwidth progressively more and more and therefore receive less feedback. Learner-regulated KR is also very effective, especially for adults. Because learners generally ask for KR only when they actually need the feedback, they do not receive too much and feel a greater sense of control over the learning situation.

The importance of appropriate extrinsic feedback cannot be overemphasized. More often than not, movement educators provide extrinsic feedback too frequently or too soon, without realizing the negative effects this has on both short- and long-term retention. Just like practice, feedback should be designed around the learner and the task.

ONLINE LEARNING

Visit the web resource at www.HumanKinetics.com/MotorLearningAndDevelopment for an accompanying lab activity, video clips, and exercises from the chapter.

LEARNING AIDS

Supplemental Activities

1. Many variables influence the effectiveness of extrinsic feedback, including the skill level and age of the learner and the difficulty of the task. Practitioners should consider the type of feedback that would be most appropriate, as well as the frequency at which to provide the feedback. Answer the following questions in regard to these important considerations:
    a. What are the benefits of providing extrinsic feedback?
    b. When might extrinsic feedback not be needed?
    c. When might extrinsic feedback enhance skill acquisition?
    d. When can extrinsic feedback be counterproductive—that is, degrade skill acquisition?
    e. Counter the misconceptions listed in table 17.3. Explain why each is a misconception.

2. If you were teaching someone a new motor skill, how would you incorporate feedback into your program? Provide a progression of feedback instruction from the initial instruction to skill refinement. You could design this feedback schedule for any motor skill, from teaching striking skills to a child to teaching an adult how to walk following an injury. Describe the motor skill you are teaching and the characteristics of the learner. Be sure to include a timeline for this progression.

Glossary

absolute frequency of KR—The number of trials in which KR was provided.

attention-directed cues—Cues that direct attention to the most important aspects of the movement pattern.

attention-focusing cues—Cues that not only direct attention to specific aspects of the movement pattern but also include error-correcting suggestions.

average feedback—Feedback that includes only the average performance error(s), or the essence of the performances.

bandwidth feedback—Feedback given only when the performance is outside a particular range.

biofeedback—Extrinsic feedback that provides concurrent kinematic information related to physiological processes.

concurrent feedback—Feedback received during the movement.

descriptive feedback—Feedback that describes the nature of a performance error.

error correction stage—Stage 3 of the video learning stages, in which learners are able to identify their errors and in some cases understand the causes.

error detection stage—Stage 2 of the video learning stages, in which learners are comfortable viewing their performances. Attention-focused cues should be used to help them detect their errors during this stage.

extrinsic feedback—Feedback that comes from an external source, additional to sensory information.

faded feedback—Feedback based on the skill level of the learner; beginners receive high-frequency feedback initially and progressively less feedback with improvement.

feedback delay interval—The time between the completion of a performance attempt and the presentation of feedback.

guidance hypothesis—The hypothesis that the benefits of high-frequency KR can be deceiving because learners tend to perform better initially than they would if they had received lower-frequency KR.

independence stage—The final stage of the video feedback learning stages, in which learners require minimal to no video supplementation by an instructor.

interresponse interval—The period between two performance attempts.

intrinsic feedback—Feedback that is received from sensory sources before, during, and after a movement.

kinematic feedback—Feedback on the observable aspects of the movement, such as the space–time properties of a performance.

kinetic feedback—Feedback on the underlying processes of the movement, such as force.

knowledge of performance (KP)—Feedback that provides information about the characteristics of the movement pattern produced.

knowledge of results (KR)—Terminal feedback that describes the outcome of the movement.

learner-regulated feedback—A feedback schedule that puts learners in control of feedback by allowing them to decide how often to receive extrinsic feedback, and after which trials.

negative reinforcement—Feedback that elicits unpleasant feelings that the learner will want to avoid.

positive reinforcement—Feedback following a movement that promotes the recurrence of the same movement pattern.

postfeedback delay interval—The time between the presentation of extrinsic feedback and the subsequent performance attempt.

prescriptive feedback—Feedback that provides suggestions for correcting performance errors.

relative frequency of KR—The percentage of performance attempts for which KR is provided.

shock stage—Stage 1 of the video learning stages, in which learners are often more focused on their visual appearance on video than on their movement patterns or performances.

summary feedback—Feedback provided on all attempts following a set number of performance attempts.

terminal feedback—Feedback provided following the movement.

DEVISING A PLAN

Chapter Objectives

After reading this chapter, you should be able to do the following:

- List physical factors that instructors can manipulate.
- Develop ecological task analyses.
- Analyze case studies and develop appropriate practice and feedback schedules by manipulating the task and environment to teach motor skills for each scenario.

In this textbook you have learned about many concepts related to motor learning and motor development. You have learned how to classify motor skills, which is particularly helpful for creating appropriate practice and feedback schedules. You have also learned how to measure learning and maximize performance and, most important, long-term retention based on variables such as the complexity and duration of the motor skill and the developmental and skill levels of the learner by manipulating the task and the environment. You will now put all of these concepts together by using ecological task analyses in particular case studies.

Ecological Task Analysis

Traditional task analysis is a method of analyzing movement performance by comparing learners' movement patterns to a correct model. This approach has several problems. The main one is that comparing learners with a model, or correct form, assumes that the structural constraints of the learner are similar to those of the model—in other words, that the learner is capable of moving like the model. Traditional task analysis is also problematic because everyone is placed on a continuum of performance ranging from incorrect to correct. The instructor observes the learner and corrects the movements that deviate from the correct form. Refer to chapter 14 for a discussion on the gold standard of movement versus variability. Each individual is built differently, with varying intrinsic dynamics, including previous movement experience, skill level, body size, and muscular strength, which cause people to solve movement challenges in different ways. Finally, the traditional task analysis model does not account for the interaction between the task and the environment.

The **ecological task analysis model**, on the other hand, accounts for learners' individual differences. This is accomplished by manipulating the environment and task

on a progression of complexity, allowing learners to increase the complexity on one or more levels of a motor skill at a time. Davis and Burton (1991) identified four major steps for designing an ecological task analysis:

1. The instructor selects the task goal and structures the environmental constraints around it. An important component in the ecological task model is the involvement of the learner in this process.

2. The instructor provides learners with movement options rather than constraining their movements by instructing them to complete the movement pattern in a particular way (as in the traditional task analysis model). The instructor may even provide equipment options, such as different-sized balls. Learners may decide to make the task more or less challenging, depending on the size or bounciness of the ball. Learners who are presented with choices are likely to take more ownership of the learning process and remain motivated.

3. After learners have attempted the movement pattern, the instructor manipulates the environment, task, or both, to enhance performance.

4. The instructor then gives learners augmented feedback.

Creating an ecological task analysis for a motor skill involves three steps. The first is making a list of all the constraints associated with performing the motor skill. For playing basketball, important constraints are coordination, balance, agility, strength, and control. Once the individual constraints are established, the second step is to list the interactions between the task and the environment. In other words, How can the task of playing basketball be simplified? The equipment can be modified for smaller children, such as using a smaller or lighter ball, to account for constraints such as height and strength. The hoop could be lowered, and the court size could be decreased. A beginner would likely practice shooting balls while stationary to decrease the balance and coordination constraints. The third step is to develop a range from simple to complex for each task and environmental constraint. Keep in mind that large changes in performance can result from small variations in a constraint (Haywood & Getchell, 2014). Task analyses are also helpful in therapeutic situations by providing patients with multiple options and progressions as they improve.

Task analysis can be an easy way for both instructors and learners to manipulate the task and the environment, and it helps in the creation of individualized programs even in group settings. For instance, one learner could be at the lowest level for all six factors in the catching example in table 18.1, whereas another may be using a medium-sized, heavy ball that is traveling at a slow speed (a relatively complex catching task). Learners who are given the opportunity to manipulate the task conditions often find the activity more interesting and rewarding.

Ecological task analysis is a method of outlining several possible task and environmental constraints at various levels of difficulty. Once an ecological task analysis is developed, it can become a tool for both the instructor (or therapist) and the learner (or client) to use to manipulate the complexity of the task and assess the level of the learner or client. Ecological task analysis allows for easy comparisons across individuals by comparing learners' levels for each factor rather than by evaluating product outcomes (e.g., distance or accuracy). Product outcomes are limiting given that some learners adopt unorthodox techniques to throw farther. For example, a learner who catches more balls than another learner (product outcome) may be using his chest in the catch (poor technique).

Table 18.1 Ecological Task Analysis for Catching

	Factors					
	Size of object being caught	Distance for object being thrown	Weight of object being caught	Speed at which ball is coming	Predictability of trajectory of object being caught	Anticipation of ball coming and getting hands ready
Level of difficulty: simple	Large	Short	Light	Slow	Along the ground	Hands up when it gets close
Level of difficulty: moderate	Medium	Medium	Moderate	Moderate	Bounced along the ground	Hands up when it's on its way
Level of difficulty: complex	Small	Long	Heavy	Fast	In the air	Hands up before ball is thrown

Case Studies

Now that you understand how to develop an ecological task analysis and have an understanding of motor behavior concepts across the life span, you are invited to take these concepts and apply them to the following case studies. These case studies are written with varying perspectives: as a therapist, as an instructor, or as an athlete. For each case study, summarize the situation and describe the constraints (learner, task, and environment) and develop an ecological task analysis. See figure 18.1 for a model of the constraints. Then develop a specific and measurable goal that includes a timeline. Using motor learning concepts, develop a practice schedule to achieve this goal. Your practice schedule can include variable practice, part versus whole practice, mental practice, or distribution of practice (or a combination of these). Be specific in how you recommend administering that type of practice, and describe your rationale for choosing that practice

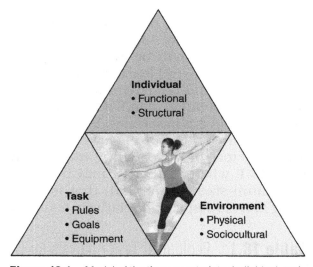

Figure 18.1 Model of the three constraints: individual, task, and environment.

schedule (i.e., factors such as the type of motor skill, the complexity of skill, and learner characteristics). Finally, develop a feedback schedule including the type, frequency, and amount of feedback. Describe your rationale for choosing that feedback schedule.

Case Study 1

Physical Therapy After a Bicycle Accident

Rachel is 45 years old and experienced major head trauma during her cycling training for a triathlon one week ago.

She incurred a closed head injury with a hematoma and has hemiplegia affecting her left side, which means that she has minimal function and control on that side. She currently cannot walk or use her left arm to feed herself or write, and she is left handed. She will require therapy to improve her function on the left side, including increasing her control of her left side and ultimately being able to walk and write with her left hand. Currently, she can move from a standing position to a sitting position and can get onto a bed using her unimpaired arm. She needs help taking steps and cannot balance her weight on her impaired leg. In your case study, discuss the patient, tasks that could be used to improve her movement control, and how the environment can be manipulated. Consider the motor learning principles discussed throughout this book in your explanations. Create a goal and explain how you will help Rachel obtain it through your practice and feedback schedules. Be very specific about practice and feedback schedules, and include a rationale for each based upon motor learning principles.

Case Study 2
Motor Development Screening

Omar is a five-year-old boy who is right arm and right leg dominant. He was referred for a screening for possible entry into an early intervention program for children with perceptual motor delays. When Omar throws, he rotates his entire body and releases the ball in an unpredictable manner. At times, his head moves with his trunk. When instructed to catch a ball, he turns his head away, closes his eyes, and holds his arms out. Omar gallops when asked to skip or slide, even following a demonstration. He kicks in an upright position, takes a small step forward, pulls his leg back in a straight position, and makes contact with the ball with his toes. He dribbles by slapping the ball and maintaining focus on the ball, and can dribble only with his right hand. When instructed to leap, Omar runs and then takes a large step. During the screening process, you provided multiple demonstrations. Omar was well behaved but needed multiple reminders and often lost attentional focus. What are Omar's biggest rate limiters for performing fundamental motor

skills? What strategies might improve Omar's attentional focus and motor skills? Consider the motor learning principles discussed throughout this book in your explanations. Create a goal and explain how you will help Omar obtain it through your practice and feedback schedules. Be very specific about practice and feedback schedules, and include a rationale for each based upon motor learning principles.

Case Study 3
Varsity Swimmer Who Can't Drop Time

Shira is a senior in high school and is struggling with her swim times. She goes to every practice offered, works hard, listens to her coaches, and makes the appropriate adjustments, yet she is making no improvements, meet after meet. For two years, Shira has been struggling with her times and continues to get frustrated. Before her meets, she is anxious, and after her meets, she beats herself up over her performances. What factors might be affecting Shira's lack of improvement? What does she need to do to begin to see improvements again? Create a goal and explain how you will help Shira obtain it through practice and feedback schedules. Be very specific about practice and feedback schedules, and include a rationale for each based upon motor learning principles.

Case Study 4
Adolescent With Sensory Impairments

Darnell is a 13-year-old with sensory impairments, including blindness and a residual loss of hearing. Unfortunately, he has not learned many fundamental motor skills, which is in part due to the lack of appropriate activities taught in physical education class that are modified to include him. Darnell is usually told to walk around the gym or participate in a sedentary activity while the rest of the class participates in a sport or other physical activity. When he runs, he does not have a flight phase. Technically, this means that he is actually just walking quickly rather than running. Darnell does not leap prior to kicking a ball. He does not extend his leg back very far, and he kicks the ball at the top of his foot. Darnell's slide and gallop appear the same because he is unsure of the difference. Darnell's poor performances in these fundamental motor skills are not the result of physical limitations. Given his inability to see other students running, throwing, and jumping, Darnell must learn the movement patterns in other ways. He also has not had many opportunities to practice motor skills that most children acquire by the age of seven. Considering that Darnell is a now a teenager, how can you teach him these fundamental motor skills? Is it possible for him to advance to the same level as his peers? Consider the motor learning principles discussed throughout this book in your explanations. Create a goal and explain how you will help Darnell obtain it through practice and feedback schedules. Be very specific about practice and feedback schedules, and include a rationale for each based upon motor learning principles.

Case Study 5

Older Adult With Multiple Conditions

Ida, an 82-year-old, came to a fitness center to begin an exercise program on her doctor's advice. She had a medical release from her doctor and during her initial screening disclosed that she has osteoarthritis in her knees and her left shoulder, mild osteoporosis, cataracts, blood pressure around 140/90 mmHg, and some hearing loss. Her right hip was replaced seven years ago, and she had gone to physical therapy. Ida's goals for her program were to increase her strength and improve her balance to decrease her risk of falls. What are some of the considerations in developing Ida's program? What types of activities should she avoid because of her conditions? Also, what instructional strategies would help when instructing

Ida on the exercises? Consider the motor learning principles discussed throughout this book in your explanations. Create a goal and explain how you will help Ida obtain it through practice and feedback schedules. Be very specific about practice and feedback schedules, and include a rationale for each based upon motor learning principles.

Case Study 6

Develop Your Own Case Study

Develop your own case study, perhaps using a personal experience of a motor skill, sport, or activity. Describe the learner(s), the situation, and the motor skill, sport, or activity.

Summary

This final chapter provided additional tools to use to examine a situation and devise a plan based on the motor behavior concepts described throughout this book. Movement professionals must have a solid understanding of these concepts to prepare the environment and instruct learners, whether they are athletes, students, classes, patients, or clients, based on their individual constraints. The task and environment should be modified to design the most effective practice sessions for individuals or groups.

LEARNING AIDS

Glossary

ecological task analysis model—A method of analyzing movement performance that accounts for individual differences by manipulating the environment and task on a progression of complexity, allowing learners to increase complexity on one or more levels of a skill at a time.

traditional task analysis—A method of analyzing movement performance by comparing the movement pattern to a correct model.

REFERENCES

Chapter 1

Adams, D.L. (1999). Develop better motor skill progressions with Gentile's taxonomy of tasks. *Journal of Physical Education, Recreation and Dance, 70* (8), 35.

Argyle, M., & Kendon, A. (1967). The experimental analysis of social performance. In L. Berkowitz (Ed.), *Advances in experimental social psychology.* New York: Academic Press.

Bernstein, N. (1967). *The co-ordination and regulation of movement.* London: Pergamon Press.

Brace, D.K. (1927). *Measuring motor ability.* New York: A.S. Barnes.

Calvo-Merino, B., Glaser, D.E., Grezes, J., Passingham, R.E., & Haggard, P. (2005). Action observation and acquired motor skills: An fMRI study with expert dancers. *Cerebral Cortex, 15,* 1243-1249.

Clark, J.E., & Whitall, J. (1989). What is motor development? The lessons of history. *Quest, 41,* 183-202.

Cohen, R.G., & Rosenbaum, D.A. (2004). Where objects are grasped reveals how grasps are planned: Generation and recall of motor plans. *Experimental Brain Research, 157,* 486-495.

Darwin, C. (1859). *On the origin of species by means of natural selection, or the preservation of favoured races in the struggle for life* (1st ed.). London: John Murray.

Darwin, C. (1871). *The descent of man, and selection in relation to sex* (1st ed.). London: John Murray.

Darwin, C. (1872). *The origin of species by means of natural selection, or the preservation of favoured races in the struggle for life* (6th ed.). London: John Murray.

Fitts, P., & Posner, M.I. (1967). *Human performance.* Belmont, CA: Brooks/Cole.

Fleishman, E.A. (1962). The description and prediction of perceptual motor skill learning. In R. Glasser (Ed.), *Training research and education* (pp. 137-175). Pittsburgh: University of Pittsburgh Press.

Fleishman, E.A. (1964). *The structure and measurement of physical fitness.* Englewood Cliffs, NJ: Prentice Hall.

Gallahue, D.L., Ozmun, J.C., & Goodway, J.D. (2012). *Understanding motor development* (7th ed.). New York: McGraw-Hill.

Gentile, A.M. (2000). Skill acquisition: Action, movement and neuromotor processes. In J.H. Carr & R.B. Shepherd (Eds.), *Movement science: Foundations for physical therapy in rehabilitation* (2nd ed., pp. 111-187). Rockville, MD: Aspen.

Gesell, A. (1928). *Infancy and human growth.* New York: Macmillan.

Gesell, A. (1954). The ontogenesis of infant behavior. In L. Carmichael (Ed.), *Manual of child psychology* (2nd ed.). New York: Wiley.

Halverson, L.E. (1970). *Research in motor development: Implications for program in early childhood education.* Paper presented at the Midwest Association for Health, Physical Education and Recreation, Chicago.

Henry, F.M. (1968). Specificity vs. generality in learning motor skills. In R.C. Brown & G.S. Kenyon (Eds.), *Classical studies on physical activity* (pp. 331-340). Englewood Cliffs, NJ: Prentice Hall.

Hirsiger, S., Pickett, K., & Konczak, J. (2012). The integration of size and weight cues for perception and action: Evidence for a weight-size illusion. *Experimental Brain Research, 223,* 137-147.

Honeybourne, J. (2006). *Acquiring skill in sport: An introduction.* London: Routledge.

Kandel, S., & Perret, C. (2015). How do movements to produce letters become automatic during writing acquisition? Investigating the development of motor anticipation. *International Journal of Behavioral Development, 39* (2), 113-120.

Kenyon, L. K. & Blackinton, M.T (2011) Applying motor-control theory to physical therapy practice: A case report, *Physiotherapy Canada, 63,* 345–354.

Knapp, B. (1963). *Skill in sport.* London: Routledge & Kegan Paul.

Lashley, K.S. (1951). The problem of serial order in behavior. In L.A. Jeffress (Ed.), *Cerebral mechanisms in behavior* (pp. 112-131). New York: Wiley.

McGraw, M. (1935). *Growth: A study of Johnny and Jimmy.* New York: Appleton-Century-Crofts.

McGraw, M.B. (1940). Signals of growth. *Child Study, 18,* 8-10.

McGraw, M.B. (1969). *The neuromuscular maturation of the human infant.* New York: Hafner. (Original work published 1945)

Ribadi, H., Rider, R., & Toole, T. (1987). Comparison of static and dynamic balance in congenitally blind, sighted, and sighted blindfolded adolescents. *Physical Activity Quarterly, 4,* 220-225.

Rosenbaum, D.A. (2010). *Human motor control* (2nd ed.). Amsterdam: Academic Press.

Schmidt, R.A., & Lee, T.D. (2014). *Motor learning and performance* (5th ed.). Champaign, IL: Human Kinetics.

Sparrow, W.A. (1992). Measuring changes in coordination and control. In J.J. Summers (Ed.), *Approaches to the study of motor control and learning* (pp. 147-162). Amsterdam; New York: North-Holland.

Spirduso, W.W., Francis, K.L., & MacRae, P.G. (2005). *Physical dimensions of aging* (2nd ed.). Champaign, IL: Human Kinetics.

Talović, M., Hodžić, M., Bajramović, I., Jeleškovič, E., & Alić, H. (2009). Influence of the motor and functional abilities to the efficiency of football techniques elements performance. *Homo Sporticus, 11* (1), 41-44.

Thelen, E., Fisher, D.M., Ridley-Johnson, R., & Griffin, N.J. (1982). Effects of body build and arousal on newborn infant stepping. *Developmental Psychobiology, 15* (5), 447-453.

Turvey, M.T. (1990). Coordination. *American Psychologist, 45* (8), 938-953.

Chapter 2

Adams, R., & Dijkstra, S. (1966). Short-term memory for motor responses. *Journal of Experimental Psychology, 71,* 314-318.

Allen, P.A., Smith, A.F., Vires-Collins, H., & Sperry, S. (1998). The psychological refractory period: Evidence for age differences in attentional time-sharing. *Psychology and Aging, 13,* 218-229.

Atkinson, R.C., & Shiffrin, R.M. (1968). Human memory: A proposed system and its control processes. In K.W. Spence & J.T. Spence (Eds.), *The psychology of learning and motivation: Advances in research and theory* (Vol. 2, pp. 89-197). New York: Academic Press.

Baddeley, A.D. (1986). *Working memory.* New York: Oxford University Press.

Baddeley, A.D. (1995). Working memory. In M.S. Gazzaniga (Ed.), *The cognitive neurosciences* (pp. 755-764). Cambridge, MA: MIT Press.

Cherry, E.C. (1953). Some experiments on the recognition of speech, with one and with two ears. *The Journal of the Acoustical Society of America, 25* (5), 975-979.

Easterbrook, J.A. (1959). The effect of emotion on cue utilization and the organization of behavior. *Psychological Review, 66,* 183-201.

Freudheim, A.M., Wulf, G., Madureira, F., Pasetto, S.C., & Correa, U.C. (2010). An external focus of attention results in greater swimming speed. *International Journal of Sports Science and Coaching, 5,* 533-542.

Gallahue, D.L., Ozmun, J.C., & Goodway, J.D. (2012). *Understanding motor development: Infants, children, adolescent and adults* (7th ed.). Boston: McGraw-Hill.

Haywood, K.M., & Getchell, N. (2014). *Life span motor development* (6th ed.). Champaign, IL: Human Kinetics.

Helsen, W., & Pauwels, J.M. (1993). The relationship between expertise and visual information processing in sport. In J.L. Starkes & F. Allard (Eds.), *Cognitive issues in motor expertise* (pp. 109-134). Amsterdam: Elsevier Science.

Hick, W.E. (1952). On the rate of gain of information. *Quarterly Journal of Experimental Psychology, 4,* 11-26.

Ille, A., & Cadopi, M. (1999). Memory for movement sequences in gymnastics: Effects of age and skill level. *Journal of Motor Behavior, 31,* 290-300.

Kahneman, D. (1973). *Attention and effort.* Englewood Cliffs, NJ: Prentice Hall.Landers, D.M., & Arent, S.M. (2010). Arousal-performance relationships. In J.M. Williams (Ed.), *Applied sport psychology: Personal growth to peak performance* (6th ed., pp. 221-226). Dubuque, IA: McGraw-Hill.

Leavitt, J.L. (1979). Cognitive demands of skating and stick handling in ice hockey. *Canadian Journal of Applied Sport Science, 4,* 46-55.

Li, K., Su, W., Fu, H., & Pickett, K.A. (2015). Kinethetic deficit in children with developmental coordination disorder. *Research in Developmental Disabilities, 38,* 125-133.

Magill, R., & Anderson, D. (2013). *Motor learning and control: Concepts and applications* (10th ed.). New York: McGraw-Hill.

Marieb, E.N., Wilhelm, P.B., & Mallatt, J.B. (2017). *Human anatomy* (8th ed.). London: Pearson Education.

McNevin, N.H., Shea, C.H., & Wulf, G. (2003). Increasing the distance of an external focus of attention enhances learning. *Psychological Research, 67,* 22-29.

Miller, G.A. (1956). The magical number seven plus or minus two: Some limits on our capacity for processing information. *Psychological Review, 63,* 81-97.

Nideffer, R.M. (1976). Test of attentional and interpersonal style. *Journal of Personality and Social Psychology, 34,* 394-404.

Perreault, M.E., & French, K.E. (2015). External-focus feedback benefits free-throw learning in children. *Research Quarterly for Exercise and Sport, 86*, 422-427.

Schmidt, R.A. & Lee, T.D. (2011). *Motor control and learning: A behavioral emphasis.* (5th ed.). Champaign, IL: Human Kinetics.

Schrauf, M., Wist, E.R., & Ehrenstein, W.H. (1999). Development of dynamic vision based on motion contrast. *Experimental Brain Research, 124,* 469-473.

Smith, M.C. (1967). Theories of the psychological refractory period. *Psychological Bulletin, 67,* 202-213.

Starkes, J.L., Deakin, J.M., Lindley, S., & Crisp, F. (1987). Motor versus verbal recall of ballet sequences by young expert dancers. *Journal of Sport Psychology, 9,* 222-230.

Vance, J., Wulf, G., Töllner, T., McNevin, N., & Mercer, J. (2004). EMG activity as a function of the performer's focus of attention. *Journal of Motor Behavior, 36,* 450-459.

Visser, J., & Geuze, R.H. (2000). Kinaesthetic acuity in adolescent boys: A longitudinal study. *Developmental Medicine & Child Neurology, 42,* 93-96.

Weinberg, R.S., & Gould, D. (2015). *Foundations of sport and exercise psychology* (6th ed.). Champaign, IL: Human Kinetics.

Wickens, C.D. (1980). The structure of processing resources. In R. Nickerson (Ed.), *Attention and performance VII* (pp. 239-257). Hillsdale, NJ: Erlbaum.

Wickens, C.D. (1992). *Engineering psychology and human performance* (2nd ed.). New York: HarperCollins.

Wulf, G. (2013). Attentional focus and motor learning: A review of 15 years. *International Review of Sport and Exercise Psychology, 6,* 77-104.

Wulf, G., & Dufek, J.S. (2009). Increased jump height with an external focus due to enhances lower extremity joint kinetics. *Journal of Motor Behavior, 41,* 401-409.

Wulf, G., Dufek, J.S., Lozano, L., & Pettigrew, C. (2010). Increased jump height and reduced EMG activity with an external focus. *Human Movement Science, 29*(3), 440-448.

Wulf, G., Höß, M., & Prinz, W. (1998). Instructions for motor learning: Differential effects of internal versus external focus of attention. *Journal of Motor Behavior, 30,* 169-179.

Wulf, G., & Lewthwaite, R. (2010). Effortless motor learning? An external focus of attention enhances movement effectiveness and efficiency. In B. Bruya (Ed.), *Effortless attention: A new perspective in the cognitive science of attention and action* (pp. 75-101). Cambridge, MA: The MIT Press.

Wulf, G., McNevin, N.H., & Shea, C.H. (2001). The automaticity of complex motor skill learning as a function of attentional focus. *The Quarterly Journal of Experimental Psychology, 54A,* 1143-1154.

Wulf, G., & Su, J. (2007). An external focus of attention enhances golf shot accuracy in beginners and experts. *Research Quarterly for Exercise and Sport, 78,* 384-389.

Wulf, G., Wächter, S., & Wortmann, S. (2003). Attentional focus in motor skill learning: Do females benefit from an external focus? *Women in Sport and Physical Activity Journal, 12,* 37-52.

Chapter 3

Adolph, K.E., Eppler, M.A., & Gibson, E.J. (1993). Crawling versus walking infants' perception of affordances for locomotion over sloping surfaces. *Child Development, 64* (4), 1158-1174.

Clark, J.E., & Whitall, J. (1989). What is motor development? The lessons of history. *Quest, 41,* 183-202.

Ennis, C. (1992). Reconceptualizing learning as a dynamical system. *Journal of Curriculum and Supervision, 7*(2), 115-130.

Fitts, P.M. (1954). The information capacity of the human motor system in controlling the amplitude of movement. *Journal of Experimental Psychology, 47,* 381-391.

Fitts, P., & Posner, M.I. (1967). *Human performance.* Belmont, CA: Brooks/Cole.

Gibson, J.J. (1966). *The senses considered as perceptual systems.* Boston: Houghton Mifflin.

Gibson, J.J. (1977). The theory of affordances. In R. Shaw & J. Bransford (Eds.), *Perceiving, acting and knowing: Toward an ecological psychology.* Hillsdale, NJ: Erlbaum.

Gibson, J.J. (1979). *The ecological approach to visual perception.* Boston: Houghton Mifflin.

Henry, F.M., & Rogers, D.E. (1960). Increased response latency for complicated movements and the "memory drum" theory of neuromotor reaction. *Research Quarterly, 31,* 448-458.

Keele, S.W. (1973). *Attention and human performance.* Pacific Palisades, CA: Goodyear.

Kenyon, L.K., & Blackinton, M.T. (2011). Applying motor control theory to physical therapy practice: A case report. *Physiotherapy Canada, 63* (3), 345-354.

Kugler, P.N., Kelso, J.A.S., & Turvey, M.T. (1982). On the control and coordination of naturally developing systems. In J.A.S. Kelso & J.E. Clark (Eds.), *The development of movement control and coordination* (pp. 5-78). New York: Wiley.

Marteniuk, R.G. (1976). *Information processing in motor skills.* New York: Holt, Rinehart & Winston.

Michaels, C.F., & Carello, C. (1981). *Direct perception.* Englewood Cliffs, NJ: Prentice Hall.

Newell, K.M. (1986). Constraints on the development of coordination. In M.G. Wade & H.T.A Whiting (Eds.), *Motor development in children: Aspects of coordination and control* (pp. 341-360). Dordrecht, The Netherlands: Martinus Nijhoff.

Polit, A., & Bizzi, E. (1978). Processes controlling arm movements in monkeys. *Science, 201* (4362), 1235-1237.

Rival, C., Olivier, I., & Ceyte, H. (2003). Effects of temporal and/or spatial instructions on the speed-accuracy trade-off of pointing movements in children. *Neuroscience Letters, 336,* 65-69.

Schmidt, R.A. (1975a). *Motor skills.* New York: Harper & Row.

Thelen, E., & Ulrich, B.D. (1991). Hidden skills: A dynamical systems analysis of treadmill stepping during the first year. *Monographs of the Society for Research in Child Development, 56,* (1, Serial No. 223).

Warren, W.H. Jr. (1984). Perceiving affordances: Visual guidance of stair climbing. *Journal of Experimental Psychology: Human Perception and Performance, 10,* 683-703.

Woodworth, R.S. (1899). The accuracy of voluntary movement. *Psychological Review, 3* (Suppl. 2), 1-114.

Chapter 4

Arutyunyan, G.A., Gurfinkel, V.S., & Mirskii, M.L. (1968). Study of taking aim at a target. *Biophysics, 13,* 536-538.

Arutyunyan, G.A., Gurfinkel, V.S., & Mirskii, M.L. (1969). The organization of movements in human execution of a task involving exactness of post. *Biophysics, 14,* 1162-1167.

Bernardi, N., Darainy, M., & Ostry, D.J. (2015). Somatosensory contributions to the initial stages of human motor learning. *The Journal of Neuroscience, 35* (42), 14316 -14326.

Bernstein, N. (1967). *The co-ordination and regulation of movement.* London: Pergamon Press.

Chow, J.Y., Davids, K., Button, C., & Koh, M. (2008). Coordination changes in a discrete multi-articular action as a function of practice. *Acta Psychologica, 127,* 163-176.

Clark, J.E. (2007). On the problem of motor skill development. *Journal of Physical Education, Recreation and Dance, 78* (5), 39-44.

Clark, J.E., & Metcalf, J.M. (2002). The mountain of motor development: A metaphor. In J.E. Clark & J.H. Humphrey (Eds.), *Motor development: Research and reviews* (Vol. 2, pp. 163-190). Reston, VA: National Association for Sport and Physical Education.

Drost, D.K, Brown, K., Wirth, C.K., & Greska, E.K. (2015). Teaching elementary-age youth catching skills using theoretically based motor-development strategies. *Journal of Physical Education, Recreation, and Dance, 86* (1), 30-35.

Fitts, P., & Posner, M.I. (1967). *Human performance.* Belmont, CA: Brooks/Cole.

Gallahue, D.L., Ozmun, J.C., & Goodway, J.D. (2012). *Understanding motor development: Infants, children, adolescent and adults* (7th ed.). Boston: McGraw-Hill.

Gentile, A.M. (1972). A working model of skill acquisition with application to teaching. *Quest, 17,* 3-23.

Gentile, A.M. (1987). Skill acquisition: Action, movement and neuromotor processes. In J.H. Carr, R.B. Shepherd, J. Gordon, A.M. Gentile, & J.M. Held (Eds.), *Movement science: Foundations for physical therapy in rehabilitation* (pp. 93-154). Rockville, MD: Aspen.

Gentile, A.M. (2000). Skill acquisition: Action, movement and neuromotor processes. In J.H. Carr & R.B. Shepherd (Eds.), *Movement science: Foundations for physical therapy in rehabilitation* (2nd ed., pp. 111-187). Rockville, MD: Aspen.

Goodway, J.D., Ozmun, J.C., & Gallahue, D.L. (2012). Motor development in young children. In O. Saracho & B. Spodek (Eds.), *Handbook of research on the education of young children.* London: Routledge.

Haibach, P.S., Daniels, G., & Newell, K.M. (2004). Coordination changes in the early stages of learning to cascade juggle. *Human Movement Science, 23,* 185-206.

Ko, Y.G., Challis, J.H., & Newell, K.M. (2003). Learning to coordinate redundant degrees of freedom in a dynamic balance task. *Human Movement Science, 22,* 47-66.

Konczak, J., Velden, H.V., & Jaeger, L. (2009). Learning to play the violin: Motor control by freezing, not freeing degrees of freedom. *Journal of Motor Behavior, 41,* 243-252.

Newell, K.M. (1984). In Jerry Thomas (Ed.), *Motor development during childhood and adolescence* (pp. 106–120). Minneapolis: Burgess.

Newell, K.M. (1986). Constraints on the development of coordination. In M.G.Wade & H.T.A Whiting (Eds.), *Motor development in children: Aspects of coordination and control* (pp. 341-361). Amsterdam: Martinus Nijhoff Publishers.

Newell, K.M., Kugler, P.N., van Emmerik, R.E.A., & McDonald, P.V. (1989). Search strategies and the acquisition of coordination. In S.A. Wallace (Ed.), *Perspectives on the coordination of movement* (pp. 85-122). Amsterdam: North-Holland.

Newell, K.M., & Vaillancourt, D.E. (2001). Dimensional change in motor learning. *Human Movement Science, 20* (4-5), 695-715.

Newell, K.M., & van Emmerik, R.E.A. (1989). The acquisition of coordination: Preliminary analysis of learning to write. *Human Movement Science, 8,* 17-32.

Rose, D.J., & Christina, R.W. (2006). *A multilevel approach to the study of motor control and learning* (2nd ed.). San Francisco: Pearson Benjamin Cummings.

Seefeldt, V. (1980). Developmental motor patterns: Implications for elementary school physical education. In C. Nadeau, W. Holliwell, K. Newell, & G. Roberts (Eds.), *Psychology of motor behavior and sport* (pp. 314–323). Champaign, IL: Human Kinetics.

Shank, M.D., & Haywood, K.M. (1987). Eye movements while viewing a baseball pitch. *Perceptual and Motor Skills, 64,* 1191-1197.

Stodden, D.F., & Goodway, J.D (2007). The dynamic association between motor skill development and physical activity. *Journal of Physical Education, Recreation and Dance, 78,* 33-49.

Stodden, D.F., Goodway, J.D., Langendorfer, S.J., Roberton, M.A., Rudisill, M.E., Garcia, C., & Garcia, L.E. (2008). A developmental perspective on the role of motor skill competence in physical activity: An emergent relationship. *Quest, 60,* 290-306.

Stodden, D., Ture, L.K., Langendorfer, S.J., & Gao, Z. (2013). Associations among selected motor skills and health-related fitness: Indirect evidence for Seefeldt's proficiency barrier in young adults. *Research Quarterly for Exercise and Sport, 84,* 397-403.

Vereijken, B. (1991). *The dynamics of skill acquisition.* Unpublished doctoral dissertation, Free University, Amsterdam.

Vereijken, B., van Emmerik, R.E.A., Whiting, H.T.A., & Newell, K.M. (1992). Free(z)ing degrees of freedom in skill acquisition. *Journal of Motor Behavior, 24* (1), 133-142.

Verrel, J., Pologe, S., Manselle, W., Lindenberger, U., & Woollacott, M. (2013). Coordination of degrees of freedom and stabilization of task variables in a complex motor skill: Expertise-related differences in cello bowing. *Experimental Brain Research, 224* (3), 323-334.

Zanone, P.G., & Kelso, J.A.S. (1994). The coordination dynamics of learning: Theoretical structure and experimental agenda. In S. Swinnen, H. Heuer, J. Massion, & P. Casaer (Eds.), *Interlimb coordination: Neural, dynamical, and cognitive constraints* (pp. 461-490). San Diego: Academic Press.

Chapter 5

Almond, L. (1986). Primary and secondary rules. In R. Thorpe, D. Bunker, & L. Almond (Eds.), *Rethinking games teaching* (pp. 38-40). Loughborough, UK: University of Technology, Loughborough.

Anderson, J.R. (1993). *Rules of mind.* Hillsdale, NJ: Erlbaum.

Asher, J.J. (1964). Vision and audition in language learning. *Perceptual and Motor Skills, 19,* 255-300.

Bebko, J.M., Demark, J.L., Im-Bolter, N., & MacKewn, A. (2005). Transfer, control, and automatic processing in a complex motor task: An examination of bounce juggling. *Journal of Motor Behavior, 37,* 465-474.

Beilock, S.L., Bertenthal, B.I., McCoy, A.M., & Carr, T.H. (2004). Haste does not always make waste: Expertise, direction of attention, and speed versus accuracy in performing sensorimotor skills. *Psychonomic Bulletin & Review, 11* (2), 373-379.

Bransford, J.D., Franks, J.J., Morris, C.D., & Stein, B.S. (1979). Some general constraints on learning and memory research. In L.S. Cermak & F.I.M. Craik (Eds.), *Levels of processing in human memory* (pp. 331-354). Hillsdale, NJ: Erlbaum.

Coker, C.A. (2013). *Motor learning and control for practitioners* (3rd ed.). Scottsdale, AZ: Holcomb Hathaway.

Cook, V.J. (1997). L2 users and English spelling. *Journal of Multilingual and Multicultural Development, 18,* 474-488.

Figueredo, L. (2006). Using the known to chart the unknown: A review of first-language influence on the development of English-as-a-second-language spelling skill. *Reading and Writing, 19,* 873-905.

Fitts, P., & Posner, M.I. (1967). *Human performance.* Belmont, CA: Brooks/Cole.

Forrester, L.W., Wheaton, L.A., & Luft, A.R. (2008). Exercise-mediated locomotor recovery and lower-limb neuroplasticity after stroke. *Journal of Rehabilitation Research & Development, 45* (2), 205.

Haibach, P.S., Daniels, G.L., & Newell, K.M. (2004). Coordination changes in the early stages of learning to cascade juggle. *Human Movement Science, 23,* 185-206.

Hopper, T., & Bell, R. (1999). Games classification system: Teaching strategic understanding and tactical awareness. *California Association for Health, Physical Education, Recreation and Dance, 66* (4), 14-19.

Howard, R.W. (2014). Learning curves in highly skilled chess players: A test of the generality of the power law of practice. *Acta Pscychologica, 151,* 16-23.

Loy, J. (1968). The nature of sport: A definitional effort. *Quest, 10,* 1-15.

Majed, L., Heugas, A.-M., Chamon, M., & Siegler, I.A. (2012). Learning an energy-demanding and biomechanically constrained motor skill, racewalking: Movement reorganization and contribution of metabolic efficiency and sensory information. *Human Movement Science, 31,* 1598-1614.

Morris, L. (2001). Going through a bad spell: What the spelling errors of young ESL learners reveal about their grammatical knowledge. *Canadian Modern Language Review, 58,* 273-286.

Mount, J. (1996). Effect of practice of a throwing skill in one body position on performance of the skill in an alternate position. *Perceptual and Motor Skills, 83,* 723-732.

Neumann, O. (1984). On controlled and automatic processes. In W. Prinz & A. Sanders (Eds.), *Cognition and motor processes* (pp. 225-295). New York: Springer.

Newell, K.M., Liu, Y.T., & Mayer-Kress, G. (2006). Human learning: Power laws or multiple characteristic time scales? *Tutorials in Quantitative Methods for Psychology, 2,* 66-76.

Newell, K.M., & Rosenbloom, P.S. (1981). Mechanisms of skill acquisition and the law of practice. In J.R. Anderson (Ed.), *Cognitive skills and their acquisition* (pp. 1-55). Hillsdale, NJ: Erlbaum.

Rink, J. (1998). Teaching concepts and content-specific pedagogy. In *Teaching physical education for learning* (pp. 281-292). Boston: McGraw-Hill.

Rose, D.J., & Christina, R.W. (2006). *A multilevel approach to the study of motor control and learning* (2nd ed.). San Francisco: Pearson Benjamin Cummings.

Schmidt, R.A. & Lee, T.D. (2011). *Motor control and learning: A behavioral emphasis.* (5th ed.). Champaign, IL: Human Kinetics.

Siedentop, D. (2012). *Introduction to physical education fitness and sport* (8th ed.). New York: McGraw-Hill.

Snoddy, G.S. (1926). Learning and stability: A psychophysical analysis of a case of motor learning with clinical applications. *Journal of Applied Psychology, 10,* 1-36.

Thorndike, E.L. (1914). *Educational psychology.* New York: Columbia University.

Thorpe, R., Bunker, D., & Almond, L. (1986). *Rethinking games teaching.* Loughborough, UK: University of Technology, Loughborough.

Voss, D.E., Ionta, M.K., & Myers, B.J. (1985). *Proprioceptive neuromuscular facilitation* (3rd ed.). Philadelphia: Harper & Row.

Werner, P., & Almond, L. (1990). Models of games education. *Journal of Physical Education, Recreation and Dance, 61* (4), 23-27.

Chapter 6

Abernathy, B., Kippers, V., Mackinnon, L.T., Neal, R.J., & Hanrahan, S. (1996). *The biophysical foundations of human movement.* Melbourne: Macmillan Education Australia.

Adolph, K.E. (1997). Learning in the development of infant locomotion. *Monographs of the Society for Research in Child Development, 62* (3, Serial No. 251).

Adolph, K.E. (2008). Learning to move. *Current Directions in Psychological Science, 17,* 213-218.

Adolph, K.E., & Berger, S.E. (2006). Motor development. In W. Damon & R.M. Lerner (Series Eds.) & D. Kuhn & R.S. Siegler (Vol. Eds.), *Handbook of child psychology: Vol. 2: Cognition, perception, and language* (6th ed., pp. 161-213). New York: Wiley.

Aicardi, J., & Bax, M. (1992). Cerebral palsy. In J. Aicardi (Ed.), *Diseases of the nervous system in childhood* (2nd ed., pp. 210-239). London: Mac Keith Press.

American Academy of Pediatrics Task Force on Infant Positioning and SIDS. (1992). Positioning and SIDS. *Pediatrics, 89,* 1120-1126.

Angulo-Barroso, R., Burghardt, A.R., Lloyd, M., & Ulrich, D. (2007). Physical activity in infants with Down syndrome receiving a treadmill intervention. *Infant Behavior and Development, 31, 2,* 255-269.

Bayley, N. (2006). *Bayley Scales of Infant Development.* New York: Psychological Corporation.

Burton, A.W., & Miller, D.E. (1998). *Movement skill assessment.* Champaign, IL: Human Kinetics.

Campos, A.C., Rocha, N.A.C.F., & Savelsbergh, G.J.P. (2009). Reaching and grasping movements in infants at risk: A review. *Research in Developmental Disabilities, 30,* 819-826.

Campos, J.J., Witherington, D., Anderson, D.I., Frankel, C.I., Uchiyama, I., & Barbu-Roth, M.A. (2008). Rediscovering development in infancy. *Child Development, 79* (6), 1625-1632.

Carmichael, L. (1946). The onset and early development of behavior. In L. Carmichael (Ed.), *Manual of child psychology* (pp. 43-166). New York: Wiley.

Carr, J. (1970). Mental and motor development in young Mongol children. *Journal of Mental Deficiency Research, 14,* 205-220.

Cintas, H.L. (1995). Cross-cultural similarities and differences in development and the impact of parental expectations on motor behavior. *Pediatric Physical Therapy, 7,* 103-111.

Creighton, D.E., & Sauve, R.S. (1988). The Minnesota Infant Development Inventory in the developmental screening of high-risk infants at eight months. The Canadian Journal of Behavioural Science, *20* (4), 424 – 433.

Dusing, S.C., & Harbourne, T.H. (2010). Variability in postural control during infancy: Implications for development, assessment, and intervention. *Physical Therapy, 90* (12), 1838-1849.

Eimas, P.D. (1975). Auditory and phonetic coding of the cues for speech: Discrimination of the [r-l] distinction by young infants. *Perception & Psychophysics, 18,* 341-347.

Evans, P.M., & Alberman, E. (1985). Recording motor deficits of children with cerebral palsy. *Developmental Medicine and Child Neurology, 27,* 401-406.

Frantz, R.L. (1963). Pattern vision in newborn infants. *Science, 140* (3564), 296-297.

Gabbard, C. (2011). *Lifelong motor development* (6th ed.). San Francisco: Benjamin Cummings.

Gesell, A. (1946). The ontogenesis of infant behavior. In L. Charmichael (Ed.), *Manual of child psychology* (pp. 295-331). New York: Wiley.

Gesell, A., & Ames, L.B. (1940). The ontogenetic organization of prone behavior in human infancy. *Journal of Genetic Psychology, 56,* 247-263.

Gibson, E.J., & Pick, A.P. (2000). An ecological approach to perceptual development. In E.J. Gibson & A.P. Pick (Eds.), *An ecological approach to perceptual learning and development* (pp. 14-25). New York: Oxford University Press.

Hadders-Algra, M. (2000). The neuronal group selection theory: A framework to explain variation in normal motor development. *Developmental Medicine and Child Neurology, 42,* 566-572.

Hadders-Algra, M. (2013). Typical and atypical development of reaching and postural control in infancy. *Developmental Medicine and Child Neurology, 55,* 5-8.

Harlow, H.F. (1949). The formation of learning sets. *Psychological Review, 56,* 51-65.

Haywood, K.M., & Getchell, N. (2014*). Life span motor development* (6th ed.). Champaign, IL: Human Kinetics.

Henderson, S.E. (1985). Motor skill development. In D. Lane & B. Stratford (Eds.), *Current approaches to Down syndrome* (pp. 397-405). London: Holt, Rinehart & Winston.

Henderson, S.E. (1986). Some aspects of the motor development of motor control in Down's syndrome. In H.T.A. Whiting & M.G. Wade (Eds.), *Themes in motor development* (pp. 69-92). Boston: Martinus Nijhoff.

Hogg, J., & Moss, S.C. (1983). Prehensile development in Down's syndrome and non-handicapped preschool children. *British Journal of Developmental Psychology, 1, 2,* 189-204.

Ireton, H., & Thwing, E. (1980). *Minnesota Infant Development Inventory.* Minneapolis: Behavior Science System.

Jenkins, K.J., Correa, A., Feinstein, J.A., et al. (2014). Noninherited risk factors and congenital cardiovascular defects: Current knowledge. *Circulation, 115,* 2995-3014.

Johnson, S., & Marlow, N. (2006). Developmental screen or developmental testing? Early Human Development, *82* (3), 173-183.

Kaiser, L.L., & Campbell, C.G. (2014). Practice paper of the Academy of Nutrition and Dietetics abstract: Nutrition and lifestyle for a healthy pregnancy outcome. *Journal of the Academy of Nutrition and Dietetics, 114* (9), 1447.

Karch, D., Kang, K.-S., Wochner, K., Philippi, H., Hadders-Algra, M., Pietz, J., & Dickhaus, H. (2012).

Kinematic assessment of stereotypy in spontaneous movements in infants. *Gait & Posture, 36,* 307-311.

Koshy, G., Delpisheh, A., & Brabin, B.J. (2010). Dose response association of pregnancy cigarette smoking exposure, childhood stature, overweight and obesity, *European Journal of Public Health,173,* 286-291.

Kuhl, P.K., Williams, K.A., Lacerda, F., Stevens, K.N., & Lindblom, B. (1992). Language experience alters phonetic perception in infants by 6 months of age. *Science, 255,* 606-608.

Lenke, M.C. (2003). Motor outcomes in premature infants. *Newborn and Infant Nursing Reviews, 3,* 104-109.

Libertus, K., & Landa, R.J. (2013). The early motor questionnaire (EMQ): A parental report measure of early motor development. *Infant Behavior and Development, 36,* 833-842.

Lloyd, M., Burghardt, A., Ulrich, D.A., & Angulo-Barroso, R. (2010). Physical activity and walking onset in infants with Down syndrome. *Adapted Physical Activity Quarterly, 27,* 1-16.

Lydic, J.S., & Steele, C. (1979). Assessment of the quality of sitting and gait patterns in children with Down's syndrome. *Physical Therapy, 12* (59), 1489-1494.

Lynch, T.A., & Abel, D.E. (2015). Teratogens and congenital heart disease. *Journal of Diagnostic Medical Sonography, 31* (5), 301-305.

Maitre, N.L., Slaughter, J.C., & Aschner, J.L. (2013). Early prediction of cerebral palsy after neonatal intensive care using motor development trajectories in infancy. *Early Human Development, 89* (10), 781-786.

McGraw, M.B. (1943). *The neuromuscular maturation of the human infant.* New York: Columbia University Press.

Mercer, J. (1998). *Infant development: A multidisciplinary introduction.* Pacific Grove, CA: Brooks/Cole.

Monson, R.M., Deitz, J., & Kartin, D. (2003). The relationship between awake positioning and motor performance among infants who slept supine. *Pediatric Physical Therapy, 15* (4), 196-203.

Moore, M.L. (2003). Preterm labor and birth: What have we learned in the past two decades? *Journal of Obstetric, Gynecologic, and Neonatal Nursing, 32,* 638-649.

Mullen, E.M. (1995). *Mullen: Scales of early learning (AGS edition).* Circle Pines, MN: American Guideline Service.

Newell, K.M. (1986). Constraints on the development of coordination. In M.G. Wade & H.T.A. Whiting (Eds.), *Motor development in children: Aspects of coordination and control* (pp. 341-361). Amsterdam: Nijhoff.

Newell, K.M., Liu, Y.-T., & Mayer-Kress, G. (2003). A dynamical systems interpretation of epigenetic landscapes for infant motor development. *Infant Behavior & Development, 26,* 449-472.

Newell, K.M., McDonald, P.V., & Baillargeon, R. (1993). Body scale and infant grip configurations. *Developmental Psychobiology, 26* (4), 195-205.

Palfrey, J.S., Singer, J.D., Walker, D.K., & Butler, J.A. (1986). Health and special education: A study of new developments for handicapped children in five metropolitan communities. *Public Health Reports, 101* (4), 379-388.

Piek, J. (2002). The role of variability in early motor development. *Infant Behavior and Development, 25* (4), 452-465.

Piek, J.P. (2006). *Infant motor development.* Champaign, IL: Human Kinetics.

Pollock, A.S., Durward, B.R., Rowe P.J., & Paul, J.P. (2000). What is balance? *Clinical Rehabilitation, 14* (4), 402-406.

Robinson, J.S., Moore, V.M., Owens, J.A., et al. (2000). Origins of fetal growth restriction. *European Journal of Obstetrics, Gynecology, and Reproductive Biology, 92,* 13-19.

Rosenbaum, P., Paneth, N., Leviton, A., Goldstein, M., Bax, M., Damiano, D., Dan, B., & Jacobsson B. (2007). A report: The definition and classification of cerebral palsy—April 2006. *Developmental Medicine & Child Neurology Supplement, 109,* 8-14.

Salls, J.S., Silverman, L.N., & Gatty, C.M. (2002). The relationship of infant sleep and play positioning to motor milestone achievement. *American Journal of Occupational Therapy, 56* (5), 577-580.

Shirley, M.M. (1931). *The first two years: A study of twenty-five babies. Vol 1. Locomotor development.* Minneapolis: The University of Minnesota Press.

Spencer, J.T., Clearfield, M., Corbetta, D., Ulrich, B., Buchanan, P., & Schoner, G. (2006). Moving towards a grand theory of development: In memory of Esther Thelen. *Child Development, 77* (6), 1521-1538.

Sporns, O., & Edelman, G. (1993). Solving Bernstein's problem: A proposal for the development of coordinated movement by selection. *Child Development, 64,* 960-981.

Squires, J., Bricker, D., & Potter, L. (1997). Revision of a parent-completed developmental screening tool: Ages & Stages questionnaires. Journal of Psychology, *22* (3), 313-328.

Thelen, E. (1985). Developmental origins of motor coordination: Leg movements in human infants. *Developmental Psychobiology, 18* (1), 1-22.

Thelen, E. (1992). Development as a dynamic system. *Current Directions in Psychological Science, 1,* 189-193.

Thelen, E. (1995). Motor development: A new synthesis. *American Psychologist, 50* (2), 79-95.

Thelen, E., Corbetta, D., & Spencer, J.P. (1996). The development of reaching during the first year: The role of movement speed. *Journal of Experimental Psychology: Human Perception and Performance, 22,* 1059-1076.

Thelen, E., & Ulrich, B.D. (1991). Hidden skills: A dynamic systems analysis of treadmill stepping during the first year. *Monographs of the Society for Research in Child Development, 56,* (1, Serial No. 223).

Timiras, P.S. (1972). *Developmental physiology and aging.* New York: Macmillan.

Tracy, E.E. (2013). Alcohol: An unfortunate teratogen: Fetal alcohol syndrome is entirely preventable. We need to remind ourselves and our patients of this fact. *OBG Management, 25* (1), 36-45.

Ulrich, B.D., & Ulrich, D.A. (1993). Dynamic systems approach to understanding motor delay in infants with Down syndrome. In G.J.P. Savelsbergh (Ed.), *The development of coordination in infancy.* Amsterdam: Elsevier Science.

Ulrich, B.D., Ulrich, D.A. & Collier, D.H. (1992). Alternating stepping patterns: Hidden abilities of 11-month -old infants with Down syndrome. *Developmental Medicine and Child Neurology, 34,* 233-239.

Ulrich, B.D., Ulrich, D.A., Collier, D., & Cole, E. (1993). Developmental shifts in the ability of infants with Down syndrome to produce treadmill steps. *Physical Therapy, 7* (1), 14-23.

Von Hofsten, C. (1984). Developmental changes in the organization of pre-reaching movements. *Developmental Psychobiology, 20,* 378-388.

Vouloumanos, A., & Werker, J.F. (2004). Turned to the signal: The privileged status of speech for young infants. *Developmental Status, 7,* 270-276.

Waldmeier, S., Grunt, S., Delgado-Eckert, E., Latzin, P., Steinlin M., & Fuhrer, K. (2013). Correlation properties of spontaneous motor activity in healthy infants: A new computer-assisted method to evaluate neurological maturation. *Experimental Brain Research, 227* (4), 433-446.

Chapter 7

Adolph, K.E. (2008). The growing body in action: What infant locomotion tells us about perceptually guided action. In R. Klatzky, M. Behrmann, & B. MacWhinney (Eds.), *Embodiment, ego-space, and action*: Carnegie Mellon Symposium (pp. 275-321). Mahwah, NJ: Erlbaum.

Atwater, A.E. (1979). Biomechanics of overarm throwing movements and of throwing injuries. *Exercise and Sport Sciences Reviews, 7,* 43-85.

Bayley, N. (1935). The development of motor abilities during the first three years. *Monographs of the Society for Research in Child Development, 1,* 1.

Butterfield, S.A., & Loovis, E.M. (1993). Influence of age, sex, balance and sport participation on development of throwing by children in grades K–6. *Perceptual and Motor Skills, 76,* 459-464.

Clark, J.E., & Metcalf, J.M. (2002). The mountain of motor development: A metaphor. In J.E. Clark & J.H. Humphrey (Eds.), *Motor development: Research and reviews* (Vol. 2, pp. 163-190). Reston, VA: National Association for Sport and Physical Education.

Clark, J.E., Phillips, S.J., & Peterson, R. (1989). Developmental stability in jumping. *Developmental Psychology, 25,* 929-935.

Clarke, P. (2003). *Where the ancestors walked: Australia as an aboriginal landscape.* Crows Nest, New South Wales, Australia: Allen & Unwin.

Cole, W.G., Chan, G., Vereijken, B., & Adolph, K.E. (2013). Perceiving affordances for different motor skills. *Experimental Brain Research, 225* (3), 309-319.

DeOreo, K., & Keogh, J. (1980). Performance of fundamental motor tasks. In C.B. Corbin (Ed.), *A textbook of motor development* (2nd ed., pp. 76-91). Dubuque, IA: Brown.

Eckert, H. (1987). *Motor development.* Indianapolis: Benchmark Press.

Gabbard, C. (2012). *Lifelong motor development* (6th ed.). San Francisco: Benjamin Cummings.

Gallahue, D.L., & Cleland Donnelly, F. (2003). *Developmental physical education for today's children* (4th ed.). Champaign, IL: Human Kinetics.

Gallahue, D.L., & Ozmun, J.C. (2005). *Understanding motor development: Infants, children, adolescents, adults* (6th ed.). Boston: McGraw-Hill.

Gallahue, D., Ozmun, J., & Goodway, J. (2012). *Understanding motor development: Infants, children, adolescents, adults* (7th ed.). Boston: McGraw-Hill.

Gibson, J.J. (1977). The theory of affordances. In R. Shaw & J. Bransford (Eds.), *Perceiving, acting and knowing: Toward an ecological psychology.* Hillsdale, NJ: Erlbaum.

Gutteridge, M.V. (1939). A study of motor achievements of young children. *Archives of Psychology, 244,* 1-178.

Halverson, L.E., Roberton, M.A., & Langendorfer, S. (1982). Development of the overarm throw: Movement and ball velocity changes by seventh grade. *Research Quarterly for Exercise and Sport, 53,* 198-205.

Halverson, L.E., & Williams, K. (1985). Developmental sequences for hopping over distance: A prelongitudinal screening. *Research Quarterly for Exercise and Sport, 56,* 37-44.

Haubenstricker, J.L., Seefeldt, V.D., & Branta, C.F. (1983, April). *Preliminary validation of a developmental sequence for the standing long jump.* Paper presented at the meeting of the American Alliance for Health, Physical Education, Recreation and Dance, Houston, TX.

Hayne, H., & Findlay, N. (1995). Contextual control of memory retrieval in infancy. Evidence for associative priming. *Infant Behavior and Development, 18* (2), 195-207.

Haywood, K.M., & Getchell, N. (2005). *Life span motor development* (4th ed.). Champaign, IL: Human Kinetics.

Haywood, K., & Getchell, N. (2014). *Lifespan motor development* (6th ed.). Champaign, IL: Human Kinetics.

Jones-Petranek, L. & Barton, G.V. (2011). The overarm-throwing pattern among u-14 ASA female softball players. A comparative study of gender, culture and experience. *Research Quarterly for Exercise and Sport, 82* (2), 220-228.

Kretch, K.S. & Adolph, K.E. (2015). Active vision in passive locomotion: Real-world free viewing in infants and adults. *Developmental Science, 18,* 736-750.

Leme, S., & Shambes, G. (1978). Immature throwing patterns in normal adult women. *Journal of Human Movement Studies, 4,* 85-93.

Lorson, K.M., Stodden, D.F., & Goodway, J.D. (2013). Age and gender differences in adolescent and adult overarm throwing. *Research Quarterly for Exercise and Sport, 84* (2), 239-244.

McCaskill, C.L., & Wellman, B.L. (1938). A study of common motor achievements at the pre-school ages. *Child Development, 9,* 141.

Newell, K.M. (1986). Constraints on the development of coordination. In M.G. Wade & H.T.A Whiting (Eds.), *Motor development in children: Aspects of coordination and control* (pp. 341-360). Dordrecht, The Netherlands: Martinus Nijhoff.

Owen, N., Healy, G.N., Matthews, C.E., & Dunstan, D.W. (2010). Too much sitting: the population health science of sedentary behavior. *Exercise Sport Science Review, 38* (3), 105-113.

Payne, G.V., & Isaacs, L.D. (2008). *Human life motor development: A lifespan approach* (7th ed.). New York: McGraw-Hill.

Payne, G.V., & Isaacs, L.D. (2012). *Human motor development: A lifespan approach* (8th ed.). New York: McGraw-Hill.

Rehling, S.L. (1996). *Longitudinal differences in overarm throwing velocity and qualitative throwing techniques of elementary boys and girls.* Unpublished doctoral dissertation, Arizona State University, Tucson.

Roberton, M.A. (1977). Stability of stage categorizations across trials: Implications for the "stage theory" of overarm throw development. *Journal of Human Movement Studies, 3,* 49-59.

Roberton, M.A., & Konczak, J. (2001). Predicting children's overarm throw ball velocities from their developmental levels in throwing. *Research Quarterly for Exercise and Sport, 72,* 91-103.

Runion, B., Roberton, M.A., & Langendorfer, S.J. (2003). Forceful overarm throwing: A comparison of two cohorts measured 20 years apart. *Research Quarterly for Exercise and Sport, 74,* 334-330.

Savelsbergh, G., Davids, K., van der Kamp, J., & Bennett, J. (2003). *Development of movement co-ordination in children: Applications in the field of ergonomics, health sciences and sport.* New York: Routledge.

Seefeldt, V., & Haubenstricker, J. (1975). *Developmental sequence of kicking* (Rev. ed.). Unpublished research, Michigan State University, East Lansing.

Shirley, M.M. (1931). *The first two years: A study of twenty five babies. Vol. 1: Postural and locomotor development.* Minneapolis: University of Minnesota Press.

Soska, K.C., Adolph, K.E., & Johnson, S.P. (2010). Systems in development: Motor skill acquisition facilitates three-dimensional object completion. *Developmental Psychology, 46,* 129-138.

Spencer, J.P., Perone, S., & Buss, AT. (2011). Twenty years and going strong: A dynamic systems revolution in motor and cognitive development. *Child Development Perspectives, 5* (4), 260-266.

Sutherland, D. (1997). The development of mature gait. *Gait and Posture 6.* 163-170.

Thelen, E. (1985). Developmental origins of motor coordination: Leg movements in human infants. *Developmental Psychobiology, 18,* 1-22.

Thelen, E., & Ulrich, B.D. (1991). Hidden skills: A dynamic systems analysis of treadmill stepping during the first year. *Monographs of the Society for Research in Child Development, 56* (1, Serial No. 223).

Thelen, E., Ulrich, B.D., & Jensen, J.L. (1989). The developmental origins of locomotion. In M.H. Woolacott & A. Shumway-Cook (Eds.), *Development of posture and gait across the lifespan* (pp. 25-47). Columbia, SC: University of South Carolina Press.

Thomas, J.R., Alderson J., Thomas K., Campbell A., & Elliott, B. (2010). Developmental gender differences for overhand throwing in aboriginal Australian children. *Research Quarterly for Exercise and Sport, 81* (4), 432-441.

Thomas, J.R., & French, K.E. (1985). Gender differences across age in motor performance: A meta-analysis. *Psychological Bulletin, 98,* 260-282.

Thomas, J. R., & Marzke, M. (1992). The development of gender differences in throwing: Is human evolution a factor? In R. Christina & H. Eckert (Eds.), *The academy papers: Enhancing human performance in sport* (pp. 60-76). Champaign, IL: Human Kinetics.

Ulrich, B. (2010). Opportunities for early intervention based on theory, basic neuroscience, and clinical science. *Physical Therapy Journal, 90,* 1868-1880.

Whitall, J. (2003). Development of locomotor coordination and control in children. In G. Savelsbergh, K. Davids, J. Van der Kamp, & S. Bennett (Ed.), *Development of movement co-ordination in children: Applications in the field of ergonomics, health sciences and sport* (pp. 251-270). New York: Routledge.

Wickstrom, R.L. (1983). *Fundamental motor patterns* (3rd ed.). Philadelphia: Lea & Febiger.

Wild, M. (1938). The behavior pattern of throwing and some observations concerning its course of development in children. *Research Quarterly, 9* (3), 20.

Yoshida, H., & Smith, L.B. (2008). What's in view for toddlers? Using a head camera to study visual experience. *Infancy, 13* (3), 229-248.

Chapter 8

Adrian, M.J., & Cooper, J.M. (1995). *Biomechanics of human movement* (2nd ed.). Indianapolis: Benchmark Press.

Agency for Healthcare Research and Quality and the Centers for Disease Control and Prevention (2002). Activity and older Americans: Benefits and strategies. Retrieved May 11, 2010, from www.ahrq.gov/ppip/activity.htm

AGS Panel on Persistent Pain in Older Persons. (2002). The management of persistent pain in older persons. *Journal of the American Geriatric Society, 50* (Suppl. 6), S205-S224.

Baert, V., Gorus, E., Mets, T., Geerts, C., & Bautmans, I. (2011). Motivators and barriers for physical activity in the oldest old: A systematic review. *Ageing Research Review, 10,* 464-474.

Belsky, J.K. (1984). *The psychology of aging.* Monterey, CA: Brooks/Cole.

Berger, B.G., & Hecht, L.M. (1989). Exercise, aging, and psychological well-being: The mind-body question. In A.C. Ostrow (Ed.), *Aging and motor behavior.* Indianapolis: Benchmark Press.

Berger, B.G., & McInman, A. (1993). Exercise and the quality of life. In R.N. Singer, M. Murphy, & L.K. Tennant (Eds.), *Handbook of research on sport psychology.* New York: Macmillan.

Bernard, T., Sultana, F., Lepers, R., Hauss-wirth, C., & Brisswalter, J. (2009). Age-related decline in Olympic triathlon performance: Effect of locomotion mode. *Experimental Aging Research, 36* (1), 64-78.

Bock, O., & Beurskens, R. (2010). Changes of locomotion in old age depend on task setting. *Gait & Posture, 32* (4), 645-649.

Braver, E.R., & Trempel, R.E. (2003). Are older drivers at higher risk of involvement in crashes resulting in deaths or nonfatal injuries among their passengers or other road users? *American Journal of Epidemiology, 157,* S50.

Butler, R.J., Crowell, H.P., & Davis, I.M. (2003). Lower extremity stiffness: Implications for performance and injury. *Clinical Biomechanics, 18,* 511-517.

Castro, C., Martínez, C., & Tornay, F.J. (2005). Vehicle distance estimations in nighttime driving: A real-setting study. *Transportation Research Report Part F: Traffic Psychology and Behavior, 8* (1), 31-45.

Centers for Disease Control and Prevention. (2009). U.S. physical activity statistics. Retrieved from http://apps.nccd.cdc.gov/PASurveillance/DemoCompareResultV.asp?State=0&Cat=1&Year=2007&Go=GO

Cole, K.J., Rotella, D.L., & Harper, J.G. (1999). Mechanisms for age-related changes of fingertip forces during precision gripping and lifting in adults. *Journal of Neuroscience, 19,* 3228-3247.

Comfort, A. (1979). *Aging, the biology of senescence* (2nd ed.). New York: Holt, Rinehart, Winston.

DeSimone, B. (2006, September 11). *Act II of Navratilova's career ends with a win.* Retrieved from www.espn.com/sports/tennis/usopen06/news/story?id=2578105

DiPietro, L., Williamson, D.F., Caspersen, C.J., & Eaker, E. (1993). The descriptive epidemiology of selected physical activities and body weight among adults trying to lose weight: The Behavioral Risk Factor Surveillance System Survey, 1989. *International Journal of Obesity, 17,* 69-76.

Donato, A.J., Tench, K., Glueck, D.H., Seals, D.R., Eskurza, I., & Tanaka, H. (2003). Declines in physiological functional capacity with age: A longitudinal study in peak swimming performance. *Journal of Applied Physiology, 94* (2), 764-769.

Donorfio, L.K.M., Mohyde, M., Coughlin, J., & D'Ambrosio, L. (2008). A qualitative exploration of self-regulation behaviors among older drivers. *Journal of Aging and Social Policy, 20* (3), 323-339.

Elble, R.J. (1997). Changes in gait with normal aging. In J.C. Masdeu, L. Sudarsky, & L. Wolfson (Eds.), *Gait disorders of aging: Falls and therapeutic strategies* (pp. 93-106). Philadelphia: Lippincott-Raven.

Flanagan, E.P., & Harrison, A.J. (2007). Muscle dynamics differences between legs in healthy adults. *Journal of Strength and Conditioning Research, 21,* 67-72.

Fried, L.P., Storer, D.J., King, D.E., & Lodder, F. (1991). Diagnosis of illness presentations in the elderly. *Journal of the American Geriatric Society, 39,* 117-123.

Gabbard, C.P. (2012). *Lifelong motor development* (6th ed.). London: Pearson.

Guralnik, J.M., & Simonsick, E.M. (1993). Physical disability in older Americans [Special issue]. *Journal of Gerontology, 48,* 3-10.

Halverson, L.E., Roberton, M.A., & Landendorfer, S. (1982). Development of the overarm throw: Movement and ball velocity changes by seventh grade. *Research Quarterly for Exercise and Sport, 53,* 198-205.

Hertel, J., Freidrich, N., Wittfeld, K., Pietzner, M., Budde, K., Van der Auwera, S., Lohmann, T., Teumer, A., Vo Izke, H., Nauck, M., & Jorgen Grabe, H. (2016). Measuring biological age via metabonomics: The metabolic age score. *The Journal or Proteome Research, 15,* 400-410.

Hill, A.V. (1925). The physiological basis of athletic records. *Lancet, 209* (2), 483-486.

Jagacinski, R.J., Greenberg, N., & Liao, M.J. (1997). Tempo, rhythm, and aging in golf. *Journal of Motor Behavior, 29* (2), 159-173.

Jette, A., & Branch, L. (1992). A ten-year follow-up of driving patterns among community-dwelling elderly. *Human Factors, 34,* 25-31.

Kalman, Y.M., Kavé, G., & Umanski, D. (2015). Writing in a digital world: Self-correction while typing in younger and older adults. *International Journal of Environment Research & Public Health, 12,* 12723-12734.

Kenney, W.L., Wilmore, J., & Costill, D. (2015). *Physiology of sport & exercise* (6th ed.). Champaign, IL: Human Kinetics.

Klinger, A., Masataka, T., Adrian, M., & Smith, E. (1980). *Temporal and spatial characteristics of movement patterns of women over 60.* Paper presented at the National Conference of the American Alliance for Health, Physical Education, Recreation and Dance, Detroit.

Knechtle, B., Rüst, C.A., Rosemann, T., & Lepers, R. (2012). Age-related changes In 100-km ultra-marathon running performance. *AGE, 34,* 1033-1045.

Kocaman, S.A., Cetin, M., Durakoglugil, M.E., Erdogan, T., Canga, A., & Cicek, Y. (2012). The degree of premature hair graying as an independent risk marker for coronary artery disease: A predictor of biological age rather than chronological age. *The Anatolian Journal of Cardiology, 12* (6), 457.

Lorson, K.M., Stodden, D.F., Langendorfer, S.J., & Goodway, J.D. (2013). Age and gender differences in adolescent and adult overarm throwing. *Research Quarterly for Exercise and Sport, 84,* 239-244.

Macera, C.A., Cavanaugh, A., & Bellettiere, J. (2015). State of the art review: Physical activity and older adults. *American Journal of Lifestyle Medicine, 11*(1), 42-57.

Marshall, S.C. (2008). The role of reduced fitness to drive due to medical impairments in explaining crashes involving older drivers. *Traffic Injury Prevention, 9,* 291-298.

Meltzer, D.E. (1994). Age dependence of Olympic weightlifting ability. *Medicine & Science in Sports & Exercise, 26* (8), 1053-1067.

Meng, A., & Siren, A.K. (2012). Cognitive problems, self-rated changes in driving skills, driving-related discomfort and self-regulation of driving in old drivers. *Accident Analysis & Prevention, 49,* 322-329.

Murray, M.P., Kory, R.C., & Sepic, B.C. (1970). Walking patterns of normal women. *Archives of Physical Medicine and Rehabilitation, 51,* 637-650.

National Health Interview [NHIS]. (2014). Centers for Disease Control and Prevention (CDC)/ National Center for Health Statistics (NCHS).

National Highway Traffic Safety Administration. (2000). *Traffic safety facts 2000. National Center for Statistics and Analysis, Research and Development.* Washington, DC: National Highway Traffic Safety Administration.

Nelson, C.J. (1981). *Locomotor patterns of women over 57.* Unpublished master's thesis, Washington State University, Pullman.

Payne, G.V., & Isaacs, L.D. (2016). *Human life motor development: A lifespan approach* (9th ed.). New York: McGraw-Hill.

Ranganathan, V.K., Siemionow, V., Sahgal, V., Liu, J.Z., & Yue, G.H. (2001). Skilled finger movement exercise improves hand function. *Journal of Gerontology A: Biological Science and Medical Science, 56,* M518-522.

Reider, B. (2008). Live long and prosper. *American Journal of Sports Medicine, 36* (3), 441-442.

Roberton, M.A., & Halverson, L.E. (1984). *Developing children: Their changing movement.* Philadelphia: Lea & Febiger.

Roberton, M.A., & Konczak, J. (2001). Predicting children's overarm throw ball velocities from their developmental levels in throwing. *Research Quarterly for Exercise and Sport, 72,* 91-103.

Rosenblum, S., & Werner, P. (2005). Assessing the handwriting process in healthy elderly persons using a computerized system. *Aging Clinical and Experimental Research, 18* (5), 433-439.

Schulz, R., & Curnow, C. (1988). Peak performance and age among superathletes: Track and field, swimming, baseball, tennis, and golf. *Journal of Gerontology, 43* (5), 113-120.

Shephard, R.J. (2008). *Aging, physical activity, and health.* Champaign, IL: Human Kinetics.

Spirduso, W.W., Francis, K.L., & MacRae, P.G. (2005). *Physical dimensions of aging* (2nd ed.). Champaign, IL: Human Kinetics.

Steffen, T.M., Hacker, T.A., & Mollinger, L. (2002). Age and gender-related test performance in community-dwelling elderly people: Six-minute walk test, Berg balance scale, timed up & go test, and gait speeds. *Physical Therapy, 82* (2), 128-137.

Stephens, T., & Craig, C.L. (1990). *The well-being of Canadians: Highlights of the 1988 Campbell's Soup Survey.* Ottawa: Canadian Fitness and Lifestyle Research Institute.

Thapa, P., Gideon, P., Fought, R., Kormicki, M., & Ray, W. (1994). Comparison of clinical and biomechanical measures of balance and mobility in elderly nursing home residents. *Journal of the American Geriatrics Society, 42,* 493-500.

Tseng, M.H., & Cermak, S.A. (1993). The influence of ergonomic factors and perceptual-motor abilities on handwriting performance. *American Journal of Occupational Therapy, 47,* 919-926.

U.S. Department of Health and Human Services. (2008). *2008 physical activity guidelines for Americans: Be active, healthy, and happy!* Washington, DC: U.S. Department of Health and Human Services.

U.S. Department of Health and Human Services, Administration for Community Living. (2013). Administration on aging. Retrieved from www.aoa.gov/Aging_Statistics/Profile/2013/docs/2013_Profile.pdf

Wang, L. (2008). The kinetics and stiffness characteristics of the lower extremity in older adults during vertical jumping. *Journal of Sports Science and Medicine, 7,* 379-386.

Williams, K., Haywood, K., & VanSant, A. (1990). Characteristics of older adult throwers. In J.E. Clark & J. Humphrey (Eds.), *Advances in motor development research* (Vol. 3, pp. 29-44). New York: AMS Press.

Williams, K., Haywood, K., & VanSant, A. (1991). Throwing patterns of older adults: A follow-up investigation. *International Journal of Aging and Human Development, 33* (4), 279-294.

Williams, K., Haywood, K., & VanSant, A. (1998). Changes in throwing by older adults: A longitudinal investigation. *Research Quarterly for Exercise and Sport, 66* (1), 1-10.

Willmott, M. (1986). The effect of vinyl floor surface and carpeted floor surface upon walking in elderly hospital inpatients. *Age and Ageing, 15,* 119-120.

Winter, D.A., Patla, A.E., Frank, J.S., & Walt, S.E. (1990). Biomechanical walking pattern changes in the fit and healthy elderly. *Physical Therapy, 70,* 340-347.

Wright, V.J., & Perricelli, B.C. (2008). Age-related rates of decline in performance among elite senior athletes. *American Journal of Sports Medicine, 36* (3), 443-450.

Chapter 9

Baker, J., & Davids, K. (2007). Introduction. *International Journal of Sport Psychology, 38,* 1-3.

Bogin, B. (1998, February). The tall and the short of it. *Discover,* 40-44.

Bouchard, C., An, P., Rice, T., Skinner, J.S., Wilmore, J.H., Gagnon, J., Perusse, L., Leon, A.S., & Rao, D.C. (1999). Familial aggregation of VO2 max response to exercise training: Results from the HERITAGE family study. *Journal of Applied Physiology, 87,* 1003-1008.

Clarke, H.H. (1975). Joint and body range of movement. *Physical Fitness Research Digest, 5,* 16-18.

Clark, J.E. (2007). On the problem of motor skill development. *Journal of Physical Education, Recreation and Dance, 78* (5), 39-44.Eimas, P.D. (1975). Auditory and phonetic coding of the cues for speech: Discrimination of the [r-l] distinction by young infants. *Perception & Psychophysics, 18,* 341-347.

Davids, K., & Baker, J. (2007). Genes, environment and sport performance: Why the nature-nurture dualism is no longer relevant. *Sports Medicine, 37,* 961-980.

Ericsson, K.A. (2003). Development of elite performance and deliberate practice: An update from the perspective of the expert performance approach. In J.L. Starkes & K.A. Ericsson (Eds.), *Expert performance in sports* (pp. 49-83). Champaign, IL: Human Kinetics.

Ericsson, K.A. (2007). Deliberate practice and the modifiability of body and mind: Toward a science of the structure and acquisition of expert and elite performance. *International Journal of Sport Psychology, 38,* 109-123.

Ericsson, K.A. (2013). Training history, deliberate practice and elite sports performance: An analysis in response to Tucker and Collins review—what makes champions? *British Journal of Sports Medicine, 47,* 533-535.

Ericsson, K.A. (2016). Summing up hours of any type of practice versus identifying optimal practice activities: Commentary on Macnamara, Moreau, & Hambrick (2016). *Perspectives on Psychological Science, 11,* 351-354.

Fox, P.W., Hershberger, S.L., & Bouchard, T.J. (1996). Genetic and environmental contributions to the acquisition of motor skill. *Nature, 384,* 356-358.

Gabbard, C.P. (2012). *Lifelong motor development* (6th ed.). San Francisco: Benjamin Cummings.

Gallahue, D.L., & Ozmun, J.C. (2005). *Understanding motor development: Infants, children, adolescents, adults* (6th ed.). Boston: McGraw-Hill.

Geladas, N., Koskolou, M., & Klissouras, V. (2007). Nature or nurture: Not an either-or question. *International Journal of Sport Psychology, 38,* 124-134.

Gollnick, P.D., Timson, B.F., Moore, R.L., & Riedy, M. (1981). Muscle enlargement and number of fibers in skeletal muscles of rats. *Journal of Applied Physiology, 50,* 936-943.

Haubenstricker, J., Wisner, D., Seefeldt, V., & Branta, C. (1997). Gender differences and mixed longitudinal norms on selected motor skills for children and youth. *Journal of Sport and Exercise Psychology: NASPSPA Abstracts, 19,* S63, 6.

Haywood, K.M., & Getchell, N. (2014). *Life span motor development* (6th ed.). Champaign, IL: Human Kinetics.

Howe, M.J.A., Davidson, J.W., & Sloboda, J.A. (1998). Innate talents: Reality or myth? *Behavioral and Brain Sciences, 21,* 399-442.

Joyner, M.J. (1993). Physiological limiting factors and distance running: Influence of gender and age on record performances. *Exercise and Sport Science Reviews, 21,* 103-133.

Kail, R.V., & Cavanaugh, J.C. (2016). *Human development: A lifespan view* (7th ed.). Toronto, ON: Nelson.

Kellman, P.J., & Arterberry, M.E. (1998). *The cradle of knowledge: Development of perception in infancy.* Cambridge, MA: MIT Press.

Keogh, J., & Sugden, D. (1985). *Movement skill development.* New York: Macmillan.

Klissouras, V., Geladas, N., & Koskolou, M. (2007). Nature prevails over nurture. *International Journal of Sport Psychology, 38,* 35-67.

Krogman, W.M. (1972). *Child growth.* Ann Arbor, MI: University of Michigan Press.

Kuhl, P.K., Williams, K.A., Lacerda, F., Stevens, K.N., & Lindblom, B. (1992). Language experience alters phonetic perception in infants by 6 months of age. *Science, 255,* 606-608.

Lowrey, G.H. (1986). *Growth and development of children.* Chicago: Year Book Medical.

Macnamara, B.N., Moreau, D., & Hambrick, D.Z. (2016). The relationship between deliberate practice and performance in sports: A meta-analysis. *Perspectives on Psychological Science, 11,* 333-350.

Malina, R.M. (1978). Growth of muscle tissue and muscle mass. In F. Faulkner & J.M. Tanner (Eds.), *Human growth: A comprehensive treatise.* New York: Plenum Press.

Malina, R.M., & Bouchard, C. (1991). *Growth, maturation, and physical activity.* Champaign, IL: Human Kinetics.

Malina, R.M., Bouchard, C., & Bar-Or, O. (2004). *Growth, maturation, and physical activity* (2nd ed.). Champaign, IL: Human Kinetics.

Malina, R.M. Bouchard, C., & Beunen, G. (1988). Human growth: Selected aspects of current research on well-nourished children. *Annual Review of Anthropology, 17,* 187-219.

Marisi, D.Q. (1977). Genetic and extragenetic variance in motor performance. *Acta Genetica Medica, 26,* 3-4.

Marshall, J.D., & Bouffard, M. (1994). Obesity and movement competency in children. *Adapted Physical Activity Quarterly, 11,* 297-305.

Marshall, J.D., & Bouffard, M. (1997). The effects of quality daily physical education on movement competency in obese versus nonobese children. *Adapted Physical Activity Quarterly, 14,* 222-237.

McGraw, M. (1935). *Growth: A study of Johnny and Jimmy.* New York: Appleton-Century-Crofts.

Morris, G.S. (1980). *Elementary physical education: Toward inclusion.* Salt Lake City: Brighton.

Neuman, A.C., & Hochberg, I. (1983). Children's perception of speech in reverberation. *Journal of the Acoustical Society of America, 73,* 2145-2149.

Newell, K.M. (1984). Physical constraints to development of motor skills. In J.R. Thomas (Ed.), *Motor development during childhood and adolescence* (pp. 105-120). Minneapolis: Burgess.

Payne, G.V., & Isaacs, L.D. (2008). *Human life motor development: A lifespan approach* (7th ed.). New York: McGraw-Hill.

Piek, J.P. (2006). *Infant motor development.* Champaign, IL: Human Kinetics.

Poole, C., Miller, S.A., & Booth Church, E. (2006). Ages & stages: All about body awareness. *Early Childhood Today.* Retrieved from www.scholastic.com/teachers/articles/teaching-content/ages-stages-all-about-body-awareness

Schrauf, M., Wist, E.R., & Ehrenstein, W.H. (1999). Development of dynamic vision based on motion contrast. *Experimental Brain Research, 124,* 469-473.

Shephard, R.J. (1998). Aging and exercise. In T.D. Fahey (Ed.), *Encyclopedia of sports medicine and science.* Internet Society for Sport Science. http://sportsci.org/encyc

Shulman, C. (2016). Nature-nurture controversy and its implications for infant and early childhood mental health. In *Research and practice in infant and childhood mental health* (Vol. 13, pp. 67-79). New York: Springer.

Thelen, E., & Smith, L.B. (1994). *A dynamic processes approach to development of cognition and action.* Cambridge, MA: MIT Press/Bradford.

Timiras, P.S. (1972). *Developmental physiology and aging.* New York: Macmillan.

Tucker, R., & Collins, M. (2012). What makes champions? A review of the relative contribution of genes and training to sporting success. *British Journal of Sports Medicine, 46,* 555-561.

Ulrich, D.A., Ulrich, B.D., Angulo-Kinzler, R.M., & Yun, J. (2001). Treadmill training of infants with Down syndrome: Evidence-based developmental outcomes. *Pediatrics, 108,* 84-91.

Visser, J., & Geuze, R.H. (2000). Kinaesthetic acuity in adolescent boys: A longitudinal study. *Developmental Medicine & Child Neurology, 42,* 93-96.

Vouloumanos, A., & Werker, J.F. (2004). Turned to the signal: The privileged status of speech for young infants. *Developmental Status, 7,* 270-276.

Wattam-Bell, J. (1996). Visual motion processing in one month old infants: Habituation experiments. *Vision Research, 36,* 1679-1685.

Williams, H.G. (1983*). Perceptual and motor development.* Englewood Cliffs, NJ: Prentice Hall.

Chapter 10

Akima, H., Kano, Y., Enomoto, Y., et al. (2001). Muscle function in 164 men and women aged 20-84 years. *Medicine & Science in Sports & Exercise, 33,* 220-226.

Baptista de Oliveira Medeiros, H., Sardinha Mendes Soares de Araújo, D., & Gil Soares de Araújo, C. (2013). Age-related mobility loss is joint-specific: An analysis from 6,000 Flexitest results. *Age, 35* (6), 2399-2407. doi: 10.1007/s11357-013-9525-z

Barbour, K.E., Helmick, C.G., Boring, M.A., & Brady, T.J. (2017 March 7). Vital signs: Prevalence of doctor-diagnosed arthritis and arthritis-attributable activity limitation—United States, 2013–2015. *Morbidity and Mortality Weekly Report* [Epub ahead of print].

Barzilai, N., & Gabriely, I. (2010). Genetic studies reveal the role of the endocrine and metabolic systems in aging. *The Journal of Clinical Endocrinology & Metabolism, 95* (10), 18-29.

Bassey, E.J., Fiatarone, M.A., O'Neill, E.F., Kelly, M., Evans, W.J., & Lipsitz, L.A. (1992). Leg extensor power and functional performance in very old men and women. *Clinical Science, 82,* 321-327.

Bemben, D.A. & Bemben, M.G. (2011). Dose-response effect of 40 weeks of resistance training on bone mineral density in older adults. *Osteoporosis International, 22,* 179-186. doi: 10.1007/s00198-010-1182-9

Blair, S.N. (2009). Physical inactivity: The biggest public health problem of the 21st century. *British Journal of Sports Medicine, 43,* 1-2.

Bradley, E.G. (2007). Nursing management: Hypertension. In S.L. Lewis, M.M. Heitkemper, S.R. Dirksen, P.G. O'Brien, and L. Bucher (Eds.), *Medical-surgical nursing* (7th ed., pp. 761-783). St. Louis: Mosby Elsevier.

Coker, C.A. (2013). *Motor learning and control for practitioners* (3rd ed.). Scottsdale, AZ: Holcomb Hathaway.

Corso, J.F. (1987). Sensory-perceptual processes and aging. *Annual Review of Gerontology and Geriatrics, 7,* 29-55.

Dempsey, J.A., & Seals, D.R. (1995). Aging, exercise and cardiopulmonary function. In D.R. Lamb, C.V Gisolfi, & E. Nadel (Eds.), *Perspectives in exercise science and sports medicine: Vol. 8. Exercise in older adults* (pp. 237-297). Indianapolis: Benchmark Press.

DeStefano, F., Coulehan, J., & Wiant, M. (1979). Blood pressure survey on the Navajo Indian reservation. *American Journal of Epidemiology, 109* (3), 335-345.

Eskurza, I., Donato, A.J., Moreau, K.L., Seals, D.R., & Tanaka, H. (2002). Changes in maximal aerobic capacity with age in endurance-trained women: 7 year follow-up. *Journal of Applied Physiology, 92,* 2303-2308.

Evans, S.L., Davy, P., Stevenson, E.T., & Seals, D.R. (1995). Physiological determinants of 10-km performance in highly trained female runners of different ages. *Journal of Applied Physiology, 78,* 1931-1941.

Fagard, R., Thijs, L., & Amery, A. (1993). Age and the hemodynamic response to posture and to exercise. *American Journal of Geriatric Cardiology, 2* (2), 23-30.

Faulkner, J.A., & Brooks, S.V. (1995). Muscle fatigue in old animals. Unique aspects of fatigue in elderly humans. *Advancements in Experimental Medicine and Biology, 384,* 471-480.

Faulkner, J.A., Larkin, L.M., Claflin, D.R., & Brooks, S.V. (2007). Age-related changes in the structure and function of skeletal muscles. *Clinical and Experimental Pharmacology and Physiology, 34,* 1091-1096.

Fazzi, E., Lanners, J., Ferrari-Ginevra, O., Achille, C., Luparia, A., Signorini, S., & Lanzi, G. (2002). Gross motor development and reach on sound as critical tools for the development of the blind child. *Brain and Development, 24,* 269-275.

Finkelstein, J.S., Lee, M.L., Sowers, M., Ettinger, B., Neer, R.M., Kelsey, J.L., Cauley, J.A., Huang, M.H., & Greendale, G.A. (2002). Ethnic variation in bone density in premenopausal and early perimenopausal women: Effects of anthropometric and lifestyle factors. *Journal of Clinical Endocrinology and Metabolism, 87,* 3057-3067.

Foroughi, C., Monfort, S.S., Paczynski, M., McKnight, P.E., & Greenwood, P.M. (2016). Placebo effects in cognitive training. *Proceedings of the National Academy of Sciences of the United States of America, 113* (27), 7470-7474. doi: 10.1073/pnas.1601243113

Gabbard, C.P. (2012). *Lifelong motor development* (6th ed.). San Francisco: Benjamin Cummings.

Gallahue, D.L., & Ozmun, J.C. (2012). *Understanding motor development: Infants, children, adolescents, adults* (7th ed.). Boston: McGraw-Hill.

Garzia, R., & Trick, L. (1992). Vision in the 90's: The aging eye. *Journal of Optometric Vision Development, 23* (1), 4-41.

Goodpaster, B.H., Park, S.W., Harris, T.B., et al. (2006). The loss of skeletal muscle strength, mass, and quality in older adults: The health, aging and body composition study. *Journals of Gerontology: Biological Sciences and Medical Sciences, 61,* 1059-1064.

Hagberg, J.M. (1988). Effect of exercise and training on older men and women with essential hypertension. In W.W. Spirduso & H.M. Eckert (Eds.), *The academy papers: Physical activity and aging* (pp. 187-191). Champaign IL: Human Kinetics.

Hashizume, K., Suzuki, S., Takeda, T., Shigematsu, S., Ichikawa, K., & Koizumi, Y. (2006). Endocrinological aspects of aging: Adaptation to and acceleration of aging by the endocrine system. *Geriatrics & Gerontology International, 6,* 1-6.

Haywood, K.M., & Getchell, N. (2014). *Life span motor development* (6th ed.). Champaign, IL: Human Kinetics.

Hernandez, J. (2008). Prehypertension: Why should we worry? *Advance for Nurse Practitioners, 16* (1), 65-73.

Hyde, T.E., & Gengenbach, M.S. (2007). *Conservative management of sports injuries* (2nd ed., p. 845). Sudbury, MA: Jones & Bartlett.

Kanis, J.A., Johnell, O., Oden, A., et al. (2000). Long-term risk of osteoporotic fracture in Malmo. *Osteoporosis International, 11,* 669.

Kannel, W., Sorlie, P., & Gordon, T. (1980). Labile hypertension: A faulty concept? The Framingham Study. *Circulation, 61* (6), 1183-1187.

Kasch, F.W., Wallace, J.P., Van Camp, S.P., & Verity, L. (1988). A longitudinal study of cardiovascular stability in active men aged 45-65 years. *Physician and SportsMedicine, 16* (1), 117-126.

Kenshalo, D.R. (1977). Age changes in touch, vibration, temperature, kinesthesis, and pain sensitivity. In J.E. Birren & K.W. Schaie (Eds.), *Handbook of the psychology of aging* (pp. 562-579). New York: Van Nostrand Reinhold.

Lazarus, N.R., & Harridge, S.D.R. (2010). Exercise, physiological function, and the selection of participants for aging research. *Journals of Gerontology, Series A: Biological Sciences and Medical Sciences, 65A*, 854-857.

Lee, T. (2010). Intrepid exploring: Looking past fears of short-term memory loss in aging to deploy the brain's long-term memories and-wisdom. *Journal of Aging, Humanities, and the Arts, 4*, 18-29. doi: 10.1080/19325610903551541.

Lexell, J. (1995). Human aging, muscle mass, and fiber type composition. *Journals of Gerontology: Biological Sciences and Medical Sciences, 50* (Special Issue), 11-16.

Lexell, J., Taylor, C.C., & Sjostrom, M. (1988). What is the cause of the ageing atrophy? Total number, size and proportion of different fiber types studied in whole vastus lateralis muscle from 15- to 83-year-old men. *Journal of Neurological Science, 84*, 275-294.

Linton, A.D. (2007). Age-related changes in the special senses. In A.D. Linton & H.W. Lach (Eds.), *Matteson & McConnell's gerontological nursing* (3rd ed., pp. 600-627). St. Louis: Saunders Elsevier.

McArdle, W., Katch, F., & Katch, V. (2001). *Exercise physiology: Energy, nutrition, and human performance* (5th ed.). Philadelphia: Lippincott Williams & Wilkins.

Millodot, M. (1977). The influence of age on the sensitivity of the cornea. *Investigative Ophthalmology & Visual Science, 16* (3), 240-242.

Morgan, D.W., & Craig, M. (1992). Physiological aspects of running economy. *Medicine & Science in Sports & Exercise, 24*, 456-461.

National Center for Health Statistics. (2011). Health, United States, 2010: With Special Feature on Death and Dying. Hyattsville, MD. https://www.cdc.gov/nchs/data/hus/hus10.pdf

National Institutes of Health. (2014). 8th Report of the Joint National Committee on the Prevention, Detection, Evaluation, and Treatment of High Blood Pressure. Retrieved from https://www.guideline.gov/summaries/summary/48192/2014-evidence-based-guideline-for-the-management-of-high-blood-pressure-in-adults-Report-from-the-panel-members-appointed-to-the-Eighth-Joint-National-Committee-JNC-8 .

Niinimaa, V., & Shephard, R.J. (1978). Training and exercise conductance in the elderly. II. The cardiovascular system. *Journal of Gerontology, 35*, 672-682.

Nillsson, B.E., & Westlin, N.E. (1971). Bone density in athletes. *Clinical Orthopaedics, 77*, 179-182.

Nouchi, R., Taki, Y., Takeuchi, H., Hashizume, H., Akitsuki, Y., Shigemune, Y., Sekigushi, A., Kotozaki, Y., Tsukiura, T., Yomogida, Y., & Kawashima, R. (2012). Brain training game improves executive functions and processing speed in the elderly: A randomized controlled trial. *PLOS One, 7* (1), e29676. doi:10.1371/journal.pone.0029676

Owsley, C., & Ball, K. (1993). Assessing visual function in the older driver. *Clinics in Geriatric Medicine, 9* (2), 389-401.

Paterson, D.H., Cunningham, D.A., & Babcock, M.A. (1989). Oxygen kinetics in the elderly. In G.D. Swanson, F.S. Grodins, & R.L. Hughson (Eds.), *Respiratory control: A modelling perspective* (pp. 171-178). New York: Plenum Press.

Pimentel, A.E., Gentile, C.L., Tanaka, H., Seals, D.R., & Gates, P.E. (2003). Greater rate of decline in maximal aerobic capacity with age in endurance-trained than in sedentary men. *Journal of Applied Physiology, 94* (6), 2406-2413.

Ratey, J.J. (2001). *A user's guide to the brain: Perception, attention, and the four theaters of the brain.* New York: Vintage Books.

Reeve, J., Walton, L.J., Lunt, M., Wolman, R., Abraham, R., et al. (1999). Determinants of the first decade of bone loss after menopause at spine, hip, and radius. *Quarterly Journal of Medicine, 92*, 261-273.

Sachs, C., Hamberger, B., & Kaijser, L. (1985). Cardiovascular responses and plasma catecholamines in old age. *Clinical Physiology, 5*, 239-249.

Saxon, S.V., Etten, M.J., & Perkins, E.A. (2010). *Physical change & aging: A guide for the helping professions* (5th ed.). New York: Springer.

Schieber, F. (1992). Aging and the senses. In J.E. Birren, R.B. Sloane, & G.D. Cohen (Eds.), *Handbook of mental health and aging* (2nd ed., pp. 252-306). San Diego: Academic Press.

Schultheis, L. (1991). The mechanical control system of bone in weightless spaceflight and in aging. *Experimental Gerontology, 26*, 203-214.

Schwartz, R. (1990). Body fat distribution in healthy young and older men. *Journal of Gerontology, 46* (6), 181-185.

Shank, M.D., & Haywood, K.M. (1987). Eye movements while viewing a baseball pitch. *Perceptual and Motor Skills, 64*, 1191-1197.

Sharma, A., Flom, P.L., Rosen, C.J., & Schoenbaum, E.E. (2015). Racial differences in bone loss and relation to menopause among HIV-infected and uninfected women. *Bone, 77*, 24-30.

Shephard, R.J. (1991). Fitness and aging. In C. Blais (Ed.), *Aging into the twenty-first century* (pp. 22-35). Downsview, ON: Captus University.

Shephard, R.J. (1993). *Health and aerobic fitness.* Champaign, IL: Human Kinetics.

Shephard, R.J. (1997). *Aging, physical activity, and health.* Champaign, IL: Human Kinetics.

Shephard, R.J. (1998). Aging and exercise. In T.D. Fahey (Ed.), *Encyclopedia of sports medicine and science.* Internet Society for Sport Science. http:// sportsci.org.

Shephard, R.J. (2008). Aging, physical activity and health. *International Encyclopedia of Public Health,* 61-69. doi: 10.1016/B978-012373960-5.00627-4

Snowdon, D.A. (2003). Healthy aging and dementia: Findings from the nun study. *Annals of Internal Medicine, 139* (5), 450-454.

Spirduso, W.W., Francis, K.L., & MacRae, P.G. (2005). *Physical dimensions of aging* (2nd ed.). Champaign, IL: Human Kinetics.

Svänborg, A., Eden, S., & Mellstrom, D. (1991). Metabolic changes in aging as predictors of disease: The Swedish experience. In D.K. Ingram, G.T. Baker, & N.W. Shock (Eds.), *The potential for nutritional modulation of aging* (pp. 81-90). Trumbull, CT: Food & Nutrition Press.

Tanaka, H., & Seals, D.R. (2003). Dynamic exercise performance in Masters athletes: Insight into the effects of primary human aging on physiological functional capacity. *Journal of Applied Physiology, 95,* 2152-2162.

Tate, C., Hyek, M., & Taffet, G. (1994). Mechanisms for the response of cardiac muscle to physical activity in old age. *Medicine & Science in Sports & Exercise, 26* (5), 561-567.

Van Norman, K. (1995). *Exercise programming for older adults.* Champaign, IL: Human Kinetics.

Weale, R. (1963). New light on old eyes. *Nature, 198,* 944-946.

Wilson, T.M. & Tanaka, H. (2000). Meta-analysis of the age-associated decline in maximal aerobic capacity in men: Relation to training status. *American Journal of Physiology-Heart and Circulatory Physiology, 278* (3), 829-834.

Yen, P. (2004). Nutritional treatment of coronary artery disease. *Geriatric Nursing, 25* (4), 246-247.

Zerzawy, R. (1987). Hämodynamische Reaktionen unter verschiedenen Belastungsformen [Hemodynamic reactions to different types of work]. In R. Rost & F. Webering (Eds.), *Kardiology im Sport [Cardiology in sport].* Cologne: German Sports Medicine Federation.

Chapter 11

Abernethy, B. (1991). Visual search strategies and decision-making in sport. *International Journal of Sport Psychology, 22,* 189-210.

Atkinson, J., & Braddick, O. (2012). Visual attention in the first years: Typical development and developmental disorders. *Developmental Medicine and Child Neurology 54,* 589-595.

Bjorklund, D.F., & Douglas, R.N. (1997). The development of memory strategies. In N. Cowan (Ed.), *The development of memory in childhood* (pp. 201-246). Hove, UK: The Psychology Press.

Brown, A.L. (1975). The development of memory: Knowing, knowing about knowing, and knowing how to know. In H.W. Reese (Ed.), *Advances in child development and behavior* (Vol. 10). New York: Academic Press.

Brown, A.L. (1978). Knowing when, where, and how to remember: A problem of metacognition. In R. Glaser (Ed.), *Advances in instructional psychology.* Hillsdale, NJ: Erlbaum.

Chase, W.G., & Simon, H.A. (1973). Perception in chess. *Cognitive Psychology, 4,* 55-81.

Chi, M.T.H. (1978). Knowledge structures and memory development. In R.S. Siegler (Ed.), *Children's thinking: What develops?* (pp. 73-105). Hillsdale, NJ: Erlbaum.

Chi, M.T.H. (1981). Knowledge development and memory performance. In M.P. Friedman, J.P. Das, & N. O'Connor (Eds.), *Intelligence and learning* (pp. 221-229). New York: Plenum Press.

Côté, J., Lidor, R., & Hackfort, D. (2009). ISSP position stand: To sample or to specialize? Seven postulates about youth sport activities that lead to continued participation and elite performance. *International Journal of Sport and Exercise Physiology, 9,* 7-17.

Crain, W.C. (1985). *Theories of development: Concepts and applications* (2nd ed.). Englewood Cliffs, NJ: Prentice Hall.

Cuevas, K., & Bell, M.A. (2014). Infant attention and early childhood executive function. *Child Development, 85,* 397-404.

Ericsson, K.A. (2003). Development of elite performance and deliberate practice: An update from the perspective of the expert performance approach. In J.L. Starkes & K.A. Ericsson (Eds.), *Expert performance in sports* (pp. 49-83). Champaign, IL: Human Kinetics.

Ericsson, K.A. (2013). Training history, deliberate practice and elite sports performance: An analysis in response to Tucker and Collins review—what makes champions? *British Journal of Sports Medicine, 47,* 533-535.

Fantz, R.L. (1963). Patterned vision in newborn infants. *Science, 140,* 296-297.

Fantz, R.L. (1964). Visual experience in infants: Decreased attention to familiar patterns relative to novel ones. *Science, 146,* 668-670.

Fitts, P., & Posner, M.I. (1967). *Human performance.* Belmont, CA: Brooks/Cole.

Flavell, J.H. (1979). Metacognition and cognitive monitoring: A new area of cognitive-developmental inquiry. *American Psychologist, 34,* 906-911.

Flavell, J.H., Beach, D.H., & Chinsky, J.M. (1966). Spontaneous verbal rehearsal in a memory task as a function of age. *Child Development, 37,* 283-299.

Flavell, J.H., Friedrichs, A.G., & Hoyt, J.D. (1970). Developmental changes in memorization processes. *Cognitive Psychology, 1,* 324-340.

French, K.E., Spurgeon, J.H., & Nevett, M.E. (1995). Expert-novice differences in cognitive and skill execution components of youth baseball performance. *Research Quarterly for Exercise and Sport, 66,* 194-201.

French, K.E., & Thomas, J.R. (1987). The relation of knowledge to children's basketball performance. *Journal of Sport Psychology, 9,* 15-32.

Gallagher, J.D., & Thomas, J.R. (1984). Rehearsal strategy effects on developmental differences for recall of a movement series. *Research Quarterly for Exercise and Sport, 55,* 123-128.

Ginsburg, H., & Opper, S. (1969). *Piaget's theory of intellectual development: An introduction.* Englewood Cliffs, NJ: Prentice Hall.

Hastie, P.A., Calderon, A., Rolim, R.J., & Guarino, A.J. (2013). The development of skill and knowledge during a sport education season of track and field. *Research Quarterly for Exercise and Sport, 84,* 336-344.

Hick, W.E. (1952). On the rate of gain of information. *Quarterly Journal of Experimental Psychology, 4,* 11-26.

Hoover, J.H., & Wade, M. (1985). Motor learning theory and mentally retarded individuals: A historical review. *Adapted Physical Activity Quarterly, 2,* 228-252.

Janelle, C.M., & Hillman, C.H. (2003). Expert performance in sport: Current perspectives and critical issues. In J.L. Starkes & K.A. Ericsson (Eds.), *Expert performance in sports* (pp. 19-47). Champaign, IL: Human Kinetics.

Keogh, J., & Sugden, D. (1985). *Movement skill development.* New York: Macmillan.

Kourtessis, T., & Reid, G. (1997). Knowledge and skill of ball catching in children with cerebral palsy and other physical disabilities. *Adapted Physical Activity Quarterly, 14,* 24-42.

Lefebvre, C., & Reid, G. (1998). Prediction in ball catching by children with and without a developmental coordination disorder. *Adapted Physical Activity Quarterly, 15,* 299-315.

Liu, T., & Jensen. J.L. (2011). Effects of strategy use on children's motor performance in a continuous timing task. *Research Quarterly for Exercise and Sport, 82,* 198-209.

Magill, R.A. (2017). *Motor learning and control: Concepts and applications* (11th ed.). New York: McGraw-Hill.

Ornstein, P.A., & Naus, M.J. (1978). Rehearsal processes in children's memory. In P.A. Ornstein (Ed.), *Memory development in children.* Hillsdale, NJ: Erlbaum.

Payne, G.V., & Isaacs, L.D. (2008). *Human life motor development: A lifespan approach* (7th ed.). New York: McGraw-Hill.

Piaget, J. (1976). *The child and reality* (A. Rosin, Trans.) New York: Grossman.

Reid, G. (1980a). Overt and covert rehearsal in short-term motor memory of mentally retarded and nonretarded persons. *American Journal of Mental Deficiency, 85,* 69-77.

Reid, G. (1980b). The effects of memory strategy instruction in short term motor memory of the mentally retarded. *Journal of Motor Behavior, 112,* 221-227.

Reynolds, G.D., Courage, M.L., & Richards, J.E. (2013). The development of attention. In D. Reisberg (Ed.), *Oxford handbook of cognitive psychology* (pp. 1000-1013). Oxford UK: Oxford University Press.

Ryu, D., Kim, S., Abernethy, B., & Mann, D.L. (2013). Guiding attention aids the acquisition of anticipatory skill in novice soccer goalkeepers. *Research Quarterly for Exercise and Sport, 84,* 252-262.

Schneider, W., & Ornstein, P.A. (2015). The development of children's memory. *Child Development Perspectives, 9,* 190-195.

Shaffer, D. (1999). *Developmental psychology: Childhood and adolescence* (5th ed.). Pacific Grove, CA: Brookes/Cole.

Stanley, J., & Krakauer, J.W. (2013). Motor skill depends on knowledge of facts. *Frontiers in Human Neuroscience, 7,* 503.

Starkes, J.L., & Allard, F. (1991). Motor-skill experts in sports, dance, and other domains. In K.A. Ericsson & J. Smith (Eds.), *Towards a general theory of expertise: Prospects and limits* (pp. 126-152). Cambridge, UK: Cambridge University Press.

Starkes, J.L., Deakin, J.M., Lindley, S., & Crisp, F. (1987). Motor versus verbal recall of ballet sequences by young expert dancers. *Journal of Sport Psychology, 9,* 222-230.

Starkes, J.L., & Ericsson, K.A. (Eds.). (2003). *Expert performance in sports.* Champaign, IL: Human Kinetics.

Ste-Marie, D. (2003). Expertise in sport judges and referees: Circumventing information processing limitations. In J.L. Starkes & K.A. Ericsson (Eds.), *Expert performance in sports* (pp. 19-47). Champaign, IL: Human Kinetics.

Sugden, D.A. (1978). Visual motor short term memory in educationally subnormal boys. *British Journal of Educational Psychology, 48,* 330-339.

Thomas, J.R., Thomas, K.T., & Gallagher, J.D. (1993). Developmental considerations in skill acquisition. In R.N. Singer, M. Murphey, & L.K. Tennant

(Eds.), *Handbook of research on sport psychology* (pp. 73-105). New York: Macmillan.

Toner, J. (2014). Knowledge of facts mediate 'continuous improvement' in elite sport: A comment on Stanley and Krakauer (2013). *Frontiers in Human Neuroscience, 10,* 142.

Tulving, E. (1985). How many memory systems are there? *American Psychologist, 40,* 385-398.

Tulving, E. (2002). Episodic memory: From mind to brain. *Annual Review of Psychology, 53,* 1-25.

Wall, A.E., McClements, J., Bouffard, M., Findlay, H., & Taylor, J. (1985). A knowledge-based approach to motor development: Implications for the physically awkward. *Adapted Physical Activity Quarterly, 2,* 21-42.

Wall, A.E., Reid, G., & Harvey, W.J. (2007). Interface of the KB and ETA approaches. In W.E. Davis & G.D. Broadhead (Eds.), *Ecological task analysis and movement* (pp. 259-277). Champaign, IL: Human Kinetics.

Weiss, M.R. (1983). Modeling and motor performance: A developmental perspective. *Research Quarterly for Exercise and Sport, 54,* 190-197.

Wetzel, N. (2014). Development of control of attention from different perspectives. *Frontiers in Psychology, 5,* 1000.

Wickens, C.D., & and Benel, D.C.R. (1982). The development of time-sharing skills. In J.A.S. Kelso & J.E. Clark (Eds.), *The development of movement control and coordination* (pp. 253-272). New York: Wiley.

Williams, A.M., & Davids, K. (1998). Visual search strategy, selective attention, and expertise in soccer. *Research Quarterly for Exercise and Sport, 69,* 127-135.

Winther, K.T., & Thomas, J.R. (1981). Developmental differences in children's labeling of movement. *Journal of Motor Behavior, 13,* 77-90.

Chapter 12

Aiken, C.H., Fairbrother, J.T., & Post, P.G. (2012). The effects of self-controlled video feedback on the learning of the basketball set shot. *Frontiers in Psychology, 3,* 338.

Andrieux, M., Boutin, A., & Thon, B. (2016). Self-control of task difficulty during early practice promotes motor skill learning. *Journal of Motor Behavior, 48,* 57-65.

Babic, M.J., Morgan, P.J., Plotnikoff, R.C., Lonsdale, C., White, R.L., & Lubans, D.R. (2014). Physical activity and physical self-concept in youth: Systematic review and meta-analysis. *Sports Medicine, 44,* 1589-1601.

Bai, Y., Chen, S. Vazou, S., Welk, G.J., & Schaben, J. (2015). Mediated effects of perceived competence on youth physical activity and sedentary behavior. *Research Quarterly for Exercise and Sport, 86,* 406-413.

Bailey, R., Cope E.J., & Pearce, G. (2013). Why do children take part and remain involved in sport? A literature review and discussion of implications for sport coaches. *International Journal of Coaching Science, 7,* 56-75.

Balish, S.M., McLaren, C., Rainham, D., & Blanchard, C. (2014). Correlates of youth sport attrition: A review and future directions. *Psychology of Sport and Exercise, 15,* 429-439.

Bandura, A. (1997). *Self-efficacy: The exercise of control.* New York: Freeman.

Barnett, L.M., Ridgers, N.D., & Salmon, J. (2015). Associations between young children's perceived and actual ball skill competence and physical activity. *Journal of Science and Medicine in Sport, 18,* 167-171.

Bauman, A.E., Reis, R.S., Sallis, J.F., Wells, J.C., Loos, R.J.F., & Martin, B.W. (2012). Correlates of physical activity: Why are some people active and others not? *Lancet, 380,* 258-271.

Cairney, J., Kwan, M.Y.W., Velduizen, S., Hay, J., Bray, S.R., & Faught, B.F. (2012). Gender, perceived competence and the enjoyment of physical education in children: A longitudinal examination. *International Journal of Behavioral Nutrition and Physical Activity, 9,* 26.

Caprara, G.V., Pastorelli, C., & Weiner, B. (1997). Linkages between causal ascriptions, emotion, and behavior. *International Journal of Behavioral Development, 20,* 153-162.

Chase, M.A. (2001). Children's self-efficacy, motivational intentions, and attributions in physical education and sport. *Research Quarterly for Exercise and Sport, 72,* 47-54.

Chiviacowsky, S., & Wulf, G. (2005). Self-controlled feedback is effective if it is based on the learner's performance. *Research Quarterly for Exercise and Sport, 76,* 42-48.

Chiviacowsky, S., Wulf, G., de Medeiros, F.L., Kaefer, A., & Tani, G. (2008). Learning benefits of self-controlled knowledge of results in 10-year-old children. *Research Quarterly for Exercise and Sport, 79,* 405-410.

Cleary, T.J., & Zimmerman, B.J. (2001). Self-regulation differences during athletic practice by experts, non-experts and novices. *Journal of Applied Sport Psychology, 13,* 185-206.

Côté, J ., Baker, J., & Abernethy, B. (2003). From play to practice: A developmental framework for acquisition of expertise in team sports. In J.L. Starkes & K.A. Ericsson (Eds.), *Expert performance in sports* (pp. 89-113). Champaign, IL: Human Kinetics.

Crain, W.C. (1985). *Theories of development: Concepts and applications* (2nd ed.). Englewood Cliffs, NJ: Prentice Hall.

Crocker, P.R.E., Hoar, S.D., McDonough, M.H., Kowaski, K.C., & Niefer, C.B. (2004). Emotional experiences in youth sport. In M.R. Weiss (Ed.), *Developmental sport and exercise psychology: A lifespan perspective* (pp. 197-221). Morgantown, WV: Fitness Information Technology.

Deci, E.L., & Flaste, R. (1995). *Why we do what we do: The dynamics of personal autonomy.* New York: Putnam.

Deci, E.L., & Ryan, R.M. (1985). *Intrinsic motivation and self-determination in human behavior.* New York: Plenum Press.

Erikson, E.H. (1963). *Childhood and society* (2nd ed.). New York: Norton.

Feltz, D.L., Short, S.E., & Sullivan, P.J. (2008). *Self-efficacy in sport.* Champaign, IL: Human Kinetics.

Garner, P.W., & Waajid, B. (2012). Emotional knowledge and self-regulation as predictors of preschools' cognitive ability, classroom behavior, and social competence. *Journal of Psychoeducational Assessment, 30,* 330-343.

Harter, S. (1978). Effectance motivation reconsidered: Toward a developmental model. *Human Development, 21,* 34-64.

Harter, S. (1985). *Manual for the Self-perception Profile for Children.* Denver: University of Denver.

Harter, S. (1999). *The construction of self: A developmental perspective.* New York: Guilford.

Haywood, K.M., & Getchell, N. (2014). *Life span motor development* (6th ed.). Champaign, IL: Human Kinetics.

Holfelder, B., & Schott, N. (2014). Relationship of fundamental movement skills and physical activity in children and adolescents: A systematic review. *Psychology of Sport and Exercise, 15* 382-391.

Horn, T.S. (1987). The influence of teacher-coach behavior on the psychological development of children. In D. Gould & M.R. Weiss (Eds.), *Advances in pediatric sport science: Volume 2, Behavioral issues* (pp. 121-142). Champaign, IL: Human Kinetics.

Horn, T.S., & Hasbrook, C.A. (1986). *The sport competence information scale.* Oxford, OH: Miami University.

Janelle, C.M., Barba, D.A., Frehlich, S.G., Tennant, L.K., & Cauraugh, J.H. (1997). Maximizing performance feedback effectiveness through videotape replay and a self-controlled learning environment. *Research Quarterly for Exercise and Sport, 68* (4), 269-279.

Jokic, C.S., Polatajko, H., & Whitebread, D. (2013). Self-regulation as a mediator in motor learning: The effect of the cognitive orientation to occupational performance approach on children with DCD. *Adapted Physical Activity Quarterly, 29,* 103-126.

Keetch, K.M., & Lee, T.D. (2007). The effect of self-regulated and experimenter-imposed practice schedules on motor learning for tasks of varying difficulty. *Research Quarterly for Exercise and Sport, 78,* 476-486.

Kitsantas, A., & Zimmerman, B.J. (1998). Self-regulation of motoric learning: A strategic cycle view. *Journal of Applied Sport Psychology, 10,* 220-239.

Kolovelonis, A., Goudas, M., Hassandra, M., & Dermitzaki, I. (2012). Self-regulated learning in physical education: Examining the effects of emulative and self-control practice. *Psychology of Sport and Exercise, 13,* 383-389.

LeGear, M., Greyling, L., Sloan, E., Bell, R.I., Williams, B.-L., Naylor, P-J., & Temple, V. (2012). A window of opportunity? Motor skills and perceptions of competence of children in kindergarten. *International Journal of Behavioral Nutrition and Physical Activity, 9,* 29.

Leversen, I., Danielsen, A.G., Wold, B., & Samdal, O. (2012). What they want and what they get: Self-reported motives, perceived competence, and relatedness in adolescent leisure activities. *Child Development Research,* article 684157.

Lewthwaite, R., Chiviacowsky, S., Drews, R., & Wulf, G. (2015). Choose to move: The motivational impact of autonomy support on motor learning. *Psychonomic Bulletin & Review, 22,* 1383-1388.

Lloyd, M., Reid, G., & Bouffard, M. (2006). Self-regulation of sport-specific and educational problem solving tasks by boys with and without DCD. *Adapted Physical Activity Quarterly, 23,* 370-389.

Lloyd, M., Saunders, T.J., Bremer, E., & Tremblay, M.S. (2014). Long-term importance of fundamental motor skills: A 20-year follow-up study. *Adapted Physical Activity Quarterly, 31,* 67-78.

Lubans, D.R., Morgan, P.J., Cliff, D.P., Barnett, L.M., & Okely, A.D. (2010). Fundamental movement skills in children and adolescents: Review of associated health benefits. *Sports Medicine, 40,* 1019-1035.

Lubans, D.R., Plotnikiff, R.C., & Lubans, N.J. (2012). Review: A systematic review of the impact of physical activity programmes on social and emotional well-being in at-risk youth. *Child and Adolescent Mental Health, 17,* 2-13.

Maatta, S., Ray, C., & Roos, E. (2014). Associations of parental influence and 10-11-year-old children's physical activity: Are they mediated by children's perceived competence and attraction to physical activity? *Scandinavian Journal of Public Health, 42,* 45-51.

Magill, R.A. (2017). *Motor learning and control: Concepts and applications* (11th ed.). New York: McGraw-Hill.

McKiddie, B., & Maynard, I.W. (1997). Perceived competence of school children in physical education. *Journal of Teaching in Physical Education, 16,* 324-339.

Nasuti, G., & Rhodes, R.E. (2013). Affective judgement and physical activity in youth: Review and meta-analysis. *Annals of Behavioral Medicine, 45,* 357-376.

Petlichkoff, L.M. (2004). Self-regulation skills for children and adolescents. In M.R. Weiss (Ed.), *Developmental sport and exercise psychology: A lifespan perspective* (pp. 269-288). Morgantown, WV: Fitness Information Technology.

Post, P.G., Fairbrother, J.T., & Barros, J.A.C. (2011). Self-controlled amount of practice benefits learning of a motor skill. *Research Quarterly for Exercise and Sport, 82,* 474-481.

Post, P.G., Fairbrother, J.T., Barros, J.A.C., & Kulpa, J.D. (2014). Self-controlled practice with a fixed time period facilitates the learning of a basketball set shot. *Journal of Motor Learning and Development, 3,* 9-15.

Robinson, L.E. (2010). The relationship between perceived physical competence and fundamental motor skills in preschool children. *Child: Care, Health, and Development, 37,* 589-596.

Robinson, L.E., Stodden, D.F., Barnett, L.M., Lopes, V.T., Logan, S.W., Rodrigues, L.P., & D'Hondt, E. (2015). Motor competence and its effect on positive developmental trajectories of health. *Sports Medicine, 45,* 1273-1284.

Rodgers, W.M., Markland, D., Selzler, A.-M., Murray, T., & Wilson, P.M. (2014). Distinguishing perceived competence and self-efficacy: An example from exercise. *Research Quarterly for Exercise and Sport, 85,* 527-539.

Ryan, R.M., & Deci, E.L. (2000). Self-determination theory and the facilitation of intrinsic motivation, social development, and well-being. *American Psychologist, 55,* 68-78.

Sanli, E.A., Patterson, J.T., Bray, S.R., & Lee, T.D. (2013). Understanding self-controlled motor learning through the self-determination theory. *Frontiers in Psychology, 3,* 611.

Schmidt, R.A., & Lee, T.D. (2011). *Motor control and learning: A behavioral emphasis* (5th ed.). Champaign, IL: Human Kinetics.

Schmidt, R.A., & Lee, T.D. (2014). *Motor learning and performance: A situation-based learning approach* (5th ed.). Champaign, IL: Human Kinetics.

Seabra, A.C., Seabra, A.F., Mendonca, D.M., Brustad, R., Maia, J.A., Fonseca, A.M., & Malina, R.M. (2012). Psychosocial correlates of physical activity in school children aged 8-10 years. *European Journal of Public Health, 23,* 794-798.

Seligman, M. (1975). *Helplessness: On depression, development, and death.* San Francisco: Freeman.

Shaffer, D. (1999). *Developmental psychology: Childhood and adolescence* (5th ed.). Pacific Grove, CA: Brooks/Cole.

Singer, R.N. (2002). Preperformance state, routines, and automaticity: What does it take to realize expertise in self-paced events? *Journal of Sport and Exercise Psychology, 24,* 359-375.

Stodden, D.F., Gao, Z., Goodway, J.D., & Langendorfer, S.J. (2014). Dynamic relationships between motor skill competence and health-related fitness in youth. *Pediatric Exercise Science, 26,* 231-241.

Stodden, D.F., Goodway, J.D., Langendorfer, S.J., Roberton, M.A., Rudisill, M.E., Garcia, C., & Garcia, L.E. (2008). A developmental perspective on the role of motor skill competence in physical activity: An emergent relationship. *Quest, 60,* 290-306.

Sun, H., & Chen, A. (2010). A pedagogical understanding of the self-determination theory in physical education. *Quest, 62,* 364-384.

Tamminen, K.A., & Crocker, P.R.E. (2013). 'I control my own emotions for the sake of the team': Emotional self-regulation and interpersonal emotion regulation among female high-performance curlers. *Psychology of Sport and Exercise, 14,* 737-747.

Teixeira, P.J., Carraca, E.L., Markland, D., Silva, M.N., & Ryan, R.M. (2012). Exercise, physical activity, and self-determination theory: A systematic review. *International Journal of Behavioral Nutrition and Physical Activity, 9,* 78.

Vallerand, R.J. (1997). Toward a hierarchical model of intrinsic and extrinsic motivation. In M.P. Zanna (Ed.), *Advances in experimental social psychology: Vol. 2* (pp. 271-360). New York: Academic Press.

Vallerand, R.J. (2007). Intrinsic and extrinsic motivation in sport and physical activity: A review and a look at the future. In G. Tenenbaum & E. Eklund (Eds.), *Handbook of sport psychology* (3rd ed., pp. 49-83). New York: Wiley.

Van den Berghe, L., Vansteenkiste, M., Cardon, G., Kirk, D., & Haerens, L. (2014). Research on self-determination in physical education: Key findings and proposals for future research. *Physical Education and Sport Pedagogy, 19,* 97-121.

Weiner, B. (1985). An attribution theory of achievement motivation and emotion. *Psychological Review, 92,* 548-573.

Weiss, M.R., McCullagh, P., Smith, A.L., & Berlant, A.R. (1998). Observational learning and the fearful child: Influence of peer models on swimming skill performance and psychological responses. *Research Quarterly for Exercise and Sport, 69,* 380-394.

Weiss, M.R., & Williams, L. (2004). The why of youth sport involvement: A developmental perspective on motivational processes. In M.R. Weiss

(Ed.), *Developmental sport and exercise psychology: A lifespan perspective* (pp. 223-268). Morgantown, WV: Fitness Information Technology.

Wu, W.F.W., & Magill, R.A. (2011). Allowing learners to choose: Self-controlled practice schedules for learning multiple movement patterns. *Research Quarterly for Exercise and Sport, 82,* 449-457.

Wulf, G., & Toole, T. (1999). Physical assistance devices in complex motor skill learning: Benefits of a self-controlled practice schedule. *Research Quarterly for Exercise and Sport, 70,* 265-272.

Yerkes, R.M., & Dodson, J.D. (1908). The relation of strength of stimulus to rapidity of habit-formation. *Journal of Comparative Neurology and Psychology, 18,* 459-482.

Zimmerman, B.J. (2000). Attaining self-regulation: A social cognitive perspective. In M. Boekaerts, P.R. Pintrich, & M. Zeidner (Eds.), *Handbook of self-regulation* (pp. 13-39). San Diego: Academic Press.

Zimmerman, B.J., & Kitsantas, A. (1997). Developmental phases in self-regulation: Shifting from process goals to outcome goals. *Journal of Educational Psychology, 89,* 29-36.

Zimmerman, B.J., & Kitsantas, A. (1999). Acquiring writing revision skill: Shifting from process to outcome self-regulatory goals. *Journal of Educational Psychology, 91,* 241-250.

Chapter 13

Ajzen, I. (1985). From intentions to actions: A theory of planned behaviour. In J. Kuhl & J. Beckman (Eds.), *Action control: From cognition to behavior* (pp. 11-39). Heidelberg, Germany: Springer.

Ajzen, I. (1991). The theory of planned behavior. *Organizational Behavior and Human Decision Processes, 50* (2), 179-211.

Bandura, A. (1997). *Self-efficacy: The exercise of control.* New York: Freeman.

Bert, H., Petrie, T.A., MacIntire, M.M., & Jones, G. (2010). The influences of skill level, anxiety, and psychological skills use on amateur golfers' performances. *Journal of Applied Sport Psychology, 22* (2), 123-133.

Bherer, L., Kramer, A.F., & Peterson, M.S. (2008). Transfer effects in task-set cost and dual-task cost after dual-task training in older and younger adults: Further evidence for cognitive plasticity in attentional control in late adulthood. *Experimental Aging Research, 34,* 188-219.

Bickmore, T.W., Caruso, L., Clough-Gorr, K., & Heeren, T. (2005). "It's just like you talk to a friend" relational agents for older adults. *Interacting with Computers, 17,* 711-735.

Biddle, S., Fox, K., & Boutcher, S. (2000). *Physical activity and psychological well-being.* London: Routledge.

Ceria-Ulep, C.D., Serafica, R.C., & Tse, A. (2011). Filipino older adults' beliefs about exercise activity. *Nursing Forum, 46* (4), 240-250.

Chogahara, M., O'Brien Cousins, S., & Wankel, L.M. (1998). Social influences on physical activity in older adults: A review. *Journal of Aging and Physical Activity, 6* (1), 1-17.

Cobb-Clark, D.A., Kassenboehmer, S.C., & Schurer, S. (2014). Healthy habits: The connection between diet, exercise, and locus of control. *Journal of Economic Behavior & Organization, 98,* 1-28.

Craik, F.I.M. (1986). A functional account of age differences in memory. In F. Flix & H. Hagendorf (Eds.), *Human memory and cognitive capabilities, mechanisms, and performance* (pp. 409-422). Amsterdam: Elsevier, North-Holland.

Crews, D.J., Lochbaum, M.R., & Karoly, P. (2000). Self-regulation: Concepts, methods and strategies in sport and exercise. In R.N. Singer, H.A. Hausenblas, & C.M. Janelle (Eds.), *Handbook of sport psychology* (2nd ed., pp. 566-581). New York: Wiley.

Dacey, M., Baltzell, A., & Zalchkowsky, L. (2008). Older adults' intrinsic and extrinsic motivation toward physical activity. *American Journal of Health Behavior, 32* (5), 570-582.

Darlow, S.D., & Xu, X. (2011).The influence of close others' exercise habits and perceived social support on exercise. *Psychology of Sport and Exercise, 12* (5), 575-578.

Deford, F. (1980, July 14). A match goes down in history. *Sports Illustrated.*

Dishman, R.K. (1994). *Advances in exercise adherence.* Champaign, IL: Human Kinetics.

Easterbrook, J.A. (1959). The effect of emotion on cue utilization and the organization of behavior. *Psychological Review, 66,* 183-201.

Eimer, M., Nattkemper, D., Schröger, E., & Prinz, W. (1996). Involuntary attention. In O. Neumann & A.F. Sanders (Eds.), *Handbook of perception and action. Vol. 3: Attention* (pp. 155-184). San Diego: Academic Press.

Erikson, E. (1980). *Identity and the life cycle.* New York: Norton.

Erikson, E.H. (1963). *Childhood and society* (2nd ed.). New York: Norton.

Gabbard, C.P. (2012). *Lifelong motor development* (6th ed.). San Francisco: Benjamin Cummings.

Gallahue, D.L., Ozmun, J.C., & Goodway, J.D. (2012). *Understanding motor development: Infants, children, adolescents, adults* (7th ed.). Boston: McGraw-Hill.

Gardner, P.J. (2011). Natural neighborhood networks—Important social networks in the lives of older adults aging in place. *Journal of Aging Studies, 25* (3), 263-271.

Gray, P.M., Murphy, M.H., Gallagher, A.M., & Simpson, E.E.A. (2016). Motives and barriers to physical activity among older adults of different socioeconomic status. *Journal of Aging and Physical Activity, 24*, 419-429.

Hausenblas, H.A., Carron, A.V., & Mack, D.E. (1997). Application of the theories of reasoned action and planned behavior to exercise behavior: A meta-analysis. *Journal of Sport and Exercise Psychology, 19*, 36-51.

Hess, T.M., Follett, K.J., & McGee, K.A. (1998). Aging and impression formation: The impact of processing skills and goals. *Journals of Gerontology: Psychological Sciences and Social Sciences, 53B*, 175-187.

Kirschenbaum, D.S. (1984). Self-regulation and sport psychology: Nurturing and emerging symbiosis. *Journal of Sport Psychology, 6*, 159-183.

Kirschenbaum, D.S. (1987). Self-regulation of sport performance. *Medicine & Science in Sports & Exercise, 19*, S106-S113.

Kitsantas, A., & Zimmerman, B.J. (2002). Comparing self-regulatory processes among novice, non-expert, and expert volleyball players: A microanalytic study. *Journal of Applied Sport Psychology, 14*, 91-105.

Kosma, M. (2012). An expanded framework to determine physical activity and falls risks among diverse older adults. *Research on Aging, 36* (1), 95-114.

Lees, F.D., Clark, P.G., Nigg, C.R., & Newman, P. (2005). Barriers to exercise behavior among older adults: A focus-group study. *Journal of Aging and Physical Activity, 13* (1), 23-33.

Lindgren De Groot, G.C., & Fagerström, L. (2011). Older adults motivating factors and barriers to exercise to prevent falls. *Scandinavian Journal of Occupational Therapy, 18*, 153-160.

Litt, M., Kleppinger, A., & Judge, J. (2002). Initiation and maintenance of exercise behavior in older women: Predictors from social learning model. *Journal of Behavioral Medicine, 25* (1), 83-97.

Locke, E.A., & Latham, G.P. (1990). *A theory of goal setting and task performance*. Englewood Cliffs, NJ: Prentice Hall.

Luo, L., & Craik, F.I.M. (2008). Aging and memory: A cognitive approach. *La Revue Canadienne de Psychiatrie, 53* (6), 346-353.

Lustig, C., & Meck, W.H. (2001). Paying attention to time as one gets older. *Psychological Science, 12* (6), 478-484.

Määttä, S., Pääkkönnen, A., Saavalainen, P., & Partanen, J. (2005). Selective attention event-related potential effects from auditory novel stimuli in children and adults. *Clinical Neurophysiology, 116*, 129-141.

Massey, M.V., Meyer, B.B. & Naylor, A.H. (2015). Self-regulation strategies in mixed martial arts. *Journal of Sport Behavior, 38* (2), 192-211.

McAuley, E. (1992). The role of efficacy cognitions in the prediction of exercise behaviour in middle aged adults. *Journal of Behavioral Medicine, 15*, 65-88.

Mihalik, B.J., O'Leary, J.T., Mcguire, F.A., & Dottavio, F.D. (1989). Sports involvement across the life span: Expansion and contraction of sports activities. *Research Quarterly for Exercise and Sport, 60* (4), 396-398.

Molander, B., & Bäckman, L. (1989). Age differences in heart rate patterns during concentration in a precision sport: Implications for attentional functioning. *Journal of Gerontology: Psychological Sciences, 44*, P80-P87.

Molander, B., & Bäckman, L. (1994). Attention and performance in miniature golf across the life span. *Journal of Gerontology: Psychological Sciences, 49* (2), P35-P41.

Motalebi, S.A., Iranagh, J.A., Abdollahi, A., & Lim, W.K. (2014). Applying of theory of planned behavior to promote physical activity and exercise. *Journal of Physical Education and Sport, 14* (4), 562-568.

Mowla, A. et al. (2007). Do memory complaints represent impaired memory performance in patients with major depressive disorder? *Depression & Anxiety, 25*, 92-96.

Nabi, R.L., & Thomas, J. (2013). The effects of reality-based television programming on diet and exercise motivation and self-efficacy in young adults. *Health Communication, 28* (7), 699-708.

Nyberg, L., Lövdén, M., Riklund, K., Lindenberger, U., & Bäckman, L. (2012). Memory aging and brain maintenance. *Trends in Cognitive Sciences, 16* (5), 292-305.

Rackow, P., Scholz, U., & Hornung, R. (2014). Effects of a new sports companion on received social support and physical exercise: An intervention study. *Applied Psychology: Health & Well-Being, 6* (3), 300-317.

Rhodes, R.E., Martin, A.D., Taunton, J.E., Rhodes, E.C., Donnelly, M., & Elliot, J. (1999). Factors associated with exercise adherence among older adults: An individual perspective. *Sports Medicine, 28* (6), 397-411.

Rook, K.S. (2000). The evolution of social relationships in later adulthood. In S.H. Qualls & N. Abeles (Eds.), *Psychology and the aging revolution*. Washington, DC: American Psychological Association.

Schaie, K.W., & Willis, S.L. (1991). *Adult development and aging* (3rd ed.). New York: HarperCollins.

Spirduso, W.W., Francis, K.L., & MacRae, P.G. (2005). *Physical dimensions of aging* (2nd ed.). Champaign, IL: Human Kinetics.

Stephens, T., & Craig, C.L. (1990). *The well-being of Canadians: Highlights of the 1988 Campbell's Soup Survey.* Ottawa: Canadian Fitness and Lifestyle Research Institute.

Thomas, D. (2009, April). Media is on demand but content is still king. *Nielsen Consumer Insight.* Retrieved from http://en-us.nielsen.com/main/insights/consumer_insight/april_2009/media_is_on_demand.

Thomas, W.H., Sorensen, K.L., & Abby. L.T. (2006). Locus of control at work: A meta-analysis. *Journal of Organizational Behavior, 27,* 1057-1087.

Valois, P., Shephard, R.J., & Godin, G. (1986). Relationship of habit and perceived physical ability to exercise behavior. *Perceptual and Motor Skills, 62,* 811-817.

Van Gerven, P.W.M. & Guerreiro, M.J.S. (2016). Selective attention and sensory modality in aging: Curses and blessings. *Frontiers in Human Neuroscience, 10,* 1-7.

Verhaeghen, P., Steitz, W.D., Sliwinski, M.J., & Cerella, J. (2003). Aging and dual-task performance: A meta-analysis, *Psychology and Aging, 18,* 443-460.

Vestergren, P., & Nilsson, L.-G. (2011). Perceived causes of everyday memory problems in a population-based sample aged 39-99. *Applied Cognitive Psychology, 25,* 641-646

Waschall, S.B., & Kernis, M.H. (1996). Level and stability of self-esteem as predictors of children's intrinsic motivation and reactions to anger. *Personality and Social Psychology Bulletin, 22,* 4-13.

Weinberg, R.S., & Gould, D. (2003). *Foundations of sport and exercise psychology* (3rd ed.). Champaign, IL: Human Kinetics.

Weiss, G., & Gould, D. (2015). *Foundations of Sport and Exercise Psychology* (6th ed.). Champaign, IL. Human Kinetics.

White, K.M., Terry, D.J., Troup, C., Rempel, L.A., Norman, P., Mummery, K., Riley, M., Posner, N., & Kenardy, J. (2012). An extended theory of planned behavior intervention for older adults with type 2 diabetes and cardiovascular disease. *Journal of Aging and Physical Activity, 20* (3), 281-299.

Williams, J.M., & Leffingwell, T.R. (1996). Cognitive strategies in sport and exercise psychology. In J.L. Van Raalte & B.W. Brewer (Eds.), *Exploring sport and exercise psychology* (pp. 51-73). Washington, DC: American Psychological Association.

Yardley, L., Donovan-Hall, M., Francis, K., & Todd, C. (2007). Attitudes and beliefs that predict older people's intention to undertake strength and balance training. *Journals of Gerontology B Psychological Sciences & Social Sciences, 62* (2), P119-P125.

Zelinski, E.M., & Kennison, R.F. (2001). The Long Beach Longitudinal Study: Evaluation of longitudinal effects of aging on memory and cognition. *Home Health Care Services Quarterly, 19* (3), 45-55.

Zinsser, N., Bunker, L.K., & Williams, J.M. (2001). Cognitive techniques for building confidence and enhancing performance. In J.M. Williams (Ed.), *Applied sport psychology: Personal growth to peak performance* (4th ed., pp. 284-311). Mountain View, CA: Mayfield.

Chapter 14

Badami, R., VaezMousavi, M., Wulf, G., & Namazizadeh, M. (2011). Feedback after good versus poor trials affects intrinsic motivation. *Research Quarterly for Exercise and Sport, 82,* 360-364.

Badami, R., VaezMousavi, M., Wulf, G., & Namazizadeh, M. (2012). Feedback about more accurate versus less accurate trails: Differential effects on self-confidence and activation. *Research Quarterly for Exercise and Sport, 83,* 196-203.

Bakerman, R., & Brownlee, J.R. (1980). The strategic use of parallel play: A sequential analysis. *Child Development 51,* 873-878.

Bandura, A. (1997). *Self-efficacy: The exercise of control.* New York: Freeman.

Beak, S., Davids, K., & Bennett, S.J. (2000). One size fits all? Sensitivity to moment of inertia information from tennis rackets in children and adults. In S.J. Haake & A. Coe (Eds.), *Tennis science and technology* (pp. 109-118). London: Blackwell.

Bergeron, M.F., Mountjoy, M., Armstrong, N., Chia, M., Côté, J., Emery, C.A., Faigenbaum, A., Hall Jr., G., Kriemler, S., Léglise, M., Malina, R.M., Pensgaard, A.M., Sanchez, A., Soligard, T., Sundgot-Borgen, J., van Mechelen, W., Weissensteiner, J.R., & Engebretsen, L. (2015). International Olympic Committee consensus statement on youth athletic development. *British Journal of Sport Medicine, 49,* 843-851.

Bloom, B.S. (Ed.). (1985). *Developing talent in young people.* New York: Ballantine.

Bunker, B., & Thorpe, R. (1986). The curriculum model. In R. Thorpe, D. Bunker, & L. Almond (Eds.), *Rethinking games teaching* (pp. 7-10). Loughborough, UK: University of Technology, Loughborough.

Buszard, T., Farrow, D., Reid, M., & Masters, R.S.W. (2014). Modifying equipment in early skill development. *Research Quarterly for Exercise and Sport, 85,* 218-225.

Butler, J., Griffin, L., Lombardo, B., & Nastasi, R. (Eds.). (2003). *Teaching games for understanding in physical education and sport: An international perspective* (pp. 1-224). Reston, VA: National Association of Sport and Physical Education.

Button, C., MacLeod, M., Sanders, R., & Coleman, S. (2003). Examining movement variability in the basketball free-throw action at different levels. *Research Quarterly for Exercise and Sport, 74* (3), 257-269.

Caine, D., DiFiori, J., & Maffulli, N. (2006). Physeal injuries in children's and youth sport: Reasons for concern? *British Journal of Sport Medicine, 40,* 749-760.

Clément-Guillotin, C., Chalabaev, A., & Fontayne, P. (2011). Is sport still a masculine domain? A psychological glance. *International Journal of Sport Psychology, 42,* 1-12.

Coakley, J. (1980). Play, games, and sport: Developmental implications for young people. *Journal of Sport Behavior, 3,* 99.

Collier, D.H. (2005). Instructional strategies for adapted physical education. In J.P. Winnick (Ed.), *Adapted physical education and sport* (4th ed., pp. 109-130). Champaign, IL: Human Kinetics.

Côté, J. (1999). The influence of the family in the development of talent in sport. *Sport Psychologist, 13,* 395-417.

Côté, J., Baker, J., & Abernethy, B. (2003). From play to practice: A developmental framework for acquisition of expertise in team sports. In J.L. Starkes & K.A. Ericsson (Eds.), *Expert performance in sports* (pp. 89-113). Champaign, IL: Human Kinetics.

Côté, J., Baker, J., & Abernethy, B. (2007). Practice and play in the development of sport expertise. In R. Eklund & G. Tenenbaum (Eds.), *Handbook of sport psychology* (3rd ed. pp. 184-202) Hoboken, NJ: Wiley.

Côté, J., Lidor, R., & Hackfort, D. (2009). ISSP position stand: To sample or to specialize? Seven postulates about youth sport activities that lead to continued participation and elite performance. *International Journal of Sport and Exercise Physiology, 9,* 7-17.

Davids, K., Button, C., & Bennett, S. (2008). *Dynamics of skill acquisition: A constraints-led approach.* Champaign, IL: Human Kinetics.

Deakin, J.M., & Cobley, S. (2003). A search for deliberate practice: An examination of the practice environments in figure skating and volleyball. In J.L. Starkes & K.A. Ericsson (Eds.), *Expert performance in sports* (pp. 115-135). Champaign, IL: Human Kinetics.

Deci, E.L., Koestner, R., & Ryan, R.M. (1999). A meta-analytic review of experiments examining the effects of intrinsic rewards on intrinsic motivation. *Psychological Bulletin, 125* (6), 627-668.

Deci, E.L., Koestner, R., & Ryan, R.M. (2000). Extrinsic rewards and intrinsic motivation in education: Reconsidered once again. *Review of Educational Research, 71* (1), 1-27.

Deci, E.L., & Ryan, R.M. (1985). *Intrinsic motivation and self-determination in human behavior.* New York: Plenum Press.

Deci, E.L., & Ryan, R.M. (2000). The "what" and "why" of goal pursuits: Human needs and the self-determination of behavior. *Psychological Inquiry, 11,* 227-268.

Dyer, S., & Moneta, G.B. (2006). Frequency of parallel, associative, and cooperative play in British children of different social status. *Social Behavior and Personality: An International Journal, 34,* 587-592.

Dewey, J. (1916). *Democracy in education.* New York: Macmillan.

Eime, R.M., Young, J A., Harvey, J.T., & Payne, W.R. (2013). A systematic review of the psychological and social benefits of participation in sport for children and adolescents: Informing development of a conceptual model of health through sport. *International Journal of Behavioral Nutrition and Physical Activity, 10,* 135.

Ericsson, K.A. (2003). Development of elite performance and deliberate practice: An update from the perspective of the expert performance approach. In J.L. Starkes & K.A. Ericsson (Eds.), *Expert performance in sports* (pp. 49-83). Champaign, IL: Human Kinetics.

Fitts, P., & Posner, M.I. (1967). *Human performance.* Belmont, CA: Brooks/Cole.

Fraser-Thomas, J.L., Côté, J., & Deakin, J. (2005). Youth sports programs: An avenue to foster positive youth development. *Physical Education and Sport Pedagogy, 10,* 19-40.

Fredricks, J.A., & Eccles, J.S. (2004). Parental influences on youth involvement in sports. In M.R. Weiss (Ed.), *Developmental sport and exercise psychology: A lifespan perspective* (pp. 145-164). Morgantown, WV: Fitness Information Technology.

Ginsburg, K.R. (2007). The importance of play in promoting healthy child development and maintaining strong parent-child bonds. *Pediatrics, 119* (1), 182-191.

Gould, D., Feltz, D., & Weiss, M.R. (1985). Motives for competing in competitive youth swimming. *International Journal of Sport Psychology, 16,* 126-140.

Grehaigne, J.F., Godbout, P., & Bouthier, D. (2001). The teaching and learning in decision making in team sports. *Quest, 53,* 59-76.

Griffin, L.L., Brooker, R., & Patton, K. (2005). Working towards legitimacy: Two decades of teaching for understanding. *Physical Education and Sport Pedagogy, 10,* 213-223.

Hardin, M., & Greer, J.D. (2009). The influence of gender-role socialization, media use and sports participation on perceptions of gender-appropriate sports. *Journal of Sport Behavior, 32,* 207-226.

Harter, S. (1978). Effectance motivation reconsidered: Toward a developmental model. *Human Development, 21,* 34-64.

Harter, S. (1981). A new self-report scale of intrinsic versus extrinsic orientation in the classroom: Motivational and informational components. *Developmental Psychology, 17,* 300-312.

Harvey, W.J., Fagan, T., & Kassis, J. (2003). Enabling students with ADHD to use self-control in physical activity. *Palaestra, 19* (3), 32-35.

Haywood, K.M., & Getchell, N. (2014). *Life span motor development* (6th ed.). Champaign, IL: Human Kinetics.

Heinze, J.E., Heinze, K.L., Davis, M.M., Butchart, A.T., Singer, D.C., & Clark, S.J. (2014). Gender role beliefs and parents' support of athletic participation, *Youth and Society*, 1-24.

Hellison, D. (1995). *Teaching responsibility through physical activity.* Champaign, IL: Human Kinetics.

Hellison, D. (2003). *Teaching responsibility through physical activity* (2nd ed.). Champaign, IL: Human Kinetics.

Henderlong, J., & Lepper, M.R. (2002). The effects of praise on children's intrinsic motivation: A review and synthesis. *Psychological Bulletin, 128* (5), 774-795.

Holt, L., Strean, W.B., & Bengoechea, E.G. (2002). Expanding the teaching games for understanding model: New avenues for future research and practice. *Journal of Teaching in Physical Education, 21* (2), 162-176.

Janelle, C.M., & Hillman, C.H. (2003). Expert performance in sport: Current perspectives and critical issues. In J.L. Starkes & K.A. Ericsson (Eds.), *Expert performance in sports* (pp. 19-47). Champaign, IL: Human Kinetics.

Kilpatrick, M., Hebert, E., & Jacobsen, D. (2002). Physical activity motivation: A practitioner's guide to self-determination theory. *Journal of Physical Education, Recreation and Dance, 73*, 36-41.

Kyllo, L.B., & Landers, D.M. (1995). Goal setting in sport and exercise: A research synthesis to resolve the controversy. *Journal of Sport and Exercise Psychology, 17*, 117-137.

Lewthwaite, R., Chiviacowsky, S., Drews, R., & Wulf, G. (2015). Choose to move: The motivational impact of autonomy support on motor learning. *Psychonomic Bulletin & Review, 22*, 1383-1388.

Lillard, A.S., Lerner, M.D., Hopkins, E.J., Dore, R.A., Smith, E.D., & Palmquist, C.M. (2013). The impact of pretend play on children's development: A review of the evidence. *Psychological Bulletin, 139*, 1-34.

McPherson, S.L., & Kernodle, M.W. (2003). Tactics, the neglected attribute of expertise. In J.L. Starkes & K.A. Ericsson (Eds.), *Expert performance in sports* (pp. 137-167). Champaign, IL: Human Kinetics.

Milteer, K.M., & Ginsburg, K.R. (2012). The importance of play in promoting healthy child development and maintaining strong parent-child bonds: Focus on children in poverty. *Pediatrics, 129* (1), e204-e213.

Nicholls, J.G. (1989). *The competitive ethos and democratic education.* Cambridge, MA: Harvard University Press.

Ntoumanis, N. (2001). A self-determination approach to the understanding of motivation in physical education. *British Journal of Educational Psychology, 71*, 225-242.

Orlick, T., & Botterill, C. (1975). *Every kid can win.* Chicago: Nelson-Hall.

Parten, M.B. (1932). Social participation among preschool children. *The Journal of Abnormal Social Psychology, 27*, 243-269.

Petitpas, A.J., Cornelius, A.E., VanRoalte, J.L. & Jones, T. (2005). A framework for planning youth sport programs that foster psychosocial development. *The Sport Psychologist, 19*, 63-80.

Piaget, J. (1976). *The child and reality* (A. Rosin, Trans.) New York: Grossman.

Sanli, E.A., Patterson, J.T., Bray, S.R., & Lee, T.D. (2013). Understanding self-controlled motor learning through the self-determination theory. *Frontiers in Psychology, 3*, 611.

Schmidt, R.A. (1975). *Motor skills.* New York: Harper & Row.

Schmidt, R.A., & Lee, T.D. (2014). *Motor learning and performance: A situation-based learning approach* (5th ed.). Champaign, IL: Human Kinetics.

Smith, P.K. (1978). A longitudinal study of social participation in preschool children: Solitary and parallel play re-examined. *Developmental Psychology, 14*, 517-523.

Soberlak, P., & Côtè, J. (2003). The developmental activities of elite ice hockey players. *Journal of Applied Sport Psychology, 15*, 41-49.

Tauer, J.M., & Harackiewicz, J.M. (2004). The effects of cooperation and competition on intrinsic motivation and performance. *Journal of Personality and Social Psychology, 86*, 849-861.

Vallerand, R.J. (1997). Toward a hierarchical model of intrinsic and extrinsic motivation. In M.P. Zanna (Ed.), *Advances in experimental social psychology: Vol. 2* (pp. 271-360). New York: Academic Press.

Vallerand, R.J. (2007). Intrinsic and extrinsic motivation in sport and physical activity: A review and a look at the future. In G. Tenenbaum & E. Eklund (Eds.), *Handbook of sport psychology* (3rd ed., pp. 49-83). New York: Wiley.

Vickers, J.N. (2007). *Perception, cognition, and decision training.* Champaign, IL: Human Kinetics.

Vygotsky, L.S. (1978). Mind in society: The development of higher psychological processes. Cambridge, MA: Cambridge University Press.

Wall, A.E., Reid, G., & Harvey, W.J. (2007). Interface of the KB and ETA approaches. In W.E. Davis & G.D. Broadhead (Eds.), *Ecological task analysis and movement* (pp. 259-277). Champaign, IL: Human Kinetics.

Weiss, M.R. (2008). 2007 C.H. McCloy lecture: "Field of Dreams": Sport as a context for youth development. *Research Quarterly for Exercise and Sport, 79*, 434-449.

Weiss, M.R., & Stuntz, C.P. (2004). A little friendly competition: Peer relationships and psychosocial development in youth sport and physical activity contexts. In M.R. Weiss (Ed.), *Developmental sport and exercise psychology: A lifespan perspective* (pp. 165-196). Morgantown, WV: Fitness Information Technology.

Weiss, M.R., & Williams, L. (2004). The why of youth sport involvement: A developmental perspective on motivational processes. In M.R. Weiss (Ed.), *Developmental sport and exercise psychology: A lifespan perspective* (pp. 223-268). Morgantown, WV: Fitness Information Technology.

Werner, P., Thorpe, R., & Bunker, D. (1996). Teaching Games for Understanding: The evolution of a model. *Journal of Physical Education, Recreation and Dance, 67* (1), 28-33.

Wulf, G., & Adams, N. (2014). Small choices can enhance balance learning. *Human Movement Science, 38*, 235-240.

Wulf, G., Chiviacowsky, S., & Cardoza, P. L. (2014). Additive benefit of autonomy support and enhanced expectations for motor learning. *Human Movement Science, 37*, 12-20.

Zimmerman, B.J. (2000). Attaining self-regulation: A social cognitive perspective. In M. Boekaerts, P.R. Pintrich, & M. Zeidner (Eds.), *Handbook of self-regulation* (pp. 13-39). San Diego: Academic Press.

Chapter 15

Adams, J.A. (1971). A closed-loop theory of motor learning. *Journal of Motor Behavior, 3*, 111-150.

Adams, J.A. (1986). Use of model's knowledge of results to increase the observer's performance. *Journal of Human Movement Studies, 12*, 89-98.

Andrieux, M., & Proteau, L. (2013). Observation learning of a motor task: Who and when? *Experimental Brain Research, 229*, 125-137.

Andrieux, M., & Proteau, L. (2014). Mixed observation favors motor learning through better estimation of the model's performance. *Experimental Brain Research, 232*, 3121-3132.

Ashford, K., Bennett, S.J., & Davids, K. (2006). Observational modeling effects for movement dynamics and movement outcome measures across differing task constraints: A meta-analysis. *Journal of Motor Behavior, 38*, 185-205.

Ashford, K., Davids, K., & Bennett, S.J. (2007). Developmental effects influencing observational modeling: A meta-analysis. *Journal of Sports Sciences, 25*, 547-558.

Avila, L.T.G., Chiviacowsky, S., & Wulf, G. (2012). Positive social-comparative feedback enhances motor learning in children. *Psychology of Sport and Exercise, 13*, 849-853.

Bandura, A. (1986). *Social foundations of thought and action: A social cognitive theory.* Englewood Cliffs, NJ: Prentice Hall.

Bandura, A. (1997). *Self-efficacy: The exercise of control.* New York: Freeman.

Blandin, Y., & Proteau, L. (2000). On the cognitive basis of observational learning: Development of mechanisms for the detection and correction of errors. *Quarterly Journal of Experimental Psychology, 53A*, 846-867.

Bouffard, M., & Dunn, J.G.H. (1993). Children's self-regulated learning of movement sequences. *Research Quarterly for Exercise and Sport, 64*, 393-403.

Boyce, B.A (1992). Effects of assigned versus participant set goals on skill acquisition and retention of a selected shooting task. *Journal of Teaching Physical Education, 11*, 220-234.

Breslin, G., Hodges, N.J., & Williams, A.M. (2009). Effect of information load and time on observational learning. *Research Quarterly for Exercise and Sport, 80*, 480-490.

Cadopi, M., Chatillon, J.F., & Baldy, R. (1995). Representation and performance: Reproduction of form and quality of movement in dance by eight- and 11-year-old novices. *British Journal of Psychology, 86*, 217-225.

Carroll, W.R., & Bandura, A. (1990). Representational guidance of action production in observational learning: A causal analysis. *Journal of Motor Behavior, 22*, 85-97.

Chiviacowsky, S., Wulf, G., & Avila, L.T.G. (2012). An external focus of attention enhances motor learning in children with intellectual disabilities. *Journal of Intellectual Disability Research, 57*, 627-634.

Darden, G.F. (1997). Demonstrating motor skills: Rethinking that expert demonstration. *Journal of Physical Education, Recreation and Dance, 68* (6), 31-35.

Domuracki, K., Wong, A., Olivieri, L., & Grierson, L.E.M. (2015). The impacts of observing flawed and flawless demonstrations on clinical skill learning. *Medical Education, 49*, 186-192.

Farrow, D., & Abernethy, B. (2002). Can anticipatory skills be learned through implicit video-based perceptual training? *Journal of Sports Sciences, 20*, 471-485.

Fitts, P., & Posner, M.I. (1967). *Human performance.* Belmont, CA: Brooks/Cole.

Gentile, A.M. (1972). A working model of skill acquisition with application to teaching. *Quest, 17*, 3-23.

Gentile, A.M. (1998). Implicit and explicit processes during acquisition of functional skills. *Scandinavian Journal of Occupational Therapy, 5*, 7-16.

Gould, D. (2006). Goal setting for peak performance. In J.M. Williams (Ed.), *Applied sport psychology: Personal growth to peak performance* (pp. 240-259). New York: McGraw-Hill.

Gould, D., & Chung, Y. (2004). Self-regulation skills in young, middle, and older adulthood. In M. Weiss (Ed.), *Developmental sport and exercise psychology: A lifespan perspective* (pp. 383-402). Morgantown, WV: Fitness Information Technology.

Goulet, C., Bard, C., & Fleury, M. (1989). Expertise differences in preparing to return a tennis serve: A visual information processing approach. *Journal of Sport and Exercise Psychology, 11,* 382-398.

Gredin, V., & Williams M. (2016). The relative effectiveness of various instructional approaches during the performance and learning of motor skills. *Journal of Motor Behavior, 48,* 86-97.

Green, T.D., & Flowers, J.H. (1991). Implicit versus explicit learning processes in probabilistic, continuous fine-motor catching task. *Journal of Motor Behavior, 23,* 293-300.

Hodges, N., & Franks, I.M. (2002). Modelling coaching practice: The role and demonstration. *Journal of Sports Sciences, 20,* 793-811.

Huff, M., & Schwan, S. (2012). The verbal facilitation effect in learning to tie nautical knots. *Learning and Instruction, 22,* 376-385.

Kitsantas, A., & Zimmerman, B.J. (1998). Self-regulation of motoric learning: A strategic cycle view. *Journal of Applied Sport Psychology, 10,* 220-239.

Kolovelonis, A., Goudas, M., & Dermitzaki, I. (2011). The effect of different goals and self-recording on self-regulation of learning a motor skill in a physical education setting. *Learning and Instruction, 21,* 355-364.

Kolovelonis, A., Goudas, M., & Dermitzaki, I. (2012). The effects of self-talk and goal setting on self-regulation of learning and new motor skill in physical education. *International Journal of Sport and Exercise Psychology, 10,* 221-235.

Kyllo, L.B., & Landers, D.M. (1995). Goal setting in sport and exercise: A research synthesis to resolve the controversy. *Journal of Sport and Exercise Psychology, 17,* 117-137.

Lago-Rodriguez, A., Cheeran, B., Koch, G., Hortobagyi, T., & Fernandez-del-Olmo, M. (2014). The role of mirror neurons in observation motor learning: An integrative review. *European Journal of Human Movement, 32,* 82-103.

Langhorne, P., Bernhardt, J., & Kwakkel, G. (2011). Stroke rehabilitation. *Lancet, 377,* 1693-1702.

Lee, T.D., Chamberlin, C.J., & Hodges, N. (2001). Practice. In R.N. Singer, H.A. Hausenblas, & C.M. Janelle (Eds.), *Handbook of sport psychology* (2nd ed., pp. 115-143). New York: Wiley.

Lee, T.D., & White, M.A. (1990). Influence of an unskilled model's practice schedule on observational learning. *Human Movement Science, 9,* 349-367.

Lefebvre, C., & Reid, G. (1998). Prediction in ball catching by children with and without a developmental coordination disorder. *Adapted Physical Activity Quarterly, 15,* 299-315.

Locke, E.A., & Latham, G.P. (1985). The application of goal setting to sports. *Sport Psychology Today, 7,* 205-222.

Magill, R.A. (2017). *Motor learning and control: Concepts and applications* (11th ed.). New York: McGraw-Hill.

Martens, R., Burwitz, L., & Zuckerman, J. (1976). Modeling effects on motor performance. *Research Quarterly, 47,* 277-291.

McCullagh, P., & Weiss, M.R. (2001). Modeling: Considerations for motor skill performance and psychological responses. In R.N. Singer, H.A. Hausenblas, & C.M. Janelle (Eds.), *Handbook of sport psychology* (2nd ed., pp. 205-238). New York: Wiley.

Meaney, K.S. (1994). Developmental modeling effects on the acquisition, retention, and transfer of a novel motor task. *Research Quarterly for Exercise and Sport, 65,* 31-39.

Newell, K.M. (1981). Skill learning. In D. Holding (Ed.), *Human skills* (pp. 203-226). New York: Wiley.

Ringenbach, S.D.R., & Lantero, D.A. (2005). Bimanual coordination preferences in adults with Down syndrome. *Adapted Physical Activity Quarterly, 22,* 83-98.

Saemi, E., Porter, J., Wulf, G., Ghotbi-Varzaneh, A., & Bakhtari, S. (2013). Adopting an external focus of attention facilitates motor learning in children with attention deficit hyperactivity disorder. *Kinesiology, 45,* 179-185.

Sanchez, D. J., & Reber, P. J. (2013). Explicit pre-training does not improve implicit perceptual-motor sequence learning. *Cognition, 126,* 341-351.

Schmidt, R.A. (1975). The schema theory of discrete motor skill learning. *Psychological Review, 82,* 225-260.

Schmidt, R.A., & Lee, T.D. (2005). *Motor control and learning: A behavioral emphasis* (4th ed.). Champaign, IL: Human Kinetics.

Schmidt, R.A., & Lee, T.D. (2011). *Motor control and learning: A behavioral emphasis* (5th ed.). Champaign, IL: Human Kinetics.

Schmidt, R.A., & Lee, T.D. (2014). *Motor learning and performance: A situation-based learning approach* (5th ed.). Champaign, IL: Human Kinetics.

Scully, D.M., & Newell, K.M. (1985). Observational learning and the acquisition of motor skills:

Towards a visual perception perspective. *Journal of Human Movement Studies, 11,* 169-186.

Sorsdahl, A.B., Moe-Neilssen, R., Kaale, H.K., Rieber, J., & Strand, L.I. (2010). Changes in basic motor abilities, quality of movement and everyday activities following intensive, goal-directed activity focused on physiotherapy in a group setting for children with cerebral palsy. *BMC Pediatrics, 10,* 26.

Ste-Marie, D.M., Law, B., Rymal, A.M., Jenny, O., Hall, C., & McCullagh, P. (2012). Observation interventions for motor learning and performance: An applied model for the use of observations. *International Review of Sport and Exercise Psychology, 5,* 145-176.

Ste-Marie, D.M., Vertes, K., Rymal, A.M., & Martini, R. (2011). Feedforward self-modeling enhances skill acquisition in children learning trampoline skills. *Frontiers in Psychology, 2,* 155.

Weeks, D.L. (1992). A comparison of modeling modalities in the observational learning of an externally paced skill. *Research Quarterly for Exercise and Sport, 63,* 373-380.

Weeks, D.L., & Anderson, L.P. (2000). The interaction of observational learning with overt practice: Effects on motor learning. *Acta Psychologica, 104,* 259-271.

Weinberg, R.S., & Gould, D. (2011). *Foundations of sport and exercise psychology* (5th ed.). Champaign, IL: Human Kinetics.

Weiss, M.R. (1983). Modeling and motor performance: A developmental perspective. *Research Quarterly for Exercise and Sport, 54,* 190-197.

Weiss, M.R., Ebbeck, V., & Wiese-Bjornstal, D.M. (1993). Developmental and psychological factors related to children's observational learning of physical skills. *Pediatric Exercise Science, 5,* 301-317.

Weiss, M.R., McCullagh, P., Smith, A.L., & Berlant, A.R. (1998). Observational learning and the fearful child: Influence of peer models on swimming skill performance and psychological responses. *Research Quarterly for Exercise and Sport, 69,* 380-394.

West, A.L., Edner, N.C., & Hastings E.C. (2013). Linking goals and aging. In E.A. Locke & G.P. Latham (Eds.), *New developments in goal setting and performance* (pp. 439-459). New York: Routledge.

Wiese-Bjornstal, D.M., & Weiss, M.R. (1992). Modeling effects on children's form kinematics, performance outcome, and cognitive recognition of a sport skill: An integrated perspective. *Research Quarterly for Exercise and Sport, 63,* 67-75.

Williams, A.M., & Davids, K. (1998). Visual search strategy, selective attention, and expertise in soccer. *Research Quarterly for Exercise and Sport, 69,* 127-135.

Williams, A.M., & Hodges, N.J. (2005). Practice, instruction and skill acquisition in soccer: Challenging tradition. *Journal of Sports Sciences, 23,* 637-650.

Williams, A.M., Ward, P., Smeeton, N.J., & Allen, D. (2004). Developing anticipation skills in tennis using on-court instruction: Perception versus perception and action. *Journal of Applied Sport Psychology, 16,* 350-360.

Williams, J.G. (1989). Visual demonstrations and movement production: Effects of timing variations in a model's action. *Perceptual and Motor Skills, 68,* 891-896.

Wrisberg, C.A., & Pein, R.L. (2002). Note of learners' control of the frequency of model presentation during skill acquisition. *Perceptual and Motor Skills, 94,* 792-794.

Wulf, G. (2013). Attention focus and motor learning: A review of 15 years. *International Review of Sport and Exercise Psychology, 6,* 77-104.

Wulf, G., Chiviacowsky, S., Schiller, E., & Avila, L.T.G. (2010). Frequent external-focus feedback enhances motor learning. *Frontiers in Psychology, 1,* 190.

Wulf, G., Raupach, M., & Pfeiffer, F. (2005). Self-controlled observational practice enhances learning. *Research Quarterly for Exercise and Sport, 76,* 107-111.

Wulf, G., & Weigelt, C. (1997). Instructions about physical principles in learning a complex skill: To tell or not to tell. . . . *Research Quarterly for Exercise and Sport, 68,* 362-367.

Zimmerman, B.J. (2000). Attaining self-regulation: A social cognitive perspective. In M. Boekaerts, P.R. Pintrich, & M. Zeidner (Eds.), *Handbook of self-regulation* (pp. 13-39). San Diego: Academic Press.

Zimmerman, B.J., & Kitsantas, A. (1996). Self-regulated learning of a motoric skill: The role of goal setting and self-monitoring. *Journal of Applied Sport Psychology, 8,* 60-75.

Zimmerman, B.J., & Kitsantas, A. (1997). Developmental phases in self-regulation: Shifting from process goals to outcome goals. *Journal of Educational Psychology, 89,* 29-36.

Chapter 16

Asa, S.K.de P., Melo, M.C.S., Piemonte, M.E.P. (2014). Effects of mental and physical practice on a finger opposition task among children. *Research Quarterly for Exercise and Sport, 85,* 308-315.

Bach, P., Allami, B.K., Tucker, M., & Ellis, R. (2014). Planning-related motor processes underlie mental practice and imitation learning. *Journal of Experimental Psychology: General, 143,* 1277-1294.

Barreiros, J., Figueiredo, T., & Godinho, G. (2007). The contextual interference effect in applied settings. *European Physical Education Review, 13,* 195-208.

Battig, W.F. (1979). The flexibility of human memory. In L.S. Cermak & F.I.M. Craik (Eds.), *Levels of processing in human memory* (pp. 23-44). Hillsdale, NJ: Erlbaum.

Bernardi, N.F., De Buglio, M., Trimarchi, P.D., Chielli, A., & Bricolo, E. (2013). Mental practice promotes motor anticipation: Evidence from skilled music performance. *Frontiers in Human Neuroscience, 7,* 451.

Bortoli, L., Spagolla, G., & Robazza, C. (2001). Variability effects on retention of a motor skill in elementary school children. *Perceptual and Motor Skills, 93,* 51-63.

Boyce, B.A., Coker, C.A., & Bunker, L. (2006). Implications for variability of practice from pedagogy and motor learning perspectives: Finding a common ground. *Quest, 58,* 330-343.

Brady, F. (1998). A theoretical and empirical review of the contextual interference effect and the learning of motor skills. *Quest, 50,* 266-293.

Brady, F. (2004). Contextual interference: A meta-analytic study. *Perceptual and Motor Skills, 99,* 116-126.

Brady, F. (2008). The contextual interference effect and sport skills. *Perceptual and Motor Skills, 106,* 461-472.

Breslin, G., Hodges, N.J., Steenson, A., & Williams, A.M. (2012). Constant or variable practice: Recreating the especial skill effect. *Acta Psychologica, 140,* 154-157.

Bryan, W.L., & Harter, N. (1897). Studies in the physiology and psychology of telegraphic language. *Psychological Review, 4,* 27-53.

Bryan, W.L., & Harter, N. (1899). Studies on the telegraphic language. *Psychological Review, 6,* 345-375.

Chan, J.S.Y., Luo, Y., Yan, J.H., Cai, L., & Peng, K. (2015). Children's age modulates the effect of part and whole practice in motor learning. *Human Movement Science, 42,* 261-272.

Cheong, J.P.G., Lay, B., Grove, J.L., Medic, N., & Razman, R. (2012). Practicing field hockey skills along the contextual interference continuum: A comparison of five practice schedules. *Journal of Sports Science and Medicine, 11,* 304-311.

Cocks, M., Moulton, C.-A., Luu, S., & Cil, T. (2014). What surgeons can learn from athletes: Mental practice in sports and surgery. *Journal of Surgical Education, 7,* 262-269.

Crossman, E.R.F.W. (1959). Theory of acquisition of speed-skill. *Ergonomics, 2,* 153-166.

Dail, T.K., & Christina, R.W. (2004). Distribution of practice and metacognition in learning long-term retention of a discrete motor task. *Research Quarterly for Exercise and Sport, 75,* 148-160.

Davids, K., Button, C., & Bennett, S. (2008). *Dynamics of skill acquisition: A constraints-led approach.* Champaign, IL: Human Kinetics.

Deakin, J.M., & Cobley, S. (2003). A search for deliberate practice: An examination of the practice environments in figure skating and volleyball. In J.L. Starkes & K.A. Ericsson (Eds.), *Expert performance in sports* (pp. 115-135). Champaign, IL: Human Kinetics.

Del Rey, P., Whitehurst, M., & Wood, J. (1983). Effects of experience and contextual interference on learning and transfer. *Perceptual and Motor Skills, 56,* 581-582.

Douvis, S.J. (2005). Variable practice in learning the forehand drive in tennis. *Perceptual and Motor Skills, 101,* 531-545.

Edwards, J.M., Elliott, D., & Lee, T.D. (1986). Contextual interference effects during skill acquisition and transfer in Down's syndrome adolescents. *Adapted Physical Activity Quarterly, 3,* 250-258.

Ericsson, K.A. (2003). Development of elite performance and deliberate practice: An update from the perspective of the expert performance approach. In J.L. Starkes & K.A. Ericsson (Eds.), *Expert performance in sports* (pp. 49-83). Champaign, IL: Human Kinetics.

Farrow, D., & Maschette, W. (1997). The effects of contextual interference on children learning forehand tennis groundstrokes. *Journal of Human Movement Studies 33,* 47-67.

Feghhi, I., Abdoli, B., & Valizadeh, R. (2011). Compare contextual interference effect and practice specificity in learning basketball free throw. *Procedia-Social and Behavioral Sciences, 15,* 2176-2180.

Feltz, D.L., & Landers, D.M. (1983). The effects of mental practice on motor skill learning and performance: A meta-analysis. *Journal of Sport Psychology, 5,* 25-57.

Fitts, P., & Posner, M.I. (1967). *Human performance.* Belmont, CA: Brooks/Cole.

Gentile, A.M. (1972). A working model of skill acquisition with application to teaching. *Quest, 17,* 3-23.

Gentile, A.M. (2000). Skill acquisition: Action, movement and neuromotor processes. In J.H. Carr & R.B. Shepherd (Eds.), *Movement science: Foundations for physical therapy in rehabilitation* (2nd ed., pp. 111-187). Rockville, MD: Aspen.

Gerson, R.F., & Thomas, J.R. (1977). Schema theory and practice variability within a neo-Piagetian framework. *Journal of Motor Behavior, 2,* 127-134.

Goode, S., & Magill, R.A. (1986). Contextual interference effects in learning three badminton serves. *Research Quarterly for Exercise and Sport, 57,* 308-314.

Green, D.P., Whitehead., J., & Sugden, D.A. (1995). Practice variability and transfer of a racket skill. *Perceptual and Motor Skills, 81,* 1275-1281.

Herbert, E.P., Landin, D., & Solmon, M.A. (1996). Practice schedule effects on the performance and learning of low- and high-skilled students: An applied study. *Research Quarterly for Exercise and Sport, 67,* 52-58.

Hird, J.S., Landers, D.M., Thomas, J.R., & Horan, J.J. (1991). Physical practice is superior to mental practice in enhancing cognitive and motor task performance. *Journal of Sport and Exercise Psychology, 13,* 281-293.

James, E.G., & Conatser, P. (2014). Effects of practice variability on unimanual arm rotation. *Journal of Motor Behavior, 46,* 203-210.

Jarus, T., & Goverover, Y. (1999). Effects of contextual interference and age on acquisition, retention, and transfer of motor skill. *Perceptual and Motor Skills, 88,* 437-447.

Jeannerod, M. (1999). To act or not to act: Perspectives on the representation of actions. *Quarterly Journal of Experimental Psychology, 52A* (1), 1-29.

Keetch, K.M., & Lee, T.D. (2007). The effect of self-regulated and experimenter-imposed practice schedules on motor learning for tasks of varying difficulty. *Research Quarterly for Exercise and Sport, 78,* 476-486.

Keetch, K.M., Schmidt, R.A., Lee, T.D., & Young, D.E. (2005). Especial skills: Their emergence with massive amounts of practice. *Journal of Experimental Psychology: Perception and Performance, 31,* 970-978.

Kerr, R., & Booth, B. (1978). Specific and varied practice of motor skill. *Perceptual and Motor Skills, 46,* 395-401.

King, A.C., & Newell, K.M. (2013). The learning of isometric force time scales is differently influenced by constant and variable practice. *Experimental Brain Research, 227,* 149.

Kolh, R.M., Ellis, S.D., & Roenker, D.L. (1992). Alternating actual and imagery practice: Preliminary theoretical considerations. *Research Quarterly for Exercise and Sport, 63,* 162-170.

Kwon, Y.H., Kwon, J.W., & Lee, M.H. (2015). Effectiveness of motor sequential learning according to practice sessions in healthy adults: Distributed practice versus massed practice. *Journal of Physical Therapy Science, 27,* 769-772.

Landin, D., & Hebert, E.P. (1997). A comparison of three practice schedules along the contextual interference continuum. *Research Quarterly for Exercise and Sport, 68,* 357-361.

Lee, T.D. (2012). Contextual interference: Generalizability and limitations. In N. Hodges & M. A. Williams (Eds.), *Skill acquisition in sport: Research, theory and practice* (pp. 79-93). New York: Routledge.

Lee, T.D., Chamberlin, C.J., & Hodges, N. (2001). Practice. In R.N. Singer, H.A. Hausenblas, & C.M.

Janelle (Eds.), *Handbook of sport psychology* (2nd ed., pp. 115-143). New York: Wiley.

Lee, T.D., & Magill, R.A. (1985). Can forgetting facilitate skill acquisition? In D. Goodman, R.B. Wilberg, & I.M. Franks (Eds.), *Differing perspectives on memory, learning and control* (pp. 3-22). Amsterdam: North-Holland.

Lee, T.D., & White, M.A. (1990). Influence of an unskilled model's practice schedule on observational learning. *Human Movement Science, 9,* 349-367.

Lin, C.-H.J., Wu, A.D., Udompholkul, P., & Knowlton, B.J. (2010). Contextual interference effects in sequence learning for young and older adults. *Psychology and Aging, 25,* 929-939.

Magill, R.A. (2017). *Motor learning and control: Concepts and applications* (11th ed.). New York: McGraw-Hill.

Magill, R. & Anderson, D. (2013). *Motor learning and control: Concepts and applications* (10th ed.). New York: McGraw-Hill.

Martin, K.A., Moritz, S.A., & Hall, C.R. (1999). Imagery use in sport: A literature review and applied model. *Sport Psychologist, 13,* 245-268.

Moradi, J., Movahedi, A., & Salehi, H. (2014). Specificity of learning a sport skill to the visual condition of acquisition. *Journal of Motor Behavior, 46,* 17-23.

Moxley, S.E. (1979). Schema: The variability of practice hypothesis. *Journal of Motor Behavior, 2,* 65-70.

Naylor, J.C., & Briggs, G.E. (1963). Effects of task complexity and task organization on the relative efficiency of part and whole training methods. *Journal of Experimental Psychology, 65,* 217-224.

Newell, K.M., & McDonald, P.V. (1992). Searching for solutions to the coordination function: Learning as exploratory behavior. *Advances in Psychology, 87,* 517-532.

Nilsen, D.M., Gillen, G., & Gordon, A.M. (2010). Use of mental practice to improve upper-limb recovery after stroke: A systematic review. *The American Journal of Occupational Therapy, 64,* 695-708.

Pease, D.G., & Pupnow, A.A. (1983). Effects of varying force production in practice schedules of children learning a discrete motor task. *Perceptual and Motor Skills, 57,* 275-282.

Pigott, R.E., & Shapiro, D.C. (1984). Motor schema: The structure of the variability session. *Research Quarterly for Exercise and Sport, 55,* 41-45.

Pollock, B.J., & Lee, T.D. (1997). Dissociated contextual interference effects in children and adults. *Perceptual and Motor Skills, 84,* 851-858.

Post, P.G., Fairbrother, J.T., & Barros, J.A.C. (2011). Self-controlled amount of practice benefits learning of a motor skill. *Research Quarterly for Exercise and Sport, 82,* 474-481.

Post, P.G., Fairbrother, J.T., Barros, J.A.C., & Kulpa, J.D. (2014). Self-controlled practice with a fixed time period facilitates the learning of a basketball set shot. *Journal of Motor Learning and Development, 3*, 9-15.

Proteau, L. (1992). On the specificity of learning and the role of visual information for movement control. In L. Proteau & D. Elliott (Eds.), *Vision and motor control* (pp. 67-103). Amsterdam: North Holland.

Proteau, L., Blandin, Y., Alain, C., & Dorion, A. (1994). The effects of the amount and variability of practice on the learning of a multi-segmented motor task. *Acta Psychologia (Amst), 85*, 61-74.

Proteau, L., Marteniuk, R.G., Girourd, Y., & Dugas, C. (1987). On the type of information used to control and learn an aiming movement after moderate and extensive training. *Human Movement Science, 6*, 181-199.

Ranganathan, R., & Newell, K.M. (2012). Changing up the routine: Intervention-induced variability in motor learning. *Exercise and Sport Sciences Reviews, 41*, 64-70.

Robertson, S.D., Tremblay, L., Anson, J.G., & Elliott, D. (2002). Learning to cross a balance beam: Implications for teachers, coaches and therapists. In K. Davids, G. Savelsbergh, S. Bennett, & J. van der Kamps (Eds.), *Dynamic interception actions in sport: Current research and practical applications* (pp. 109-125). London: Taylor and Francis.

Sanli, E.A., Patterson, J.T., Bray, S.R., & Lee, T.D. (2013). Understanding self-controlled motor learning through the self-determination theory. *Frontiers in Psychology, 3*, 611.

Schmidt, R.A. (1975). The schema theory of discrete motor skill learning. *Psychological Review, 82*, 225-260.

Schmidt, R.A., & Lee, T.D. (2005). *Motor control and learning: A behavioral emphasis* (4th ed.). Champaign, IL: Human Kinetics.

Schmidt, R.A., & Lee, T.D. (2011). *Motor control and learning: A behavioral emphasis* (5th ed.). Champaign, IL: Human Kinetics.

Schmidt, R.A., & Lee, T.D. (2014). *Motor learning and performance: A situation-based learning approach* (5th ed.). Champaign, IL: Human Kinetics.

Schmidt, R.A., & Wrisberg, C.A. (2008). *Motor learning and performance: A situation-based learning approach* (4th ed.). Champaign, IL: Human Kinetics.

Shea, J.B., & Morgan, R.L. (1979). Contextual interference effects on the acquisition, retention, and transfer of a motor skill. *Journal of Experimental Psychology: Human Learning and Memory, 5*, 179-187.

Snoddy, G.S. (1926). Learning and stability: A psychophysical analysis of a case of motor learning with clinical applications. *Journal of Applied Psychology, 10*, 1-36.

Soucy, M.-C., & Proteau, L. (2001). Development of multiple movement representations with practice: Specificity versus flexibility. *Journal of Motor Behavior, 33*, 243-254.

Spruit, E.N., Band, G.P.H., & Hamming, J.F. (2015). Increasing efficiency of surgical training: Effects of spacing practice on skill acquisition and retention in laparoscopy training. *Surgical Endoscopy, 29*, 2235-2243.

Ste-Marie, D.M., Clark, S.E., Findlay, L.C., & Latimer, A.E. (2004). High levels of contextual interference influence handwriting skill writing acquisition. *Journal of Motor Behavior, 36*, 115-126.

Thorndike, E.L. (1914). *Educational psychology: briefer course*. New York: Columbia University Press.

Thorndike, E.L., & Woodworth, R.C. (1901). The influence of improvement in one mental function upon the efficiency of other functions. II. The estimate of magnitudes. *Psychological Review, 8*, 384-395.

Tremblay, L., & Proteau, L. (1998). Specificity of practice: The case of powerlifting. *Research Quarterly for Exercise and Sport, 69*, 284-289.

Tremblay, L., & Proteau, L. (2001). Specificity of practice in a ball interception task. *Canadian Journal of Experimental Psychology, 55*, 207-218.

Vera, J.G., Alvarez, J.C., & Medina, M.M. (2008). Effects of different practice conditions on acquisition, retention, and transfer of soccer skills by 9 year old school children. *Perceptual and Motor Skills, 106*, 447-460.

Wrisberg, C.A., & Mead, B.J. (1981). Anticipation of coincidence in children: A test of schema theory. *Perceptual and Motor Skills, 52*, 599-606.

Wrisberg, C.A., & Mead, B.J. (1983). Developing coincident timing skill in children: A comparison of training methods. *Research Quarterly for Exercise and Sport, 54*, 67-74.

Wulf, G. (1991). The effect of type of practice on motor learning in children. *Applied Cognitive Psychology, 5*, 123-134.

Wulf, G., & Schimdt, R.A. (1994). Feedback-induced variability and the learning of generalized motor programs. *Journal of Motor Behavior, 26*, 348-361.

Yan, J.H., Thomas, J.R., & Thomas, K.T. (1998). Children's age moderates the effect of practice variability: A quantitative review. *Research Quarterly for Exercise and Sport, 69*, 210-215.

Yao, W.X., & DeSola, W. (2009). Variable practice versus constant practice in the acquisition of wheelchair propulsive speeds. *Perceptual and Motor Skills, 109*, 133-139.

Zetou, E., Papadakis, L., Vernadakis, N., Derri, V., Bebetsos, E., & Filippou, F. (2014). The effect of variable and stable practice on performance and learning the header skill of young athletes in soccer. *Procedia- Social and Behavioral Sciences,* *152,* 824-829.

Chapter 17

Agethan, M., & Krause, D. (2016). Effects of bandwidth feedback on the automatization of an arm movement sequence. *Human Movement Science,* *45,* 71-83.

Anderson, D.L., Magill, R.A., Sekiya, H., & Ryan, G. (2005). Support for an explanation of the guidance effect in motor skill learning. *Journal of Motor Behavior, 37* (3), 231-238.

Barclay, C.R., & Newell, K.M. (1980). Children's processing of information in motor skill acquisition. *Journal of Experimental Child Psychology, 30,* 98-108.

Bilodeau, E.A., & Bilodeau, I.M. (1958). Variable frequency of knowledge of results and the learning of a simple skill. *Journal of Experimental Psychology,* *55,* 379-383.

Bilodeau, I.M. (1966). Information feedback. In E.A. Bilodeau (Ed.), *Acquisition of skill* (pp. 225-296). New York: Academic Press.

Brucker, B.S., & Bulaeva, N.V. (1996). Biofeedback effect on electromyographic responses in patients with spinal cord injury. *Archives of Physical Medicine and Rehabilitation, 77,* 133-137.

Chiviacowsky, S., & Drews, R. (2014). Effects of generic versus non-generic feedback on motor learning in children. *PLOS One, 9* (2), e88989.

Chiviacowsky, S., & Wulf, G. (2006). Self-controlled feedback: Does it enhance learning because performers get feedback when they need it? *Research Quarterly for Exercise and Sport, 73,* 408-415.

Chiviacowsky, S., & Wulf, G. (2007). Feedback after good trials enhances learning. *Research Quarterly for Exercise and Sport, 78,* 40-47.

Chiviacowsky, S., Wulf, G., Laroque de Medeiros, F., Kaefer, A., & Wally, R. (2008). Self-controlled feedback in 10-year-old children: Higher feedback frequencies enhance learning. *Research Quarterly for Exercise and Sport, 79* (1), 122-127.

Darden, G.F. (1999). Videotape feedback for student learning and performance: A learning stages approach. *Journal of Physical Education, Recreation and Dance, 70* (9), 40-45, 62.

Dozza, M., Chiari, L., Peterka, R.J., Wall, C., &. Horak, F.B. (2011). What is the most effective type of audio-biofeedback for postural motor learning? *Gait & Posture, 34* (3), 313-319.

Fischman, M.F., & Oxendine, J.B. (2001). Motor skill learning for effective coaching and performance. In J.M. Williams (Ed.), *Applied sport psychology: Personal growth to peak performance* (pp. 13-28). Mountain View, CA: Mayfield.

Fishman, S., & Tobey, C. (1978). Augmented feedback. In W.G. Anderson & G.T. Barrette (Eds.),

What's going on in gym: Descriptive studies of physical education classes [Monograph]. *Motor Skills: Theory Into Practice, 1,* 51-62.

Flinn, N.A., & Radomski, M.V. (2002). Learning. In C.A. Trombly & M.V. Radomski (Eds.), *Occupational therapy for physical dysfunction* (5th ed., pp. 283-297). Baltimore: Lippincott Williams & Wilkins.

Gallagher, J.D., & Thomas, J.R. (1980). Effects of varying post-KR intervals upon children's motor performance. *Journal of Motor Behavior, 12,* 41-46.

Herbert, E., & Landin, D. (1997). *Videotape feedback in skill acquisition.* Paper presented at Southern District AAHPERD conference, New Orleans.

Intiso, D., Santilli, V., Grasso, M.G., Rossi, R., & Caruso, I. (1994). Rehabilitation of walking with electromyographic biofeedback in drop-foot after stroke. *Stroke, 25,* 1189-1192.

Jones, V. (2011). *Play through the foul.* First One Digital Publishing.

Kernodle, M.W., & Carlton, L.G. (1992). Information feedback and the learning of multiple-degree-of-freedom activities. *Journal of Motor Behavior, 24* (2), 187-196.

Konttinen, N., Lyytinen, H., & Viitasalo, J. (1998). Rifle-balancing in precision shooting: Behavioral aspects and psychophysiological implication. *Scandinavian Journal of Medicine and Science in Sports, 8,* 78-83.

Lai, Q., & Shea, C.H. (1999). Bandwidth knowledge of results enhances generalized motor program learning. *Research Quarterly for Exercise and Sport, 70,* 79-83.

Lambert, J., & Bard, C. (2005). Acquisition of visuomanual skills and improvement of information processing capacities in 6-to-10-year-old children performing a 2D pointing task. *Neuroscience Letters, 377,* 1-6.

Lee, T.D., & Carnahan, H. (1990). Bandwidth knowledge of results and motor learning. *Quarterly Journal of Experimental Psychology, 42,* 777-789.

Liu, Y., Cao, C., & Yan, J.H. (2013). Functional aging impairs the role of feedback in motor learning. *Geriatrics Gerontology International, 13,* 849-859.

Magill, R.A. (2001). Augmented feedback in motor skill acquisition. In R.N. Singer, H.A. Hausenbas, & C.M. Janelle (Eds.), *Handbook of sport psychology* (pp. 88-114). New York: John Wiley and Sons.

Magill, R.A. (2017). *Motor learning and control: Concepts and applications* (11th ed.). New York: McGraw-Hill.

Menickelli, J., Landin, D., Grisham, W., & Hebert, E. (2000). The effects of videotape feedback with augmented cues on the performances and thought processes of skilled gymnasts. *Journal of Sport Pedagogy, 6,* 56-72.

Mononen, K., Viitasalo, J.T., Konttinen, N., & Era, P. (2003). The effects of augmented kinematic feedback on motor skill learning in rifle shooting. *Journal of Sports Sciences, 21,* 867-876.

Newell, K.M., & Carlton, M.J. (1987). Augmented information feedback and the acquisition of isometric tasks. *Journal of Motor Behavior, 19,* 4-12.

Newell, K.M., Quinn, J.T. Jr., Sparrow, W.A., & Walter, C.B. (1983). Kinematic information feedback for learning a simple rapid response. *Human Movement Science, 2,* 255-270.

Newell, K.M., & Walter, C.B. (1981). Kinematic and kinetic parameters as information feedback in motor skill acquisition. *Journal of Human Movement Studies, 7,* 235-254.

Pèrez, P., Liana, S., Brizuela, G., & Encarnación, A. (2009). Effects of three feedback conditions on aerobic swim speeds. *Journal of Sports Science and Medicine, 8,* 30-36.

Roberts, T., & Brown, L. (2008). Learn more in less time: Fundamental aquatic skill acquisition via video technology. *Strategies, 21,* 20-31.

Rose, D.J., & Christina, R.W. (2006). *A multilevel approach to the study of motor control and learning* (2nd ed.). San Francisco: Pearson Benjamin Cummings.

Rucci, J.A. & Tomporowski, P.D. (2010). Three types of kinematic feedback and the execution of the hang power clean. *Journal of Strength and Conditioning Research, 24* (3), 771-778.

Sadowski, J., Mastalerz, A., & Niznikowski, T. (2013). Benefits of bandwidth feedback in learning a complex gymnastic skill. *Journal of Human Kinetics, 37,* 83-93.

Salmoni, A.W., Schmidt, R.A., & Walter, C.B. (1984). Knowledge of results and motor learning: A review and critical appraisal. *Psychological Bulletin, 95,* 355-386.

Schwarz, M., Olson, P.R., & Andrasik, F. (2003). A historical perspective on the field of biofeedback and applied psychophysiology. In Schwarz, M. Andrasik, F. (Eds.), *Biofeedback: A practitioner's guide* (3rd ed., pp. 3-19). New York: Guilford.

Sharma, D.A., Chevidikuunan, M.F., Khan, F.R., & Gaowgzeh, R.A. (2016). Effectiveness of knowledge of result and knowledge of performance in the learning of a skilled motor activity by healthy young adults. *Journal of Physical Therapy Science, 28* (5), 1482-1486.

Sherwood, D.E. (1988). Effect of bandwidth knowledge of results on movement consistency. *Perceptual and Motor Skills, 66,* 535-542.

Siedentop, D., & Tannehill, D. (2000). *Developing teaching skills in physical education.* Mountain View, CA: Mayfield.

Sigrist, R., Rauter, G., Riener, R., & Wolf, P. (2013). Augmented visual, auditory, haptic, and multimodal feedback in motor learning: A review. *Psychonomic Bulletin & Review, 20,* 21-53.

Sullivan, K.J., Kantak, S.S., & Burtner, P.A. (2008). Motor learning in children: Feedback effects on skill acquisition. *Physical Therapy, 88* (6), 720-732.

Swinnen, P.S., Schmidt, R.A., Nicholson, D.E., & Shapiro, D.C. (1990). Information feedback for skill acquisition: Instantaneous knowledge of results degrades learning. *Journal of Experimental Psychology: Learning, Memory and Cognition, 16,* 706-716.

Thorndike, E.L. (1931). *Human learning.* New York: Century.

Tzetzis, G., Votsis, E., & Kourtessis, T. (2008). The effect of different corrective feedback methods on the outcome and self-confidence of young athletes. *Journal of Sports Science & Medicine, 7* (3), 371-378.

Weeks, D.L., & Sherwood, D.E. (1994). A comparison of knowledge of results scheduling methods for promoting motor skill acquisition and retention. *Research Quarterly for Exercise and Sport, 65* (2), 136-142.

Winstein, C.J., & Schmidt, R.A. (1990). Reduced frequency of knowledge of results enhances motor skill learning. *Journal of Experimental Psychology: Learning, Memory, and Cognition, 16,* 677-691.

Wu, W.F.W., Young, D.E., Schandler, S.L., Meir, G., Judy, R.L.M., Perez, J., & Cohen, M.J. (2011). Contextual interference and augmented feedback: Is there an additive effect for motor learning? *Human Movement Science, 30* (6), 1092-1101.

Wulf, G., Clauss, A., Shea, C.H., & Whitacre, C. (2001). Benefits of self-control in dyad practice. *Research Quarterly for Exercise and Sport, 72,* 299-303.

Yan, J.H. & Dick, M.B. (2006). Practice effects on motor control in healthy seniors and patients with mild cognitive impairment or mild Alzheimer's disease. *Neuropsychology, Development, Cognition Section B Aging, Neuropsychology & Cognition, 13,* 385-410.

Young, D.E., & Schmidt, R.A. (1992). Augmented kinematic feedback for motor learning. *Journal of Motor Behavior, 24,* 261-273.

Chapter 18

Davis, W.E., & Burton, A.W. (1991). Ecological task analysis: Translating movement behavior theory into practice. *Adapted Physical Activity Quarterly, 8,* 154-177.

Haywood, K.M., & Getchell, N. (2014). *Life span motor development* (6th ed.). Champaign, IL: Human Kinetics.

INDEX

ABOUT THE AUTHORS

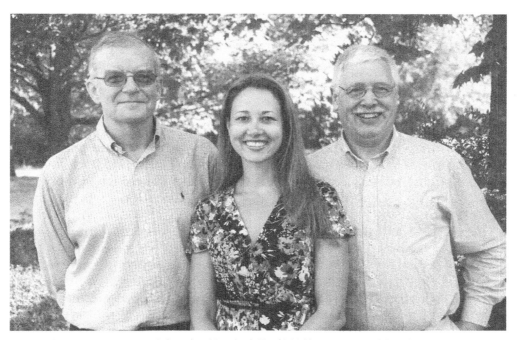

Greg Reid *(left)*, Pamela Haibach-Beach *(center)*, and Douglas Collier *(right)*. Photo is courtesy of the authors.

Pamela S. Haibach-Beach, PhD, is a professor in the department of kinesiology, sport studies, and physical education (KSSPE) at the College at Brockport, State University of New York. Haibach-Beach earned her doctorate in kinesiology with an emphasis in motor behavior from Pennsylvania State University under the advisement of Dr. Karl M. Newell. She is the coordinator of the kinesiology major and the study abroad program in the KSSPE department.

Haibach-Beach's research focuses on motor learning, motor development, and balance, including those of developing individuals, individuals with disabilities, and other special populations. Haibach-Beach regularly presents and conducts workshops at national and international conferences related to motor behavior. She is founder and codirector of the Institute of Movement Studies for Individuals With Visual Impairments (IMSVI).

Haibach-Beach serves as an elected board member for the American Kinesiology Association (AKA) and also chairs the AKA publications committee. She is a former president of the National Association for Sport and Physical Education (NASPE) Motor Development and Learning Academy and is a member of the International Federation for Adapted Physical Activity (IFAPA), the Society of Health and Physical Educators (SHAPE America), International Society of Motor Control (ISMC), and the North American Society for the Psychology of Sport and Physical Activity (NASPSPA). Active in her community, Haibach-Beach serves as a cochair for an active-community initiative called

Walk! Bike! Brockport! and is a Brockport Lions Club member.

In her free time, Haibach-Beach enjoys being physically active and spending time outdoors. She, her husband, and her two children reside in Brockport, New York. As both a researcher and a mother, she enjoys experiencing the growth and development of her two children.

Gregory D. Reid, PhD, is a professor emeritus in the department of kinesiology and physical education at McGill University in Montreal, Quebec. A former elementary school physical education teacher and longtime youth coach in ice hockey and baseball, Reid obtained his graduate education in adapted physical activity, motor learning, and special education at the University of California (UCLA) and Pennsylvania State University. As a teacher and researcher, he maintained a strong focus on theory-to-practice applications. Reid's research covered performance, learning, and development; spanned children to older adults; and included an emphasis of individuals with and without disabilities.

In addition to his teaching and research, Reid supervised practicum experiences of undergraduates teaching individuals with disabilities. He is a former undergraduate and graduate program director and chair of the department of kinesiology and physical education at McGill University.

In 1997, Reid received the G. Lawrence Rarick Research Award from AAHPERD's National Consortium for Physical Education and Recreation for Individuals with Disabilities. He was elected an international member of the American Academy of Kinesiology in 1999. He is also a fellow of the International Federation of Adapted Physical Activity (IFAPA) and the 2015 recipient of their Elly D. Friedmann Professional Contribution Award.

Reid and his wife, Carol, reside in Sainte-Adele, Quebec. They have two grown sons, Drew and Tyler. In his free time Reid enjoys hiking, bicycling, cross-country and downhill skiing, and reading novels. And he never tires of observing the motor development and learning accomplishments of his grandchildren, Jacob, Chloe, and Ethan.

Douglas H. Collier, PhD, is an associate professor in the department of kinesiology, sport studies, and physical education at the College at Brockport, State University of New York. Collier was a delegate to the Jasper talks (1985), a significant policy workshop that became the catalyst to Collier's career-long interest in motor development. For the past three decades, his research agenda has examined various facets of motor development that pertain to the education of typically developing children and those with identifiable disabilities. He is also interested in positive and proactive solutions to challenging behavior in school-age learners. Collier has presented his research at multiple national and international conferences concerned with the study of motor development and pedagogy.

Over the course of his 24-year career in higher education, Collier has served in multiple leadership positions at local, state, and national levels. He is a member of the North American Federation of Adapted Physical Activity (NAFAPA), the Society of Health and Physical Educators (SHAPE America), and the North American Society for the Psychology of Sport and Physical Activity (NASPSPA).

Collier holds a doctorate in human performance from Indiana University, where he studied under the advisement of Drs. Dale Ulrich, Beverly Ulrich, and Esther Thelen. In his free time, Collier enjoys racket sports, photography, and canoeing. He and his wife, Christine, reside in Brockport, New York. They have two grown daughters, Robin and Shannon.